RECENT ADVANCES IN MUCOSAL IMMUNOLOGY

Part A: Cellular Interactions

Recent Volumes in this Series

Volume 212
ACUTE RENAL FAILURE: Clinical and Experimental
Edited by Alberto Amerio, Pasquale Coratelli, Vito M. Campese, and Shaul G. Massry

Volume 213
MECHANISMS OF LYMPHOCYTE ACTIVATION AND IMMUNE REGULATION
Edited by Sudhir Gupta, William E. Paul, and Anthony S. Fauci

Volume 214
THE NEW DIMENSIONS OF WARFARIN PROPHYLAXIS
Edited by Stanford Wessler, Carl G. Becker, and Yale Nemerson

Volume 215
OXYGEN TRANSPORT TO TISSUE IX
Edited by I. A. Silver and A. Silver

Volume 216 A
RECENT ADVANCES IN MUCOSAL IMMUNOLOGY, Part A: Cellular Interactions
Edited by Jiri Mestecky, Jerry R. McGhee, John Bienenstock, and Pearay L. Ogra

Volume 216 B
RECENT ADVANCES IN MUCOSAL IMMUNOLOGY, Part B: Effector Functions
Edited by Jerry R. McGhee, Jiri Mestecky, Pearay L. Ogra, and John Bienenstock

Volume 217
THE BIOLOGY OF TAURINE: Methods and Mechanisms
Edited by Ryan J. Huxtable, Flavia Franconi, and Alberto Giotti

Volume 218
CORONAVIRUSES
Edited by Michael M. C. Lai and Stephen A. Stohlman

Volume 219
REGULATION OF OVARIAN AND TESTICULAR FUNCTION
Edited by Virendra B. Mahesh, Dharam S. Dhindsa, Everett Anderson, and Satya P. Kalra

---

RECENT ADVANCES IN MUCOSAL IMMUNOLOGY

Part A: Cellular Interactions

Edited by

Jiri Mestecky
Jerry R. McGhee
University of Alabama at Birmingham
Birmingham, Alabama

John Bienenstock
McMaster University
Hamilton, Ontario, Canada

and

Pearay L. Ogra
State University of New York at Buffalo
Buffalo, New York

PLENUM PRESS • NEW YORK AND LONDON

Library of Congress Cataloging in Publication Data

International Congresses on Mucosal Immunology (1986: Niagara Falls, N.Y.)
Recent advances in mucosal immunology.

(Advances in experimental medicine and biology; v. 216)
"Proceedings of the International Congress on Mucosal Immunology, held June 29-July 3, 1986, in Niagara Falls, New York"—T.p. verso.
A satellite symposium of the 6th International Congress of Immunology, held in Toronto, Ont., 1986.
Includes bibliographies and index.
1. Mucous membrane—Congresses. 2. Immunity—Congresses. 3. Mucous membrane—Diseases—Immunological aspects—Congresses. I. Mestecky, Jiri, 1941-
II. McGhee, Jerry R. III. Bienenstock, John. IV. Ogra, Pearay L. V. International Congress of Immunology VI. Series. (6th: 1986: Toronto, Ont.) VII. Title. [DNLM: 1. Mucous Membrane—immunology—congresses.
QS 532.5.M8 161r 1986]
QR185.9.M83I58 1986 611'.0187 87-14129

Proceedings of the International Congress on Mucosal Immunology,
held June 29-July 3, 1986, in Niagara Falls, New York

DOI 10.1007/978-1-4684-5344-7

A Division of Plenum Publishing Corporation
233 Spring Street, New York, N.Y. 10013

DEDICATION

This volume is dedicated to the memory of three colleagues who are no longer with us: Dr. Henry G. Kunkel, Dr. Eva Orlans, and Dr. Richard M. Rothberg. Their contribution to the field of mucosal immunology and their participation in past meetings are deeply appreciated by all of us. Original studies of Dr. Rothberg in the area of oral immunization with protein antigens, assays of immune responses, and in milk immunology were of considerable significance to many subsequent investigations. Dr. Orlans will be remembered for her discoveries in developmental immunology and hepatobiliary transport of IgA. Much has been written about Dr. Kunkel's contributions to immunology since his untimely death. He himself, wrote a short summary of his contributions to immunology in the evening prior to his death. We are deeply grateful to his wife, Betty, for making this unique document available to us. He did not mention his contributions to IgA immunology which included many pioneering immunochemical and cellular studies and many investigators who have participated at this series of meetings were trained in his laboratory. Perhaps in the future his contribution to this area will be fully evaluated.

Accomplishments - Henry G. Kunkel

I. Liver Disease work: This was the initial research work begun at the Rockefeller Institute. Clinical studies dominated and three significant papers were written on the progression of a few cases of acute hepatitis to a more chronic disease. Two liver disease syndromes were described for the first time and continue to be recognized today. The one was chronic liver disease in young females with a distinct hormone element and with marked hypergammaglobulinemia. This was sometimes associated with arthritis and positive lupus tests. The other was given the name of primary biliary cirrhosis and was associated with hyperlipidemia and sometimes xanthomata.

II. Studies of SLE and Rheumatoid Arthritis: This work stemmed directly from the liver disease syndromes described above which had some manifestations of SLE. It was soon apparent that SLE was an entirely different disease without liver manifestations. We were intrigued with the L.E. cell phenomenon in this disease and demonstrated that it was an antibody-mediated reaction. This finding led to the first description of DNA antibodies in this disease as well as many other antibodies including those to nucleoprotein, histones, microsomes, and mitochondria. Sm antibodies were also described. A role for certain of these antibodies in the renal disease was demonstrated, primarily by their recognition in the kidney by fluorescence and by their elution at high concentration from autopsy kidneys. Immune complex disease was first described and SLE was designated as the prototype.

Studies of rheumatoid factor from rheumatoid arthritis patients showed that this was a 19S antibody and not some obscure factor. It existed in the serum as a complex with 7S IgG. These complexes could be visualized in the ultracentrifuge. Other complexes involving Igs also were described, particularly IgG - IgG complexes involving IgG rheumatoid factor. These were shown to be especially apparent in joint fluids of these patients.

The chief accomplishment in these diseases was to demonstrate for the first time that unusual antibodies are present and that they frequently circulate as immune complexes, some of which are involved in at least kidney damage. Our initial evidence that these "factors" were antibodies received considerable resistance even from immunologists. However, our simultaneous work on classical antibodies and their many different types placed us in a position of knowing more about human antibodies than anyone else and acceptance of our proposals soon ensued.

III. Basic Immunology: Immunoglobulin work: The high gammaglobulin levels in liver disease and especially in the studies of young girls led to an investigation of this serum component in great detail. The extreme abnormality in multiple myeloma immediately attracted our attention but these proteins were thought to be abnormal proteins. It was possible to demonstrate for the first time that these proteins were closely related to normal immunoglobulins; cross reactions clearly showed this, especially with antibodies to normal gammaglobulin. As a result we decided to use these homogenous myeloma proteins as models for individual immunoglobulins or antibodies. This theme was dominant in all our subsequent work and that of the people who trained with us. Perhaps our most important discovery was the finding that these proteins possessed individual antigenic specificity or idiotypic specificity as it was subsequently termed. This was evident in the early myeloma studies and later was similarly defined for isolated antibodies. Antibodies could be raised against the V regions of these proteins that helped define these V regions, study their genetics, and diversity. It became a dominant branch of immunology. Cross-idiotypic specificity relating to antigen binding was described first, which also developed into a major subfield.

Myeloma proteins also aided greatly in defining the many different types of immunoglobulins. The discovery of two types of light chains, kappa and lambda, and the definition of four subclasses of heavy chains, as well as the heavy and light chains themselves, primarily ensued from our laboratory. The genetics of human Igs was largely worked out with homogenous myeloma proteins and the heavy chain linkage group was delineated.

The IgM proteins were defined for the first time as a distinct class of Igs which contained multiple antibodies. This class was distinguished clearly on the basis of its antigenic specificity in addition to high carbohydrate content. It had previously been thought to represent a polymer of ordinary IgG proteins.

Cellular Immunology: Our work gradually shifted from serum antibodies to the cells that produce these antibodies as well as those regulating their production. Membrane Igs on B lymphocytes were clearly shown to be primarily IgM and IgD. These two proteins were shown to have identical V regions as demonstrated by anti-idiotypic antibodies. Two major discoveries were made in the cellular histocompatibility area. The DR system primarily represented on B cells was delineated and clearly separated from the classical HLA system. Secondly, the complement system was related to the histocompatibility system. The second component of complement, C2, was inherited in close linkage with the HLA system. Both of these discoveries opened up new fields of investigation.

IV. Miscellaneous Accomplishments:

Electrophoresis: Zone electrophoresis was developed into a major method of protein separation. Block electrophoresis in various supporting media was originated, particularly through the use of starch and polyvinyl supports. The theory of zone electrophoresis was developed.

Density Gradient Ultracentrifugation: This technique that had been used for cell separation was first employed for separation of proteins, notably Igs.

Hbg A_2: This normal hemoglobin was described for the first time. Quantitation of this component showed its elevation in thalassemia and was utilized diagnostically.

Immune Deficiency: A number of significant observations were made. Firstly, gene defects were described where specific subclass gene products were missing in multiple family members. Secondly, absence of B cells in many cases was first described. Thirdly, and most recently, reversal of various types of immune deficiency *in vitro* with products of T cell hybridomas was achieved.

Co-workers: All these accomplishments were carried out with a brilliant group of collaborators. Those who participated in the projects listed are as follows: Robert Slater, Alexander Bearn, Edward Ahrens, Gerald Edelman, Halstead Holman, Edward Franklin, Hans Müller-Eberhard, Ralph Williams, Mart Mannik, William Yount, Shu Man Fu, and Robert Winchester.

PREFACE

Increasing interest in the immunology of mucosal surfaces is obvious from the number of publications in scientific journals and from the frequency of national and international symposia devoted to this subject. Particularly encouraging are the large numbers of young investigators who have chosen to work in this area of theoretical immunology with profound practical implications.

The two volumes represented here are the result of an International Congress Of Mucosal Immunology held at the Niagara Falls Convention Center and the Niagara Falls Hilton on June 29 - July 3, 1986. This satellite meeting of the International Congress of Immunology placed emphasis on all aspects of the Mucosal Immune System. This included the regulation of differentiation of mucosal lymphocytes, mucosa-associated lymphoreticular tissue and lymphocyte homing, the immunology of mucosa-associated tissues and glands, effector functions in mucosal immunity, and the effects of environmental antigens on the immune response, all of which are included in Volume I. The second volume has emphasized studies of the immune response and effector functions, IgA biosynthesis and transport, IgA proteases and effector functions, developmental aspects and immunodeficiency, the immunopathology of IgA and mucosal immunoprophylaxis. A total of 218 papers are included in these two volumes and a comparison to past meetings held at four to five year intervals indicates the explosive growth of mucosal immunology. A total of 50 papers were presented at the 1973 meeting and 81 reports were given at the 1977 meeting, both of which were held in Birmingham, Alabama and were published in the current series by Plenum Press. The third meeting in this series, held in 1982 in New York City contained 113 contributions. Clearly, the Mucosal Immune System has come of age.

The hosting of a Congress of this magnitude and the compilation of two Volumes of publications obviously necessitates our sincere thanks for the efforts of many individuals and groups. The secretarial staffs of the Editors of these Volumes are gratefully acknowledged. These volumes would not have been possible without the expert skill and dedication of Ms. Yvonne A. Noll, who corrected and retyped all papers in this series. We also acknowledge financial support from the following:

Abbott Laboratories, North Chicago, Illinois
Dr. J. Claude Bennett, Department of Medicine, University of Alabama At Birmingham
Dr. Charles A. McCallum, Office of the President, University of Alabama At Birmingham
Dr. James Pittman, School of Medicine, University of Alabama At Birmingham
Procter and Gamble, Co., Cincinnati, Ohio
Dr. Leonard Robinson, School of Dentistry, University of Alabama At Birmingham
Ross Laboratories, Columbus, Ohio

The Editors
February, 1987

ANAMNESTIC RESPONSE

All who work in the area of Mucosal Immunology realize the importance of memory or recall for local immune responses. As you proceed to read the papers in these volumes, it is most appropriate for us to pay a special tribute to a very talented person who worked for several months on these Proceedings. Ms. Yvonne A. Noll retyped all of our manuscripts, and at the same time converted them to the standard format. We all received copies for our corrections, and she patiently made the necessary changes which also came from the Editors. Other time was spent in obtaining new Figures and in some cases retyping manuscripts which were redone by some authors. This monumental task was performed mainly during the period of October, 1986 through February, 1987. On behalf of all of those who contributed to these two volumes we pay our wholehearted thanks to Yvonne.

CONTENTS VOLUME 1

SESSION IV: EFFECTOR FUNCTIONS IN MUCOSAL IMMUNITY

CONTENTS VOLUME 2

SESSION VI: IMMUNE RESPONSE AND EFFECTOR FUNCTIONS

SESSION IX: DEVELOPMENTAL ASPECTS AND IMMUNODEFICIENCY

INTRODUCTORY ADDRESS

In this series of Mucosal Immunology Symposia, a distinguished colleague has been chosen to deliver the opening address. At the present meeting Dr. John J. Cebra was selected because of his outstanding contributions to both humoral and cellular aspects of mucosal immunology. In this function, he joins the previously chosen speakers listed below.

Past Speakers

1. Dr. J.F. Heremans, "The IgA System in Connection with Local and Systemic Immunity," Adv. Exp. Biol. Med. Volume 45, 1, 1974, Plenum Press, NY.

2. Dr. T.B. Tomasi, Jr., "New Areas Arising from Studies of Secretory Immunity," Adv. Exp. Biol. Med. Volume 107, 1, 1978, Plenum Press, NY.

3. Dr. L.Å. Hanson, "Mucosal Immunity," Annals of the New York Academy of Sciences, Volume 409, 1, 1983.

PERTURBATIONS IN PEYER'S PATCH B CELL POPULATIONS INDICATIVE OF PRIMING FOR A SECRETORY IgA RESPONSE

J.J. Cebra, P.M. Griffin, D.A. Lebman and S.D. London

Department of Biology,
University of Pennsylvania
Philadelphia, PA USA

INTRODUCTION

Many years after Johann Peyer described localized accumulations of lymphoid cells in the mammalian intestinal mucosa (Peyer's patches, PP) (1) we proposed a special role for them in the development of secretory IgA responses (2). Initially we found that rabbit PP cells were enriched sources of precursors for IgA-plasma cells and could repopulate the spleen and intestinal lamina propria of irradiated recipients with such plasma cells much more effectively than could lymphoid cells from other sources (2). This was a somewhat accidental finding made while trying to elucidate the mechanism for transporting IgA from lamina propria plasma cells into the gut lumen. Jose O'Daly had been following up the detection of secretory component (SC) in glandular epithelial cells (3) and observed that many of the apparently nonspecialized epithelial cells lining the Lieberkühn crypts contained numerous cytoplasmic granules that stained positively for both IgA and SC (4). The issue became the direction of flow - were the granules the result of endocytosis of sIgA from the intestinal fluid in the crypt lumen or were they formed at the plasma membrane on the basal side of the cells from IgA dimer secreted by the proximal plasma cells? At this time Asher Frensdorff had been using lymphoid cells from rabbits heterozygous at the Ig kappa chain locus (b locus) to analyze for functional allelic exclusion in B lymphocytes by transferring them into irradiated recipients of yet a different kappa allotype (5). Fluorescent anti-allotype reagents were used to detect the plasma cell progeny of these lymphocytes. When O'Daly proposed that the direction of granular transport in crypt cells could be solved by re-populating the lamina propria around some crypts with donor-derived cells of one allotype while leaving IgA cells of a different, host allotype, around other crypts, an adoptive transfer of the Frensdorff sort was suggested, but into sub-lethally irradiated recipients. The only caveat was to identify a source of B lymphocyte precursors for IgA plasma cells. Susan Craig attempted such adoptive transfers with lymphoid cells from many sources, including PP, which she had learned about while attending seminars in the Gastroenterology Division, Johns Hopkins Medical School. Her transfer of PP cells to successfully repopulate lamina propria with IgA plasma cells (2) has stimulated much subsequent experimental work. Our own findings that the immediate precursors of IgA plasma cells had a surface phenotype that is sIgM-negative, sIg-positive (6) suggested that isotype 'switching' may take place in PP, where the microenvironment appears to favor IgA-commitment. We have since sought to understand the role of PP in B cell differentiation. This paper will describe some of the cellular perturbations in PP that correlate with priming for a secretory IgA response and some of the properties of IgA-memory cells that appear at these mucosal sites.

MATERIALS AND METHODS

T-lymphocyte dependent B cell clones were grown _in vitro_ in splenic fragment cultures following transfer of limiting numbers of a particular specificity of B cells from PP and other sources to carrier-primed, lethally irradiated recipient mice (7,8). B cells enriched on films of haptenated gelatin for a given specificity were grown in microculture (10 μl) in the presence of appropriate 'filler', 'feeder', and/or T-helper (Th) cells (9,10). The isotypes of antibody expressed by B cell clones was determined qualitatively and quantitatively by radioimmunoassay (11).

RESULTS

Cellular correlates of priming for a specific IgA response

Cell transfers between allotype congenic, histocompatible inbred mouse strains (BALB/c and CB20) confirmed the preeminence of PP as a source of precursors that can effectively repopulate the intestinal lamina propria of irradiated recipients with IgA-plasma cells (12). Pat Gearhart sought to identify the functional properties of the PP B cells that could account for their greater potential to generate IgA-plasma cells than B cells from other sources (8). She tested the isotype potential of single precursor B cells as expressed over many (8-10) generations in the form of specific antibodies secreted by their clones in response to thymus-dependent (TD) antigens in splenic fragment cultures. Her findings (8) led to the operational definition of IgA-committed murine memory B cells as those which generate clones exclusively secreting IgA in response to specific TD antigens. Such clonal precursors, specific for certain antigenic determinants such as phosphocholine (PC), β2→1 fructosyl (In, inulin), β-galactosyl (β-gal) and α1-3 glucosyl (dex) but not others, such as trinitrophenyl (TNP), fluoresceinyl (Flu) and those of cholera toxin (TXN), are prevalent in PP of young adult, conventionally reared mice (8,13). These IgA-committed precursors arise naturally in PP, but appear to lag behind an earlier rise in frequency of B cells of the corresponding specificity. For instance, PC-specific B cells increase sharply in frequency between 8-12 days of neonatal life (14) and In-specific B cells between 3-5 weeks of age (15) while Table 1 indicates that young adult levels of IgA-committed B cells of these specificities are not found in PP until mice reach 8-11 weeks of age. We have proposed that the natural colonization of the intestine with commensal bacteria during neonatal life may provide the stimulus for increases in frequency of B cells of certain specificities (vs. 'environmental' determinants) and could also specifically drive B cell development in PP leading to the accumulation of IgA-committed cells in mucosal sites. Young adult mice were maintained germ-free for up to one year, or colonized with normal gut commensals at 4 months and assayed 8 months later (16). Our findings were that frequencies of anti-PC and anti-In remained considerably lower than normal in the year-old germ-free mice. The deliberately colonized mice showed both increased frequencies of these specificities in all lymphoid tissues tested and gradients of IgA committed cells from largest proportions in PP to lowest in distal lymphoid tissues (16). Thus colonization of young adult mice with natural bacterial flora could reproduce quantitatively and qualitatively the perturbation in the populations of two specificities of B cells that is normally observed during neonatal development. Again, two further experiments using deliberate bacterial colonization of germ-free mice summarized in Table 2 show that rises in frequencies of anti-In B cells precede by some weeks the selective accumulations of IgA-committed B cells in PP. Such observations suggest that chronic antigenic stimulation of the gut mucosa primes specific B cells - increases their frequency - and eventually leads to isotype 'switching' and IgA-commitment. A model for this process

Table 1. IgA-committed B cells specific for PC- or In- determinants do not become prevalent in Peyer's patches until 8-11 weeks after birth

specificity:	$\bar{a}$ PC		$\bar{a}$ In	
age of donor:	5 wks	8-11 wks	5 wks	8-11 wks
% clones expressing:				
IgA only	7	35	5	61
some IgA	11	50	45	78
IgM only	71	38	20	22
some IgM	93	65	75	33
some IgG	14	23	35	11
# clones	28	26	20	18

Table 2. Isotype patterns expressed by clones from In-specific B cells taken from formerly germ-free mice at varying times after colonization[a]

	time after colonization			
	1 wk	2 wks	3 wks	3-18 wks
splenic clones expressing (%):				
A only	0	0	0	29
M only	70	54	9	0
some M	100	92	100	18
# clones	10	24	44	45
freq./10^6 B cells[b]	8	22	39	41
Peyer's patch clones expressing (%):				
A only	0	20	5	42
M only	50	0	0	0
some M	100	40	89	31
# clones	4	5	18	19
freq./10^6 B cells[b]	11	34	100	92

[a]Mice were colonized 1-3 wks with lactobacilli/streptococci or 3-18 wks with Schaedler's commensals.

[b]Germ-free frequencies: spleen 2-7/10^6; PP 4-<13/10^6.

is based on the central premise that the gene-segment rearrangements responsible for isotype switching and IgA commitment are dependent on antigen-driven B cell division in PP (13). Thus we sought to duplicate the rather slow natural process attributed to chronic gut mucosal stimulation using acute stimulation with nominal antigens. Cholera toxin, a non-replicating antigen with a binding specificity for GM1-ganglioside, and reovirus 1, a replicating enteric virus which preferentially binds to the dome epithelial cells (M cells) overlaying PP, were delivered to mice either intraduodenally (i.d.) or intraperitoneally (i.p.) (London et al., this volume). Both antigens, delivered by either route, resulted in a rapid rise in TD specific B cells in all tissues within 10-14 days ($\sim$1-2/10^6 to 4-30/10^6). However, only animals receiving antigen intraduodenally showed a high proportion of IgA-committed memory cells and these were always most prevalent in PP (17, Table 3). In the case of the TXN antigen given i.d. vs. i.p., a direct correlation was found between the rise in IgA-committed precursors in PP, as scored upon secondary stimulation _in vitro_ in splenic fragment culture, and the secondary _in vivo_ response to i.d. restimulation, as estimated from the IgA anti-TXN containing cells that appeared in gut lamina propria (17). Thus, efficacious priming for a gut mucosal IgA response seems related to tissue-binding properties of the antigen delivered i.d. and can be correlated with the rise of frequency of IgA-committed B cells in PP. Finally, the especial effectiveness of TXN appears to depend on both the binding and pharmacologic activities of the molecule. The B subunit does increase the frequency of specific PP B cells but does not generate as many IgA-committed memory cells as the holotoxin (18). On the other hand, holotoxin given i.d. appears to non-specifically affect pre-existing memory cells of other specificities in PP, such that their resultant clones become more likely to express IgA following specific antigen-stimulation _in vitro_ (18). The elucidation of the mechanism for this 'bystander' effect of holotoxin should prove relevant to understanding the general process of IgA-commitment occurring in PP.

Properties of IgA-committed B cells and the role of PP germinal centers in their development

Most lymphoid tissues show the development of histologically obvious germinal centers (GC) only after acute or chronic antigenic stimulation, especially proximal to draining lymph nodes (19). However, the PP of conventionally reared mice display chronically active germinal centers containing about 15% of the total B cells, including most of the dividing

10%. These structures contain a circumferential region of $sIgD^+$ B cells and a large core of B cells that bind high levels of peanut agglutinin (PNA^{hi}), are $sIgD^-$ and have low surface densities of Ig ($s\kappa^{lo}$) (20). Finally, the roughly 10% of PP B cells that bear surface IgA ($sIgA^+$) are distributed between the $PNA^{hi}s\kappa^{lo}$ and $PNA^{lo}s\kappa^{hi}$ subsets (see Fig. 1), their relative abundance shifting from the former to the latter with age. The GC have been implicated in the development of memory B cells (19) and those of PP appear to be sites of both B cell division and isotype 'switching' to the expression of sIgA or sIgG (20,21, see Fig. 1). Since the permanently active GC in PP are likely the result of chronic stimulation by environmental antigens we tested for memory B cells specific for In-, PC-, and β-gal determinants in subsets of PP cells resolved by fluorescence-activated cell sorting (FACS). Table 4 shows that anti-PC IgA clonal precursors are enriched in the $sIgD^-$ and markedly depleted in the $sIgD^+$ subsets respectively. Anti-In precursors are enriched in frequency in the $sIgA^+$ subset and clones of all specificities derived from these cells exclusively secreted IgA. Thus, we have provided the first direct formal proof that sIgA-positivity is indicative of the isotype potential of IgA-memory cells. When germinal center B cells ($PNA^{hi}s\kappa^{lo}$) were compared with small, resting B cells ($PNA^{lo}s\kappa^{hi}$), the latter subset accounted for almost all the antigen-dependent clonal precursors, including the IgA-memory cells

Table 3. Acute intraduodenal stimulation with cholera toxin or reovirus 1 increases frequencies and proportions of specific IgA-committed B cells

	Specificity:				
	anti-toxin[a]		anti-reovirus 1		
Tissue:	PP	Spl	PP[b]	PP[c]	Spl[c]
clones expressing (%):					
IgA only	50	38	40	64	50
some IgA	77	62	40	73	61
some IgM	4	38	0	18	33
# clones	22	13	10	11	18
freq./10^6[d]	4.4	12	25	33	31

[a] 14 d after priming.
[b] 10 d after priming.
[c] 27 d after priming.
[d] Preimmunization frequencies <1-2/10^6 for both specificities.

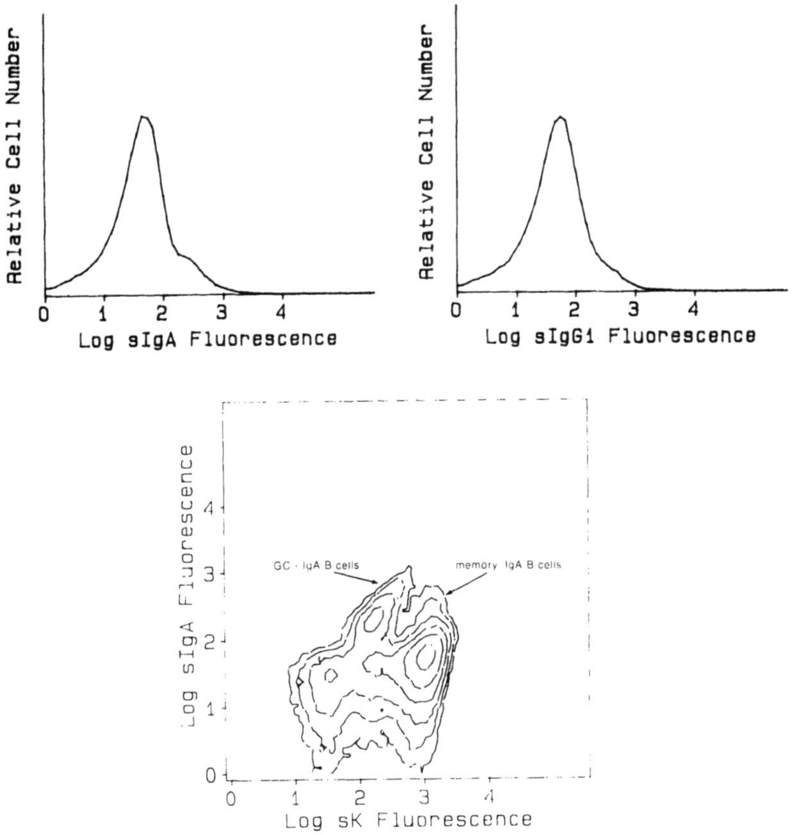

Figure 1. sIgA and sIgG1 B cells in Peyer's patches. Peyer's patches contain both $sIgA^+$ and $sIgG1^+$ B cells. The $sIgA^+$ B cells occur in both the $s\kappa^{lo}$ (germinal center) and $s\kappa^{hi}$ (memory populations).

(Table 5). Some of the splenic fragment cultures of GC cells did secrete Ig but these were antigen-independent, usually made only IgM in very small amounts and the antibodies were highly cross-reactive and of low avidity for any determinant with which they cross-reacted. We analyzed the functional potential of these PP subsets of B cells by two other methods: a) content of mRNA for alpha chain of IgA by semi-quantitative dot-blotting; and b) active synthesis of cytoplasmic IgA by incorporation of ^{35}S-methionine into alpha chain. The bulk of both mRNA for and synthesis of alpha chain given by PP could be accounted for by cells with the surface phenotype $PNA^{hi}sIgA^+$. In some instances a $PNA^{hi}s\kappa^{hi}$ subset could be resolved from the PNA^{hi} fraction and this appeared most active in synthesizing alpha chain. On the basis of our observations we would suggest the following process occurs in PP leading to IgA-committed memory B cells. Antigen stimulates specific B cell proliferation in GC leading to loss of sIgD, acquisition of the $s\kappa^{lo}$ phenotype, and isotype switching, including

Table 4. Surface immunoglobulin (sIg) phenotype correlates with isotype potential of Peyer's patch B cells

	Exp. 1 (ā PC)[b]			Exp. 2 (ā PC, ā In, ā TNP)		
	unfract. PP	sIgM,sIgD +ve	sIgM,sIgD −ve	unfract. PP	sIgA +ve	sIgA −ve
total clones	20	20	5	74	14	31
Isotype expressed (%):						
IgM only	5	20	0	8	0	3
IgM + IgG	18	10	0	0	0	0
IgM + IgA	5	10	20	7	0	16
IgM, IgG, IgA	27	40	0	1	0	22
IgG + IgA	9	10	0	19	0	19
IgG only	0	5	20	0	0	0
IgA only	36	5	60	65	100	39
freq./10^6 B cells[a]	--	--	--	27	65	9

[a]ā In only.

[b]Adapted from (32).

Table 5. Thymus-dependent, antigen-sensitive clonal precursors from Peyer's patches are $PNA^{lo}/s\kappa^{hi}$ (memory cells)

				$PNA^{lo}/s\kappa^{hi}$ (memory cells)			
				% clones expressing:			
Phenotype of B cell	total inoculum tested(x10^{-6})	total clones	freq/10^6 injected cells	IgM only	some IgM	some IgA	IgA only
$PNA^{lo}s\kappa^{hi}$	134	107	0.8	19	59	72	22
PNA^{hi}(all)	34	48[a]	1.4[a]	90	94	8	2

[a]High estimates, many 'clones' conted more than once due to cross- reactions among ā PC-, ā β-Gal, ā In-, and ā TNP specificites; most secreted antibody of low avidity, IgM isotype, and antigen-independent for expression.

expression of sIgA. Such cells may further diversify to pre-memory and pre-plasmablast cells but the former require 8-14 days to become restimulable by antigen to generate clones exclusively secreting IgA. This is the time span required to generate IgA memory cells following acute primary i.d. stimulation with cholera toxin or reovirus 1 (17, Table 3). The pre-plasmablasts likely account for the antigen-independent, Ig-positive cultures from PNA^{hi} B cells. These cells, having received an initial stimulation in vivo by environmental antigen, may undergo a few divisions and secrete cross-reactive IgM antibodies in the supportive splenic fragment culture. Plasma cells from lamina propria account for the bulk of the mRNA for alpha chain and the synthesis of cytoplasmic IgA. Further, these cells probably account for the preponderance of the mRNA for the secreted form of alpha chain found in PP cells by Word et al. (22). The IgA-committed memory B cells that respond to antigen by generating an IgA-secreting clone are found predominantly in the small, resting $s\kappa^{hi}$, $sIgD^{-}$ population outside GC. These IgA memory cells appear to have a long half-life and remain at highest frequency in PP up to 12 weeks after initial mucosal priming with TXN (23). They and their putative precursors in GC (PNA^{hi}, $s\kappa^{lo}$, $sIgA^{+}$) would likely account for the subset of PP cells enriched by panning on anti-IgA coated plates by Woloschak, who found them to contain mainly the mRNA for membrane form of IgA (24).

To support the above postulates the following would be required: (1) to demonstrate clonal culture in vitro the acquisition of antigen-responsiveness by $PNA^{hi}s\kappa^{lo}$ GC cells and to determine whether many of their clones exclusively make IgA. The latter would support IgA-commitment already occurring at the GC stage and would provide evidence against reversible isotype switching, a process that could occur through synthesis of polycistronic mRNAs allowing cells to express sIgA without becoming isotype restricted (24); (2) to determine whether diversification of IgA-committed B cells into pre-memory or pre-plasmablast cells takes place while they are still in GC; (3) to determine the major route by which putative $sIgA^{+}$ progenitors of IgA-committed memory cells pass from GC to arrive in regions of small, resting B cells in PP. Pre-plasmablasts can be tracked to the mesenteric lymph nodes (25), then thoracic duct lymph (26) before they selectively lodge in lamina propria (26,27). IgA-committed memory cells also can be detected in peripheral blood following gut mucosal priming (23). However, it is not known whether pre-memory cells for IgA-precursors pass from GC into the circulation or move directly into regions of small, resting B cells in PP; (4) to identify any peculiar cellular or molecular stimuli required to trigger an IgA-memory cell to generate a clone secreting IgA-antibodies.

Antigen-specific T cell clones bearing Fc receptors for IgA (FcR) have been grown from primed PP cells and these appear to enhance the number of IgA-secreting cells *in vitro* (28). Their targets appear to be $sIgA^+$ B cells which have already undergone isotype switching (29). Soluble factors from T-T hybridomas and T cell clones have also been reported to enhance numbers of IgA secreting cells and IgA secretion respectively (30,31). Thus far, none of these up-regulating stimuli for IgA production have been applied to clonal B cell cultures. Thus, the precise stage of susceptibility of the B cells, the type of effect - to enhance proliferation or secretion - and the isotype specificity corresponding to these stimuli remain unknown. A promising antigen-dependent clonal B cell culturing procedure for testing the requirements for expression of secreted IgA is the microculturing (10 μl) of enriched, single antigen-specific B cells (9). The enrichment on haptenated-gelatin has already been shown to isolate IgA-committed B cells and the microculture has already been used to analyze antigen-driven isotype switching (10). Recently, B cells primed *in vivo* to switch to expression of IgG isotypes have been enriched for a particular specificity, pulsed with antigen and co-cultured with carrier-specific T helper cell lines to give clones secreting IgG antibodies in the absence of detectable IgM. Thus, these procedures may be applicable for determining the requirements for stimulating single IgA-committed B cells to generate antibody secreting clones *in vitro*.

ACKNOWLEDGEMENTS

We thank Ethel R. Cebra, Alvan Chaney, Jennifer Kennedy and Katherine Paschetto for their excellent technical assistance. This work was supported by grants AI-17997, CA-15822 and AI-18554.

REFERENCES

1. Gillespie, C.G. (Ed.), Dir. of Sci. Biography, 10, 567, 1974.
2. Craig, S.W. and Cebra, J.J., J. Exp. Med. 134, 188, 1971.
3. Tomasi, T.B., Jr., Tan, E.M., Solomon, A. and Prendergast, R.A., J. Exp. Med. 121, 101, 1965.
4. O'Daly, J.A., Craig, S.W. and Cebra, J.J., J. Immunol. 106, 286, 1971.
5. Frensdorff, A., Jones, P.P., Berwald-Netter, Y., Cebra, J.J. and Mage, R., Science 171, 391, 1971.

6. Jones, P.P., Craig, S.W., Cebra, J.J. and Herzenberg, L.A., J. Exp. Med. 140, 452, 1974.
7. Klinman, N.R., J. Exp. Med. 136, 241, 1972.
8. Gearhart, P.J. and Cebra, J.J., J. Exp. Med. 149, 216, 1979.
9. Nossal, G.J.V. and Pike, B.L., J. Immunol. 120, 145, 1978.
10. Cebra, J.J., Cebra, E.R., Kotloff, D.B., Lebman, D.A., Schweitzer, P.A. and Shahin, R.D., Biochem. Soc. Symp. 51, 159, 1986.
11. Hurwitz, J.L., Tagart, V.B., Schweitzer, P.A. and Cebra, J.J., Eur. J. Immunol. 12, 342, 1982.
12. Cebra, J.J., Gearhart, P.J., Kamat, R., Robertson, S.M. and Tseng, J., Cold Spring Harbor Symp. Quant. Biol. 41, 201, 1977.
13. Cebra, J.J., Fuhrman, J.A., Gearhart, P.J., Hurwitz, J.L. and Shahin, R.D., in Recent Advances in Mucosal Immunity, (Edited by Strober, W., Hanson, L.A. and Sell, K.W.), p. 155, Raven Press, New York, 1982.
14. Sigal, N.H., Pickard, A.R., Metcalf, E.S., Gearhart, P.J. and Klinman, N.R., J. Exp. Med. 146, 933, 1977.
15. Shahin, R.D. and Cebra, J.J., Infect. Immunity 32, 211, 1981.
16. Cebra, J.J., Gearhart, P.J., Halsey, J.F., Hurwitz, J.L. and Shahin, R.D., J. Reticuloendothelial Soc. 28:(suppl), 61, 1980.
17. Fuhrman, J.A. and Cebra, J.J., J. Exp. Med. 153, 534, 1981.
18. Cebra, J.J., Fuhrman, J.A., Lebman, D.A. and London, S.D., in Vaccines 86, (Edited by Brown, F., Chanock, R.M. and Lerner, R.A.), p. 129, Cold Spring Harbor Laboratory, Cold Spring Harbor, 1986.
19. Coico, R.F., Bhogal, B.S. and Thorbecke, G.J., J. Immunol. 131, 2254, 1983.
20. Butcher, E.C., Rouse, R.V., Coffman, R.L., Nottenburg, C.N., Hardy, R.R. and Weissman, I.L., J. Immunol. 129, 2698, 1982.
21. Kraal, G., Weissman, I.L. and Butcher, E.C., Nature 298, 377, 1982.
22. Word, C.J., Mushinski, J.F. and Tucker, P.W., EMBO J. 2, 887, 1983.
23. Cebra, J.J., Fuhrman, J.A., Griffin, P., Rose, F.V., Schweitzer, P.A. and Zimmerman, D., Annals of Allergy 53, 541, 1984.
24. Woloschak, G.E., Molec. Immunochem. 23, 581, 1986.
25. Husband, A.J., Monie, H.J. and Gowans, J.L., in Immunology of the Gut, Ciba Foundation Symposium 46, Elsevier, New York, p. 29, 1977.
26. Pierce, N.F. and Gowans, J.L., J. Exp. Med. 142, 1550, 1975.
27. Husband, A.J., J. Immunol. 128, 1355, 1982.
28. Kiyono, H., McGhee, J.R., Mosteller, L.M., Eldridge, J.H., Koopman, W.J., Kearney, J.F. and Michalek, S.M., J. Exp. Med. 156, 1115, 1982.
29. Kiyono, H., Cooper, M.D., Kearney, J.F., Mosteller, L.M., Michalek, S.M., Koopman, W.J. and McGhee, J.R., J. Exp. Med. 159, 798, 1984.

30. Kiyono, H., Mosteller-Barnum, L.M., Pitts, A.M., Williamson, S.I., Michalek, S.M. and McGhee, J.R., J. Exp. Med. 161, 731, 1985.

31. Coffman, R.L., Bond, M.W., Carty, J. and Mosmann, T.R., Progress in Immunology 6, Abs. 3.13.16, p. 267, 1986.

32. Gearhart, P.J., Hurwitz, J.L. and Cebra, J.J., Proc. Natl. Acad. Sci. USA 77, 5424, 1980.

RABBIT IgA HEAVY CHAIN GENES: CLONING AND IN VITRO EXPRESSION

R.C. Burnett, R.D. Schneiderman and K.L. Knight

Department of Microbiology and Immunology, University
of Illinois College of Medicine at Chicago
Chicago, IL USA

INTRODUCTION

Southern blot analysis of rabbit germline DNA showed the rabbit genome contained at least 10 Cα genes (1). This observation was of particular interest since both mouse and human have only one and two Cα genes, respectively. Genomic blot data are consistent with studies of rabbit IgA heavy chain allotypes which suggested the existence of multiple IgA isotypes (2-4). To further examine the complexity and genetic control of rabbit IgA, we have undertaken molecular and genetic studies of the IgA heavy chains.

RESULTS

Cloning of IgA heavy chain genes

Recombinant cosmid and phage libraries, prepared from rabbits homozygous for the IgA heavy chain allotypes, were screened with a rabbit Cα cDNA probe (5). A 770 bp fragment from the 3' end of the cDNA which encodes the CH2 and CH3 domains and contains 3' untranslated sequence was used as a probe. The identified clones were restriction mapped and examined for overlapping segments of DNA. The results of the mapping studies identified two clusters of Cα genes (Fig. 1). The first cluster contains four Cα genes and spans approximately 55 kb of DNA. The second cluster contains three

Cα genes and spans 35 kb of DNA. In each cluster, the Cα genes are separated by approximately 12 kb of DNA. The orientation of each gene was established by differential hybridization with the CH2-CH3 probe and with a CH1 probe. Within each cluster, all genes had the same orientation relative to one another. The two Cα gene clusters have not been linked by overlapping clones to one another or to the remainder of the heavy chain chromosomal region which contains the genes encoding JH, Cμ, Cγ, and C_{ϵ} (1).

Genomic blot analysis of rabbit DNA revealed 10 Bam HI fragments which hybridized to the Cα cDNA probe (Fig. 2). The seven cloned Cα genes represent the 12 kb, 9.3 kb, 8.0 kb, 7.9 kb, 7.8 kb, 6.2 kb, and 2.8 kb hybridizing fragments. Based on this analysis, the genes residing on the 23 kb, 17 kb and 2.1 kb fragments have yet to be cloned.

In vitro expression of four Cα genes

To test for expressibility of the cloned Cα genes, the Cα1, Cα2, Cα3, and Cα4 genes were cloned into a eukaryotic expression vector and then transfected into the murine plasmacytoma cell line, J558L. J558L is a heavy chain loss variant which produces lambda light chains in the absence of heavy chains (6). A pSV2gpt derived vector was kindly provided by Dr. V.T. Oi (Becton Dickinson Monoclonal Ct., Mt. View, California). This vector contains a rearranged murine VDJ gene and the murine heavy chain enhancer region (Fig. 3). Stable transfectomas were selected in mycophenolic acid. The exogenous heavy chains associate with the light chains and are then secreted into the culture medium. Expression of chimeric heavy chains containing murine VH and rabbit Cα was assayed by solid phase radiobinding analysis of culture supernatant fluids. Transfectomas resulting from each of the four constructs were shown to secrete molecules which reacted with goat anti-rabbit Fcα antibody in the solid phase radiobinding assay. Thus, all four Cα genes can be expressed in vitro.

SDS-polyacrylamide gel electrophoresis analysis of Ig molecules immunoprecipitated from lysates of each transfectoma was used to determine the nature of the IgA molecules produced by these transfectomas. Immunoprecipitations were performed with anti-rabbit Fcα and anti-mouse lambda light chain antibodies. Each antibody precipitated both heavy and light chains, confirming the expectation that the heavy and light chains would associate in vitro (Fig. 4). Two different sized heavy chains were observed; the

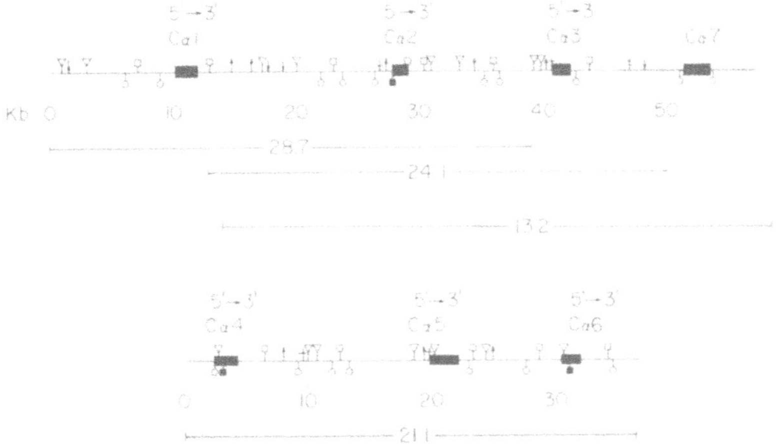

Figure 1. Organization of two clusters of Cα genes based on restriction mapping of individual or overlapping cosmid clones. The seven Cα genes are indicated by solid boxes. The enzyme symbols are: (ɗ), Bam HI; (Ÿ), Hind III; (♀), Kpn I; (↓), Eco RI; (ǂ), Sac II; (+), Bal I; (↑) Sal I; and (↓) Xho I.

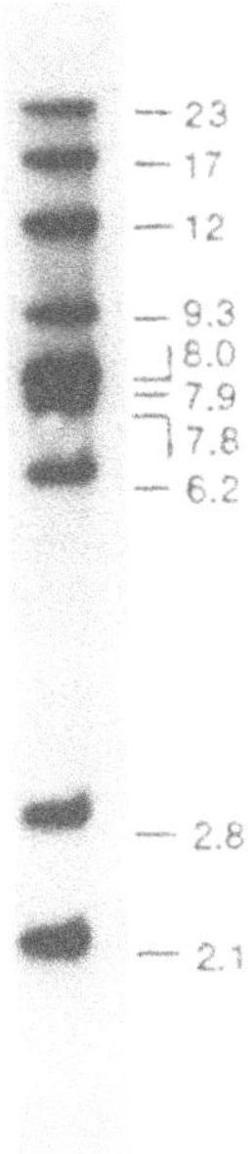

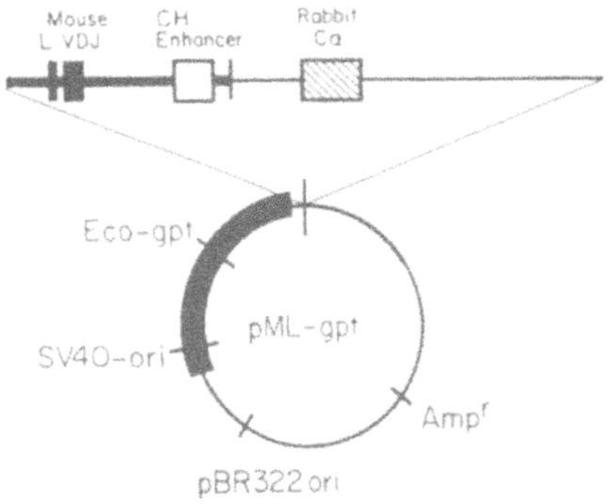

Figure 2 (left). Southern blot analysis of rabbit sperm DNA restricted with BamHI. ^{32}P-Cα cDNA was used as a probe; hybridization was performed in 40% formamide, 10% dextran sulfate, 0.6 M NaCl, and 0.06 M sodium citrate at 42°C. The size (in kilobase pairs) of each hybridizing fragment is designated.

Figure 3 (right). Map of vector containing murine VDJ and rabbit Cα gene. The vector contains a VDJ from a dansyl-binding hybridoma, murine heavy chain enhancer, Eco-gpt gene with the SV40 promoter, and the gene for ampicillin resistance. The site for cloning the various rabbit Cα genes is designated by a vertical bar downstream of the CH enhancer.

heavy chains from the α2 and α4 constructs were 55 kd and from the α3 and α1 constructs, 60 kd (data for α1 not shown). The biochemical basis for these molecular weight differences has yet to be determined.

Phylogenetic analysis of Cα gene amplification

Since the domestic rabbit has so many Cα genes, we decided to investigate other lagomorphs to determine the phylogeny of Cα gene amplification. Southern blot analyses were conducted on DNA from cottontail rabbit (genus: *Sylvilagus*) and jackrabbit (genus: *Lepus*) both of which belong to the same family (*Leporidae*) as the domestic rabbit (genus: *Orytolagus*). Liver DNA from a cottontail rabbit and a jackrabbit were kindly provided by M. Weil and W.J. Mandy (Univ. of Texas, Austin, TX). As observed in domestic rabbit, both the cottontail and jackrabbit have multiple (10 to 14) DNA fragments which hybridize with the Cα probe, indicating that they have multiple Cα genes (Fig. 5). Some of the bands may reflect restriction site polymorphisms between allelic genes and thus, the actual number of genes could be less than the number of hybridizing bands. Some of the larger hybridizing fragments of the jackrabbit were quite intense, suggesting that these fragments contain more than one Cα gene. Although the exact number of genes in these animals has not been demonstrated, it is clear that they all possess multiple Cα genes. Thus, amplification of the Cα genes presumably occurred before divergence of the three genera. It will be important to investigate the other family of lagomorphs, to which pikas belong (*Ochotonidae*), to determine if the Cα gene duplications occurred before divergence of the two families.

DISCUSSION

Serologic data obtained with anti-allotype antisera have clearly identified multiple IgA isotypes in rabbit serum and colostrum (2-4). A molecular approach to study rabbit IgA has been undertaken in order to determine the complexity of rabbit Cα genes and to examine the regulatory mechanisms which control their expression. Although we have cloned seven Cα genes, there are at least three Cα genes which have yet to be cloned. Screening of additional recombinant libraries will be necessary in order to clone the remaining genes and to complete the restriction map of the heavy chain chromosomal region.

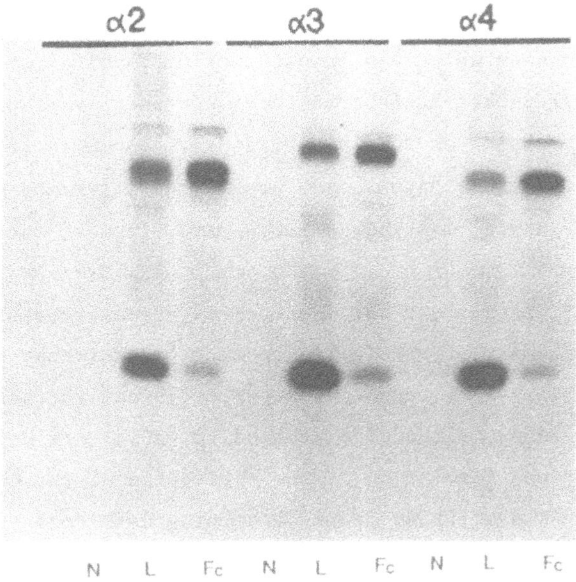

Figure 4. SDS-PAGE analysis of immunoprecipitates of biosynthetically labeled IgA from J558L cells transfected with vector constructs containing either the Cα2 (α2), Cα3 (α3), or Cα4 (α4) gene. Transfectomas were labeled in vitro with ^{35}S-methionine for 4 hours and the biosynthetically labeled IgA molecules were immunoprecipitated with goat anti-rabbit Fcα (Fc) or rabbit anti-mouse light chain (L); precipitation with normal rabbit serum (N) was used as the negative control. The immunoprecipitates were dissolved in 0.2% SDS with 0.5% 2-mercaptoethanol and electrophoresed on 10% polyacrylamide in 0.001% SDS.

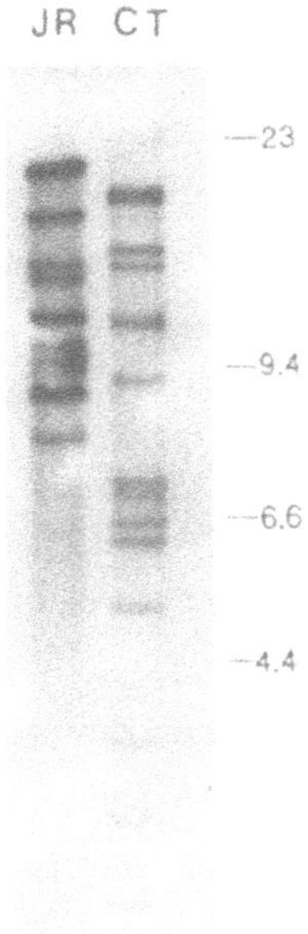

Figure 5. Southern blot analysis of BamHI digested cottontail (CT) and jackrabbit (JR) liver DNA using ^{32}P-labeled rabbit Cα encoding cDNA as a probe. The hybridizations were performed as described in Figure 2. The size standards are of Hind III digested lambda phage DNA.

The expression of individual Cα genes *in vitro* provides a source of monoclonal α-heavy chains which can be used for biochemical and serologic analyses. Monoclonal rabbit Ig isotypes have not been available due to the lack of rabbit myelomas or stable hybridomas. The monoclonal heavy chains produced by the transfectomas can now be characterized with respect to their primary structure, isotypy, allotypy and effector functions.

The fact that the first four Cα genes tested are expressible, suggests that the actual complexity of rabbit IgA is much greater than had been identified serologically. We cannot, however, rule out the possibility that some of the Cα genes, although expressed *in vitro*, are not expressed *in vivo*. To examine the regulation of the expression of the Cα genes, isotype specific DNA and antibody probes are being developed. The DNA probes will be used to detect mRNA transcripts of the various genes *in vivo*, and the antibody probes will be used to detect the protein products of each gene.

Nucleotide sequencing of the cloned Cα genes will allow us to compare the primary structures of α-heavy chains of the various IgA isotypes. One of the important structural features of IgA is its ability to bind secretory component (SC). Rabbit IgA can be divided into two populations, one which binds SC covalently and another which binds SC through non-covalent interactions. These interactions with IgA are known to occur through the α-heavy chain, but the precise amino acids involved in this binding have not been established. Nucleotide sequencing of one Cα cDNA, which encodes a molecule which binds SC non-covalently, encodes serine residues at positions 299 and 311 of the α-heavy chain. Human and mouse α-chains, which bind SC covalently, have cysteine residues at these positions. We propose that these cysteines are involved in the interchain disulfide bonds between α-heavy chains and SC (5). Correlation of the amino acid residues at positions 299 and 311 with the ability of each isotype to bind SC covalently or non-covalently should allow us to determine if this proposal is correct.

Rabbits have more Cα genes than any other mammal examined thus far. This raises the question as to the immunologic significance of multiple Cα genes. Three genera within the family *Leporidae* have multiple Cα genes. Examination of DNA from pikas, a member of the other family of lagomorphs, will determine if the amplification is common to all lagomorphs. If so, we will perform southern blot analysis on DNA from various mammals. If some animals are found to have multiple Cα genes, we could begin to search for a physiologic similarity between these animals and lagomorphs; such studies might provide information as to the biologic significance of multiple IgA isotypes.

SUMMARY

Screening of recombinant cosmid and phage libraries with a rabbit Cα cDNA probe has identified a total of seven Cα genes organized into two clusters; one cluster contains four genes and the other cluster, three genes. Southern blot analysis of genomic DNA indicates that the rabbit genome contains a minimum of ten Cα genes; at least three genes remain to be cloned.

Four of the seven cloned Cα genes have been tested for their ability to be expressed _in vitro_. Each gene was cloned 3' to a rearranged murine VDJ gene, and the chimeric gene was then transfected into J558L plasmacytoma cells. Stable transfectants were selected, and each transfectoma was shown to express a chimeric α-heavy chain. These chimeric α-heavy chains were of two sizes, 55 kd and 60 kd. Each of the four transfectomas secreted chimeric heavy chains in association with endogenous murine lambda light chains. All four Cα genes tested were expressible, indicating that the rabbit may have multiple IgA subclasses or isotypes. This is in marked contrast to mouse and human which have only one and two subclasses of IgA, respectively.

ACKNOWLEDGEMENTS

This work was supported by PHS grant AI 11234.

REFERENCES

1. Knight, K.L., Burnett, R.C. and McNicholas, J.M., J. Immunol. 134, 1245, 1985.
2. Conway, T.P., Dray, S. and Lichter, E.A., J. Immunol. 102, 544, 1969.
3. Conway, T.P., Dray, S. and Lichter, E.A., J. Immunol. 103, 622, 1969.

4. Muth, K.L., Hanly, W.C. and Knight, K.L., Molec. Immun. 20, 989, 1983.
5. Knight, K.L., Martens, C.L., Stoklosa, C.M. and Schneiderman, R.D., Nucl. Acid Res. 12, 1657, 1984.
6. Oi, V.T., Morrison, S.L., Herzenberg, L.A. and Berg, P., Proc. Natl. Acad. Sci. USA 80, 825, 1983.

IMMUNOGLOBULIN GENE EXPRESSION IN WASTED MICE

G.E. Woloschak, M. Rodriguez and C.J. Krco

Departments of Immunology, Biochemistry and Molecular Biology, and Neurology, Mayo Clinic and Foundation
Rochester, MN USA

INTRODUCTION

In 1982, Shultz et al. (1) reported the discovery of a new mouse mutation called "wasted" (wst) which is characterized by faulty DNA repair, neurologic abnormalities and immunodeficiency. The disease produced by this spontaneous autosomal recessive mutation (wst) is phenotypically manifested in homozygous wst/wst mice at three weeks of age as a neurologic abnormality. The animals develop tremor and uncoordinated movements which is followed by progressive paralysis. At that time, the animals also manifest lymphoid hypoplasia characterized by decreased thymus, lymph node and spleen to body weight. Homozygotes (wst/wst) have been reported to show decreased lymphoproliferative responses to both Con A and LPS with increasing age (2). In addition, wst/wst mice demonstrate increased susceptibility to chromosomal injury (1). The combined neurologic and immunologic dysfunction as well as an increased propensity for chromosome damage has suggested that the "wasted" mutation provides a model for ataxia telangiectasia (1,3-4).

More recent immunologic studies have demonstrated that wst/wst mice have a deficiency of secretory IgA but have normal levels of serum IgA. While surface IgA^+ cells and IgA plasma cells were present in normal numbers in splenic lymphocyte preparations, lymphocytes from Peyer's patches lacked IgA precursors (5). Because IgA responses are critical at mucosal sites, we had pursued experiments aimed at examining immunologic parameters in both secretory and systemic immune sites as well as examining the neuropathologic features of the disease. It is interesting that our studies demonstrate the B cells of Peyer's patches and IgA responses are most affected by the wst/wst mutation.

MATERIALS AND METHODS

Mice

Breeding pairs of mice bearing the wst mutation were obtained from The Jackson Laboratories (Bar Harbor, ME). Since it is possible that wst/+ heterozygotes may express immunologic abnormalities compared to wild-type (+/+), other control strains (such as B6C3) were also examined. For all experiments, affected animals 3 weeks to 4 weeks of age were used, while unaffected littermates wst/ (composed of wst/+ and +/+ mice) and the parental strain (B6C3) served as controls.

Pathologic examination

Twelve wst/wst mice and twelve wst/ (littermate) mice were examined histologically. Animals were anesthetized with pentobarbital given intraperitoneally and then sacrificed by intracardiac perfusion with 4% paraformaldehyde and 1.5% glutaraldehyde in 0.1 M phosphate buffer (pH 7.2) The spinal cords, brains, spleens, lymph nodes, thymuses, and Peyer's patches (PP) were examined. The brains were cut into six coronal sections while the spinal cords were sectioned coronally into 15-20 blocks, 1-2 mm in thickness. All the tissues were embedded in 2-hydroxyethyl methacrylate by using the JB4 system (Polysciences, Warrington, PA). Semi-thin sections were made and stained with a modified hematoxylin-eosin method.

cDNA probes

Plasmid probes used in these experiments were generously provided by the following individuals: p107αR5 from Dr. L. Hood; pαJ558, pμ (3741)[9], pγ2b(11)[7] from Dr. K. Marcu; γ3-, γ2a- and γ1-specific probes from Dr. S. Cory; κ and λ probes from Dr. J.D. Capra; IL-2 from Dr. Taniguchi; IL-2 receptor from Dr. T. Honjo; and pActin from Dr. A. Minty.

FACS studies

The percentages of cells bearing specific surface markers were determined by FACS analyses of ficoll-fractionated mononuclear cells. As controls for Fc receptor binding, cells were incubated either directly with fluorescein-labeled normal rabbit IgG or indirectly with normal goat IgG followed by fluorescein-conjugated Staph A protein. Any positive fluorescence from controls was subtracted as background during FACS analysis.

Separation of B cells

Isolation of resting B cells was done using percoll (Pharmacia) gradients. Resting B cells were purified from the 70% to 75% percoll fraction.

RNA preparation

Poly A^+ RNA was prepared as in previous work from our lab (6,7) in three steps: (1) alkaline phenol extraction, (2) precipitation from 3M sodium acetate, and (3) oligo dT cellulose column chromatography. Poly A^+ RNA was purified by oligo dT cellulose column chromatography until no unbound material absorbing at 254 nm was detected.

DNA dot blot hybridization

Standard dot blot hybridization was used to obtain relative estimates of the amounts of Ig-specific RNAs and other RNAs within each RNA preparation. This technique of dotting excess clone-specific DNA and hybridizing to ^{32}P-labeled RNA has been used previously in our lab (6-8). In all experiments, 1 μg double-stranded DNA in 1 M ammonium acetate was dotted onto nitrocellulose filters.

Poly A^+ RNA was 5'-end labeled using T4 polynucleotide kinase and 50 μCi γ-^{32}P-labeled ATP (3000 Ci/mmole). RNA was hybridized to nitrocellulose filters dotted with DNA probes at 50°C for 18 h using stringent hybridization conditions. After autoradiographs were obtained, densitometric analysis was performed for quantitative comparisons of specific hybridization using a Hirschman microdensitometer.

RESULTS

Pathology

The most striking abnormality noted on pathologic examination was extensive vacuolar degeneration of anterior horn cells (motor neurons) of the spinal cord. This was associated with similar, but less severe, abnormalities in various motor nuclei of the brain stem. Anterior horn cells showing degeneration were adjacent to neuronal cells which were normal. No inflammatory or reactive changes were seen within the central nervous system. Myelin sheaths were normal. All wst/wst animals showed neuronal vacuolar degeneration of anterior horn cells while no wst littermates (composed of wst/+ and +/+ mice) showed these abnormalities. The histologic findings of lymph organs were less specific and varied in severity. In some wst/wst animals the spleens were hypoplastic and the lymph nodes poorly developed. However, in other animals these abnormalities were less apparent. The cellularity of the thymic cortex appeared normal. Peyer's patches were well-formed in wst/wst animals and contained similar numbers of lymphoid cells as in wst littermates.

Immunology

Total percentages of B cells, T cells and macrophages in lymphocyte populations derived from Peyer's patches (PP), mesenteric lymph nodes (MLN) and spleens were determined by FACS analysis of ficoll-purified mononuclear cells by direct immunofluorescence with fluorescein-conjugated goat anti-Thy-1, anti-mouse Ig and anti-Mac-1 reagents.

The results in wst/wst mice demonstrated (Table 1) a selective decrease in percentages of Ig^+ cells in PP lymphocytes compared to control mice. Populations of lymphocytes in other tissues were relatively normal though a less significant and less reproducible decrease in the percentage of Ig^+ cells was apparent in the spleen. The decrease in Ig^+ cells in PP was not accompanied by a concomitant increase in the number of Thy-1^+ cells. In addition, since morphologic studies of wst/wst PP revealed that they contained similar numbers of lymphoid cells as in wst littermates, it is likely that a large number of Ig^-, Thy-1^- lymphoid cells resides in PP of wst/wst mice.

Table 1. FACS analysis of lymphocytes

% Positive cells[1]

Source	Spleen			MLN[2]			PP[2]		
	Thy-1	Ig	Mac-1	Thy-1	Ig	Mac-1	Thy-1	Ig	Mac-1
wst/wst	34	37	0.2	55	40	0.5	37	30	1.5
wst littermates[3]	25	52	0.2	44	49	0.2	46	61	0.6
B6C3	32	48	0.2	43	42	0.4	40	52	0.8

[1]Percentage of lymphocytes positive by FACS for each surface antigen. The FACS was calibrated for background with staining of either fluorescein-conjugated normal rabbit serum (for anti-Ig) or normal goat serum followed by fluorescein-conjugated protein A (for anti-Mac-1 and anti-Thy-1).

[2]MLN=mesenteric lymph nodes; PP=Peyer's patches.

[3]wst littermates should be composed of 67% wst/+ and 33% +/+ mice.

Further studies using FACS analysis of percoll-purified B cell examined the intensity of immunofluorescence (i.e., the amount of fluorescein-conjugated antibody bound per cell) in wst/wst and control mice. These results demonstrated an increase in the number of "very bright" B cells (Fig. 1). This was evident in both Peyer's patches and spleen (though data only for splenic B cells are shown in Fig. 1) but was not apparent in MLN B cell populations.

DNA-excess dot blot hybridizations of total tissue Poly A^+ RNA to cloned DNA immobilized on nitrocellulose filters were performed. These experiments examined RNA derived from total tissue rather than from purified B cell and T cell populations. Control levels of IL-2 and IL-2 receptor specific mRNAs in spleens and MLN of wst/wst mice were observed (Table 2). On the other hand, Ig-specific mRNAs (especially μ, γ2a, γ2b, α) were markedly depressed (50%) in PP and splenic B cells of wst/wst mice compared to littermate controls. MLN lymphocytes of wst/wst mice, expressed control levels of most

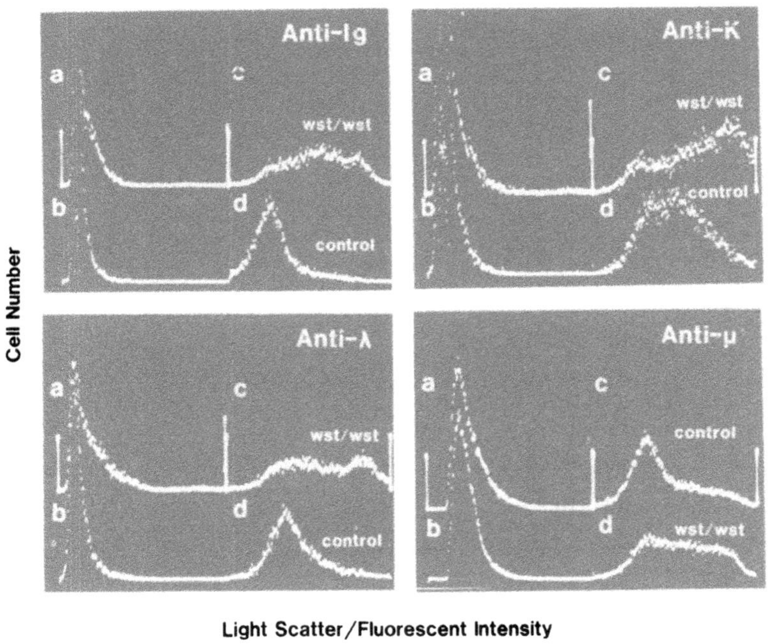

Figure 1. FACS profiles of splenic B cells derived from wst/wst mice and wst littermate controls. (a-b) Plot of light scatter against cell number. (c-d) Plot of fluorescent intensity against light scatter. wst/wst and control littermate curves are labeled. Ig^+ cells: wst littermates = 9.3%; wst/wst = 63.0%; κ^+ cells: wst littermates = 8.4%; wst/wst = 3.4%; λ^+ cells: wst littermates = 11.5%; wst/wst = 42.5%.

Table 2. mRNA expression in wst/wst and wst littermate mice [1]

	wst/· PP	wst/wst PP	wst/· MLN	wst/wst MLN	wst/· spleen	wst/wst spleen
μ	1.1(.2)	.7(.1)	0.5(0.1)	2.5(.4)	6.8(.2)	1.5(.2)
γ3	6.7(.4)	1.2(.1)	1.4(0.2)	1.2(.2)	3.4(.3)	6.3(.2)
γ1	2.7(.1)	1.7(.2)	0.2(0)	0.3(.1)	1.8(.1)	1.1(.3)
γ2b	1.1(.1)	HND	0.4(.1)	0.1(.1)	2.1(.1)	HND[2]
γ2a	1.7(.3)	HND	0.2(0)	0.4(.1)	2.4(.3)	HND
α	2.6(.3)	HND	3.3(.3)	0.4(.2)	5.5(.2)	HND
k	2.9(.4)	1.0(.1)	1.8(.3)	0.3(.2)	9.8(.8)	1.7(.1)
λ	1.6(.2)	1.0(.1)	1.2(.2)	0.8(.3)	4.9(.2)	2.7(.2)
actin	1.0(.1)	.9(.1)	1.0(.1)	1.1(.1)	0.9(.1)	1.1(.1)
IL-2	4.1(.5)	NT[2]	1.7(.4)	1.9(.2)	2.3(.3)	2.5(.1)
IL-2 receptor	5.6(.7)	NT	4.0(.5)	4.4(.4)	2.2(.4)	3.0(.8)
pACYC	HND	HND	HND	HND	HND	HND

[1]Expression was determined by DNA-excess dot blot hybridization. Autoradiographs were analyzed by microdensitometry. Figures represent comparisons to levels of actin-specific RNA present in spleens of control animals (which is set at 1.0). Numbers in parentheses represent standard errors.

[2]HND=Hybridization not detected. NT=Not tested.

Ig-specific mRNAs with the exception of α and κ mRNA. Littermate controls (wst/+ and +/+) were similar to B6C3 parental mice (data not shown). These results suggest a compartmental defect that is somewhat tissue-restricted with IgA responses being most affected.

DISCUSSION

We have identified several immunologic abnormalities in wst/wst animals including high percentages of "very bright" Ig^+ cells and low levels of splenic Ig-specific mRNA compared to littermate controls and the B6C3 parental strain. In addition, our results have established a selected deficiency in Ig^+ cells evident in PP lymphocyte populations not apparent when examining lymphocytes from other tissues. Morphologically, PP are intact and demonstrated relatively normal numbers of lymphocytes.

B cells of wst/wst mice are enriched in a population that bears large amounts of surface Ig per cell. In addition, wst/wst B cells of spleen and PP express lower levels of most Ig-specific mRNAs than control mice while T cell specific mRNAs are expressed at control levels. This apparent paradox of low Ig-specific mRNA in the presence of high numbers of "very bright" Ig^+ cells can be explained by (a) high ratios of membrane Ig to secreted Ig, perhaps as a result of inappropriate response to activation signals; (b) low rates of conversion of B cells into actively secreting plasma cells; and/or (c) poor secretion of existing Ig protein. We favor a model in which wst/wst B cells have a defect in "switching" from membrane to secreted Ig. This model is supported by (a) low levels of Ig-specific mRNA, since B cells express only very high levels of Ig mRNA once they have differentiated into Ig-secreting cells and (b) the high numbers of Ig^+ "very bright" cells. This is consistent with other recent work from our laboratory demonstrating low serum Ig levels for most heavy chain isotypes and normal mitogenic responses to T and B cell mitogens. The defect could be attributed to a deficiency in B cell differentiation factors or to an intrinsic defect within the B cells or a B cell subset in wst/wst mice.

The immunologic defect appears to be compartmentalized so that PP and splenic B cells are affected more than MLN B cells. MLN B cells were defective in expression of κ and α-mRNA but not other Ig-specific mRNAs. In addition, large numbers of "very bright" Ig^+ cells were not observed in MLN populations. These results suggest tht IgA responses may be more affected than other Ig isotypes and that the immunologic abnormality is more apparent in PP and spleen cell populations than in MLN. Low IgA levels correlate with a report by Kaiserlian et al. (5) documenting the absence of IgA precursors in PP.

Our results suggest that the wst mutation does not provide a perfect model for a known human disease. While neuropathologic findings in "wasted" mice are consistent with motor neuron disease, the immunologic abnormalities are not those of human amyotrophic lateral sclerosis. In addition, the immunologic abnormalities reported here simulate neither adenosine deaminase deficiency (9) nor ataxia telangiectasia (1). The significance for studying this model relates to the fact that it provides a mechanism of studying relationships between the immune and nervous systems.

CONCLUSIONS

1. "Wasted" mice have a deficiency in Ig^+ cells that is primarily compartmentalized to PP lymphoid populations though it is expressed slightly in spleen and is not apparent in MLN populations.

2. B cell populations from PP and spleens of wst/wst mice but not from MLN have high percentages of "very bright" Ig^+ cells.

3. Levels of Ig-specific mRNA for all Ig isotypes (except $\gamma 3$) are reduced significantly in spleens and PP of wst/wst mice. MLN exhibit a more complex picture with increased μ-mRNA, decreased α- and light chain-mRNA and control levels of all other isotypes.

4. The immunodeficiency of wst/wst mice is unusual because it is more evident in mucosal than systemic immune sites, and it affects IgA expression more than other Ig isotypes.

ACKNOWLEDGEMENTS

The authors wish to thank Kathy Jensen for typing this manuscript and Mary Jane Doerge for her technical assistance. We also wish to thank Elizabeth Howie and Mabel Pierce for their help in morphologic experiments. This work was supported in part by American Cancer Society Grant #IM-348, Fraternal Order of Eagles Grant #72 and the Mayo Foundation.

REFERENCES

1. Shultz, L.D., Sweet, H.O., Davisson, M.J., Coman, D.R., Nature 297, 402, 1982.
2. Goldowitz, D., Shipman, P.W., Porter, J.F. and Schmidt, R.R., J. Immunol. 135, 1806, 1985.
3. Swift, M., in Ataxia-Telangiectasia--A Cellular and Molecular Link Between Cancer, Neuropathology and Immune Deficiency, (Edited by Bridges, B. and Harnden, D.G.), pp. 355-361, 1982.
4. Bridges, B.A., Lenoir, G. and Tomatis, L., Cancer Research 45, 3979, 1979.
5. Kaiserlian, D., Delacroix, D. and Bach, J.R., J. Immunol. 135, 1126, 1985.
6. Woloschak, G.E., Molec. Immunol. 23, 581, 1986.
7. Woloschak, G.E., Tomasi, T.B. and Liarakos, C.D., Molec. Immunol. 23, 645, 1986.
8. Woloschak, G.E., Dweald, G., Bahn, R.S., Kyle, P.R., Greipp, P.R. and Ash, R.C., J. Cell. Biochem., 32, 23, 1986.
9. Dobner, P.R., Kawasaki, Z.S., Yu, L.-Y. and Bancroft, F.C., Proc. Natl. Acad. Sci. 78, 2230, 1986.

MOLECULAR ASPECTS OF T CELL REGULATION OF B CELL ISOTYPE DIFFERENTIATION

M.C. Sneller, D.Y. Kunimoto and W. Strober

Mucosal Immunity Section, Laboratory of Clinical Investigation, National Institute of Allergy and Infectious Diseases, NIH, Bethesda, Maryland USA

INTRODUCTION

One of the questions which has fascinated mucosal immunologists is why the mucosal B cell, i.e., the B cells developing in mucosal lymphoid follicles such as Peyer's patches, have a greater tendency to become IgA B cells, than B cells in other developmental areas. One theory is based on the supposition that surface IgM-bearing (mIgM-bearing) B cells in the mucosal follicles are more subject to antigen stimulation than cells in other areas and therefore undergo more rounds of cell division. This, in turn, is accompanied by progressive deletion of heavy chain constant region genes and thus the acquisition of IgA because the IgA heavy chain constant region is, at least in the mouse, the ultimate gene in the Ig heavy chain constant region (1,2).

Another theory is that B cell development in the Peyer's patch is governed by special T cells which direct the B cells into an IgA pathway. On the one hand, such T cells may act to influence the differentiation of uncommitted mIgM-bearing B cells and the other hand, T cells may act to expand B cell populations already committed to a particular isotype and bearing that isotype on its surface. Evidence for the existence of the form or "switch" T cells is inherent in the work of Kawanishi et al. (3) in the murine system and Mayer et al. (4) in the human system. These workers have shown that cloned T cell lines derived from Peyer's patches or circulating malignant T cells derived from patients with Sezary syndrome can induce IgM-positive B cell population to differentiate into cells expressing the IgG or IgA isotype. The cloned Peyer's patch T cell appeared to be IgA-specific in its regulatory role, whereas the circulating malignant T cells induced both IgG and IgA differentiation.

Evidence for T cell acting after isotype commitment (post-switch) comes from the work of Kiyono et al. (5) who showed that clonal T cells bearing IgA-Fc receptor have the capacity to expand B cells already bearing IgA on their surface; such cells appear to act via the release of factors that bind to cell surface IgA. It is still unclear if other factors of non-specific nature are also involved in the same process.

In recent years we have initiated studies of isotype regulation in entirely clonal systems to better elucidate that molecular mechanisms involved in B cell-isotype differentiation in general and IgA B cell isotype differentiation in particular. In the studies to be described we show that a clonal T cell population can induce a clonal pre-B cell population to activate downstream Ig heavy chain constant region genes, and thus provide additional evidence that T cells can act at the switch level of B cell isotype differentiation.

T cell regulation of isotype expression of clonal B cells

Various clonal B cell populations were studied as to their ability to undergo isotype differentiation under the influence of T cells. Ultimately, it was found that the well-known pre-B cell lymphoma, 70Z/3, which expresses surface IgM (mIgM), but not other Ig isotypes had such ability. In particular, it was found that 70Z/3 B cells when cultured alone without any stimulants express only small amounts of IgM and when cultured with LPS (1μg/ml) express a marked increase in an IgM. In either instance, however, no IgG appeared on the cell membrane. In constrast, when 70Z/3 B cells are co-cultured with a T cell hybridoma termed HAJ-3 [derived by fusing murine Peyer's patch T cell (BALB/c) with the HAT-sensitive T cell lymphoma BW 5147 (AKR)] while the cells manifest only a slight increase in surface IgM, there is now the appearance of surface IgG (mIgG). The latter was detected using a $F(ab')_2$ anti-IgG antibody in FACS analysis and in culture systems that did or did not contain LPS. Further studies disclosed that: (a) mIgG expression occurred even if the cells were exposed to mitomycin-C in doses sufficient to block cell proliferation and that such expression occurred on several different sub-clones of 70Z/3 B cells; (b) most, if not all of the B cells expressing mIgG were also expressing mIgM, but did not secrete either of these immunoglobulins; (c) co-culture of 70Z/3 B cells with active EL-4 supernatants (shown to contain BSF-1, IL-2 and BCGF-II in separate assays) did not induce mIgG expression and finally (d) subclass analysis of the mIgG on the 70Z/3 B cells following co-culture with HAJ-3 T cells with $F(ab')_2$ anti-Ig subclass antibodies disclosed that only one subclass was present, namely IgG2b. Various attempts to bring about surface IgG2b expression in 70Z/3 B cells with supernatants of HAJ-3 T cells were unsuccessful.

Molecular events occurring during induction of IgG2b expression in 70Z/3 B cells

In initial molecular studies we determined the species of Ig heavy chain mRNA in variously treated 70Z/3 B cells by northern blot analysis. It was found that 70Z/3 B cells contain μ-specific mRNA whether the cells were unstimulated, stimulated with LPS or co-cultured with HAJ-3 T cells; this finding is, of course, consistent with the fact that 70Z/3 B cells in each of these cases is expressing mIgM. Of greater interest is the fact that while unstimulated 70Z/3 B cells express low levels of γ2b-specific mRNA which is mainly of a small size characteristic of sterile transcripts, both LPS-stimulated and HAJ-3 co-cultured 70Z/3 B cells contained abundant γ2b-specific mRNA having both a small size and a larger size characteristic of membrane mRNA. These data are compatible with the view that whereas LPS stimulated 70Z/3 B cells markedly increased the quantity of IgG2b mRNA, a T cell influence is nevertheless necessary for the occurrence of mRNA that can be translated into membrane immunoglobulin.

In further studies, we determined whether or not the expression of downstream immunoglobulin (mIgG2b) in a cell concomitantly expressing surface IgM occurs in the presence or absence of C_H gene rearrangement or deletion. In these studies we analyzed DNA from unstimulated, LPS stimulated and HAJ-3 T cells co-cultured 70Z/3 B cells by Southern blotting techniques, utilizing a combination of restriction enzyme digests and C_H gene probes that would detect switch region rearrangement in the 70Z/3 B cells, if any had occurred. In the relevant studies it was shown that using Eco R1 or other appropriate restriction enzymes, the Ig genes in 70Z/B cells, even after LPS treatment or co-cultured with HAJ-3 were in a germline configuration.

In a further study of Cμ gene deletion in 70Z/3 B cells following co-culture with HAJ-3 T cells, the cultured cells were depleted of T cells (by anti-Thy 1.2 plus complement treatment) and the B cells were stained with fluorescein-labeled anti-IgG, following which the brightest 5% of cells were collected and cloned by FACS. Five of the clones thus obtained were expanded and examined for the presence of surface Ig. All five were found to express only mIgM with little or no mIgG2b; therefore, in the absence of T cells the 70Z/3 B cells isolated on the basis of their capacity to express mIgG2b, revert to cells that express only mIgM; thus they continue to have intact and active Cμ genes.

In all, the data are consistent with the view that 70Z/3 B cells can be induced to co-express mIgM and mIgG2b by a T cell clone in the absence of gene rearrangement or deletion.

Overview of T cell-induced isotype differentiation

In the studies described above it was shown that clonal T cell populations (a hybridoma derived from the Peyer's patches) could be induced to express "downstream" Ig heavy chain expression, in this case of the γ2b constant region gene, in the absence of heavy chain rearrangement or deletion. These data are thus consistent with the switch model proposed by Yoaita et al. (6) in which downstream Ig activation and expression was proposed to occur prior to switch recombination and deletion. A further point of interest is that the LPS-induced γ2b-specific mRNA synthesis occurs in the absence of IgG2b expression on the cell membrane. Thus the T cell influence in this case is not the only signal capable of causing γ2b gene activation, but is one necessary for production of mRNA capable of being translated into a membrane-expressed immunoglobulin.

A similar analysis of isotype switch was explored by Stavnezer (7) using the I.29 B cell lymphoma. In this case the B cell expressing IgM on its surface was induced to produce IgA as well as IgG2b and IgG3 following stimulation with LPS but not Con A-activated T cells. Here, the expression of downstream Ig heavy chain genes was accompanied by switch recombination and there was hypomethylation of the genes encoding for the expressed isotypes, implying pre-activation of these genes. I.29 B cells therefore appear to be pre-programmed cells that rapidly undergo switch re-combination upon LPS stimulation. These studies are not contradictory to those described above since it is possible that the I.29 B cell is one that may have become "frozen" at a stage following the reception of a T cell differentiation signal whereas the 70Z/3 B cell is a cell that is at an earlier stage of differentiation. If one takes both the data discussed above and the Stavnezer data into consideration it appears that T cells provide a signal which leads to heavy chain gene activation and that results in downstream gene expression but not switch recombination and deletion. A second signal, perhaps one derived from a different kind of T cell, then causes further differentiation and actual switch recombination and deletion.

These studies leave open the question of the class-specificity of the T cell signal: is the T cell signal merely influencing a cell pre-programmed to activate a certain Ig heavy chain gene as a result of another non-T cell influence or does the T cell signal actually direct which Ig heavy chain gene will be activated? This question cannot be answered definitively until a variety of clonal T cells and differentiable clonal B cells are at hand. At the moment evidence for both pathways can be mustered. Thus, in the Stavnezer studies (7) co-culture of I.29 with a T cell supernatant containing the B cell growth factor BSF-1 led to expression and production of IgG1, an IgG isotype never induced when cells are exposed to LPS alone. Thus, in this situation a T cell-derived factor has changed the course of B cell isotype differentiation. These data intermesh nicely with other previous data showing that BSF-1 induces LPS-unstimulated B cells to produce IgG1 and IgE rather than IgG3 (8,9). In contrast, Mayer et al. (4) showed that coculture of T cells derived from patients with Sezary syndrome (already mentioned above) and B cells from patients with hyper-IgM syndrome, that the B cells induced could switch to both IgG and IgA expression or only IgG expression. This suggests that whereas T cells are necessary for switch recombination, the precise pathway of differentiation is still determined by an internal B cell mechanism.

Accepting the fact that T cells do induce B cell switches the question arises as to the molecular mechanisms involved. Recent studies of Ig gene activation may provide a hint to the answer to this question. In such studies it has been shown that cells contain trans-acting factors which lead to gene activation, perhaps by causing the occurrence of accessible DNA sites and hypomethylation (10). It remains to be shown that such trans-acting factors can act in an isotype-specific fashion. A second possibility relates to the fact that isotype differentiation necessarily involves recombinases that cause gene recombination and deletion. However, if the isotype-specific step of isotype differentiation does not involve recombination as implied in the studies recounted above, this possibility becomes less likely. Obviously, further work will be necessary to resolve this issue.

In the studies of putative switch T cells by Kawanishi et al. (3), it was obsèrved that the switch T cells led to B cells bearing IgA in their surface rather than fully differentiated plasma cells producing IgA. In follow-up studies it was determined that T cells or T cell factors were necessary to induce terminal differentiation (11). A similar note was struck in the human switch T cell studies conducted by Mayer et al. (4). Thus, the available data is compatible to the view that switch T cell effects are distinct from T cell effects on B cell proliferation or terminal differentiation. In summary, it is quite clear that T cells are active in B cell isotype differentiation at several levels of the differentiative process. However, much additional work will be necessary to define the intracellular molecular processes that are involved in such T cell control.

REFERENCES

1. Cebra, J.J., Fuhrman, J.A., Gearhart, P.J., Horwitz, J.L. and Shahin, R.D., in Recent Advances in Mucosal Immunity, (Edited by Strober, W., Hanson, L.A. and Sell, K.W.), p. 155, Raven Press, New York, 1982.
2. Strober, W. and Jacobs, D., in Advances in Host Defense Mechanisms, Vol. 4, Mucosal Immunity, (Edited by Gallin, J.I. and Fauci, A.S.), p. 1, Raven Press, New York, 1985.
3. Kawanishi, H., Saltzman, L. and Strober, W., J. Exp. Med. 157, 433, 1983.
4. Mayer, L., Kwan, S.P., Thompson, C., Ko, H.S., Chiorazzi, N., Waldmann, T.A. and Rosen, R., N. Eng. J. Med. 314, 409, 1986.
5. Kiyono, H., Mosteller-Barnum, L.M., Pitts, A., Williamson, S., Michalek, S.M. and McGhee, J.R., J. Exp. Med. 161, 731, 1985.
6. Yaoita, Y., Kumajar, Y., Okumura, K. and Honjo, T., Nature 297, 697, 1982.
7. Stavnezer, J., in Mucosal Immunity and Infections and Mucosal Surfaces, (Edited by Strober, W., Lamm, M., McGhee, J.R. and James, S.P.), Oxford University Press, New York (in press).
8. Noma, Y., Sideras, P., Naito, T., Bergstedt-Lindquist, S., Aguma, C., Severinson, E., Tanabe, T., Kinashi, T., Matsuda, F., Yaoita, Y. and Honjo, T., Nature 314, 640, 1986.

9. Coffman, R.L., Ohara, J., Bond, M.W., Carty, J., Zlotnick, A. and Paul, W.E., J. Immunol. 136, 4538, 1986.
10. Sen, R. and Baltimore, D., Cell 46, 705, 1986.
11. Kawanishi, H., Saltzman, L. and Strober, W., J. Exp. Med. 158, 649, 1983.

SWITCH T CELL LINE, ST, INDUCES AN Ig CLASS SWITCH IN SURFACE ISOTYPE

L. Mayer

Division of Clinical Immunology, The Mount Sinai
School of Medicine of the University of New York
New York, NY USA

INTRODUCTION

We have previously demonstrated that T cells, Trac, isolated from a patient with Sezary's/mycosis fungoides was capable of inducing an Ig class switch in B cells derived from patients with immunodeficiency and hyper-IgM (1,2). Previously, it had been postulated that the defect in these patients was intrinsic to the B cell, being incapable of switching from μ to γ or α (3,4). However, we have now studied 13 such patients with 11 able to secrete IgG alone or in conjunction with IgA, in the presence of Trac and pokeweed mitogen (2). Despite these findings, two major areas remain to be elucidated: (a) the mechanism of T cell induction of the class switch and (b) determination of the normal counterpart of the malignant Trac cell.

In order to approach these issues an IL-2 dependent T cell line was established from Tac^+ Trac cells. Using this cell line, we demonstrate that the initial signal from these cells results in a switch in surface isotype in the absence of PWM, and that additional signals (BCDF) are required for terminal maturation and secretion. In addition, cell-cell contact appears to be important in the initiation of this process.

MATERIALS AND METHODS

Cell separation and culture

Heparinized venous blood was used as a source of peripheral blood mononuclear cell (PBMC) as previously described (1). T/B separation was achieved using neuramindase treated SRBC (1). All cells were cultured in RPMI 1640 (Hazelton-Dutchland, Denver, PA), 1% penicillin/streptomycin (Gibco, Grand Island, NY) and 2 mM glutamine (Gibco) henceforth termed culture medium (CM). For some experiments PWM (Gibco - 1/100 dilution) was used to stimulate B cell differentiation.

Immunofluorescence staining and antibodies

OKT3, T4, T8, and M1 were obtained from Ortho Diagnostics (Raritan, NJ). Anti-Tac was kindly provided by Dr. Thomas Waldman (NCI, Bethesda, MD). VG2, an anti-Ia framework monoclonal antibody was kindly provided by Dr. Shu Man Fu (Oklahoma Medical Center, Oklahoma City, OK). Fluorescein conjugated, affinity purified, $F(ab')_2$ rabbit anti-human IgG, IgA, IgM and goat anti-mouse Ig were obtained from Cappel Laboratories (Cochranville, PA). HB52 (αIgG) and HB70 (αIgM) were obtained from ATCC (Rockville, MD). All reagents were tested to ensure lack of cross reactivity on human myelomas (ELISA) or EBV transformed B cell lines. Staining was performed and analyzed as previously described (5).

Anti-LFA-1 monoclonal antibody was a kind gift of Dr. Steven Burakoff (Dana Farber Cancer Institute, Boston, MA).

ELISA for antibody secretion

ELISA for specific isotypes was performed using culture supernatants as previously described (2). Reagents used did not demonstrate cross-isotype reactivity as judged using myeloma proteins as standards.

Generation of IL-2 dependent line, ST

T cells isolated from patient Rac (Trac) were noted to contain 30% cells which stained with the monoclonal antibody anti-Tac (1). These cells were isolated by an indirect rosetting technique (1) and placed in macrowell cultures at 10^5 cells/well without feeder cells in CM containing 10% IL-2 (Electronucleonics, Silver Springs, MD). Cultures were fed 3 times/week for a period of 3-4 months at which time several wells demonstrated positive growth. Selected wells were expanded and maintained without feeder cells in the same medium in T25 flasks (Falcon, Oxnard, CA). Removal of IL-2 resulted in cell death within 4 days.

RESULTS AND DISCUSSION

Characterization of ST line

The fact that the ST line grew without feeder cells in medium containing IL-2 suggested that this cell might be the malignant cell derived from our patient Rac. These cells were dependent only upon the presence of IL-2 in the medium. In contrast to Trac initially isolated, the ST line was $T4^-$, $T8^-$, although intermittent weakly positive staining was noted with OKT8. Surface staining of ST revealed it to be $T3^+$, Tac^+, $LFA\text{-}1^+$, sIg^-, $M1^-$, $T6^-$, 9.3^- cells with relative uniformity.

Addition of ST cells to B cells from patients with hyper-IgM induces a switch in surface isotype

Graded doses of ST cells were added to B cells (with and without PWM) from patients with the hyper-IgM syndrome. In contrast to the response seen with Trac and PWM (IgG and IgA secretion), no Ig secretion was noted (data not shown). However, when B cells were stained after 48 hours of co-culture with 10^5 ST cells, the presence of sIgG was noted using either polyvalent or monoclonal antibodies (Table 1). No IgG staining was noted on these B cells from cultures with normal allogeneic T cells. Of note is the fact that PWM was not required for this effect, suggesting that the requirement for PWM with Trac cells was to allow for factor generation by non-switch T cells for terminal maturation and Ig secretion. This possibility is further strengthened by the finding that secretion can be induced with exogenous BCDF.

Table 1. T cell line, ST, induces an isotype switch in surface Ig expression

		% Positive[a]		
B cells	T cell source	sIgG	sIgA	sIgM
Coluc	0	ND[b]	ND	9.6
Coluc	Tallo	ND	ND	10.9
Coluc	ST	1.7	ND	8.9

[a]1 x 10^6 B cells are cultured for 48 hours with either 1 x 10^5 Tallo cells, a normal allogeneic IL-2 dependent T cell line or ST with or without PWM. Quantitation of surface Ig is obtained by indirect immunofluorescence.

[b]Not detectable.

Similar data were obtained using 3 other B cell preparations from patients with the hyper-IgM syndrome. It is of interest, however, that no sIgA staining was ever detected, even at 96-120 hours. This finding may relate to a more specific signal (isotype restricted) given by the ST cells or due to the production of a relatively weak signal that does not promote switching further downstream.

Anti-LFA-1 blocks the switch signal

LFA molecules represent "adhesion" molecules that enhance cell-cell contact and potentially regulatory interactions (6). We have previously been unable to demontrate the presence of secreted "switch" factor from our Trac cells. Multiple attempts at T cell fusion have been unsuccessful as well. To attempt to determine whether the switch signal was indeed factor-mediated, monoclonal anti-LFA-1 was added in varying concentrations to cultures of Trac and B cells (Table 2). In the presence of anti-LFA-1 no IgG or IgA secretion was noted, suggesting that cell-cell contact may be important in the switch process. These data do not rule out the possibility of a short range lymphokine, a possibility that would also be consistent with our inability to generate factors from Trac or ST cells.

The ability of α-LFA-1 to block switch to IgG and IgA induced by Trac was also seen with the ST line. Here no sIgG was noted after co-culture with anti-LFA-1 (data not shown).

Loss of sIgD after exposure to Trac on ST

One of the hallmarks of the hyper-IgM B cell is the presence of significant amounts of sIgD. Coico et al. (7) have recently described T cells

Table 2. α-LFA blocks switch T cell signal

Target cell	T cell source	α-LFA	ng/ml IgG	ng/ml IgA	ng/ml IgM
B (hyper IgM)	-	-	<0.5	<0.5	11.6
B (hyper IgM)	-	+	<0.5	<0.5	12.8
B (hyper IgM)	T_{rac}	-	7.3	1.6	25.3
B (hyper IgM)	T_{rac}	+	<0.5	<0.5	18.6
B (hyper IgM)	T_{con}^{+}	-	<0.5	<0.5	65.6
B (hyper IgM)	T_{con}^{+}	+	<0.5	<0.5	69.7

bearing the Fcδ receptor which appear to augment primary IgG responses. Although there is no direct evidence for induction of an Ig class switch, it is postulated that such Fcδ^+ T cells may play a role in isotype regulation. In conjunction with these findings we have evaluated the expression of sIgD on hyper-IgM B cells after exposure to either Trac or ST cells. As seen in Table 3, beginning at 2 hours there is a dramatic decrease in sIgD which is almost complete by 8 hours of culture. Such a decrease is not seen when these B cells are co-cultured with normal allogeneic T cells and is not seen in 1 patient where switching does not occur (data not shown). These data suggest that the initial signal to switch may relate to IgD translation. Conceivably, a signal to stop IgD production may allow for switching further downstream. Although we have no evidence

Table 3. Loss of sIgD following exposure to Trac

		% Staining		
	Time (hours)	sIgM	sIgD	Ia
B (hyper-IgM) + Trac	0	7.6	11.3	94.6
B (hyper-IgM) + Trac	2	7.9	10.8	97.2
B (hyper-IgM) + Trac	4	8.5	5.6	93.2
B (hyper-IgM) + Trac	6	7.1	3.1	95.3
B (hyper-IgM) + Trac	8	8.0	<0.1	98.1

that our Trac or ST cells are Fcδ^+, such studies are currently underway. In addition, it will be of interest to determine whether T cells from patients with the hyper-IgM syndrome are incapable of generating Fcδ^+ T cells and whether Fcδ^+ T cells induced in normals are capable of inducing an Ig class switch in these patients.

ACKNOWLEDGEMENTS

The authors wish to acknowledge Chris Thompson for his expert technical assistance, Steve Burakoff for the α-LFA-1 antibody and Hyacinth Fyffe for help in preparing this manuscript.

This work was supported by a US PHS grant CA 41583. Dr. Mayer is a recipient of the Iram T. Hirschl Trust Career Development Award.

REFERENCES

1. Mayer, L., Posnett, D.N., Kunkel, H.G., J. Exp. Med. 161, 134, 1985.
2. Mayer, L., Kwan, S.P., Thompson, C., Ko, H.S., Chiorazzi, N., Waldmann, T.A. and Rosen, F., N. Engl. J. Med. 314, 409, 1986.
3. Geha, R.S., Hyslop, N., Alami, S., Farah, F., Schneeberger, E.E. and Rosen, F.S., J. Clin. Invest. 64, 385, 1979.
4. Levitt, D., Haber, P., Rich, K. and Cooper, M.D., J. Clin. Invest. 72, 1650, 1983.
5. Mayer, L., Fu, S.M., Cunningham-Rundles, C. and Kunkel, H.G., J. Clin. Invest. 74, 2115, 1984.
6. Golde, W.T., Kappler, J.W., Greenstein, J., Malissen, B., Hood, L. and Marrack, P., J. Exp. Med. 161, 635, 1985.
7. Coico, R.F., Xue, B., Wallace, D., Siskind, G.W. and Thorbecke, G.J., J. Exp. Med. 162, 1852, 1985.

REGULATORY T CELL NETWORKS IN THE SECRETORY IMMUNE SYSTEM

J.H. Eldridge, H. Kiyono, I. Suzuki, K. Kitamura, T. Kurita, K.W. Beagley, M.L. McGhee, S.M. Michalek, D.R. Green* and J.R. McGhee

Departments of Microbiology, Oral Biology and Preventative Dentistry, the Institute of Dental Research, The University of Alabama at Birmingham, University Station, Birmingham, AL USA; and *Department of Immunology, Faculty of Medicine, University of Alberta, Edmonton, Alberta, Canada T6G 2H7

INTRODUCTION

The mucosal surfaces of man and other mammals are in direct continuity with the external environment. As such, they are continually exposed to antigens from the environment and represent the major bodily site of antigenic exposure and recognition. In the case of ingested antigens, there is selective uptake into the Peyer's patches (PP), which are distinct aggregates of lymphoreticular nodules along the anti-mesenteric aspect of the gastrointestinal (GI) tract and a major component of the gut-associated lymphoreticular tissues (GALT). The PP contain a large subpopulation of B lymphocytes that are committed to IgA synthesis (1), macrophages (2), dendritic accessory cells (3) and regulatory T lymphocytes of the T-helper (Th), T suppressor (Ts) and T contrasuppressor (Tcs) subsets (4-7). Overlying the PP is a lymphoepithelium which contains microfold cells (M cells; also termed follicular-associated epithelial cells) with highly developed pinocytotic channels which allow sampling of antigens from the gut lumenal contents, and transport of these antigens to the underlying lymphoreticular cells (8,9). The oral administration of antigen leads to the stimulation of both the B lymphocyte (follicular) and T lymphocyte (parafollicular) zones within the PP, but B lymphocyte maturation to the plasma cell stage does not occur in this tissue. Rather, the predominantly IgA B lymphoblasts extravasate from the PP and are observed first in the mesenteric lymph nodes, later in the spleen and finally in the lamina propria of the GI tract where final differentiation to IgA secreting plasma cells take place (10,11). In addition to recirculating to the GI tract, the GALT-derived IgA precursor B lymphocytes also home to mucosal sites distant to the gut and contribute to the production of secretory IgA (sIgA) antibodies in bronchial secretions, colostrum, milk, saliva and tears (12-15).

Although it is clear that the PP are an inductive site for sIgA antibody responses to enterically-encountered antigens, the oral administration of large doses of soluble proteins (16) or the continuous feeding of particulate T cell dependent (TD) antigens (17,18) can induce a state of systemic unresponsiveness termed oral tolerance (19). Several mechanisms, including immune complexes (20), anti-idiotypic antibodies (21), and Ts cells (22-25) have been proposed for the maintenance of this state. However, the majority of work to date indicates that excessive or prolonged antigenic stimulation in GALT leads to the induction of Ts cells which home to systemic lymphoid tissues and mediate this unresponsiveness (21-25). In addition, it has been shown that the oral administration of antigen can result in the induction of Th cell dependent IgA responses at the mucosa concurrent with a state of Ts cell mediated systemic unresponsiveness (21,24). Thus, it is apparent that there is a striking duality in the interaction of GALT-derived regulatory T cells with the immune system which allows the induction and maintenance of an immune response of essentially a single isotype in specific anatomic sites.

The two major questions posed by these findings involve the cellular and molecular mechanisms which: (1) predispose the PP to the induction of an immune response which is dominated by IgA; and (2) maintain the IgA response despite the presence of strong T cell mediated suppression. Of relevance to the first point is the work of Kawanishi et al. (25), which demonstrated that clones of Con A induced, IL-2 dependent T cells could be derived from murine PP. These clones, when added to cultures of LPS-stimulated surface IgM positive B lymphocytes could induce the expression of surface IgA, but could not support their differentiation to IgA secretion. This IgA "switch" T cell provides an explanation for the high IgA precursor frequency in the PP. Our own studies have centered around the regulatory T cells which support antigen-driven differentiation of B lymphocytes to IgA secretion.

RESULTS

IgA isotype specific Th cells and T-T hybridomas

Antigen specific T cell clones were derived from C3H/HeJ mice which had been orally immunized with sheep erythrocytes (SRBC) by isolating the PP T cells and culturing them in the presence of antigen, irradiated feeder cells and IL-2 (26). Twenty-one of 63 clones which expressed Th activity were capable of supporting the development of IgA anti-SRBC plaque-forming cells (PFC) in cultures of unprimed, T cell depleted spleen or PP cells. Phenotypic characterization of the IgA supporting PP Th cell (PP Th A) clones by fluorescence microscopy showed that they were Thy-1.2^{+}, Lyt-1^{+}, 2^{-}, I-A^{k-} and Ig^{-}. In addition, when analyzed by rosetting with immunoglobulin coated erythrocytes, the PP Th A clones all expressed Fc receptors specific for IgA (FcαR), but not for IgM or IgG (Table 1). In contrast, those clones which did not support IgA responses were FcαR^{-}. This result suggested that the FcαR on the cloned PP Th A cells conferred functional specificity in their action. Further, it indicated that the specificity was mediated through the recognition of IgA on the B cell cytoplasmic membrane.

In order to test this supposition, several of the PP Th A clones were tested for their ability to support PFC responses when cultured with B cells which had been fractionated into surface IgA positive (IgA^{+}) and IgA^{-} populations by panning or by using a fluorescence-activated cell sorter (FACS) (27). IgA^{-} PP B cells cultured with cloned PP Th A cells and antigen produced a greatly reduced number of specific PFC of the IgA class relative to unfractionated B cells, while the IgM response was unaffected (Table 2). Conversely, the IgA^{+} B cells produced an augmented IgA anti-SRBC PFC response in the presence of the PP Th A cells, and the IgM response in these cultures was severely depressed in comparison to the cultures containing unfractionated B cells. Similar results were obtained whether spleen or PP were used as the source for the isolation of IgA^{+} and IgA^{-} B cells, and the FACS or panning were equally effective as separation procedures. The conclusion that the FcαR on the PP Th A cells functioned as a recognition structure for their selective interaction with IgA^{+} B cells was further supported by the demonstration that IgA, but not IgM or IgG, was able to block IgA-specific helper function (28), and that the ontogenetic development of B cells capable of collaborating with the PP Th A cells paralleled the appearance of IgA^{+} cells (27).

In order to facilitate studies of the FcαR at the molecular level, two PP Th A clones were fused with a HAT-sensitive variant of the R1.1

Table 1. Isotype-specific Fc receptors on cloned Peyer's patch Th cells which support IgA responses[a]

PP Th A clone	Percent positive for rosette formation[b]		
	IgM	IgG2a	IgA
1	<1	0	88
5	<1	0	90
7	0	0	92
9	0	0	96
11	<1	0	97
14	0	0	89

[a]Monoclonal IgM, IgG2a or IgA anti-DNP antibodies were reacted with TNP conjugated SRBC at a subagglutinating dose. Following extensive washing the immunoglobulin coated erythrocytes were reacted with the PP Th A cells. At least 1,500 lymphoid cells were scored for each test.

[b]Values represent the mean percent positive in two separate experiments.

Table 2. Cloned PP Th A cells collaborate with surface IgA^+ B cells to produce IgA PFC[a]

Cells cultured[b]		Anti-SRBC PFC/Microculture[c]	
PP Th A clone	PP B cells	IgM	IgA
1	Total	62 ± 2	182 ± 7
1	IgA^-	57 ± 8	28 ± 2
1	IgA^+	11 ± 1	308 ± 65
9	Total	30 ± 3	97 ± 13
9	IgA^-	27 ± 2	17 ± 2
9	IgA^+	8 ± 2	234 ± 84

[a]PP B cells were prepared from mice which had received 0.075 ml rabbit anti-mouse thymocyte serum 48 h before sacrifice. Following isolation, the PP cells were further depleted of T cells by treatment with monoclonal rat anti-Thy-1, Lyt-1 and Lyt-2, followed by rabbit anti-rat $F(ab')_2$ and C.

[b]IgA^+ and IgA^- PP B cells were isolated by staining with FITC-labeled goat anti-mouse α and separated into positive and negative populations using a FACS. B cells were cultured (1×10^5) with the indicated PP Th A cells (1×10^3) and SRBC (5×10^4). IgM and IgA anti-SRBC PFC were assessed on day 5 of culture.

[c]Values are the mean anti-SRBC PFC numbers ± SEM from duplicate cultures per experiment and three separate experiments.

thymoma (29). Supernatants from wells exhibiting hybridoma growth were screened for their ability to support IgA PFC development in SRBC-immunized cultures of lipopolysaccharide-triggered splenic B cells. Sixteen T-T hybridomas which supported IgA responses (Th HA) were identified and characterized as Thy 1.2^{+}, Lyt-1^{-},2^{-} and I-A^{k-}. As in the case of the parent PP Th A clones, there was an absolute correlation between the expression of FcαR by the Th HA lines and their ability to support IgA PFC development. In addition, the PP Th HA lines elaborated into their culture supernatant an activity which was able to regulate IgA PFC responses in an antigen unrestricted fashion in vitro (29). Passage of the supernatants from the Th HA lines over solid phase absorbents revealed that the active principle was removed by IgA, but not IgM or IgG, and indicated that the activity was due to an IgA immunoglobulin binding factor (IBFα) (Fig. 1). IgA promoting activity could be recovered from the solid-phase IgA by acid elution, and titration of this purified IBFα into cultures of whole PP cells undergoing secondary challenge with SRBC showed that low concentrations augmented, but that high concentrations profoundly suppressed, IgA/PFC development. IBFα with similar properties has been extracted from the cytoplasmic membrane fraction of the Th HA lines.

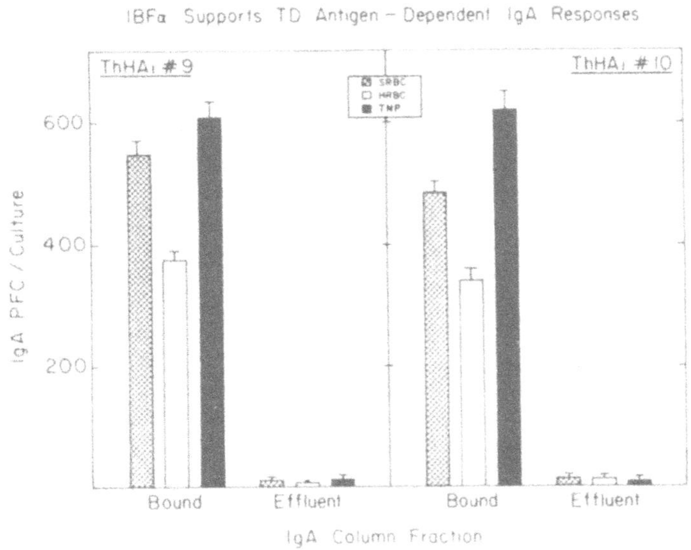

Figure 1. Detection of IBFα in PP Th HA supernatants. Supernatants (35-40 ml) from PP Th HA lines 9 and 10 grown in FCS-free HB 102 medium were passed over a solid-phase bound MOPC 315 column. The effluent and acid eluates were tested for their ability to support IgA PFC development in cultures of PP B cells immunized with SRBC (▨), HRBC (□) or TNP-SRBC (■).

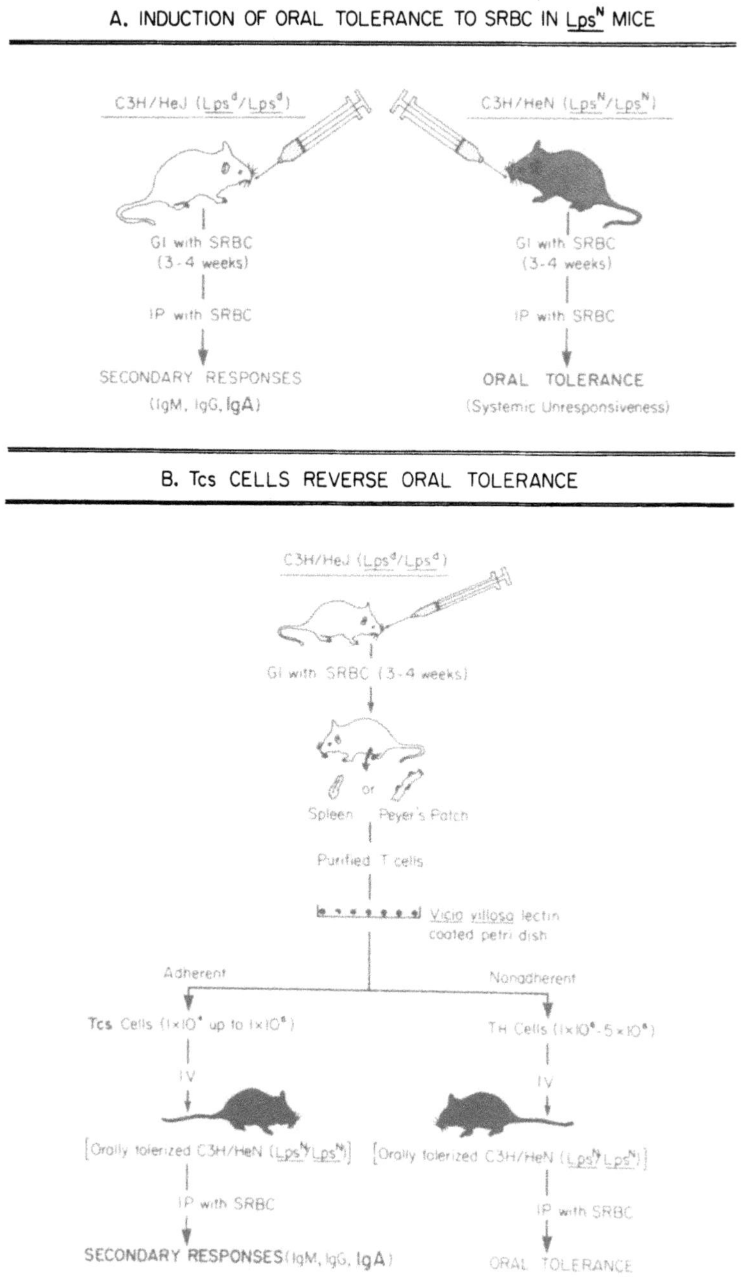

Figure 2. (A) Experimental protocol for the induction of oral tolerance to SRBC in C3H/HeN mice, and for demonstrating the resistance of C3H/HeJ mice to this mode of tolerance induction. (B) Experimental protocol for the demonstration of functional Tcs in the PP of C3H/HeJ mice following prolonged oral immunization with SRBC.

Peyer's patch T contrasuppressor cells selective for IgA responses

The C3H/HeJ mouse strain is nonresponsive to the biologic effects of bacterial lipopolysaccharide (LPS), and one manifestation of this mutation is that these mice are resistant to the induction of oral tolerance by the prolonged feeding of SRBC (30,31), (Fig. 2A). Based on the finding that C3H/HeJ mice exhibited Th cell activity after this immunization regimen, while syngeneic LPS-responsive C3H/HeN mice showed dominant Ts cell activity, we initially postulated that LPS stimulation was required for Ts cell maturation in the PP. However, the recent description of Tcs cell activity within the PP provided an alternative interpretation of those results, i.e., Tcs activity is heightened in C3H/HeJ mice and allows the expression of Th cell activity despite the presence of antigen-specific Ts cells (32). In order to test for the presence of active Tcs cells in C3H/HeJ mice with the capacity to abrogate Ts cell mediated oral tolerance, we designed an experimental model which made use of the binding of Tcs cells to the lectin of *Vicia villosa* (V.v.) (33). V.v. adherent (V.v.$^+$) and V.v.$^-$ T cells were prepared from the spleens and PP of C3H/HeJ mice following 21-28 d of oral immunization with SRBC. The existence of strong Tcs cell activity in C3H/HeJ mice following prolonged oral immunization with SRBC was demonstrated by the ability of 5 x 10^4 V.v.$^+$ PP or spleen T cells to allow splenic anti-SRBC PFC development in orally tolerized C3H/HeN mice when transferred prior to systemic challenge (34) (Fig. 2B). Experiments using monoclonal antibodies plus C to cytolytically remove T cell subsets demonstrated that the effector Tcs cells which mediate this abrogation of oral tolerance are Thy 1.2$^+$, V.v.$^+$, Lyt 1$^+$,2$^-$ and L3T4$^-$ (Table 3). This result indicates that these Tcs cells are phenotypically distinct from both Th (L3T4$^+$) and Ts (Lyt-2$^+$) cells (35). In addition, when the Tcs activity from the PP was analyzed at the isotype level, it was found to be 3 to 4-fold more efficient at allowing IgA, relative to IgM or IgG, PFC development (Table 4). In contrast, the Tcs cells isolated from the spleens of the same mice did not show as strong a preference for IgA and were more effective at allowing IgM and IgG responses.

Table 3. The T constrasuppressor cells which abrogate oral tolerance are distinct from T helper (L3T4$^+$) and T suppressor (Lyt-2$^+$) cells[a]

Adoptively transferred T cells[b]		Anti-SRBC PFC/10^7 Spleen Cells		
Treatment[c]	Number	IgM	IgG	IgA
-	1×10^6	743 ± 176	338 ± 135	946 ± 203
Anti-Thy 1.2 + C	1×10^6	87 ± 15	66 ± 8	49 ± 17
-	5×10^4	697 ± 102	363 ± 119	894 ± 203
Anti-Thy 1.2 + C	5×10^4	69 ± 21	41 ± 11	91 ± 10
Anti-Ly-1 + C	5×10^4	79 ± 19	60 ± 20	49 ± 9
Anti-Ly-2 + C	5×10^4	526 ± 51	456 ± 104	826 ± 129
Anti-L3T4 + C	5×10^4	625 ± 37	467 ± 85	752 ± 64
C3H/HeN Recipients		61 ± 20	72 ± 19	78 ± 15
C3H/HeJ Donors		589 ± 42	390 ± 33	768 ± 81

[a]Groups of C3H/HeN and C3H/HeJ mice were orally immunized with 0.25 ml of a 50% SRBC suspension on 28 consecutive days. Seven days after the final immunization, T cells and their subsets were purified from the spleens of the C3H/HeJ mice and adoptively transferred to groups of orally tolerized C3H/HeN mice. One hour after adoptive transfer the mice were immunized i.p. with SRBC.

[b]T cells were purified by the removal of adherent cells (37°C, 2 h) and treatment with anti-Ig plus C.

[c]Anti-Thy 1.2 (HO-13-4) and anti-L3T4 (GK 1.5) were used for direct cytotoxic treatments. Anti-Ly-1 (53-7.313) and anti-Lyt-2 (53-6.72) were used for indirect cytotoxic treatments in conjunction with a rabbit antiserum specific for mouse $F(ab')_2$.

Table 4. Tcs from spleens and Peyer's patches of orally-immunized C3H/HeJ mice abrogate oral tolerance in C3H/HeN mice[a]

Source of Tcs	Anti-SRBC PFC/10^7 Spleen Cells			Ratio	
	IgM	IgG	IgA	IgA/IgM	IgA/IgG
None	130 ± 12	150 ± 21	68 ± 11	-	-
Spleen	454 ± 68	490 ± 48	675 ± 69	1.49	1.38
Peyer's patch	267 ± 31	207 ± 23	895 ± 76	3.35	4.32

[a]Lyt-1$^+$, V.v.$^+$ Peyer's patch or spleen T cells from C3H/HeJ mice administered SRBC via gastric intubation for 28 consecutive days, were transferred (5×10^4 cells/mouse) to orally tolerant C3H/HeN mice. One hour after transfer the mice were challenged by i.p. injection with SRBC. IgM, IgG and IgA anti-SRBC PFC were determined 4 d later.

DISCUSSION

The isolation of cloned antigen-specific cell lines from the PP of orally immunized mice which preferentially support the development of IgA PFC in cultures of unprimed B cells indicates that isotype-specific T cells play an important role in regulating mucosal immune responses. The inability of these PP Th A clones to effectively collaborate with IgA^- B cells suggests they have no, or very limited, capacity to stimulate an isotype "switch" to IgA commitment and indicates they function through the selective clonal expansion and differentiation of B cells precommitted to IgA production. Characterization of T-T hybridomas derived from the cloned PP Th A cells further strengthens the correlation between FcαR expression on T cells and their ability to specifically regulate IgA responses. This absolute correlation supports the proposal that the FcαR functions as the recognition structure which governs the selective interaction of the isotype-restricted PP Th A cells with IgA^+ B cells. Further, the detection of functional activity in the form of an IBFα from solubilized cytoplasmic membranes and in cell-free culture supernatants suggests that a secreted form of the FcαR may play a role in regulating the IgA immune response. An additional level of isotype-specific regulation of the mucosal immune system is indicated by the observation that oral immunization induces Tcs cell development in the PP. These PP Tcs effector cells selectively abrogate T cell mediated suppression of IgA isotype responses. Thus, it appears that a network of isotype-specific regulatory T cells within the PP accounts for the induction and maintenance of a predominant IgA immune response to enterically encountered antigens: T "switch" cells provide an enriched IgA committed precursor pool; IgA specific Th cells expand the antigen stimulated B cells from this pool and Tcs cells which selectively abrogate Ts cell activity against IgA B cells function to preferentially maintain the IgA response.

ACKNOWLEDGEMENTS

Experimental results discussed in this paper were supported by U.S.P.H.S. grants AI 19674, AI 18958, AI 21774, DE 04217, AI 21032 and DE 02670.

REFERENCES

1. Craig, S.W. and Cebra, J.J., J. Exp. Med. 134, 188, 1971.
2. Kiyono, H., McGhee, J.R., Wannemuehler, M.J., Frangakis, M.V., Spalding, D.M., Michalek, S.M. and Koopman, W.J., Proc. Natl. Acad. Sci. (USA) 79, 596, 1982.
3. Spalding, D.M., Koopman, W.J., Eldridge, J.H., McGhee, J.R. and Steinman, R.M., J. Exp. Med. 157, 1646, 1983.
4. Kiyono, H., Babb, J.L., Michalek, S.M. and McGhee, J.R., J. Immunol. 125, 732, 1980.
5. Green, D.R., Gold, J., St. Martin, S., Gershon, R. and Gershon, R.K., Proc. Natl. Acad. Sci. (USA) 79, 889, 1982.
6. Suzuki, I., Kiyono, H., Kitamura, K., Green, D.R. and McGhee, J.R., Nature (London) 320, 451 1986.
7. Suzuki, I., Kitamura, K., Kiyono, H., Kurita, T., Green, D.R. and McGhee, J.R., J. Exp. Med. 164, 501 (1986).
8. Bockman, D.E. and Cooper, M.D., Am. J. Anat. 136, 455 (1973).
9. Owen, R.L., Gastroenterology 72, 440, 1977.
10. Bazin, H., Levi, G. and Doria, G., J. Immunol. 105, 1049, 1970.
11. Crabbe, P.A., Nash, D.R., Bazin, H., Eyssen, H. and Heremans, J.F., J. Exp. Med. 130, 723, 1969.
12. Mestecky, J., McGhee, J.R., Arnold, R.R., Michalek, S.M., Prince, S.J. and Babb, J.L., J. Clin. Invest. 61, 731, 1978.
13. Michalek, S.M., McGhee, J.R., Mestecky, J., Arnold, R.R. and Bozzo, L., Science 192, 1238, 1976.
14. Montgomery, P.C., Rosner, B.R. and Cohn, J., Immunol. Comm. 3, 143, 1974.
15. Hanson, L.A., Ahlstedt, S., Carlsson, B., Kaijser, B., Larsson, P., Mattsby-Baltzer, I., Sohl Akerlund, A., Svanborg-Eden, C. and Svennerholm, A.M., Adv. Exp. Med. Biol. 1007, 165, 1978.
16. Richman, L.M., Chiller, J.M., Brown, W.R., Hanson, D.G. and Vaz, N.M., J. Immunol. 121, 2429, 1978.
17. Kiyono, H., McGhee, J.R., Wannemuehler, M.J. and Michalek, S.M., J. Exp. Med. 155, 605, 1982.
18. Michalek, S.M., Kiyono, H., Wannemuehler, M.J., Mosteller, L.M. and McGhee, J.R., J. Immunol. 128, 1992, 1982.
19. Tomasi, T.B., Jr., Transplantation (Balt.) 29, 353, 1980.
20. Andre, C., Heremans, J.F., Vaerman, J.P. and Cambiaso, C.L., J. Exp. Med. 142, 1509, 1975.
21. Richman, L.K., Graeff, A.S., Yachoan, R. and Strober, W., J. Immunol. 126, 2079, 1981.

22. Mattingly, J.A. and Waksman, B.H., J. Immunol. 121, 1878, 1978.

23. Mattingly, J.A., Kaplan, J.M. and Janeway, C.A., Jr., J. Exp. Med. 152, 545, 1980.

24. Challacombe, S.J. and Tomasi, T.B., Jr., J. Exp. Med. 152, 1459, 1980.

25. Kawanishi, H., Saltzman, L.E. and Strober, W., J. Immunol. 129, 475, 1982.

26. Kiyono, H., McGhee, J.R., Mosteller, L.M., Eldridge, J.H., Koopman, W.J., Kearney, J.F. and Michalek, S.M., J. Exp. Med. 156, 1115, 1982.

27. Kiyono, H, Cooper, M.D., Kearney, J.F., Mosteller, L.M., Michalek, S.M., Koopman, W.J. and McGhee, J.R., J. Exp. Med. 159, 798, 1984.

28. Kiyono, H., Phillips, J.O., Colwell, D.E., Michalek, S.M., Koopman, W.J. and McGhee, J.R., J. Immunol. 133, 1087, 1984.

29. Kiyono, H., Mosteller-Barnum, L.M., Pitts, A.M., Williamson, S.I., Michalek, S.M. and McGhee, J.R., J. Exp. Med. 161, 731, 1985.

30. Michalek, S.M., Kiyono, H., Wannemuehler, M.J., Mosteller, L.M. and McGhee, J.R., J. Immunol. 128, 1992, 1982.

31. Kiyono, H., McGhee, J.R., Wannemuehler, M.J. and Michalek, S.M., J. Exp. Med. 155, 605, 1982.

32. Green, D.R., Gold, J., St. Martin, S., Gershon, R. and Gershon, R.K., Proc. Natl. Acad. Sci. USA 79, 889, 1982.

33. Green, D.R. and Ptak, W., Immunol. Today 7, 81, 1986.

34. Suzuki, I., Kitamura, K., Kiyono, H., Kurita, T., Green, D.R. and McGhee, J.R., J. Exp. Med. 164, 501, 1986.

35. Kitamura, K., Kiyono, H., Eldridge, J.H., Green, D.R. and McGhee, J.R., J. Immunol. (submitted for publication).

NOVEL REGULATORY MECHANISMS OF IgA SYNTHESIS: RESPECTIVE ROLES OF NEUROPEPTIDES AND CELLS OF THE ANTI-SUPPRESSOR CIRCUIT

P.B. Ernst, A.M. Stanisz, R. Scicchitano, F. Paraskevas*, D. Payan** and J. Bienenstock

Department of Pathology and Intestinal Disease Research Unit, McMaster University, Hamilton, Ontario, Canada; and *Department of Immunology, University of Manitoba, Winnepeg, Manitoba, Canada; and **Department of Medicine, University of California at San Francisco, San Francisco, CA, USA

INTRODUCTION

IgA has been recognized as the predominant class of antibody in mucosal secretions even though it constitutes a relatively small percentage of serum immunoglobulin. There are several mechanisms that contribute to IgA making up such a large proportion of the antibody in intestinal secretions (reviewed in ref. 1) including: a high frequency of IgA B cell precursors in Peyer's patches (2); T cells which facilitate an isotype switch from IgM to IgA (so called switch T cell) (3); IgA-specific helper T cells (4); a propensity of these cells to traffic selectively to mucosal surfaces (1); and the existence of a specific mechanism to facilitate the transport of IgA across the epithelium into secretions (5). In this paper, we report our data concerning two other mechanisms that may be capable of enhancing IgA production, namely neuropeptides and the antisuppressor regulatory circuit.

MATERIALS AND METHODS

Animals

CBA/J mice from 6-15 weeks of age were supplied from Jackson Laboratories (Bar Harbor, ME) and housed under conventional conditions. Age and sex matched animals were used in all experiments.

Examination of the effect of neuropeptides. The techniques used for the studies of neuropeptides have been described in detail elsewhere (6). Briefly, cell suspensions were prepared from the gut associated lymphoid tissue (GALT) of CBA/J mice including the Peyer's patches (PP) and mesenteric lymph nodes (MLN) which was studied and compared to spleen (SPL). Cell proliferation was studied by measuring incorporation of ^{3}H-thymidine by cells cultured in the presence of concanavalin A and the neuropeptides (NP), substance P (SP), somatostatin (SOM) and vasoactive intestinal polypeptide (VIP). In other experiments, the effect of NP on immunoglobulin synthesis was determined by a solid-phase inhibition-type radioimmunoassay for the quantitation of IgM, IgG or IgA.

In view of the observations to be presented that these neuropeptides indeed are capable of modulating cell proliferation and antibody production, studies were undertaken to determine the presence of receptors for two of these NP (SP or SOM) on lymphoid cells. In these studies, cell suspensions from PP or SPL were fractionated into T cell or B cell enriched populations by nylon wool columns or antibody and complement mediated cytolysis, respectively. These cells were then incubated with either SP or SOM labeled with diachlortriazinylamine (DTAF; SP*, SOM*) and specific fluorescence was detected by flow cytometry. The distribution of NP receptors on distinct lymphocyte subsets was determined by dual parameter flow cytometry: by staining for one particular lymphocyte subset (Thy 1^+, Lyt 1^+, Lyt 2^+, IgM^+, IgG^+, or IgA^+) followed by staining with labeled neuropeptide (7).

The specificity of NP binding was evaluated in an independent system involving a competitive radiolabeled ligand binding assay. The amount of ^{125}I-labeled SP or SOM which bound to intact cells was determined in the absence and presence of an excess of unlabeled (cold) NP (8).

Examination of the effect of antisuppressor cells. The antisuppressor pathway is a model of the earliest interaction of macrophages, T cells and B cells that ultimately gives rise to antigen-specific antibody responses. This is evidenced by the fact that the activity of the T cells involved in this circuit can be detected within 6 hours of immunization.

Studies involving the antisuppressor pathway included examination of two cells (an initiating and an effector cell) involved at the onset of the response, using methods described in detail elsewhere (Ernst et al. submitted; and reviewed by Paraskevas et al., 9,10). The Lyt 1^+ initiating cell (Tasi) produces a factor which can be demonstrated in serum within 6 hours of immunizing a naive animal (11). This factor (antisuppressor initiating factor, asiF) facilitates the formation of a complex which contains antigen and antibody molecules which binds to and activates an Lyt 2^+ effector cell (Tase). The factor or activated effector cells can be added to suppressed cultures to test for their ability to enhance antigen and isotype specific responses. Briefly, our assay system was set up as follows: SPL cells were immunized in vitro with SRBC and a normal range of SRBC-specific IgG and IgA response was established using the modified Cunningham plaque-forming cell (PFC) assay. Antigen-specific suppressor cells were generated as previously described (12-14) and added to these cultures, and IgG or IgA specific responses were then determined in the presence or absence of various elements of the antisuppressor network.

The demonstration of the antisuppressor network in GALT was carried out as follows. To detect Lyt 1^+ initiating cells, intraepithelial leukocytes (IEL), mesenteric lymph node (MLN), PP or SPL cells were used to reconstitute mice that were lacking initiating cells due to prior irradiation with 850 rads. These reconstituted animals were then immunized with SRBC and bled 6 hours later for the detection of the antisuppressor initiating factor which activates the antisuppressor pathway. This factor was initially detected using a rosetting assay (11) to identify the complex bound to antisuppressor effector cells in lamina propria (LP), IEL, MLN, PP or SPL (13,14). Subsequently, the functional activity of this factor was also tested as follows. Serum containing the factor was added directly to suppressed cultures or was incubated with Lyt 2^+ effector cells which were thereby activated and then added to suppressed cultures. The IgG and IgA specific PFC were then determined and expressed as PFC/ml of cultured cells.

RESULTS

Studies on the effect of NP on proliferation

SPL and PP cells were cultured alone or in the presence of NP at concentrations ranging from 10^{-7} - 10^{-12} M and the percent change in ^{3}H-thymidine incorporation was recorded. In both PP and SPL, SP increased while VIP and SOM inhibited the ^{3}H-thymidine incorporation compared to controls (Fig. 1). The effect of these NP on cell proliferation was dose dependent.

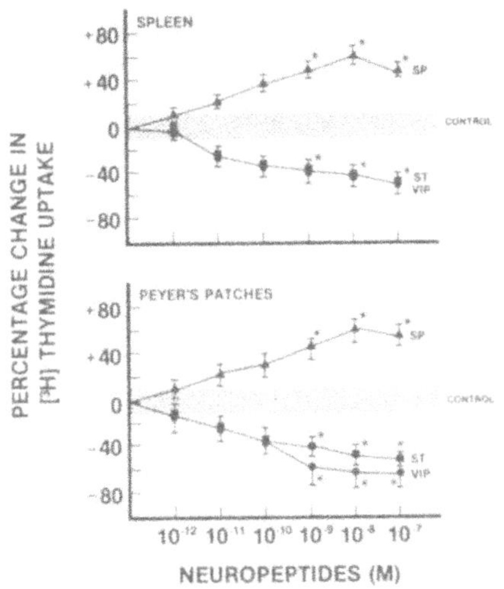

Figure 1. Proliferative responses of lymphocytes from SPL and PP stimulated with Con A (1 μg/ml) and incubated with 10^{-7} to 10^{-12}M concentration of VIP (●), SP (▲) or SOM (■). Data are presented as a percentage change in (^{3}H) thymidine uptake (control ± SD) (n=12). *$p < 0.05$.

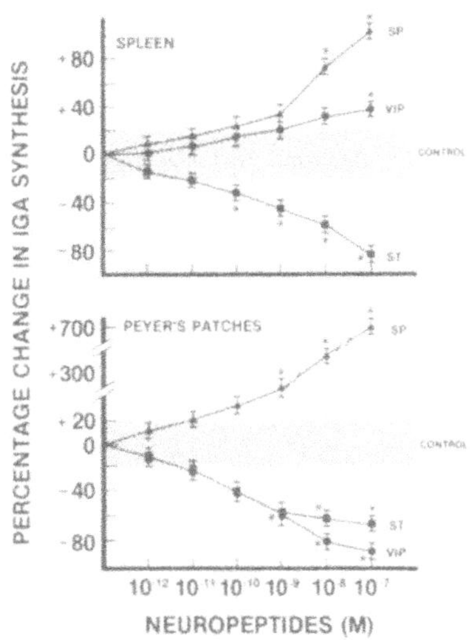

Figure 2. The effect of different neuropeptides (10^{-7} to 10^{-12}M) on IgA synthesis by lymphocytes from SPL and PP stimulated with Con A (1 μg/ml) and incubated with VIP (●), SP (▲) or SOM (■). Data are presented as percentage change in IgA concentration in supernatants of 7 day cultures *$p < 0.05$.

The effect of NP on IgA production. The total amounts of each class of immunoglobulin produced in the presence or absence of different concentrations of NP was also determined. Figure 2 shows that in both SPL and PP cultures, SP enhanced IgA production. This was particularly obvious in cultures of PP cells where there was a 300% increase over controls while in SPL cultures the increase was only 80%. SOM inhibited IgA production by both tissues while VIP enhanced production in SPL and inhibited it in PP. Again, the effects of these NP were dose-dependent. Using a fixed dose of NP (10^{-8}M), the effect of SP on IgA production was shown to be selective since this NP had little effect on IgA and only slightly increased IgM (Fig. 3). SOM decreased the production of all classes although its effect on IgA was the most pronounced (data not shown).

Binding of SP and SOM by lymphocytes. The binding of these NP to lymphocytes was first examined by preparing T and B cell enriched populations from PP and SPL and studying the binding of DTAF labeled NP (NP*) using flow cytometry. Approximately 65% of both T and B cells were shown to bind either NP*. The binding of the two NP* to distinct subsets of B (IgM^+, IgG^+ or IgA^+) and T (Thy 1^+, Lyt 1^+, Lyt 2^+) lymphocytes was assessed using dual parameter flow cytofluorometry. Table 1A shows that binding of SOM* or SP* could be demonstrated in all major subsets of T and B cells in approximately similar proportions.

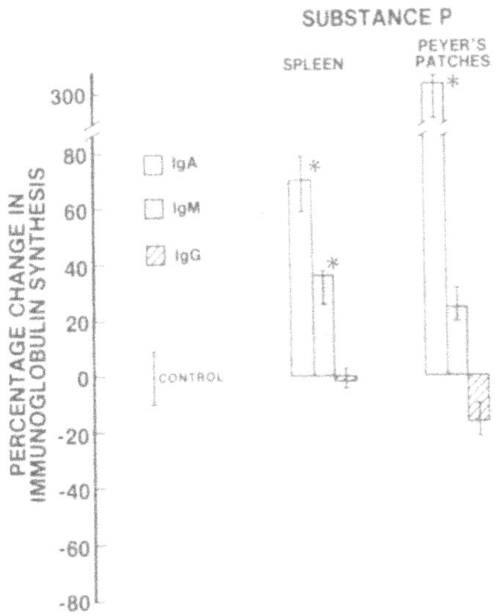

Table 3. Modulation of immunoglobulin isotype by SP (10^{-8}M). IgA, IgM and IgG concentrations of culture supernatants were determined by solid phase inhibition-type radioimmunoassay.

Table 1A. Dual parameters FACS analysis of neuropeptide binding by Peyer's patch T and B cell subsets

Surface marker	Substance P	Somatostatin
Thy 1.2	76 ± 2	84 ± 3
Lyt 1	66 ± 4	83 ± 2
Lyt 2	70 ± 3	94 ± 4
IgA	72 ± 16	94 ± 3
IgM	97 ± 1	92 ± 2
IgG	62 ± 4	83 ± 1

Values expressed as the mean percentages of cells positive (± SEM) for a particular surface marker, which also bound DTAF-labeled neuropeptide.

Specificity of NP binding. Using ^{125}I-NP, NP specific binding was determined by a competitive binding assay. In Table 1B, about 75-80% of labeled SP binding to SPL and PP was shown to be inhibitable by cold SP present in high concentrations (10^{-5} M). Similarly, approximately 90% of the labeled SOM binding was inhibited by cold SOM. These data suggest that SOM and PP bind to lymphocytes via specific receptors and studies are underway to characterize these receptors.

Studies of antisuppression in GALT

Distribution of the initiating and effector cells. The different sites in GALT were examined for the presence of cells of the antisuppressor circuit and compared to SPL which is known to contain these cells (9,10). The initiating cell which is capable of reconstituting the ability of irradiated mice to form the antisuppressor initiating factor was detected in PP, MLN but not IEL (Table 2). The cells in LP were not examined since insufficient numbers were isolated to reconstitute an animal. In other experiments, the presence of the effector cell was detected by the ability of cells in the different compartments of GALT to bind asiF. By this assay, the effector cell was demonstrated in PP and LPL but not MLN or IEL (Table 2). Thus, the PP was similar to SPL in that it contained both the initiating and effector cell and was, therefore, the tissue that was used for the subsequent studies.

Table 1B. Specificity of ^{125}I-NP binding to spleen and Peyer's patch whole cell populations

	SPL			PP		
	CPM[b] bound	Unlabeled + NP (10^{-5}M)	% Specific binding	CPM bound	Unlabeled + NP (10^{-5}M)	%Specific[c] binding
SP	793 ± 21[a]	200 ± 35	75	650 ± 15	136 ± 18	79
SOM	1685 ± 172	185 ± 27	89	2199 ± 193	169 ± 18	92

(a) = Mean ± SEM; (b) = per 10^6 cells; (c) = Specific binding defined as: CPM bound in absence cold ligand - CPM bound in presence cold (10^{-5}M) ligand.

Table 2. Distribution of the initiating and effector cells of antisuppression

Tissue	Presence	
	Tasi	Tase[a]
SPL	+++	+++
PP	+++	+++
MLN	+++	-
LP	NT	++
IEL	-	-

[a]Tasi were present (+++) if the cell preparation could reconstitute the ability of an irradiated mouse to form antisuppressor complexes as detected by complex binding to SPL Tase. Similarly, Tase were detected by the ability of the different preparations to bind the complex from normal mice. NT = not tested.

Functional evidence of antisuppression. As described in Materials and Methods, SRBC were used to stimulate SPL cell cultures in the presence or absence of antigen specific suppressor cells and the IgG and IgA specific PFC were determined. To the suppressed cultures, the components of the antisuppressor pathway were added in order to assess their functional activity. Table 3 shows that the serum collected 6 hours after immunization of mice reconstituted with PP (PP asiF) or SPL (SPL asiF), was capable of restoring the PFC response to normal levels and, therefore, contained the

Table 3. Evidence for isotype selection in vitro by the antisuppressor circuit

Culture	SRBC Specific PFC/ml[a] IgG	IgA	IgA/IgG
(1) SPL	1198	934	.8
(2) SPL + Ts	0	0	0
(3) SPL + Ts + SPL asiF	782	934	1.2
(4) SPL + Ts + PP asiF	363	967	2.7
(5) SPL + Ts + SPL Tase + SPl asiF	1442	990	.7
(6) SPl + Ts + SPL Tase + PP asiF	165	241	1.5
(7) SPL + Ts + PP Tase + SPL asiF	330	1244	3.8
(8) SPL + Ts + PP Tase + PP asiF	165	967	5.9

[a]Mean of 3 replicates from a representative experiment.

Cultures were antisuppressed by addition of serum containing the antisuppression initiating factor (asiF) alone or nylon wool column nonadherent, Lyt 1 depleted effector cell (Tase) activated in advance by asiF. Comparison of cultures 3 and 4, 5 and 6, and 7 and 8 show the effect due to the source of asiF while 5 and 7 and 6 and 8 show the effect due to the source of Tase.

antisuppressor initiating factor (experiments 3,4). Similarly, the Lyt 2^+ effector cell of antisuppression in PP could be activated by the initiating factor from either source to mediate antisuppression (experiments 7,8). Thus, as suggested by the data in Table 3, PP resembled SPL in that they both contained the initiating and effector cells of antisuppression.

The effect of antisuppression on IgA production. In addition, Table 3 shows the isotype-specific mediated by antisuppressor cells of PP, SPL or mixtures of the two (i.e., initiating factor from 1 tissue plus effector cell from other tissues). For example, when SPL antisuppressor effector cells were activated with the factor from SPL-derived initiating cells, the response was not just restored to normal levels, but normal IgA/IgG ratios were obtained. However, when the effector cell from SPL was activated by the initiating factor produced by PP, the IgA/IgG ratio favored IgA (experiment 6). More dramatic evidence of the role of antisuppression in modulating isotype expression was seen when the effector cell from PP activated by the factor from initiating cells from SPL or PP, markedly selected for IgA. The data also show that the highest IgA/IgG ratio was obtained when both the initiating cell and effector cell were derived fromm PP, and which suggests that this selectivity is a property of both of these cells. Other experiments have shown that differences in the ratio of IgA/IgG caused by the source of antisuppressor initiator or effector cells are statistically significant ($p < 0.05$) using the Wilcoxon Rank test (Ernst et al., submitted).

DISCUSSION

Data presented in this paper identify two novel mechanisms, namely neuropeptides and the antisuppressor circuit, which can be added to the growing list of mechanisms which regulate IgA production at mucosal surfaces.

The involvement of the nervous system in the direct and indirect regulation of the immune response is now well-documented (15-23). A number of hormones and neurotransmitters, including neuropeptides, have been shown to modulate immunity in vitro (21,22) and some of these actions appear to be mediated by the specific receptors present on lymphocytes and other immune cells (8,19,20,23). In particular, it has been demonstrated that the NP, somatostatin, substance P and VIP which are present in the intestine in high concentrations, can affect lymphocyte function (18,24,25), and specific receptors for these NP have been described on murine and human lymphocytes (8,19,24).

Our data show that the NP, VIP, SOM and SP can affect cell proliferation and immunoglobulin synthesis by immune splenic and Peyer's patch lymphocytes. Of particular interest, we found that there were isotype-specific differences in the effects of these NP: the effect was greatest on IgA synthesis, less on IgM synthesis while IgG synthesis was virtually unchanged. There was also an organ-specific effect in that SP dramatically enhanced IgA synthesis by PP lymphocytes.

One possible explanaton for this isotype- and organ-specific effect is that NP receptors may be present on distinct T and B lymphocyte subpopulations: VIP and SP receptors occur predominantly on murine and human T lymphocytes, respectively, and in the latter situation, mainly on T helper cells (24,26). However, we found that both B and T murine lymphocytes bind SOM* and SP* and there was no preference for a particular subpopulation to do so. Therefore, we conclude that differential expression of SOM and SP receptor by the major lymphocyte subsets is not the reason for the isotype-specific effects of these NP on immunoglobulin synthesis.

Neuropeptides may act at different levels of the immune network. We suggest that the modulatory effect of neuropeptides is likely to be mediated by direct interaction with both T and B cells and that the net effect may reflect the cell population present in a particular tissue and the degree and nature of local cell-cell interaction. Therefore, it is not surprising that SP enhanced IgA synthesis by Peyer's patch lymphocytes to a greater degree than splenic lymphocytes, in view of the relatively higher proportion of T (Tα helper and T Switch) cells and B cells in PP which are committed to IgA synthesis or its promotion.

Another mechanism by which IgA can be selected is the antisuppressor cells. The antisuppressor pathway represents the earliest interactions among antigen presenting cells, B cells and T cells, that results in the initiation of antigen-specific immune responses (9,10). The T cells involved in this pathway, which up to now has only been described in SPL, are functioning within hours of a primary immunization. In this paper, we showed that this pathway was present in GALT and both the initiating and effector cells supports the hypothesis that the PP are in fact, the primary site for the introduction of antigen to the intestinal mucosal immune system but we do not rule out that early events in immune activation could also occur elsewhere, for example, in the lamina propria.

The antisuppressor cells in PP were strikingly similar to those in SPL in several respects including their ability to reconstitute antisuppressor function in irradiated animals, produce the initiating factor, bind the initiating factor (suggesting the presence of effector cells) as well as to function as antisuppressor <u>in vitro</u>. The most surprising observation was the fact that the antisuppressor cells from the PP selected for IgA compared to those from the SPL. The data suggested both cells (the initiator and the effector) in PP can contribute to IgA production. This is quite dramatic in view of the fact that these are functional T-T interactions that occur within only 6 hours of immunization. Clearly, this is a novel concept involving very early events in the initiation of isotype-specific regulation by the immune system. This mechanism of isotype-specific regulation may be a key for the initiation of these responses and facilitate the activation of other T cells involved in the regulation of IgA.

CONCLUSIONS

1. Neuropeptides were capable of modulating both cell proliferation and immunoglobulin production by murine splenic and Peyer's patch lymphocytes.

2. SP selectively enhanced the production of IgA, particularly by PP lymphocytes.

3. Cells associated with the antisuppressor pathway are present in GALT.

4. Both the initiating cell and the effector cell from PP selected for IgA production compared to SPL which selected for IgG.

ACKNOWLEDGEMENTS

These investigations were supported by MRC Canada, the Banting Foundation and the Canadian Foundation for Ileitis and Colitis.

REFERENCES

1. Ernst P.B., Scicchitano, R., Underdown, B.J. and Bienenstock, J., in Immunology of the Gastrointestinal Tract and Liver, (Edited by Jones, R., Heyworth, M. and Owen, R.), Raven Press, New York (in press).
2. Craig, S.W. and Cebra, J.J., J. Exp. Med. 134, 188, 1971.
3. Kawanishi, H., Saltzman, L.E. and Strober, W., J. Exp. Med. 157, 433, 1983.
4. Kiyono, H., Cooper, M.D., Kearney, J.F., Mosteller, L.M., Michalek, S.M., Koopman, W.J. and McGhee, J.R., J. Exp. Med. 159, 798, 1984.
5. Underdown, B.J. and Schiff, J.M., Ann. Rev. of Immunol. 4, 389, 1986.
6. Stanisz, A.M., Befus, A.D. and Bienenstock, J., J. Immunol. 136, 152, 1986.

7. Payan, D.G., Brewster, D.R., Missirian-Bastian, A. and Goetzl, E.J., J. Clin. Invest. 74, 1532, 1984.

8. Payan, D.G., Brewster, D.R. and Goetzl, E.J., J. Immunol. 133, 3260, 1984.

9. Paraskevas, F., Lee, S.-T. and Al-Maghazachi, A., Lymphokines 9, 201, 1984.

10. Paraskevas, F., ee, S.-T. and Al-Maghazachi, A., Surv. Immunol. Res. 3, 15, 1984.

11. Orr, K.R. and Paraskevas, F., J. Immunol. 110, 456, 1973.

12. Paraskevas, F., Lee, S.-T., Maeba, J. and David, C.S., Cell. Immunol. 92, 53, 1985.

13. Lee, S.-T., Paraskevas, F. and Maeba, J., Cell. Immunol. 92, 64, 1985.

14. Paraskevas, F., Lee, S.-T. and Maeba, J., Cell. Immunol. 92, 74, 1985.

15. Bhathena, S.J., Lovie, J., Schecheter, G.P., Redman, R.S., Wahl, L. and Recant, L., Diabetes 30, 127, 1981.

16. Ottaway, C.A. and Greenberg, G.R., J. Immunol. 132, 417, 1984.

17. Besedovsky, H.O., Rey, A.E. and Sorkin, E., Immunol. Today 4, 342, 1983.

18. Rayan, D.G., Hess, C.A. and Goetzl, E.J., Cell. Immunol. 84, 422, 1984.

19. Ottaway, C.A., Bernaerts, C., Chan, B. and Greenberg, G.R., Can. J. Physiol. Pharmacol. 61, 664, 1983.

20. Danek, A., O'Dorisio, M.S., O'Dorisio, T.M. and George, J.M., J. Immunol. 131, 1173, 1983.

21. Johnson, H.M., Smith, E.M., Torres, B.A. and Blalock, J.E., Proc. Natl. Acad. Sci. USA 79, 4171, 1982.

22. Gilman, S.C., Schwartz, J.M., Milner, R.J., Bloom, F.E. and Feldman, J.D., Proc. Natl. Acad. Sci. USA 79, 4226, 1982.

23. Hartung, H.P., Wolters, K. and Toyka, K.V., J. Immunol. 136, 3856, 1986.

24. Ottaway, C.A., J. Exp. Med. 160, 1054, 1986.

25. Payan, D.G., Brewster, D.R. and Goetzl, E.J., J. Immunol. 131, 1613, 1983.

26. Payan, D.G., Brewster, D.R., Missirian-Bistra, A. and Goetzl, E.J., J. Clin. Invest 74, 1532, 1984.

Fc-SPECIFIC SUPPRESSOR T CELLS

A. Mathur, B. Van Ness and R.G. Lynch

Departments of Pathology, Biochemistry and Microbiology
University of Iowa College of Medicine
Iowa City, Iowa USA

INTRODUCTION

BALB/c mice bearing IgA-secreting plasmacytomas exhibit large numbers of Thy-1^+, Ly-2^+ lymphocytes with surface membrane receptors specific for IgA (Tα cells) (1). These lymphocytes have several characteristics of immunoregulatory T cells (2) and develop in response to the high circulating levels of polymeric IgA as evidenced by: a) their failure to develop in mice bearing IgA non-secreting variant plasmacytomas (1) and (b) their occurrence in normal mice infused daily with high concentrations of polymeric IgA (3). When suppressor Tα cells were transferred to orally-immunized mice the recipient mice exhibited a marked suppression of the IgA component, but not the IgM or IgG components, of an immune response to an orally administered antigen (4). These findings identify an immunoregulatory circuit in which IgA secreting cells are simultaneously effector cells and regulatory cells. Secreted IgA antibody, in addition to its antigen-specific effector function, can provide an inductive signal for the IgA-binding suppressor T cells which in turn can inhibit further IgA secretion. Enhanced expression of IgA receptors on suppressor T cells requires polymeric forms of IgA which suggests that IgA-Fc receptor crosslinking is a necessary step in the induction process. Under physiological conditions it may be that receptor crosslinking is mediated by the polyvalent arrays of Fc determinants that occur in immune complexes. To determine whether enhanced FcR expression on regulatory T cells was a general occurrence or was restricted to IgA, mice bearing plasmacytomas and hybridomas secreting other classes of immunoglobulin were examined.

RESULTS

We have observed that mice bearing IgG or IgM-secreting hybridomas and plasmacytomas develop splenic $L3T4^-$, $Ly2^+$ T cells that express FcR specific for the heavy chain class of the secreted monoclonal Ig. Thus, mice bearing IgG-secreting hybridomas developed increased numbers of T cells bearing Fc receptors specific for IgG ($T\gamma$) while showing no changes in the frequencies of T cells bearing FcR for either IgM ($T\mu$) or IgA ($T\alpha$) (Table 1). Similarly, mice bearing IgM-secreting hybridomas and plasmacytomas developed increased numbers of $T\mu$ cells, with no alterations in the frequencies of either $T\gamma$ or $T\alpha$ cells (Table 1). It was further shown that mice bearing non-secreting variants of the IgG (GNP-1) and IgM (MNP-1) tumors did not develop increased numbers of $T\gamma$ and $T\mu$ cells (Table 1), suggesting that high levels of circulating IgG and IgM were responsible for the enhanced expression of $T\gamma$ and $T\mu$ cells, respectively. The increased expression of $T\mu$ cells may be caused by the pentameric monoclonal IgM in mice with IgM-secreting tumors. It is possible, but not proven, that the increased expression of $T\gamma$ cells in mice with IgG-secreting tumors is triggered by aggregated forms of the monoclonal IgG.

Mice with IgE-secreting hybridomas (B53) develop large numbers of $T\varepsilon$ cells that are $L3T4^-$, $Thy\text{-}1^+$, $Ly2^+$ (5). A non-secreting variant of the B53 hybridoma (ENP-1) fails to induce elevated numbers of $T\varepsilon$ cells. Mice infused daily with IgE-rich ascites fluid from hybridoma-bearing mice develop large numbers of $T\varepsilon$ cells (5), while infusion of ascites fluid from mice with IgE non-secreting variant hybridomas fails to elicit an enhanced expression of ε-Fc receptor (Table 1). As in the case of IgG, aggregated forms of the IgE may have been the inductive signal for enhanced ε-FcR expression but this remains to be tested. Preliminary studies indicate that the various FcR are present on normal T cells on the $L3T4^+$, $Ly2^-$ and the $L3T4^-$, $Ly2^+$ subsets. The enhanced expression of FcR on $L3T4^-$, $Ly2^+$ cells in response to forms of immunoglobulin capable of cross-linking receptors is an active process but the relative contributions of receptor synthesis, redistribution and stabilizaton are yet to be determined.

As has already been shown for $Ly2^+$ $T\alpha$ cells, the $L3T4^-$, $Ly2^+$ $T\varepsilon$ cells in B53-tumor bearing mice may be functional suppressor cells. This is suggested by the pattern of IgE secretion by the hybridoma cells as they proliferate <u>in vivo</u>. During the first four days of growth the serum IgE concentration progressively increases and this is followed by a steady

Table 1. T cells with Fc Receptors in mice with immunoglobulin-secreting tumors

Tumor	% splenic T cells bearing FcαR[a]			
	IgG	IgM	IgA	IgE
HDP1 (γ,κ)[c]	35 ± 3[b]	14 ± 3	3 ± 1	-
GNP-1[c]	17 ± 2	13 ± 2	2 ± 1	-
MOPC 104E (μ,λ)[c]	11 ± 3	30 ± 4	3 ± 1	-
MNP-1[c]	16 ± 2	14 ± 2	2 ± 2	-
B53 (ε,κ)[d]	19 ± 4	15 ± 2	3 ± 2	33 ± 1
ENP-1[d]	15 ± 2	13 ± 4	2 ± 1	0.1 ± 0.1
None[e]	14 ± 5	15 ± 4	3 ± 1	0.1 ± 0.1

[a]Single cell spleen suspensions from mice were passaged over nylon-wool columns to obtain nylon wool nonadherent populations that were found to contain 95% Thy 1^+ cells, less than 5% s-Ig^+ cells, and less than 5% monocytes. Nylon wool non-adherent cells were assayed for the presence of FcR for IgG, IgM, IgA and IgE, respectively, using isotype-specific rosette assays described earlier (5).

[b]Data are expressed as the percent of total splenic nylon wool non-adherent T cells that form rosettes (RFC) in the isotype-specific rosette assays. Data are shown as mean RFC ± S.E.M., four experiments per group.

[c]10^6 HDP1, GNP-1, MOPC 104E or MNP-1 hybridoma cells were injected subcutaneously on day 0 into normal 8-12 wk old female BALB/c mice. The mice were sacrificed and their nylon wool non-adherent spleen cells were examined for the presence of FcR for IgG, IgM and IgA, on consecutive days beginning from day 2 until day 20 at which time the mice generally succumbed to the tumor. Representative data from mice on day 14 following hybridoma cell implantation are presented in this table.

[d]2×10^6 B53 or ENP-1 hybridoma cells were injected i.p. on day 0 into normal 8-12 wk old female BALB/c mice. The mice were sacrificed on days 2, 4, 6 and 8 and their nylon wool non-adherent spleen cells were examined for the presence of FcR for IgG, IgM, IgA and IgE. Representative data from mice on day 6 following hybridoma cell implantation are presented in this table.

[e]Normal 8-12 wk old tumor free female BALB/c mice were sacrificed and their nylon wool non-adherent spleen cells were examined for the presence of FcR for IgG, IgM, IgA and IgE. Data are expressed as the percent of total splenic nylon wool non-adherent cells ± S.E.M., 20 experiments per group.

increase in the frequency of suppressor T cells that express surface $Fc\varepsilon$ receptors. However, after day four serum IgE levels fell and on a per cell basis we found about a seven-fold decrease in IgE secretion between day four and day eight of in vivo growth. The inhibition of IgE production by hybridoma cells did not occur in nude mice or in normal mice pre-treated with anti-Ly2 antibody and neither of these mice develop $T\varepsilon$ cells (Mathur and Lynch, manuscript in preparation). It appears that the decreased IgE secretion results, at least in part, from a selective inhibition of ε-mRNA production in the hybridoma cells (Mathur, Van Ness and Lynch, manuscript submitted).

DISCUSSION

For each heavy chain class there appears to be a corresponding FcR expressed on immunoregulatory T cells. In response to the surge of monoclonal antibody that occurs in mice with immunoglobulin secreting tumors there is a marked enhancement of FcR expression on $L3T4^-$, $Ly2^+$ cells. In each instance the enhanced FcR matches the heavy chain class of the monoclonal immunoglobulin.

Increased expression of FcR on immunoregulatory T cells in mice with plasmacytomas and hybridomas may be an exaggerated, but otherwise normal, immunoregulatory response. Other types of lymphoid tumors commonly exhibit excessive functional activities that lead to conspicuous alterations in the lymphoid system of the host. Examples include the hypogammaglobulinemia and hypergammaglobulinemia that occur with certain T and B cell tumors, and the distinctive patterns of immune deficiency that occur in patients with multiple myeloma, chronic lymphocytic leukemia, and Hodgkin's Disease. In addition to elaborating immunoregulatory signals, plasmacytoma and hybridoma cells are responsive to immunoregulatory signals. For example, it has been shown that the proliferation and differentiation of antigen-binding murine plasmacytomas can be regulated by conventional idiotype-specific and antigen-specific T cells (reviewed in ref. 6). In the studies mentioned above the production of IgE by hybridoma cells in vivo was progressively diminished following the appearance of large numbers of suppressor T cells bearing IgE Fc receptors. The IgE decrease could reflect the activation of an isotype-specific regulatory circuit. The possibility that T cells participate in this process is currently being tested.

Their clonal nature and ability to induce and respond to regulatory signals make Ig producing tumors useful models for identifying and dissecting components of immunoregulatory mechanisms.

CONCLUSIONS

1. Immunoglobulin secreting tumors induce a marked enhancement of FcR expression on host immunoregulatory T cells.

2. The specificity of the T cell FcR matches the heavy chain class of the secreted monoclonal immunoglobulin. This has been shown for IgA, IgE, IgM, IgG and IgD (7) secreting tumors.

3. Investigations of the Fc receptor-expressing T cells in mice bearing plasmacytomas and hybridomas may provide additional insights into autoregulatory mechanisms that control the quality and quantity of immunoglobulin expressed during immune responses.

ACKNOWLEDGEMENTS

These studies were supported by U.S.P.H.S. grant CA 32277, GM 37687 and a Basil O'Connor Research grant to BVN.

REFERENCES

1. Hoover, R.G. and Lynch, R.G., J. Immunol. 125, 1280, 1980.
2. Hoover, R.G., Dieckgraefe, B., Lake, J., Kemp, J.D. and Lynch, R.G., J. Immunol. 129, 2329, 1982.
3. Hoover, R.G., Dieckgraefe, B.K. and Lynch, R.G., J. Immunol. 127, 1560, 1982.
4. Hoover, R.G. and Lynch, R.G., J. Immunol. 130, 521, 1983.
5. Mathur, A., Maekawa, S., Ovary, Z. and Lynch, R., Molec. Immunol. 23, 1193, 1986.
6. Hanley-Hyde, J.M. and Lynch, R.G., Ann. Rev. Immunol. 4, 621, 1986.

7. Coico, R.F., Xue, B., Wallace, D., Pernis, B., Siskind, G.W. and Thorbecke, G.J., Nature 316, 744, 1985.

ISOTYPE-SPECIFIC IMMUNOGLOBULIN BINDING FACTORS OF IgA AND IgE

J. Yodoi, M. Takami, T. Doi*, T. Kawabe, K. Yasuda, M. Adachi and N. Noro

Institute for Immunology and *Department of Pathology, Kyoto University Faculty of Medicine, Yoshida Sakyo-ku, Kyoto 606, Japan

INTRODUCTION

Growing evidence has shown the importance of Fc receptors (FcRs) and immunoglobulin binding factors (IBFs) specific for various immunoglobulin classes in human as well as murine immune systems (1-7). IBFs for IgA (8-13) and IgE (14-18) are particularly important because of the clinical diseases involving the abnormalities of these systems. In selective IgA deficiency and IgA nephropathy, FcR/IBF for IgA is altered (19). In atopic as well as non-atopic hyper-IgE syndromes, expression of the FcR for IgE (FcεR) is up-regulated (3,4,20).

Our previous studies on IgA-IBFs (IgA-BFs) have shown that murine splenic T cells and T hybridoma cells bearing FcαR could produce suppressive IgA-BF acting on both murine and human lymphocytes (9-11). In this paper, we demonstrate human IgA-BF produced by a natural killer (NK)-like cell line (YT) (22).

Using a monoclonal antibody (H107) recognizing human lymphocyte FcR for IgE (FcεR) (20,23), we purified FcεR and IgE-IBF (IgE-BF) to homogeneity. The relationship between soluble H107 antigen and IgE-BF produced by a B lymphoblastoid cell line, RPMI 8866 is discussed.

RESULTS

Human IgA-BF from a NK cell line (YT) and from patients with IgA nephropathy

A human large granular lymphocyte (LGL) cell line (YT) derived from the pericardial effusion of a 14 year old boy has a NK-like cytotoxic activity and an IL-2R which can be regulated (22). YT cells were positive for T9, T11 (weak), OKIa, Leu-9, Leu-11 and were negative for T1, T3, T4 and T8. Unlike mature T cells, YT cells had the germ line configuration of the T cell receptor T_{beta} chain gene. The presence of normal LGL cell population without T_{beta} gene rearrangement was suggested by the analysis of the Leu-11^{+} cells sorted from normal PBL.

As was the case with murine T cell lines producing IBFs for multiple classes (14,24), YT cells expressed FcRs for IgG, IgA and IgE. Upon stimulation with IgA, YT cells produced IgA-BF, which was specifically purified by using an IgA-affinity column. YT-derived IgA-BF suppressed pokeweed mitogen induced IgA antibody production of human PBL in vitro as determined by reversed plaque formation (Fig. 1) and ELISA assay. Neither IgG nor IgM responses were affected by IgA-BF. These results suggest that not only mature T cells but LGL/NK cells may physiologically be involved in the regulation of isotype-specific humoral immune responses. Although the data are not shown, IgA-BF from the YT cells also suppressed the enhanced IgA production of PWM-stimulated cultures of PBL from patients with IgA nephropathy.

Purification of IgE-BF by using anti-FcεR monoclonal antibodies (H107)

Using H107 moAb recognizing cell surface FcεR on human T and B lymphocytes, we tried to detect soluble H107 antigens in the culture supernatant of lymphoid cell lines, which expressed FcεR and H107 antigens at high density. The presence of soluble H107 antigens was determined by the sandwich RIA assay for the H107 antigens using rabbit anti-RPMI 8866 antibody and ^{125}I-H107 moAb as well as the inhibition assay for the binding of ^{125}I-H107 moAb to the H107^{+} FcεR^{+} RPMI 8866 B lymphoblastoid cell line. Soluble H107 antigens were detected in the culture supernatant of RPMI 8866 and RPMI 1788 B cell lines, both of which expressed H107 antigen/FcεR. There was no detectable soluble H107 antigen production by the cell lines bearing no H107 antigen/FcεR.

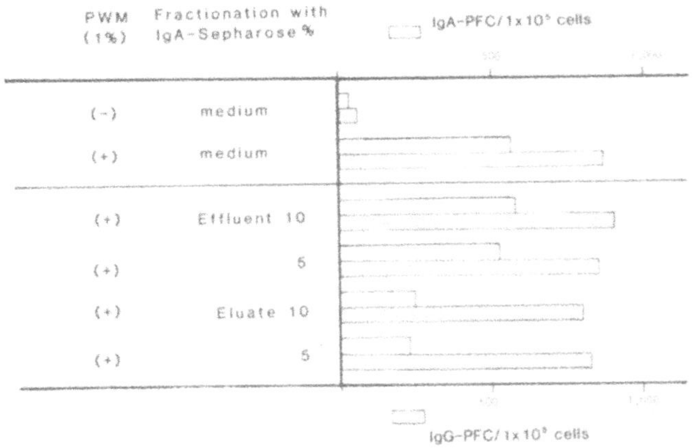

Figure 1. Suppression of IgA response by IgA-BF from YT cells. YT cells were cultured with 300 µg/ml of MOPC 315 IgA at 37°C for 18 h. The cells were washed and cultured at 5 x 10^6/ml for 24 hr in IgA-free culture medium consisting of RPMI 1640 with 10% heat-inactivated fetal calf serum with antibiotics to obtain culture supernatant. IgA binding factor was purified from the 50-fold concentrated culture supernatant by using an IgA-Sepharose column. The effluent and the acid eluate of the column were added to the culture of normal human PBL in the presence of 10 µg/ml of PWM at the concentration of 5 or 10%. After 6 days in culture, IgA and IgG antibody production was determined by a reverse plaque forming cell (PFC) assay. Results are expressed as the number of PFC per 1 x 10^5 cells.

Upon gel filtration analysis of RPMI 8866 culture supernatant, H107 antigen was eluted at approximately 20-25 Kd. After purification with the H107-Sepharose column, two adjacent protein bands were detected at ~25 Kd on SDS-PAGE with silver staining. Western blot hybridization studies showed that these 25 Kd proteins reacted with H107 moAb. In contrast, H107 antigens recovered from the RPMI 8866 cell lysates with neutral detergent (NP40) was approximately 43 Kd, consistent with the previous report on the size of FcεR on lymphocytes. Western blot analysis of both 43 Kd cell-bound H107 antigen and 25 Kd soluble H107 antigen is shown in Figure 2.

Affinity purified 25 Kd H107 antigens were fractionated with FPLC system using a gel filtration column (Superose). The H107 antigen determined by ELISA, the activity to inhibit IgE rosette formation of RPMI 8866 cells and the in vitro IgE enhancing activity in PWM-stimulated cultures of normal PBL all co-fractionated at approximately 20 Kd on Superose.

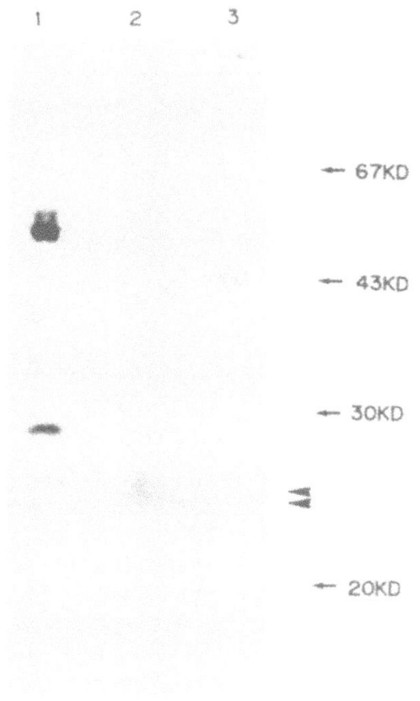

Figure 2. Western blotting of the affinity-purified cell-bound and soluble H107 antigens. Samples were analyzed with 13% SDS-PAGE under non-reducing conditions. After electroblotting to nitrocellulose membranes, the membrane was incubated with H107 antibody followed by anti-mouse IgG conjugated with horse radish peroxidase. Lane 1: mouse H107 moAb (IgG_{2b}) as a control; Lane 2: soluble H107 antigen obtained from the culture supernatant of RPMI 8866 cells purified with H107-Sepharose; Lane 3: H107 antigen purified from the lysate of RPMI 8866.

CONCLUSIONS

1. A human NK cell line (YT) without T cell receptor beta chain rearrangement expressed multiple isotype-specific FcRs and could produce suppressive IgA-BF.

2. H107 moAb reacts with two forms of H107 antigens: H107 antigen on the $Fc\varepsilon R^+$ RPMI 8866 cells has the size of 43 Kd and is associated with FcεR. Soluble H107 antigen in the culture superantant of the cell line cells has the size of 25 Kd.

3. 25 Kd soluble H107 antigens have the characteristics of enhancing IgE-BF.

ACKNOWLEDGEMENTS

The continued encouragement and advice of Drs. Y. Hamashima and H. Yoshida for this work are deeply appreciated. This work was partly supported by the Grant-in-Aid for Scientific Research from the Ministry of Education, Science and Culture of Japan.

REFERENCES

1. Gisler, R.H. and Fridman, W.H., J. Exp. Med. 142, 507, 1975.
2. Neauport-Sautes, C., Raboundin-Combin, C. and Fridman, W.H., Nature 277, 656, 1979.
3. Yodoi, J., Ishizaka, T. and Ishizaka, K., J. Immunol. 123, 455, 1979.
4. Spiegelberg, H.L., O'Connor, R.D., Simon, R.A. and Mathison, D.A., J. Clin. Invest 64, 714, 1979.
5. Hoover, R.G., Dieckgraefe, B.K. and Lynch, R.G., J. Immunol. 127, 1560, 1982.
6. Yodoi, J., Adachi, M. and Masuda, T., J. Immunol. 128, 888, 1982.
7. Hoover, R.G. and Lynch, R.G., J. Immunol. 125, 1280, 1981.
8. Yodoi, J., Adachi, M. and Noro, N., Int. Rev. Immunol. 2, 117, 1987.
9. Yodoi, J., Adachi, M., Teshigawara, K., Miyama-Inaba, M., Masuda, T. and Fridman, W.H., J. Immunol. 131, 303, 1983.
10. Adachi, M., Yodoi, J., Noro, N., Masuda, T. and Uchino, H., J. Immunol. 133, 65, 1984.
11. Noro, N., Aachi, M., Yasuda, K., Masuda, T. and Yodoi, J., J. Immunol. 136, 2910, 1986.
12. Kiyono, H., Cooper, M.D., Kearney, J.F., Mosteller, L.M., Michalek, S.M., Koopman, W.J. and McGhee, J.R., J. Exp. Med. 159, 798, 1984.
13. Kiyono, H., Mosteller-Barnum, L.M., Pitts, A.N., Williamson, S.I., Michalek, S.M. and McGhee, J.R., J. Exp. Med. 161, 731, 1986.
14. Yodoi, J. and Ishizaka, K., J. Immunol 124, 1322, 1980.
15. Yodoi, J., Hirashima, M. and Ishizaka, K., J. Immunol. 126, 877, 1981.
16. Suemura, M., Shiho, O., Deguchi, H., Yamamura, Y., Böttcher, I. and Kishimoto, T., J. Immunol. 127, 465, 1981.
17. Ishizaka, K., Yodoi, J., Suemura, M. and Hirashima, M., Immunology Today 4, 192, 1983.
18. Huff, F., Yodoi, J., Uede, T. and Ishizake, K., J. Immunol. 132, 406, 1984.

19. Adachi, M., Yodoi, J., Masuda, T., Takatsuki, K. and Uchino, H., J. Immunol. 131, 1246, 1983.
20. Nagai, T., Adachi, M., Noro, N., Yodoi, J. and Uchino, H., Clinical Immunol. Immunopathol. 35, 261, 1985.
21. Adachi, M., Okumura, K., Watanabe, N., Noro, N., Masuda, T. and Yodoi, J., Immunogenetics 22, 77, 1985.
22. Yodoi, J., Teshigawara, K., Nikaido, T., Fukui, K., Noma,T., Honjo, T., Takigawa, M., Sasaki, M., Minato, N., Tsudo, M., Uchiyama, T. and Maeda, M., J. Immunol. 134, 1623, 1985.
23. Noro, N., Yoshioka, A., Adachi, M., Yasuda, K., Masuda, T. and Yodoi, J., J. Immunol. 137, 1258, 1986.
24. Yodoi, J., Adachi, M., Teshigawara, K., Masuda, T. and Fridman, W.H., Immunology 48, 551, 1983.

ISOTYPE SPECIFIC IMMUNOREGULATION: ROLE OF $Fc\alpha R^+$ T CELLS AND $IBF\alpha$ IN IgA RESPONSES

T. Kurita, H. Kiyono*, M.L. McGhee and J.R. McGhee

Departments of Microbiology, *Oral Biology and Preventive Dentistry, The Institute of Dental Research, University of Alabama at Birmingham Birmingham, AL USA

INTRODUCTION

T cell subsets which express Fc receptors for immunoglobulin (FcR) are important in isotype-specific regulation of B cell responses (1). These FcR^+ T cells secrete isotype-specific immunoglobulin binding factors (IBF) which recognize specific Fc regions of immunoglobulin (Ig) and IBF can up or down regulate B cell antibody synthesis in these Ig classes. In this regard, allo-activated T cells which bear Fc receptors for IgG ($Fc\gamma R$) and the T2D4 T cell line ($Fc\gamma R^+$ and $Fc\alpha R^+$) release IgG binding factor ($IBF\gamma$) and suppress this isotype for in vitro responses (2). In the IgE system, Fc receptors for IgE ($Fc\varepsilon R$) occur on T cells which regulate this isotype response via production of either enhancing or suppressive IgE binding factors ($IBF\varepsilon$) (3). Both potentiating and suppressive $IBF\varepsilon$ are similar in size (Mr ~15,000). They contain a common protein core, and the degree of glycosylation determines whether $IBF\varepsilon$ enhances or suppresses the IgE responses.

The role of Fc receptors for IgA ($Fc\alpha R$) on T cells in isotype-specific immunoregulation was first suggested by the finding of high frequencies of suppressor $Fc\alpha R^+$ T cells in mice bearing IgA myeloma (4). These $Fc\alpha R^+$ T cells inhibited specific IgA responses in vivo (5). Additional support for down regulation of IgA responses by $Fc\alpha R^+$ T cells was provided by studies with the $Fc\gamma R^+$ and $Fc\alpha R^+$ T2D4 T cell line and with Con A activated murine $Fc\alpha R^+$ splenic T cells, which upon incubation with IgA, released ($IBF\alpha$) that suppressed in vitro PWM driven IgA synthesis (6,7). These murine $IBF\alpha$

are approximately 56,000 MW and preferentially act on surface IgA bearing ($SIgA^+$) B cells to suppress their secretion of antibody across the MHC and species barriers (8). On the other hand, subsets of $Fc\alpha R^+$ T cells can enhance the IgA response, since FACS isolated $Fc\alpha R^+$ T cells from human peripheral blood, which contain mainly $T4^+$ helper cells, supported in vitro IgA synthesis (9,10).

Our own interest in isotype-specific immunoregulation derived from our earlier studies that oral immunization in mice with T cell dependent (TD) antigens induce a unique population of Th cells in gut-associated lymphoreticular tissue (GALT), or Peyer's patches (PP), which mainly support IgA responses (11-13). We further isolated and cloned these unique Th cell subsets which express FcαR and preferentially act on $sIgA^+$ B cells for induction of final differentiation and secretion of IgA antibodies (14-16). In this paper, we briefly characterize FcR expression on isotype-specific T cells with emphasis on the relationship between solubilized FcαR (sFcαR) from cell membrane and the secreted form of IBFα.

Characterization of $Fc\alpha R^+$ T cells and IBFα for regulation of IgA responses

In order to examine the role of FcαR and IBFα in isotype-specific regulation, a panel of T cell lines were derived from fusion of PP Th cell clones for IgA with the R1.1 T lymphoma and the resulting T-T hybridomas were designated Th HA cells (17). Since expression of FcR on the T cell is an important feature in isotype-specific regulation, we have extensively studied FcαR expression by four different assays including immunocytoadherence, colloidal gold (CG)-immunoelectron microscopy (IEM), flow cytometry (FACS) and enzyme-linked immunoabsorbent assay (ELISA) (18,19). Immunocytoadherence of Th HA cells with IgA (MOPC 315) and TNP-conjugated erythrocytes showed that Th HA cells were $Fc\alpha R^+$; however, no rosettes were seen using monoclonal IgM or IgG (17-19). When Th HA cells were incubated with IgA followed by CG-labeled anti-IgA, an even distribution of CG was observed on the cell membrane. Furthermore, incubation of Th HA cells and IgA, followed by staining with CG-labeled TNP-human serum albumin resulted in the pattern of CG distribution and confirmed the expression of FcαR on Th HA cells (19).

When these cell lines were analyzed by FACS using IgA, IgM or IgG1 and FITC-labeled anti-heavy chain specific antibodies, approximately 60% of cultured Th HA cells expressed FcαR and interestingly, approximately

15% also expressed FcμR; however, no $Fc\gamma_1R$ was detectable on Th HA cells (19). The use of ELISA with Th HA cells as coating antigen confirmed the FACS analyses and demonstrated the expression of FcαR and the presence of less FcμR on these cells (18,19). Each assay allowed quantitative analysis of FcαR on Th HA cells and confirmed the expression of FcμR on these isotype-specific T cell lines.

Culture supernatants from these $Fc\alpha R^+$ Th HA cells (Th HA_1 #9 and #10) supported IgA responses in PP B cell cultures in the presence of TD antigens, e.g., sheep erythrocytes (SRBC). Since passage of these culture supernatants over an IgA column removed the IgA promoting activity and the low pH eluate from this column restored the IgA response, it was concluded that IgA responses were due to an IBFα (17). In addition, the IBFα was shown to either enhance or suppress antigen-dependent IgA responses, and the response seen was dependent on the amount of IBFα added to <u>in vitro</u> cultures. These results clearly indicated that FcαR expression and IBFα production are both characteristics of Th HA cells.

A key question which still remains in isotype-specific regulation is whether the FcαR on isotype-specific T cells is identical to the secreted IBFα which is found in the culture supernatant. In order to answer this question, our initial studies determined whether FcαR on Th HA cells regulate IgA responses. Soluble membrane fractions were obtained following detergent lysis of Th HA_1 #9 and #10 cells, high speed centrifugation and sonic treatment of the pelleted membrane fraction (19). This soluble membrane fraction possessed FcαR as determined by ELISA (Table 1). Interestingly, this lysate fraction also contain FcμR; however; ELISA FcμR values were three to four times lower than FcαR (19).

Addition of solubilized membrane fractions to PP B cell cultures immunized with SRBC resulted in good IgA responses, comparable to those obtained with IBFα (Table 1) (19). The biologic activity of the membrane fraction was due to sFcαR, because passage of this fraction over an IgA column removed this biologic activity and detectable FcαR as shown by ELISA. The low pH eluate from this IgA column, when added to PP B cell cultures immunized with SRBC, supported <u>in vitro</u> IgA anti-SRBC PFC responses (Table 1) (19). It is tempting to suggest that IBFα is the released form of FcαR on the membrane of isotype-specific T cells and is structurally similar to the FcαR. These results clearly indicated that FcαR and IBFα are important molecules in regulation of IgA antibody production. In addition, these molecules may also play an important role in isotype-specific T cell

Table 1. Soluble FcαR from cell membrane fractions of Th HA cells possess IBFα-like activity

Cell used	Fraction tested[a]	IgA anti-SRBC PFC/culture[b]	Detection of FcαR (ELISA O.D. 414 nm)[c]
	sFcαR (Unfractionated)	825 ± 43	0.342 ± 0.029
	IgA column bound	442 ± 47	0.437 ± 0.024
Th HA_1 #9			
	IgA column unbound	24 ± 6	0.028 ± 0.007
	IBFα	515 ± 36	0.343 ± 0.011
	sFcαR (Unfractionated)	576 ± 48	0.343 ± 0.011
	IgA column bound	321 ± 42	0.312 ± 0.029
Th HA_1 #10			
	IgA column unbound	18 ± 5	0.067 ± 0.001
	IBFα	582 ± 39	0.232 ± 0.021

[a]Detergent (NP-40) treated sFcαR fraction was chromatographed over an IgA column, and the effluent was collected. The bound fractions were eluted with low pH glycine HCl buffer. IBFα was obtained from culture supernatants of Th HA cells by using an IgA affinity column.

[b]PP B cells (2.5 x 10^6/well) were cultured and immunized with SRBC in the presence of sFcαR or IBFα. IgA anti-SRBC PFC responses were assessed on day 5 of culture.

[c]EIA plates were coated with solubilized membrane fractions and were next incubated with MOPC 315 IgA. β-galactosidase-labeled goat anti-mouse was added to wells, the plates were incubated overnight, color was developed with substrate and the OD was determined.

networks, e.g., interactions between isotype-specific Th cell and contrasuppressor T cells (see Kitamura et al. in this volume).

Generation and characterization of monoclonal antibody to FcαR/IBFα.

In order to facilitate studies on the molecular and immunobiological characteristization of FcαR and IBFα, we generated a panel of rat monoclonal antibodies (mAb) which recognized mouse FcαR. In these studies, Fischer rats were immunized with $Fc\alpha R^+$ Th HA cells or solubilized cell membrane and these immunized rat spleen cells were fused with the non-Ig-producing X63-Ag 8.563 murine myeloma cell line. Supernatant fluids from culture wells displaying hybrid growth were initially screened by inhibition of IgA binding to FcαR on Th HA cells or solubilized cell membrane using ELISA for the presence of antibody reactive with FcαR. Hybridomas that produced antibodies specific for FcαR were subcloned by limiting dilution. Selected subclones were expanded in vitro and were grown as ascites in pristane treated mice. Thus far, preliminary studies indicate that four mAbs (all rat IgG_{2c}) inhibit 50-80% of IgA binding to FcαR on Th HA cells - or solubilized cell membrane-precoated ELISA plates. When $Fc\alpha R^+$ Th HA cells were treated with these mAbs prior to incubation with IgA (MOPC 315) followed by TNP-erythrocytes, 85-100% inhibition of rosette formation was observed. FACS analysis of Th HA cells incubated with appropriate dilutions of mAb followed by FITC-anti-rat $F(ab')_2$ showed approximately 30-50% of cells stained as positive. This degree of staining was very similar to that obtained when Th HA cells were first incubated with IgA and stained with FITC-anti-α (19). Since rat IgG_{2c} can fix complement upon reaction with antigen, a direct cytotoxicity assay was also employed for further characterization of these mAbs. Approximately 20% of Th HA cells were lysed by these mAbs in the presence of complement. When the fusion partner, R1.1 T lymphoma ($Fc\alpha R^-$) was reacted with these mAb and tested for mAb specificity as described above, each assay was negative. These results clearly indicated that all four rat mAbs recognize FcαR or a closely associated structure on Th HA cells. Currently, we are further characterizing these mAbs using SDS-PAGE gel analysis and Western blotting. We plan to use these mAbs for the study of the molecular and immunobiological relationship between the FcαR and IBFα.

SUMMARY

Fcα receptor $(Fc\alpha R)^+$ T cell hybridomas (Th HA cells) were derived from fusion of Peyer's patch T helper cells (PP Th A cell) which preferentially select $sIgA^+$ B cells and support IgA responses, with the R1.1 T lymphoma cell line. Expression of FcαR on Th HA cells was extensively characterized by several methods, i.e., immunocytoadherence, colloidal gold-immunoelectron microscopy, FACS and ELISA. All four assays clearly demonstrated expression of FcαR on Th HA cells. The use of FACS and ELISA also suggested the expression of FcαR as well as the presence of lower amounts of FcμR on these cell lines. The significance of coexpression of FcαR and FcμR is currently under extensive investigation in our group.

Solubilized membrane fractions derived from Th HA cells were tested for the presence of FcαR on ELISA and for their ability to support *in vitro* IgA responses. Both FcαR and FcμR were detected in cell membrane fractions of Th HA cells. The cell membrane fraction which contained FcαR, supported *in vitro* IgA anti-SRBC PFC responses when added to PP B cell cultures in the presence of SRBC. This activity was removed by adsorption to an IgA affinity column. On the other hand, the bound fraction contained sFcαR and supported IgA anti-SRBC PFC responses in PP B cell cultures, a response pattern that was similar to those obtained with IBFα.

Taken together, these results suggest that FcαR and IBFα are similar molecules and both exhibit functional activity. To further characterize the relationship between FcαR and IBFα, four mAb which recognize the FcαR were generated by immunization of rats with Th HA cells or cell membrane fractions. Preliminary results indicate that these mAb are IgG_{2c} and recognize FcαR on Th HA cells. Currently, intensive investigations are underway to completely characterize these mAbs.

ACKNOWLEDGEMENTS

Experimental results discussed in this paper were supported by U.S. Public Health Service grants AI 18958, AI 21032, AI 19674, DE 04217 and DE 02670.

REFERENCES

1. Daeron, M. and Fridman, W.H., Ann. Inst. Pasteur/Immunol. 136, 383, 1985.
2. Fridman, W.H., Rabourdin-Combe, C., Neauport-Sautes, C. and Gisler, R.H., Immunol. Rev. 56, 51, 1981.
3. Ishizaka, K., Ann. Rev. Immunol. 2, 159, 1984.
4. Hoover, R.G. and Lynch, R.G., J. Immunol. 125, 1280, 1981.

5. Hoover, R.G. and Lynch, R.G., J. Immunol. 130, 521, 1983.

6. Yodoi, J., Adachi, M., Teshigawara, K., Miyama-Inaba, M., Masuda, T. and Fridman, W.H., J. Immunol. 131, 303, 1983.

7. Adachi, M., Yodoi, J., Noro, N., Masuda, T. and Uchino, H., J. Immunol. 133, 65, 1984.

8. Noro, N., Adachi, M., Yasuda, K., Masuda, T. and Yodoi, J., J. Immunol. 136, 2910, 1981.

9. Endoh, M., Sakai, H., Nomoto, H., Tomino, Y. and Kaneshige, H., J. Immunol. 127, 2612, 1981.

10. Suga, T., Endoh, H., Sakai, H., Miura, T., Tomino, T. and Nomoto, Y., J. Immunol. 134, 1327, 1985.

11. Kiyono, H., Babb, J.L., Michalek, S.M. and McGhee, J.R., J. Immunol. 125, 732, 1980.

12. Kiyono, H., McGhee, J.R., Wannemuehler, M.J., Frangakis, M.V., Spalding, D.M., Michalek, S.M. and Koopman, W.J., Proc. Natl. Acad. Sci. USA 79, 596, 1982.

13. Kiyono, H., Mosteller, L.M., Eldridge, J.H., Michalek, S.M. and McGhee, J.R., J. Immunol. 131, 2616, 1983.

14. Kiyono, H., McGhee, J.R., Mosteller, L.M., Eldridge, J.H., Koopman, W.J., Kearney, J.F. and Michalek, S.M., J. Exp. Med. 156, 1115, 1982.

15. Kiyono, H., Cooper, M.D. Kearney, J.F., Mosteller, L.M., Michalek, S.M., Koopman, W.J. and McGhee, J.R., J. Exp. Med. 159, 798, 1984.

16. Kiyono, H., Phillips, J.O., Colwell, D.E., Michalek, S.M., Koopman, W.J. and McGhee, J.R., J. Immunol. 133, 1087, 1984.

17. Kiyono, H., Mosteller-Barnum, L.M., Pitts, A.M., Williamson, S.I., Michalek, S.M. and McGhee, J.R., J. Exp. Med. 161, 731, 1985.

18. Kurita, T., Kiyono, H., Michalek, S.M. and McGhee, J.R., J. Immunol. Meth. 85, 269, 1985.

19. Kurita, T., Kiyono, H., Komiyama, K., Grossi, C.E., Mestecky, J. and McGhee, J.R., J. Immunol. 136, 3953, 1986.

AUTOREACTIVE T CELLS REGULATING B CELL GROWTH AND DIFFERENTIATION IN MURINE PEYER'S PATCHES

H. Kawanishi and S. Mirabella

Gut Mucosal Immunity Laboratory, SUNY at Stony Brook;
and Veterans Administration Medical Center at Northport,
New York USA

INTRODUCTION

The IgA isotype expression in an immune response is a unique feature of the gut mucosal immune system. Mechanisms governing regulation and expression of the IgA response are of key importance to an understanding of intestinal mucosal immunity (1,2).

A number of model systems (3) have been employed to examine the sequence of events involved in triggering B cell activation, proliferation and differentiation, some being involved in Ig heavy chain switching (4-6). Despite such extensive investigation, the previous studies of B cell development in the gut mucosal immune system have been limited and fragmentary and a number of important question remain to be solved.

The autologous (syngeneic) mixed lymphocyte culture (MLR) is an immunoregulatory circuit found in both animals and humans (4). It is generally defined as T cell proliferation in response to autologous (syngeneic) Ia^{+}, non-T cells. During the course of an autologous MLR, several immunologic events occur, including the T cell-dependent isotype switch of B cells.

In this communication, we examined a possible important role of autoreactive (AUT) T cells and their secreted products (lymphokines) in the regulation of B cell development in murine Peyer's patches (PP).

MATERIALS AND METHODS

Animals used

Male BALB/c (H-2d) mice, 3-4 months old.

Stimulants, including mitogens and immunologic agents

For generations of autoreactive (syngeneic, Ia activated) T cells, we used irradiated (2,500 R) or mitomycin C (50 μg/ml at 37°C, 60 min), pretreated syngeneic B cells and/or adherent cells (macrophages) from PP and the spleen (SPN). Lipopolysaccharide, E. coli 0111: B4 (LPS, optimal 20 μg/ml; suboptimal 0.2 μg/ml) was also used to stimulate B cells in vitro. Three monoclonal antibodies, anti-Thy 1.2 (HO-13-4), anti-Lyt-1 (53-7.313), anti-L3T4 (GK1.5; rat IgG_{2b}) and anti-Lyt 2 (53-6.72) were produced from hybridoma cells. In addition, a monoclonal antibody reactive to $I\text{-}A^d$ (MK-D6; IgG 2a K) was used. Monoclonal antibodies were purified from the culture supernatant or ascites of each above hybridoma cell line by isotype-specific affinity column chromatography. After elution from the column by 0.2 M glycine hydrochloride at pH 3.0, each elute was tested for its specificity. Fluoresceinated and non-fluoresceinated goat or rabbit chromatographically purified polyclonal and monospecific anti-mouse $F(ab')_2$ antibodies (μ, γ, α) were used for identification and separation of B cells and their subsets.

Preparations of single cell suspensions of adherent cells and/or lymphocytes from Peyer's patches (PP) and SPN

PP and SPN cell suspensions were made, as described previously (5).

Fractionation of cell populations (5,9)

(a) T cells (Thy 1.2); (b) B cells (sIg); (c) T cell subsets ($L3T4^+$, $Lyt\text{-}2^-$ vs. $Lyt\text{-}2^+$); (d) B cell subsets (sIgM-bearing vs. non-sIgM-bearing); (e) high density (HD) (resting) and low density (LD) (blast) B cell subsets, bearing sIgM or non-sIgM, by two subsequent discontinuous density Percoll gradients.

Cell proliferation assay was done by ^{3}H-thymidine uptake as described elsewhere (5).

Microcultures for in vitro Ig production

Using flat-bottomed 96 well microtiter plates in a final volume of 0.25 ml culture medium, 5×10^4 - 2×10^5 cells/well, were incubated for 7 days (10).

Quantitative measurement of isotype-specific antibodies secreted in microcultures were done using enzyme linked immunosorbent assay (ELISA) (10).

Direct and indirect immunofluorescence was as previously described(5).

Preparation of autoreactive PP and SPN T cells

AUT T (blast) cells were enriched by the above Percoll gradient method from fresh L3T4$^+$ T cells stimulated by mitomycin C-pretreated or postirradiated Ia$^+$ B/macrophages.

Preparation of culture supernatants containing BSF and its cofactors (IL-2) produced by culturing autoreactive PP or SPN T cells for 5 days has been described elsewhere (11).

In vitro assay for IL-2 activity (mitogenic assay), was done by using an IL-2 dependent cell line (CTLL) (10).

In vitro assay for B cell growth factor (BCGF) activity (proliferative assay of activated B cells)

Anti-IgM synergy assay and dextran sulfate (DxSO4) synergy assay were carried out as described elsewhere (3).

In vitro assay for class-specific B cell switch factor (BSWF) activity, using sIgM B cells

sIgM $\rightarrow$ sIgA BSWF-alpha and sIgM $\rightarrow$ sIgG BSWF-gamma activities were measured, as described previously (5).

In vitro assay for B cell differentiating factor (BCDF) activity was done by measuring Ig production by B cells by ELISA (3,12).

Preparation and selection of BSF-producing hybridoma cell lines

T cell hybridomas used in the experiments were produced by fusing the autoreactive L3T4$^+$ (Lyt-1$^+$, Lyt-2$^-$) PP and SPN T cells with the BW5147 AKR thymoma T cell partner. When the colonies became macroscopically visible in the 96-well cluster plates, their supernatants were tested for BCAF, BCGF, BSWF, BCDF and IL-2, as described above. Hybridoma cell cloning was carried out by limiting dilution.

Production of BSF from T cell hybridomas developed

Appropriate uncloned/cloned hybridoma cell lines were expanded *in vitro* for collection of B cell factors-enriched bulk supernatants.

RESULTS AND DISCUSSION

First, we determined the effect of in vitro induced PP AUT T cells on class specific Ig production by PP sIgM B cells in the presence or absence of LPS (Table 1). In the presence of the AUT T cells, but in the absence of LPS, the sIgM B cells produced large amounts of IgA (2.7 x more than IgG). The experiments with the AUT T cells in the presence of LPS resulted in a decrease in IgA production, but an increase in IgG production. This evidence suggests that the AUT T cells themselves possess the capability of PP B cells to assist their growth, probably heavy chain switch and terminal differentiation to IgA-producing plasma cells.

Second, we developed PP/SPN-derived AUT L3T4$^+$ (Lyt-2$^-$) T cell hybridoma cell lines, producing B cell stimulatory factors (BSF)(Table 2). The supernatants from two uncloned cell lines from PP (PP CF-13) and SPN (SPN CF-4) were selectively shown here; these lines possessed BCGF activity (Fig. 1). The supernatants also had both BSWF (tentative) and BCDF, determined by analyzing class-specific Ig produced by PP/SPN sIgM and non-sIgM (sIgG/sIgA) B cells (Fig. 2).

Third, two cloned PP (CF-13, A-9) and SPN (CF-4, C-6) AUT T cell hybridomas were representatively tested in the present studies; these supernatants exhibited the BSWF activity, the former (PP) eliciting an expression

Table 1. Effect of Peyer's patch (PP) autoreactive T cells on class specific immunoglobulin production by Peyer's patch sIgM B cells in the presence or absence of lipopolysaccharide (LPS)[a]

Culture condition	Ig Synthesis (ng/ml)[b]		
	IgM	IgG	IgA
PP-derived sIgM B cells ($5x10^4$/w)	60	30	10
+LPS (20 μg/ml)	25,478±1.751	3,608±155	10
+Autoreactive PP T cells (5×10^4/w) (1:1)	4,526±799	1,879±192	5,010±273
+Autoreactive PP T cells + LPS	28,073±2,048	4,090±322	3,290±168

[a]Cultured for 7 days.
[b]Mean ± SEM in three experiments.

Table 2. Immunoregulatory autoreactive (L3T4$^+$, Lyt$^-$, Ia reactive) T cell hybridomas developed and under study

			Selected Cloned Hybridomas to be Studied
Uncloned	1) PPTh(B*) (CF-4) 2) PPTh(B*) (CF-13) 3) PPTh(B*) (CF-14) 4) SPNTh(B*) (CF-4) 5) SPNTh(B*) (CF-5) 6) SPNTh(B*) (CF-14)		
Cloned	1)PPTh(B*) (CF-13)	15 clones/192 wells (0.5 cell/well)	E-7(BCGF); D-1(BCGF); A-9(BSWFα + BCDF, IL-2); A-7(BSWFγ+ BCDF); B-8(BSWFγ+ BCDF); B-2(BSWFγ+ BCDF); D-8(BSWFγ+ BCDF)
	2)PPTh(B*) (CF-14)	7 clones/96 wells (0.5 cell/well)	F-7(BSWFα+ BCDF)
	3)SPNTh(B*) (CF-4)	5 clones/144 wells (0.5 cell/well)	C-6(BSWF γ+ BCDF)
	4)SPNTh(B*) (CF-5)	10 clones/192 wells (0.5 cell/well)	C-4(BCGF);E-12(BCAF ± ;BSWFα+ BCDF,IL-2 ±); G-12(BSWF γ+ BCDF)
	5)SPNTh(B*) (CF-14)	11 clones/192 wells (0.5 cell/well)	A-7(BSWF γ+ BCDF);B-4(BCDF μ?)

PP, Peyer's Patch-derived; SPN, Spleen-derived

of sIgM → sIgA and the latter (SPN) that of sIgM → sIgG on B cells (Tables 3 and 4). In addition, the supernatants also had a BCDF activity (Table 4).

Finally, the development of PP-derived sIgM-bearing HD and LD B cells was examined <u>in vitro</u>, using Amicon ultrafiltrates (PM10) (x8) of three selected cloned AUT T cell hybridoma supernatants. CF-13 PP Th (B*) E-7, which contained BCGF, and both CF-14PP Th (B*) F-7 and CF-5 SPN Th (B*) E-12, which contained tentative BSWF alpha and BCDF, presented little augmentation of each class-specific Ig production by both sIgM-bearing HD and LD B cells (data not shown). In the presence of a suboptimal dose of LPS (0.2 μg/ml) and the above T cell hybridoma secretions each class-specific Ig synthesis and secretion by LD B cells was considerably altered (Fig. 3). A concentrated CF-13 PP Th (B*) E-7 supernatant increased the production of IgM and IgG in moderate amounts (2.6 and 5 times as much as LPS alone, respectively), while IgA production was also enhanced, but only to a minor extent. In contrast, both CF-14 PP Th (B*) F-7 and CF-5 SPN Th(B*) E-12 supernatants enhanced to a rather marked extent all class-specific Ig, in particular IgA, exceeding the other two Ig isotypes. The results suggest that CF-14 PP Th (B*) F-7 and CF-5 SPN Th (B*) E-12

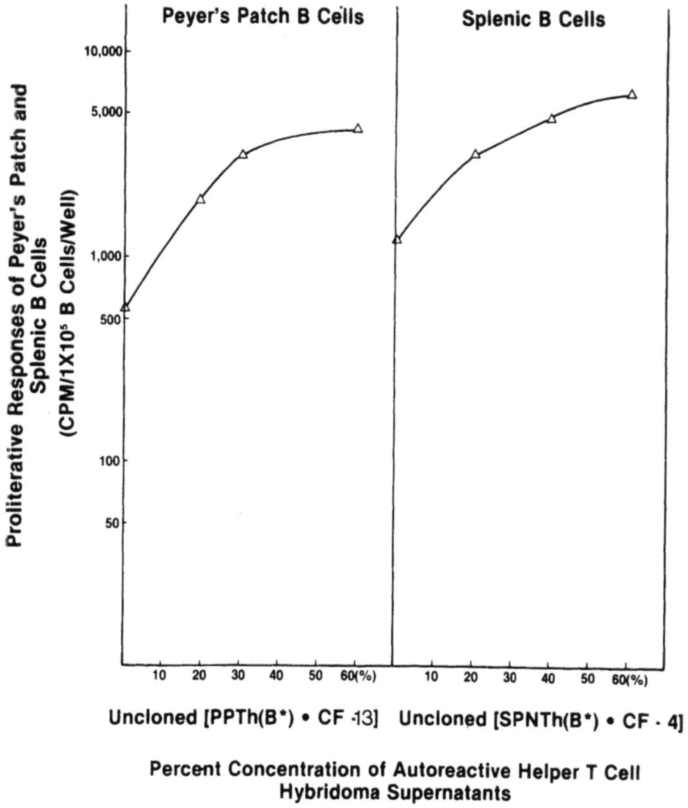

Figure 1. BCGF activity of two uncloned hybridoma supernatants from PP and SPN.

hybridoma supernatants contain at least BSWF alpha and BCDF. This study alone does not exclude an additional possibility of BSWF gamma in these hybridoma supernatants. Further studies were conducted to investigate the effect of concentrated CF-14 PP Th (B*) F-7 and CF-5 SPN Th (B*) E-12 hybridoma supernatants on the subsequent development of sIgM-bearing LD B cells in the presence of a concentrated CF-13 PP Th (B*) E-7 derived supernatant (Fig. 4). The former two supernatants (F-7 and E-12) indeed had BSWF alpha and BCDF, inducing marked augmentation of IgA production, but not IgG production. To determine BCGF activity in these three supernatants, proliferative reactivities of PP derived HD B cells were tested in the presence of a B cell activator, dextran sulfate (40 μg/ml) or anti-sIgM Ab (5 μg/ml) and the serial concentrations of the supernatants. Only one of these supernatants, CF-13 PP Th (B*) E-7 hybridoma supernatant, possessed the BCGF activity. These results clearly indicate that the AUT T cell indeed regulates B cell development in PP, and these regulatory mechanisms are mediated by a variety of BSF produced by the AUT T cell, as seen in non-GALT (3). The T-B interaction, thus, appears to be a B cell receptor-mediated interaction between the AUT T and B cell populations in GALT. It is also suggested that the functions presented here by the

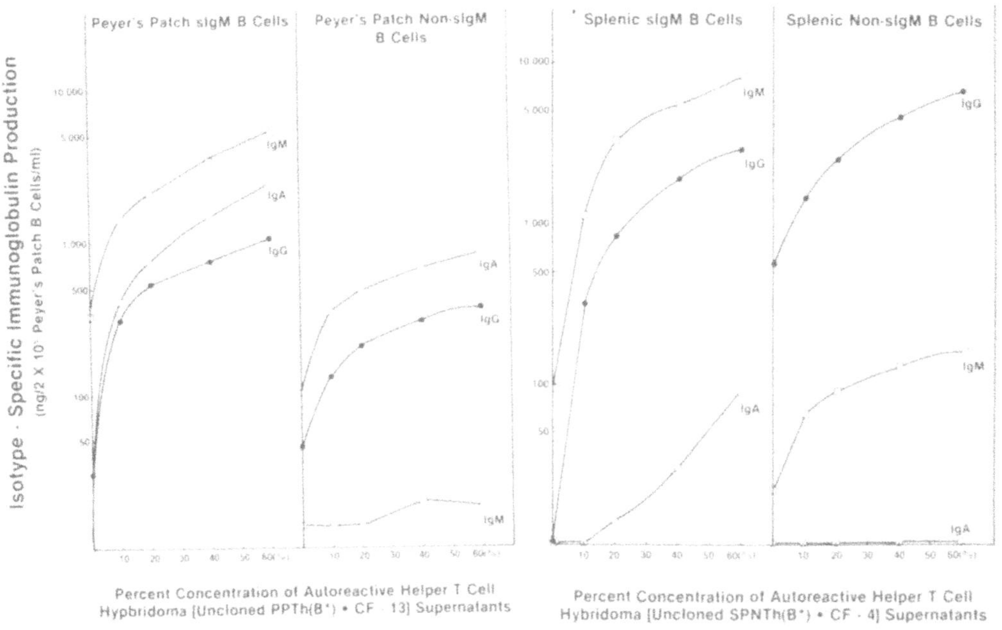

Figure 2. BSWF and BCDF activities of two uncloned hybridoma supernatants from PP and SPN.

AUT T cell is an important feature of the B cell immunoregulatory network, including T cell-directed Ig heavy chain switching processes.

CONCLUSIONS

The PP AUT T cell possesses B cell stimulatory functions regulating B cell development in the PP microenvironment by producing a variety of BSF and its cofactors. These factors include BCAF (tentative), BCGF, BSWF (tentative) and BCDF, as well as IL-2. Thus, the B cell immunoregulatory activity of the AUT T cell in PP is mediated by their BSF lymphokines.

Table 3. Effect of cloned autoreactive L3T4$^+$, Lyt-1$^+$, Lyt-2$^-$ T cell hybridoma supernatants on heavy chain switching of sIgM B cells, determined by isotype specific surface immunofluorescence

sIgM B cells pretreated with anti-IgM[a]	Percent distribution of post-treated isotype-specific Peyer's patch B cells			Percent distribution of post-treated isotype-specific Splenic B cells		
	IgM	IgG	IgA	IgM	IgG	IgA
Medium alone	96-98	0-1	0-2	95-98	0-3	0-1
+CF-13 PPTh(B*)A- 9SUP (20%)	67-72	2-5	25-27	65-71	1-2	24-28
+CF-4SPNTh(B*)C-6SUP(20%)	68-75	20-26	0-1	60-75	21-25	0-1

[a]sIgM B cells, pretreated with 20 μg/ml anti-IgM for 6 hours, prior to exposure to the hybridoma supernatants; PP, Peyer's patches; SPN, spleen.

Table 4. Effect of supernatants from Peyer's patch and spleen-derived cloned autoreactive L3T4$^+$, Lyt-1$^+$, Lyt-2$^-$ T cell hybridoma cells [PP Th (B*) CF-13-A9; SPN Th (B*) CF-4-C6] on class specific immunoglobulin production by Peyer's patch sIgM B cells

Culture condition[a]	Ig Synthesis (ng/ml)		
	IgM	IgG	IgA
PP-derived sIgM B cells ($5x10^4$/well)	220±16[b]	36±9	17±4
+ PP Th (B*) (CF-13-A9) (20%)	288±42	132±19	435±58
+ SPN Th (B*) (CF-4-C6) (20%)	323±39	477±57	12±2
+ LPS (20 μg/ml)	52330±5860	25157±3366	32±5

[a]Cultures of 7 days.
[b]Mean ± SEM in three experiments.

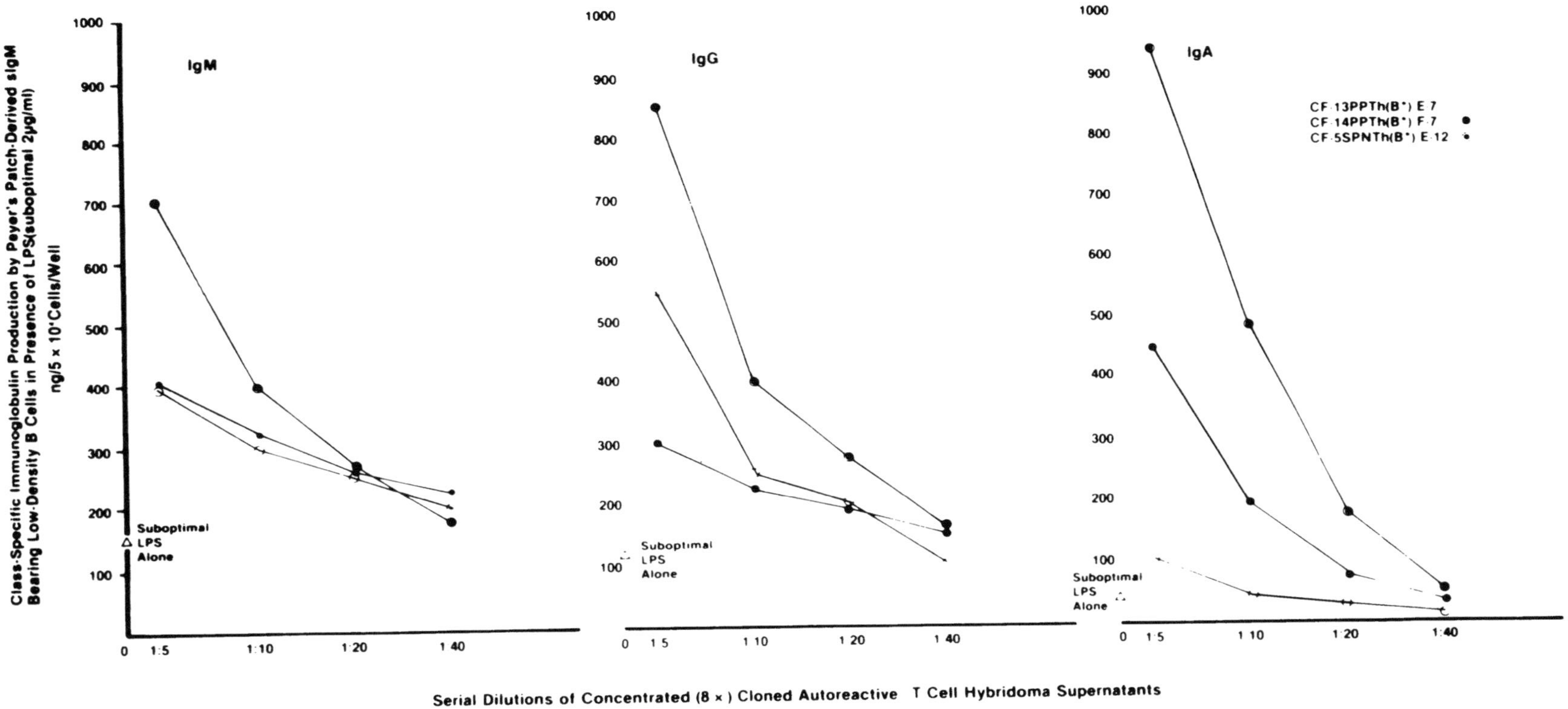

Figure 3. Effect of three cloned hybridoma supernatants on Ig production by PP-derived LD B cells in the presence of suboptimal LPS (0.2 μg/ml).

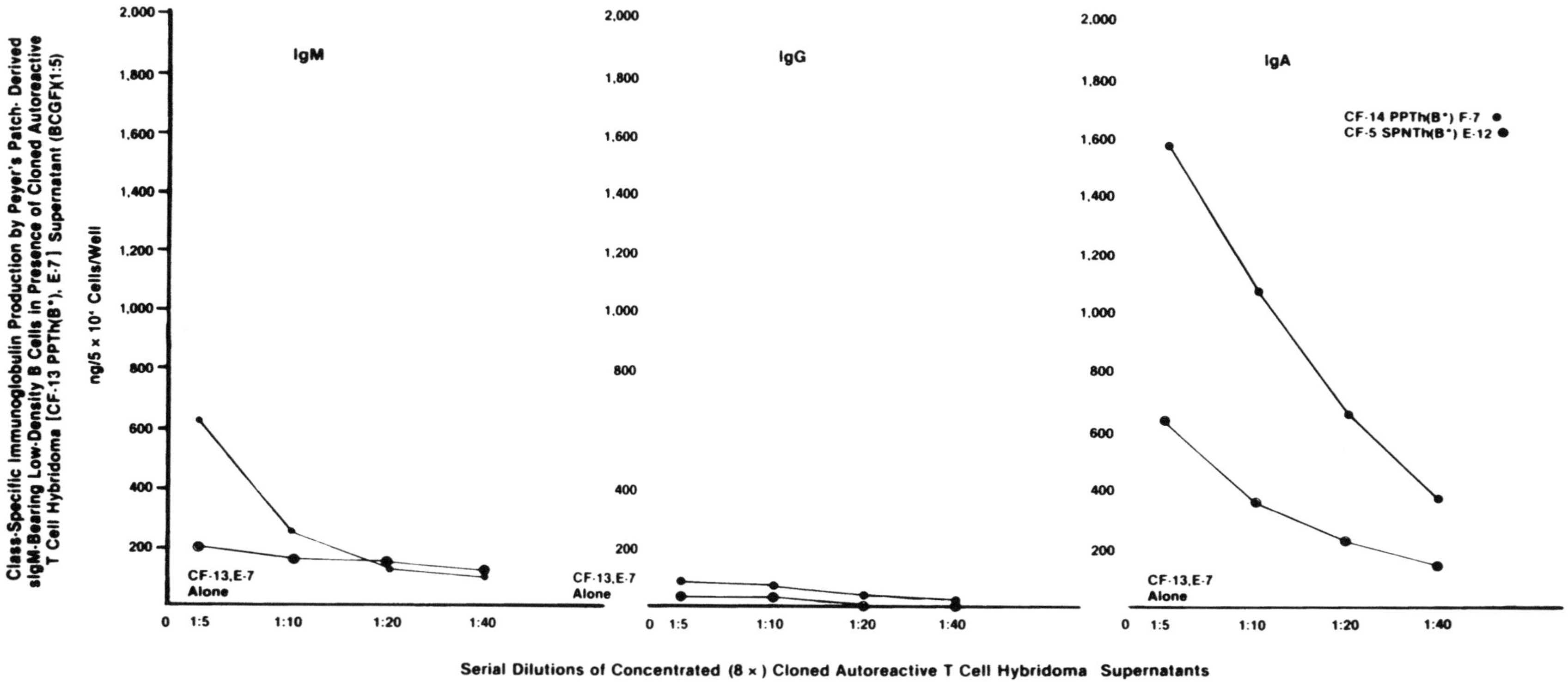

Figure 4. Effect of two cloned hybridoma supernatants on Ig production by PP-derived sIgM LD B cells in the presence of a BCGF-containing cloned hybridoma supernatant.

ACKNOWLEDGEMENTS

The authors wish to thank Ms. Ida Giannantonio for assistance in the preparation of this manuscript.

REFERENCES

1. Craig, S.W. and Cebra, J.J., J. Exp. Med. 134, 188, 1971.
2. Bienenstock, J., Befus, D, McDermott, M., Mirski, S. and Rosenthal, K., Federation Proceedings 12, 3213, 1984.
3. Howard, M., Nakahishi, K. and Paul, I.W., Immunol. Rev. 78, 185, 1984.
4. Isakson, P.C., Pure, E., Vitetta, E.S. and Krammer, P.H., J. Exp. Med. 158, 735, 1982.
5. Kawanishi, H., Saltzman, L.E. and Strober, W., J. Exp. Med. 157, 433, 1983.
6. Clayberger, C., Dekruyff, R.H. and Cantor, H., J. Immunol. 134, 691, 1985.
7. Weksler, M.E., Moody, C.E., Jr. and Kozak, R.W., Adv. Immunol. 31, 271, 1980.
8. Finnegan, A., Needleman, B. and Hodes, R.J., J. Immunol. 133, 78, 1984.
9. Kawanishi, H., Ozato, K. and Strober, W., J. Immunol. 134, 3586, 1985.
10. Kawanishi, H. and Ihle, J.N., Scand. J. Immunol. (in press).
11. Kawanishi, H. and Kieley, J., Gastroenterology 88, 1441 (Abstract), 1985.
12. Kawanishi, H., Saltzman, L.E. and Strober, W., J. Exp. Med. 158, 649, 1983.

T CELL CLONES THAT HELP IgA RESPONSES

J.M. Phillips-Quagliata and A.A. Maghazachi

Department of Pathology and Kaplan Cancer Center
New York University Medical Center
New York, New York USA

INTRODUCTION

The predominance of IgA in mucosal secretions contrasting with that of IgG in serum, is commonly thought to reflect the unique life history of lamina propria IgA plasma cell precursors in the mucosa-associated lymphoid tissue (MALT), especially the gut-associated lymphoid tissue (GALT). GALT lymphoid nodules seem to provide a milieu in which commitment of B cells to IgA production is especially favored. While many aspects of this milieu could theoretically contribute to promoting IgA at the expense of other isotypes, one of the more attractive hypotheses is that GALT lymphoid nodules contain higher numbers, relative to other lymphoid organs, of T cells capable of producing factors necessary for switching, proliferation, or differentiation of IgA B cells.

Work with T cell clones and hybridomas has demonstrated the existence of T cells that help the appearance of surface IgA (sIgA) on sIgA-negative B cells (1-3), that help downstream switching of B cells to IgG and IgA (4), and that help the differentiation of post-switch, IgA-committed B cells (5-8). There is, however, rather little proof that such T cells are more prevalent in GALT than elsewhere. Support for the idea that they are, comes from observations that (a) concanavalin A (Con A)-activated Peyer's patch (PP) T cells induce B cells cultured with lipopolysaccharide (LPS) to yield larger amounts of IgA relative to the other isotypes than do similarly activated T cells originating in spleen or other lymphoid organs (9); (b) supernatants of Con A-activated PP cells support generation of higher IgA:IgG plaque-forming cell (PFC) ratios from hapten-primed splenic B cells cultured with haptenated sheep red blood cells (SRBC) than do supernatants of similarly activated T cells from other sources (10); (c) antigen-reactive PP cell populations responding to their homologous antigen provide more bystander support for generation of IgA PFC to other antigens than do such T cells from other lymphoid tissues (10). Evidence against the idea that T cells especially capable of helping IgA responses are more abundant in GALT than elsewhere is provided by direct comparisons of the helper activity of SRBC-specific T cell populations from mesenteric lymph nodes (MN) and peripheral lymph nodes (PN) and PP. These do not differ in the amount of help they provide for IgA relative to that for other isotypes (10).

It is well known that T helper clones propagated from PN cell populations often support high IgA responses (12-14), but the frequency with which clones capable of helping IgA can be generated from this or other sources as compared to GALT has not been examined. In this paper we describe two sets of T cell clones propagated from PP and other lymphoid organs. One set was established from keyhole limpet hemocyanin (KLH) - primed T cell populations and was assessed in cognate interaction with 2,4,6 trinitrophenyl (TNP)-primed splenic B cells in the presence of TNP-KLH. The other was established from Con A-activated T cell populations and the clone supernatants were assessed for their ability to support high IgA responses by TNP-primed B cells in the presence of TNP-SRBC. We show here the frequency with which clones capable of helping high IgA responses can be propagated from cultures of the various organs and we present data illustrating the behaviour of some of the clones in greater detail.

MATERIALS AND METHODS

Medium

The basic medium used for growth of T cell clones and in the assay systems was RPMI-1640 supplemented with 15 mM HEPES, 100 U/ml penicillin, 100 μg/ml streptomycin, 0.5% Fungizone, 2 mM L-glutamine, 1% non-essential amino acids, and 1% sodium pyruvate (all from GIBCO, Grand Island, NY), 5×10^{-5} M 2-Mercaptoethanol (Fisher, Springfield, NJ) and 10% CLEX (Calf Clot Extract, Dextran Products, Ltd., Ontario, Canada). This latter product was superior to fetal calf serum in that backgrounds were generally lower.

Preparation and maintenance of T cell clones

All the clones were prepared from BALB/c mice (Taconic, Inc., Germantown, NY).

KLH clones. Mice were immunized with 100 μg KLH (Calbiochem, La Jolla, CA) in complete Freund's adjuvnt H37Ra (Difco, Detroit, MI) subcutaneously to prime the PN and intraperitoneally (i.p.) to prime the spleen, MN and PP. The response in the latter two sites was then boosted by intraduodenal injection (15) of 400 μg KLH in saline. Mononuclear cell suspensions, prepared from PN 1 week after priming, from spleen 3-4 weeks after priming (16), and from MN and PP 1-2 days after boosting, were enriched for T cells on nylon wool columns (17) and depleted of suppressor cells with anti-Lyt 2.2 antibody plus complement as previously described (10). They were cultured at 1×10^6 per ml in 24 well plates with 50 μg/ml KLH in the presence of 5×10^5 anti-Thy 1.2 plus C-treated, irradiated, syngeneic spleen cells, as a source of antigen-presenting cells (APC), and 20% conditioned medium from MLA 144 cells (a gift of Dr. Harvey Rabin) as a source of Interleukin 2 (IL-2). The medium was changed every 3 days and the APC every week. After 3 weeks the cells were cloned at limiting dilution from the bulk cultures in 96 well plates in the presence of antigen, APC and IL-2. Cells from wells showing good growth 3 to 4 weeks later were then transferred into 24 well plates and culture continued as above. The lines described here were isolated on plates yielding only 40% positive wells after seeding at one cell per well. There is, thus, a high probability that the lines are clonal.

Con A clones. These were propagated from normal PN, MN, PP and spleen T cells, prepared and cultured in the same way as described for KLH clones, except that 5 μg Con A was substituted for the KLH in the initial bulk cultures and this was reduced to 0.5 μg Con A in the limiting dilution cultures from which the clones were established. The lines described here were isolated from plates starting at one cell per well at which concentration only 35 to 40% of the wells were positive for growth. There is, therefore, a high probability that the lines are clonal.

Before assay of cloned cells of either type, they were first incubated in medium without KLH or Con A and without IL-2 for 2 hours. They were then washed four times with 40 ml warm medium to prevent antigen, Con A or IL-2 carry over.

Preparation of Con A supernatants

(a) Polyclonal Con A supernatant was prepared from BALB/c or CAF_1 spleen cells by the method previously described (10). This involved removing unbound Con A from the cells after 2 hours and then continuing the culture for a further 24 hours at which time the supernatants were removed, centrifuged, brought to 50 mM with methyl-α-D-mannoside (to block any residual Con A), filtered and stored at -20°C.

(b) Supernatants of T cell clones were prepared by incubating the extensively washed cells at 1×10^5/ml in the presence of 5×10^5/ml syngeneic, irradiated APC and either 5 or 0.5 μg/ml Con A. At the higher dose, supernatants had their optimal effect if collected up to 3 days after the start of the cultures; at the lower dose, supernatants were optimal if collected 7 days after the start of the culture. The cells were not washed free of Con A which was simply blocked by addition of methyl-α-D-mannoside to 50 mM as described above.

(c) Control Con A supernatants were prepared from irradiated APC stimulated with 5 μg/ml Con A for 3 days. They were also made 50 mM in methyl-α-D-mannoside.

B plus accessory cells: priming and preparation

Mice were immunized i.p. with 100 μg TNP-KLH absorbed to 2 mg aluminum hydroxide and 2×10^9 heat-killed *B. pertussis* organisms and boosted i.p. 4 to 6 weeks later with 50 μg TNP-KLH in saline. After a further 4 to 10 weeks their spleens were used as a source of B plus accessory cells. These were prepared from single cell suspensions of the immune spleens by depleting T cells with a cocktail of anti-Lyt 2.2 and anti-Thy 1.2 antibodies plus C. The effectiveness of T cell depletion from the preparations was demonstrated both by their minimal proliferative response to Con A and their failure to secrete antibody in culture in response to TNP-KLH. BALB/c B cells were used to assess the activity of the KLH clones and CAF_1 B cells to assess the activity of the Con A supernatants.

DNA-synthesis assays

(a) Proliferation of T cell clones in the presence of antigen or Con A and syngeneic or allogeneic APC was assessed by culturing 1×10^4 T cells with 5×10^5 irradiated APC and/or various concentrations of antigen in

0.2 ml of medium in flat-bottomed microwells for 2 days after which 1 µCi ^{3}H-thymidine (^{3}HT) was added. Culture was continued for a further 2 days after which the cultures were harvested and incorporation of the isotype into DNA was measured by liquid scintillation counting (18).

(b) Proliferation of B cells in the presence of T cell clones or their supernatants was assessed by culturing 1 x 10^{5} B plus accessory cells with graded numbers of irradiated (2000 rads) cloned T cells and various concentrations of antigen as above for 2 days, then adding 1 µCi ^{3}HT and measuring incorporation 18 hours later.

MiniMarbrook cultures

The ability of T cell clones or their supernatants to help splenic B cells generate PFC was assessed by culturing 3 x 10^{6} primed B plus accessory cells with varying numbers of the T cells and 1 µg TNP-KLH or various volumes of Con A supernatant and 1 x 10^{7} TNP-SRBC in MiniMarbrook chambers (19) in a total volume of 1 ml including 0.3 ml of nutrient cocktail (20). Each chamber was placed in 10 ml medium in a 60 mm tissue culture dish and the cultures were rocked at 37°C in 10% CO_2, 8% O_2 and 82% N_2 for 4 days. The number and isotype of anti-TNP PFC were then assayed. When optimal T cell or supernatant concentrations had been established, the effect of varying the antigen concentration was examined.

Plaque assay

IgM, IgG and IgA anti-TNP PFC were enumerated by a slide modification of the hemolytic plaque assay (21) using guinea pig C and TNP-horse red blood cells as indicators. IgA and IgG PFC were developed with rabbit specific anti-α and anti-γ chain antisera incorporated together with goat anti-µ chain antiserum (to inhibit IgM PFC) into the agarose.

Fcα Receptors (FcαR)

FcαR were assessed by the rosette method (22) using TNP-coupled ox red blood cells and a sub-agglutinating concentration of MOPC-315, an IgA α myeloma protein with anti-TNP activity. BALB/c normal mesenteric lymph node cells served as positive controls.

RESULTS

Help for IgA PFC was initially assayed in two kinds of cultures; (a) cultures permitting cognate interaction between primed splenic B cells and 31 KLH-propagated T cell clones in the presence of TNP-KLH; (b) cultures in which the primed B cells reacted to T cell replacing factors (TRF) (23-25) contained in the supernatants of 64 Con A propagated and activated clones in the presence of TNP-SRBC. Because some of the clones might conceivably produce an IgA switch factor, yet not support generation of PFC, most of the clones or their supernatants were tested both alone and in concert with polyclonal splenic Con A supernatant at a concentration capable of supporting modest numbers of PFC of all three major isotypes in the presence of TNP-SRBC. All our clones proved either active or inactive in terms of helping PFC generation irrespective of the presence of this supernatant, i.e., we did not see augmentation of IgA responses by clones that could not, by themselves, support PFC generation (data not shown).

T cells isolated from spleen and PP yield approximately the same incidences of clones capable of helping IgA (Table 1). Several clones helped IgM only or IgG only and one helped IgA only but was lost and could not be further studied. The majority of clones helped all three isotypes but to varying degrees. The results indicate that help for the different isotypes is influenced by discrete factors, not all of which are produced by all the clones.

Table 1. Help for IgM, IgG and IgA PFC provided by KLH- and Con A-propagated T cell clones

	KLH clone cells			Con A clone supernatants			
	Spleen	MN	PP	Spleen	PN	MN	PP
Total clones examined	7	4	20	8	8	5	43
No help for any isotype	3	1	2	4	3	2	27
Help for IgM + IgG + IgA	1	1	8	4	3	0	12
Help for IgM + IgG	0	1	3	0	1	0	0
Help for IgM + IgA	1	0	2	0	0	0	0
Help for IgG + IgA	0	1	0	0	0	0	1
Help for IgM only	1	0	1	0	1	3	3
Help for IgG only	1	0	3	0	0	0	0
Help for IgA only	0	0	1	0	0	0	0
Help for IgA/all +ve	2/4	2/3	11/18	4/4	3/5	0/3	13/16

Four PP-derived KLH-propagated clones (8.46, 8.48, 8.77 and 8.78), 2 spleen-derived Con A-propagated clones (4.52 and 4.65), and 2 PP-derived Con A-propagated clones (3.60 and 3.116) were selected for further study. All 4 KLH-propagated clones and 3 of the 4 Con A clones helped all isotypes with high IgA; the fourth Con A-propagated clone (3.60) helped IgG and IgA without IgM (Tables 2 and 3).

The ability of the cloned T cells or their supernatant to support B cell proliferation was next assessed. In pilot studies done at 100 μg KLH/ml, the optimal numbers of KLH-propagated irradiated T cells for a standard number of B cells was individually determined for each clone. This number of irradiated T cells of each clone was then tested on both primed and unprimed B cells in the presence of tenfold dilutions of KLH and TNP-KLH ranging from 100 μg/ml down to 0.001 μg/ml. The data obtained at the 100 μg and 0.01 μg/ml antigen concentrations with primed B cells are shown in Table 4.

Table 2. Anti-TNP PFC responses generated by 3 x 10^6 primed B cells in the presence of KLH-propagated cloned T cells and 1 μg/ml TNP-KLH

B cells	TNP-KLH	T Cell Clone	PFC/Culture[a]		
			IgM	IgG	IgA
+	-	-	18 ± 13	3 ± 2	2 ± 1
+	+	-	32 ± 15	49 ± 15	48 ± 14
-	+	+	0	0	0
+	+	8.46[b]	236 ± 82	316 ± 70	570 ± 111
+	+	8.78	445 ± 128	263 ± 8	423 ± 38
+	+	8.48	260 ± 66	819 ± 349	735 ± 281
+	+	8.77	687 ± 216	502 ± 210	688 ± 282

[a]Mean ± SE in 3-7 experiments with each clone.

[b]Each clone was tested at both 1 x 10^5 and 2.5 x 10^5 per culture. Data obtained with T cell numbers yielding the higher number of plaques are shown (2.5 x 10^5 cells of clones 8.46, 8.78 and 8.48; 1 x 10^5 cells of clone 8.77).

Table 3. Anti-TNP PFC responses generated by 3 x 10^6 primed B cells in the presence of 0.3 ml Con A supernatant from selected Con A-propagated cloned T cells and 1 x 10^7 TNP-SRBC

Source of Con A Sup	TNP-SRBC	PFC per culture IgM	IgG	IgA
0 (B cells alone)	-	68 ± 34[a]	99 ± 26	67 ± 19
0 (B cells alone)	+	85 ± 16	60 ± 12	17 ± 9
Spleen cells	+	724 ± 175	679 ± 228	519 ± 162
Spleen clone 4.52	+	1073[b]	1202	2897
Spleen clone 4.65	+	286	282	863
PP clone 3.60	+	73	258	655
PP clone 3.116	+	219	476	305

[a]Mean ± SE in the several screening experiments done with these and other clones.

[b]Geometric mean PFC in individual experiments.

The ability of the cloned T cells to proliferate in the absence of exogenous IL-2 was next assessed. Two of the KLH-propagated clones, 8.46 and 8.78, proved to be KLH specific and probably MHC-restricted in that they required the presence of both KLH and syngeneic BALB/c APC for proliferation. 8.78 could also proliferate in response to BALB.K APC alone, but not to BALB.B APC alone. The other two KLH-propagated clones, 8.48 and 8.77, and all four Con A propagated clones were autoreactive; they proliferated in the presence of BALB/c APC but not in their absence and not when BALB.B or BALB.K APC were substituted for the BALB/c APC. Addition of KLH or Con A (as appropriate) was unnecessary.

The two KLH-specific clones, 8.46 and 8.78, required the presence of KLH or TNP-KLH to make B cells proliferate but proliferation of TNP-primed B cells was enhanced by TNP-KLH especially at low concentrations (Table 4). This dose effect was not seen with unprimed B cells. We tentatively interpret this result to indicate that KLH is required to activate the cloned T cells to provide growth factors to the B cells but a sub-population of the B cells only responds to them when its antigen receptors are cross-linked by an appropriate concentration of TNP-KLH. This population is not effectively represented in unprimed B cell populations. Whether mere cross-linking

Table 4. Proliferation of TNP-primed BALB/c B cells in the presence of irradiated, KLH-propagated T cell clones

T	B	KLH		TNP-KLH		No antigen
		100[a]	0.01	100	0.01	
-	+	164 ± 51	257 ± 68	406 ± 26	73 ± 10	125 ± 28
8.46	+	1523 ± 574	781 ± 349	1820 ± 367	2917 ± 164	291 ± 10
8.78	+	2947 ± 258	2214 ± 440	3026 ± 236	5163 ± 503	339 ± 79
8.48	+	2771 ± 293	2279 ± 314	3146 ± 570	2769 ± 437	2868 ± 383
8.77	+	2151 ± 395	1355 ± 245	1809 ± 280	1851 ± 114	1992 ± 383

[a]Micrograms of antigen per ml culture.

of the B cell antigen receptors in the presence of T cells activated by KLH is sufficient to make this extra population proliferate is not clear. It could be that cognate interaction between the T cells and the B cells is required.

The two autoreactive KLH-propagated clones, 8.48 and 8.77, promoted B cell proliferation in the absence of either KLH or TNP-KLH; there was no augmenting effect of B cell receptor cross-linking by low concentrations of TNP-KLH.

The proliferative response of primed and unprimed B cells to the Con A clones or their supernatants was examined both in the presence and absence of Con A or TNP-SRBC. Three of the clones, namely 4.52, 4.65 and 3.116, supported proliferation of both primed and unprimed B cells when they or their supernatants were present in the cultures. This is illustrated by the results with clone 4.65 and primed B cells shown in Table 5.

When the cloned T cells themselves were present, they required addition of Con A to induce B cell proliferation. However, when the methyl-α-D-mannoside-blocked supernatants of Con A stimulated T cell clones were present, addition of Con A was unnecessary. This suggests that Con A induces the T cells to produce a factor which then acts on the B cells. This factor is contained in the Con A induced supernatants. The responses of both primed and unprimed B cells in the presence of either the cloned T cells

Table 5. ^{3}HT incorporation by TNP-primed B cells in the presence of Con A-stimulated T cell clone 4.65 or its supernatant

Clone	Con A[a]	TNP-SRBC[b]	Supernatant[c]	CPM ^{3}HT incorporation
-	-	-	-	326 ± 123
-	+	-	-	1339 ± 20
-	-	+	-	658 ± 51
-	+	+	-	275 ± 99
-	-	LPS[d]	-	6444 ± 607
+	-	-	-	436 ± 57
+	+	-	-	15598 ± 1049
+	+	+	-	381 ± 73
+	-	+	-	123 ± 33
-	-	-	+	31774 ± 3112
-	-	+	+	1055 ± 50

[a]0.5 μg/ml Con A.
[b]5 x 10^8/ml TNP-SRBC.
[c]25% supernatant.
[d]50 μg/ml LPS.

plus Con A or their supernatants was optimal in the absence of the rather high concentration of TNP-SRBC used in these experiments. Subsequent experiments (not shown) indicated that, while 10^5 TNP-SRBC were neither enhancing nor inhibitory, increasing concentrations of TNP-SRBC were increasingly inhibitory, complete inhibition being observed at 10^9 TNP-SRBC per culture.

Overall, the results indicate that: (a) cross-linking of B cell antigen receptors is unnecessary for them to respond to the growth factors produced by these autoreactive clones, just as it is unnecessary for them to respond to the growth stimuli provided by KLH-propagated autoreactive clones; (b) TNP-SRBC interfere with the B cell response to growth factors produced by the T cells. We believe they may absorb them. The requirement for Con A to induce B cell growth factor production by the Con A propagated autoreactive clones distinguishes them from the KLH-propagated autoreactive clones.

Table 6. Anti-TNP PFC response of TNP-primed B cells in the presence of KLH-propagated T cell clones and different antigen concentrations

T	Ag	Isotype	Antigen concentration (μg/ml) 10	0.100	0.001	0
		IgM	10 ± 5	2 ± 2	0	-
-	KLH	IgG	38 ± 20	15 ± 10	0	-
		IgA	8 ± 4	0	0	-
		IgM	30 ± 15	42 ± 21	0	-
-	TNP-KLH	IgG	33 ± 23	44 ± 24	50 ± 31	-
		IgA	2 ± 1	0	0	-
		IgM	352 ± 168	264 ± 186	131 ± 66	65 ± 12
8.46	KLH	IgA	15 ± 3	0	0	0
		IgM	822 ± 193	648 ± 13	467 ± 156	-
8.46	TNP-KLH	IgA	176 ± 61	429 ± 84	782 ± 8	-
		IgM	165 ± 19	44 ± 24	2 ± 1	31 ± 10
8.78	KLH	IgG	73 ± 51	37 ± 26	0	0
		IgA	15 ± 10	2 ± 2	0	0
		IgM	423 ± 151	357 ± 222	46 ± 19	-
8.78	TNP-KLH	IgG	1016 ± 199	1058 ± 639	456 ± 202	-
		IgA	193 ± 22	681 ± 200	890 ± 40	-
		IgM	395 ± 100	153 ± 89	258 ± 164	483 ± 95
8.77	KLH	IgA	0	0	0	0
		IgM	288 ± 135	701 ± 50	158 ± 79	-
8.77	TNP-KLH	IgA	76 ± 2	582 ± 197	1098 ± 24	-

Mean PFC/culture ± SE.

PP clone 3.60 did not support B cell proliferation either in the presence or absence of Con A and/or TNP-SRBC. Thus, this clone, which does help generation of IgG and IgA PFC but not of IgM PFC (Table 3), may be able to promote downstream switching and differentiation of B cells into PFC without inducing their proliferation.

The effect of antigen on TNP-specific PFC responses of TNP-primed B cells in the presence of the cloned T cells was next examined. The results obtained with 3 of the KLH-propagated clones at widely separated antigen concentrations are shown in Table 6.

They indicate that IgM but no IgG or IgA responses are supported in the presence of KLH; for these, the presence of TNP-KLH is essential. There are marked differences, however, in the proportions of the various isotypes produced at different TNP-KLH concentrations. The IgA responses are highest at the lowest TNP-KLH concentration, at which both the IgM and IgG responses are diminished. This result is compatible with the notion that the precursors of the IgA PFC are of higher average affinity than those of the IgM and IgG. At the highest TNP-KLH concentrations, the IgA precursors may be subject to receptor blockade or some other form of tolerance induction. It is noteworthy that clone 8.77 requires the presence of TNP-KLH to help B cells make optimal PFC responses even though it helps B cells proliferate independently of the presence of either KLH or TNP-KLH (Table 4), i.e., cross-linking of the B cell receptors for antigen <u>is</u> necessary to make the B cells differentiate into IgA and (for optimal responses) IgM PFC in the presence of this auto-reactive clone.

When the supernatants of Con A propagated autoreactive clones were tested for their ability to promote PFC responses in the presence or absence of a moderate concentration of TNP-SRBC (1×10^7) having relatively little effect on the proliferative response, it was observed (Table 7), that the effect of the antigen depended on the clone. In the case of clones 4.52 and 3.60, the IgA response was much higher in the absence of TNP-SRBC, whereas in the case of 4.65, it was higher in its presence. The IgG response showed different relationships between the particular clones and the presence or absence of TNP-SRBC. The results cannot be interpreted in a simple way. They probably indicate that multiple B cell growth and differentiation factors are produced by the different clones; some of these factors can be absorbed by TNP-SRBC and some cannot; the factors may work on different B cells with different requirements for cross-linking of their antigen receptors before they will respond. The most interesting observation is the very high IgA response promoted by clone 3.60 supernatant in the absence of TNP-SRBC. Taken in conjunction with the lack of an IgM

Table 7. ^{3}HT incorporated and PFC generated in cultures of TNP-primed B cells in the presence of supernatants of Con A stimulated clones

Supernatant	TNP-SRBC[a]	CM[a]	CPM ^{3}HT Incorp.	Anti-TNP PFC/culture IgM	IgG	IgA
-	-	-	1333 ± 483	15 ± 1	42 ± 38	15 ± 7
-	+	-	835 ± 12	20 ± 5	10 ± 2	12 ± 1
-	-	+	3782 ± 739	548 ± 128	165 ± 15	103 ± 78
4.52	-	-	26185 ± 1031	1575 ± 225	4988 ± 38	2213 ± 188
4.52	+	-	33167 ± 5427	750 ± 90	1185 ± 90	975 ± 30
4.65	-	-	25558 ± 181	608 ± 128	2783 ± 8	442 ± 143
4.65	+	-	18240 ± 1674	700 ± 96	805 ± 76	706 ± 55
3.60	-	-	1981 ± 87	98 ± 8	405 ± 150	1403 ± 23
3.60	+	-	3201 ± 1063	585 ± 165	503 ± 38	210 ± 45

[a]1 x 10^7 TNP-SRBC per culture.

[b]CM is methyl-α-D-mannoside-treated conditioned medium from irradiated APC cultured with Con A for the same period as the T cell clones plus APC used in preparation of the active supernatants.

response in the presence of this clone, the results suggest that the clone may be producing IgA switch factor, along with B cell differentiation factor(s).

Thus far, we have only examined some of the surface markers on the KLH propagated clones. All four of them are Thy 1^+, Lyt 1^+, FcαR$^-$. Three of the four are also Lyt 2^-, but surprisingly, since we depleted Lyt 2^+ cells before initiating the cultures from which the clones were derived, clone 8.46 stains to some extent with anti-Lyt-2.2 antibody.

DISCUSSION

The remarkable propensity of GALT-derived B cells to produce IgA probably reflects, at least in part, the kinds of T cells to which they are exposed in GALT. In our efforts to determine whether there is a special kind of T cell help available to the B cells only in GALT, we have examined the frequency of T cell clones capable of helping IgA that appear in cultures propagated under the influence of two agents, a specific antigen, KLH and a T cell mitogen, Con A. With neither of these methods of propagation did we find in PP versus spleen a significant difference in incidence of clones capable of helping IgA. All the lymphoid tissues examined provided some clones capable of helping IgA together with one or more other isotypes. We did find (and lose) one PP clone that helped IgA only, i.e., without other isotypes. It was present at a frequency of 1/34 among all the positive PP clones examined. To establish whether or not such clones exist at similar or lower frequencies in other lymphoid tissues would clearly be a Herculean task. The other clone that appears to us of special interest as far as the IgA response is concerned, namely 3.60, is also PP-derived. This clone produces, on stimulation with Con A, a supernatant that supports generation of IgA PFC in the absence of IgM PFC. It does not support B cell proliferation and works on primed B cells in the absence of antigen. We believe it may truly be a "switch" T cell clone that also produces B cell differentiation factor(s). Since it does support some IgG PFC, it may simply promote downstream switching, or may be more specifically capable of promoting switching to IgA. We are currently trying to hybridize this clone to BW 5147 so that we can prepare sufficient quantities of its factor for analysis.

Of the eight clones examined in detail, six turned out to be autoreactive in terms of their own proliferative response. That all four of the Con A propagated clones were autoreactive is consistent with the findings of others with similar clones (23). The six autoreactive clones can be further subdivided into three sets.

Set 1 is comprised of the two KLH-propagated clones, 8.48 and 8.77. These help cells proliferate in the absence of any stimulus other than the B cells themselves and other non-T cells in the cultures. The responding B cells do not require cross-linking of their antigen receptors to proliferate and mount an IgM PFC response although they do require it to mount IgG and IgA PFC responses. We do not yet know whether T cells of set 1 secrete B cell growth and differentiation factors into the medium or supply them directly to the B cells during cell-to-cell contact in the cultures.

Set 2, comprised of the Con A-propagated T cell clones, 4.52, 4.65 and 3.116, requires activation by Con A to make it produce B cell growth factors, which can then be detected in cell-free supernatants of the activated cells. The B cells that respond by growth and IgM PFC generation do not require cross-linking of their antigen receptors by antigen. Depending on the T cell clone, this also appears to be true for IgG and/or IgA PFC generation. The growth factors are apparently absorbed or their activity is blocked by TNP-SRBC; conceivably the factors may bind to molecules expressed not only on B cells but also, fortuitously, on SRBC. We have not yet completely resolved the question whether Con A itself could be playing some role in the B cell activation by this set of clones. We routinely block Con A in the supernatants with 50 mM methyl-α-D-mannoside which should be ample, given its affinity for this glycoside (24), but there is a theoretical possibility that multivalent binding of Con A to cell surface sugars could occur even in the presence of the blocking agent. SRBC might compete more successfully for Con A against B cells than methyl-α-D-mannoside. We are at present conducting experiments to exclude participation by Con A more rigorously. We do not think that IL-2 produced by the T cell clones is solely responsible for activating the B cell populations because we have tried the IL-2 containing MLA supernatant we use to support growth of the T cell clones and it does not support PFC generation by the B cells in the presence or absence of TNP-SRBC.

Set 3, comprised of Con A propagated clone 3.60, does not support B cell growth.

It is obvious that the way in which we have chosen to select the clones accounts for the kinds we have obtained. We may well have discarded, from among the KLH-propagated clones, set 2-type clones requiring stimulation by Con A to make them help B cells make IgA. Similarly, we may have discarded, from among the Con A-propagated clones, set 1-type clones that may interact directly with the B cells and produce relatively little supernatant factor.

Not all our T cell clones help the IgA isotype to equivalent degrees. One explanation could be that they produce different amounts of IgA specific switch factors (1-3) and/or differentiation factors that act in an IgA specific way on B cells already committed to that isotype (5-7). Alternatively, they may produce different amounts of well-defined factors such as IL-2 and interferon γ that can act synergistically with other T cell derived B cell stimulatory factors in promoting B cells committed to IgA (25). Our previous observation (10) that supernatants of Con A stimulated

PP T cells provide more help for IgA responses than do similarly stimulated splenic T cells is consistent with the idea that it is the combined products of many different kinds of T cells that give an advantage to PP in terms of helping IgA. No single T cell clone is necessarily unique to PP.

An additional feature of GALT that may well contribute to the preponderance of IgA produced at that site could be the limit imposed by proteolytic degradation in the gut on the amount of antigen actually reaching the lymphoid tissues. Our data indicate that IgA responses by primed B cells are favored in the presence of extremely low antigen concentrations. Higher concentrations seem to turn off the IgA response and turn on IgM and/or IgG responses. At present, we favor the notion that the IgA precursors are to be found among the higher affinity cells in a primed B cell population.

ACKNOWLEDGEMENTS

This work was supported by a grant from the National Institutes of Health AI 20786.

REFERENCES

1. Kawanishi, H., Saltzman, L. and Strober, W., J. Immunol. 129, 475, 1982.
2. Kawanishi, H., Saltzman, L. and Strober, W., J. Exp. Med. 157, 433, 1983.
3. Kawanishi, H., Ozato, K. and Strober, W., J. Immunol. 134, 3586, 1985.
4. Mayer, L., Posnett, D.N. and Kunkel, H.G., J. Exp. Med. 161, 134, 1985.
5. Kiyono, H., McGhee, J.R., Mosteller, L.M., Eldridge, J.H., Koopman, W.J., Kearney, J.F. and Michalek, S.M., J. Exp. Med. 156, 1115, 1982.
6. Kiyono, H., Cooper, M.D., Kearney, J.F., Mosteller, L.M., Michalek, S.M., Koopman, W.J. and McGhee, J.R., J. Exp. Med. 159, 798, 1984.
7. Kiyono, H., Phillips, J.O., Colwell, D.E., Michalek, S.M., Koopman, W.J. and McGhee, J.R., J. Immunol. 133, 1087, 1984.
8. Mayer, L., Fu, S.M. and Kunkel, H.G., J. Exp. Med. 156, 1860, 1982.
9. Elson, C.O., Heck, J.A. and Strober, W., J. Exp. Med. 149, 632, 1979.

10. Arny, M., Kelly-Hatfield, P., Lamm, M.E. and Phillips-Quagliata, J.M., Cell. Immunol. 89, 95, 1984.

11. Seman, M. and Morisset, J., in Recent Advances in Mucosal Immunity, (Edited by Strober, W., Hanson, L.A. and Sell, K.W.), p. 131, Raven Press, New York, 1982.

12. Asano, Y., Shigeta, M., Fathman, C.G., Singer, A. and Hodes, R.J., J. Exp. Med. 156, 350, 1982.

13. Seman, M., Zilberfarb, V., Gougeon, M.-L. and Thezè, J., J. Immunol. 129, 217, 1982.

14. Teale, J.M., J. Immunol. 131, 2170, 1983.

15. Pierce, N.F. and Gowans, J.L., J. Exp. Med. 142, 1550, 1975.

16. Rao, A., Faas, S.J., Miller, L.J., Riback, P.S. and Cantor, H., J. Exp. Med. 158, 1243, 1983.

17. Julius, M.H., Simpson, E. and Herzenberg, L.A., Eur. J. Immunol. 3, 645, 1973.

18. Shigeta, M., Takahara, S., Knox, S.J., Ishihara, T., Vitetta, E.S. and Fathman, C.G., J. Immunol. 136, 34, 1986.

19. Maizels, R.M. and Dresser, D.W., Immunology 32, 793, 1977.

20. Mishell, R.I. and Dutton, R.W., J. Exp. Med. 126, 423, 1967.

21. Dresser, D.W., in Handbook of Experimental Immunology, Vol. 2, (Edited by Weir, D.M.), p. 28.1, Blackwell Scientific, Oxford, 1978.

22. Strober, W., Hague, N.E., Lum, L.G. and Henkart, P.A., J. Immunol. 121, 2440, 1978.

23. Kawanishi, H., Ozato, K.. and Strober, W., J. Immunol. 134, 3586, 1985.

24. Loontiens, F.G., Van Wanwe, J.P., DeGussem, R. and DeBruyne, C.K., Carbohydrate Research, 30, 51, 1973.

25. Kagnoff, M.F., Arner, L.S. and Swain, S.L., J. Immunol. 131, 2210, 1983.

ANTIGEN-SPECIFIC HELPER T CELLS IN THE INTESTINE: ORIGIN AND MIGRATION

M.L. Dunkley and A.J. Husband

Faculty of Medicine
The University of Newcastle
NSW, 2308, Australia

INTRODUCTION

IgA responses are dependent on T cell cooperation (1-3) and populations of T cells which provide IgA specific help (Thα cells) have been identified in humans (4,5) and mouse (6) and have been cloned from murine Peyer's patches (PP) (7,8). The migration and distribution of these effector cells is crucial to a successful local response to antigen. Most studies of T cell migration have been undertaken with bulk populations responding to a wide range of antigens with varying tissue distributions but results from these experiments can only reflect the sum of potential influences exerted by a large number of different factors. Some studies have used cloned T cells but the fact that some cloned cells lose surface receptors and display abberrant migratory behaviour (9) is a concern with these models.

In an attempt to overcome these deficiencies experiments have been undertaken to study the migration and distribution patterns of a defined population of antigen-specific Thα cells arising as a result of immunization of gut-associated lymphoid tissue (GALT). This paper describes the generation of antigen-specific T helper cells in GALT of rats, a convenient animal model for the study of cell migration because of the relative ease of collection of cells from the thoracic duct. Rats were immunized with keyhole limpet hemocyanin (KLH) and the distribution of antigen-specific Thα cells determined by the ability of T cells from various tissues to help DNP-primed B cells in an *in vitro* response to TNP-KLH.

MATERIALS AND METHODS

Rats

Male rats of the inbred PVG strain were used at 90-100 days of age.

Immunization

Rats were immunized with KLH (Calbiochem, Sydney, Australia) by intraperitoneal (IP), intraduodenal (ID), IP+ID, intra-Peyer's patch (IPP), IPP+ID or subcutaneous (SC) routes as previously described (10). Additional rats were immunized IP with 100 μg of DNP-conjugated bovine gamma globulin (DNP-BGG) (Calbiochem) in Freund's complete adjuvant. Spleens were removed from these rats 3 weeks later to provide a source of DNP-primed B cells as indicator cells for the helper cell assays.

Assay of helper cell activity

Single cell suspensions were prepared from Peyer's patch (PP), mesenteric lymph nodes (MLN), spleen and peripheral lymph nodes (PLN) by passing tissues through a fine stainless steel mesh into phosphate buffered (pH 7.4) saline (PBS) containing 5% heat-inactivated fetal calf serum (FCS), 100 U/ml penicillin, 100 μg/ml streptomycin and 0.25 μg/ml fungizone. Intraepithelial lymphocytes (IEL) and lamina propria lymphocytes (LPL) were prepared using the method of Lyscom and Brueton (11). Thoracic duct lymphocytes (TDL) were collected after cannulation of the duct as previously described (10).

All suspensions to be assayed for helper activity, with the exception of LPL, were enriched for T cells using nylon wool columns (12). Cell recoveries from lamina propria (LP) were too low to elute on nylon wool.

Cell suspensions were assayed for the ability to help DNP-primed B cells respond to DNP-KLH *in vitro* (Fig. 1). KLH-primed T cells and DNP-primed spleen cells were cocultured at ratios of 1:1 and 2:1 (1 x 10^6 cells per culture in 200 μl RPMI-1640 culture medium (Flow Laboratories, Sydney, Australia) containing 5% FCS, 5 x 10^{-5} M 2-mercaptoethanol, 100 U/ml penicillin, 100 μg/ml streptomycin, 0.25 μg/ml fungizone, 2 mM L-glutamine and buffered with 10 mM HEPES. Cells were cultured either with or without antigen (0.1 μg/ml DNP-KLH). Cultures were fed daily with 25 μl of a

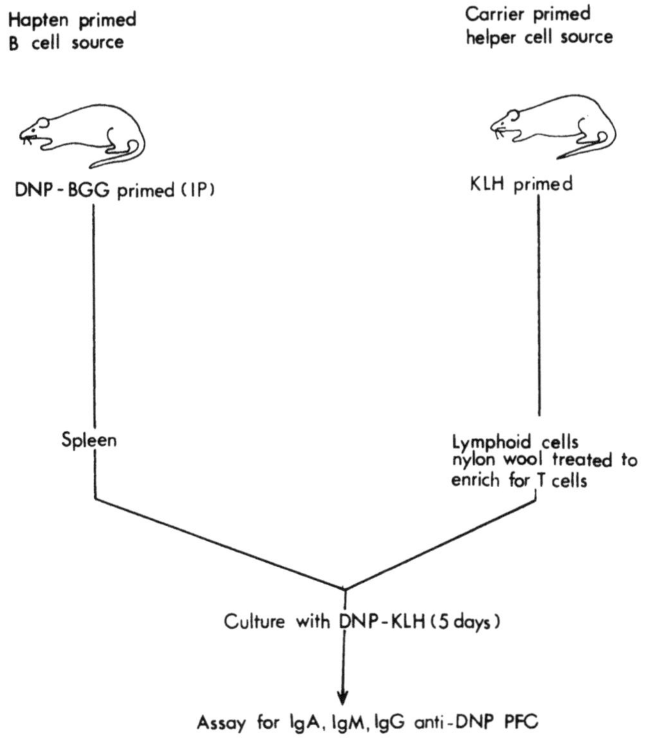

Figure 1. Antigen specific helper cell assay. Assay system to detect KLH-specific helper cell activity among T cells from various tissues of rats immunized with KLH.

nutritive cocktail (13) and after 5 d the cultured cells were washed and assayed for anti-DNP plaque forming cells (PFC) by the monolayer technique of Cunningham and Szenberg (14). Helper activity among cultured T cells was expressed as PFC/10^6 DNP-primed spleen cells cultured as described previously (10).

Previous studies verified the antigen specificity of carrier primed T cells in this assay system (10). T cells from MLN or KLH-primed rats only provide help for responses to haptenated carrier antigen of corresponding specificity when cultured with hapten-primed B cells.

RESULTS

Effect of immunization route on helper cell response

Various immunization routes were studied for their effectiveness in producing helper cells in PP, MLN and PLN. The capacity of T cells from PP and MLN to provide help for IgA anti-DNP responses in rats immunized

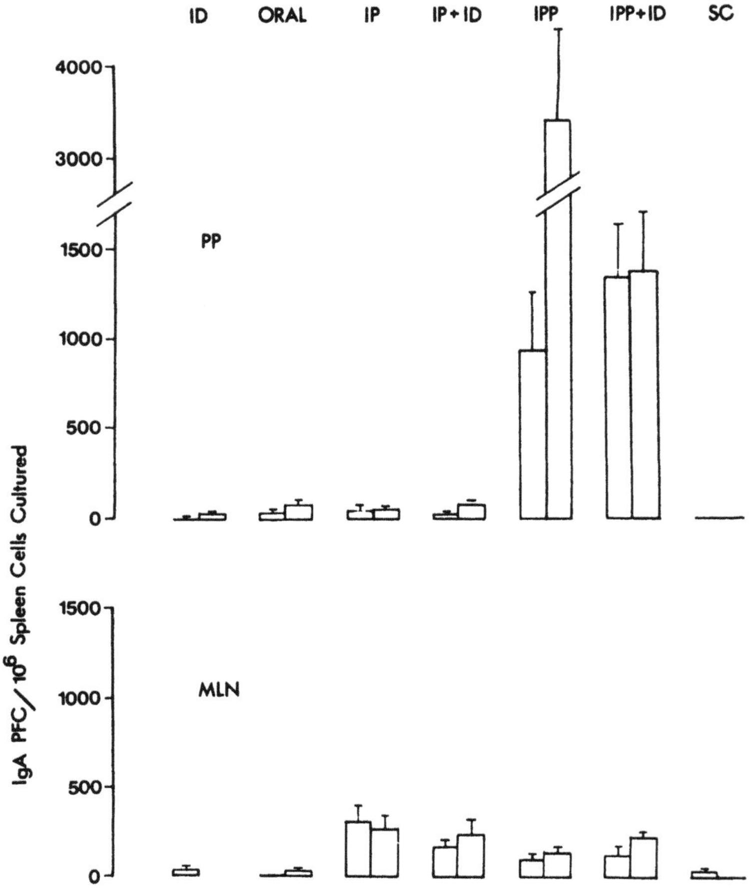

Figure 2. The effect of immunization route on the IgA helper T cell response. For each immunization route, the capacity of cells from KLH-immunized rats to help spleen cells from hapten primed rats mount an IgA-specific anti-DNP response to DNP-KLH in vitro is shown at two T cell:spleen cell ratios. The left histogram in each case is for a 1:1 ratio and the right is for a 2:1 ratio. Values are means of triplicate cultures from 4 rats (oral group), 6 rats (ID, IPP and IPP+ID groups), 8 rats (IP group) or 10 rats (IP+ID and SC groups). Vertical bars represent standard errors. (Data adapted from reference 10).

by each route is shown in Fig. 2. Oral or ID administration of KLH gave little or no response in GALT. IP and IP+ID immunizations stimulated the appearance of Thα activity in MLN but IPP immunization was the most effective route for the induction of a helper response in GALT tissues resulting in a high helper response in PP but smaller responses in MLN. An ID challenge following IPP immunization did not enhance the helper response. Systemic immunization (SC) produced no Thα response in GALT but stimulated a significant helper response in PLN (data not shown).

Phenotype of KLH-specific helper cells in PP of IPP immunized rats

The monoclonal antibody W3/25 (Sera Lab, CSL, Melbourne, Australia) has been shown to recognize helper T cells for anti-hapten antibody responses in rats (15). It was therefore of interest to determine whether the helper cells from PP of rats given IPP immunization in the present study were of the W3/25 phenotype and whether the W3/25 receptor is involved in functional help.

Initially, attempts were made to remove W3/25$^+$ cells from PP suspensions by panning (using the method described by Wysocki and Sato; 16) but this was unsuccessful due to excessive nonspecific binding of PP cells to the plates. Treatment of cell populations with W3/25 and complement was also unsuccessful probably because the antigen which W3/25 recognizes is sparsely represented on the cell membrane (17) and this monoclonal antibody does not fix complement effectively. Since addition of W3/25 antibody has been shown to inhibit in vitro MLR reactions in the rat (17) this strategy was employed to study the effects of W3/25 antibody on the help provided for anti-DNP responses in vitro when PP cells from rats primed by IPP immunization with KLH are cultured with DNP-BGG primed B cells.

The mouse ascites monoclonal antibodies W3/25 (helper/inducer) and OX8 (cytotoxic/suppressor) were added to PP helper cell cultures at a final dilution of 1/100. Figure 3 shows that W3/25 abrogated the helper response of PP cells for an IgA response to DNP whereas OX8 antibody had no effect. This confirms that KLH-specific T helper cells arising from IPP immunization are W3/25$^+$ and that the W3/25 receptor is involved in helper function.

Migration of Thα cells

Since IPP immunization produced the best helper response in GALT, this route was chosen for subsequent kinetic studies and PP, MLN, TDL and PLN were examined for helper cell activity at various times after IPP immunization (10). An IgA helper response in PP was detectable at d 2 after immunization and reached a peak at d 14, after which it again declined. A similar pattern but of lower magnitude was observed in MLN and thoracic duct although IgA-specific help was not substantial in MLN after d 3. Virtually no helper activity could be detected in PLN at any of the times studied. The kinetics of helper activity in spleen was compared with that in PP following IPP immunization (Fig. 4) and although slight helper activity was present 7 days after immunization there was no activity by d 14.

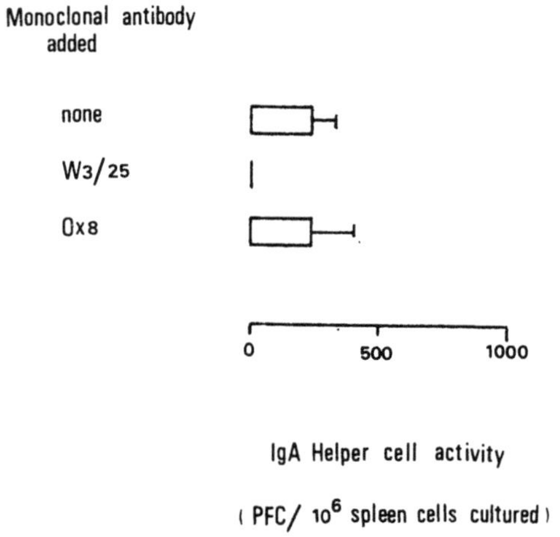

Figure 3. KLH-specific IgA helper activity among PP cells from rats 2 wk after IPP immunization. Three identical sets of cultures were established, each in triplicate, and OX8 antibody (recognizing T suppressor subset) or W3/25 antibody (recognizing T helper subset) was added to a final concentration of 1/100 of ascites and responses compared to cultures with no antibody added. Histograms represent mean IgA PFC/10^6 DNP-primed spleen cells cultured (2 experiments) and horizontal lines represent standard errors.

Thus the distribution of Thα cells following IPP immunization appears to be predominantly restricted to GALT. The presence of helper activity among TDL demonstrates that helper cells generated by GALT immunization can migrate and probably originate either in PP or MLN. To determine whether MLN contribute to the pool of Thα cells migrating via the thoracic duct the helper activity among TDL of rats from which the MLN had been removed (MLNx) several months prior to IPP immunization was examined. Helper activity among TDL or MLNx rats was essentially the same as in normal rats indicating that MLN do not contribute substantially to the migrating pool of antigen-specific helper cells and these probably originate solely from PP.

Whereas Thα cells arising in response to IPP immunization appear to originate in PP and migrate via the thoracic duct, their destination after entering the circulation is important in terms of sites of ultimate effector function. The question of whether helper cells can migrate between PP was addressed in studies in which Thα activity was compared in immunized and nonimmunized PP within individual animals. PP's in the proximal half only or distal half only were immunized and the helper activity examined in cells pooled from either proximal or distal PP. The results in Figure 5 show that substantial helper activity was detected only in

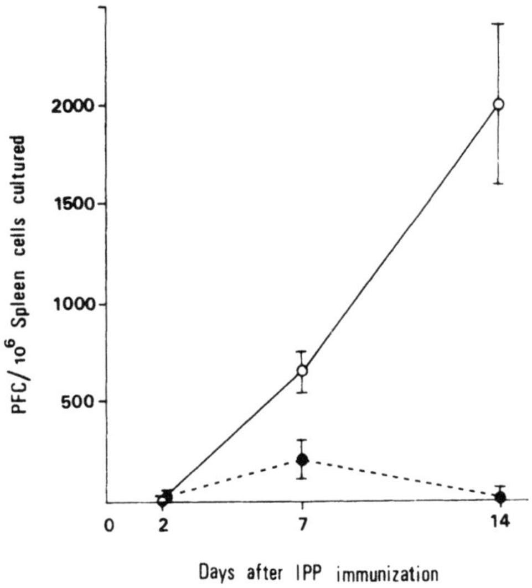

Figure 4. Kinetics of the KLH-specific IgA helper response in PP (O——O) and spleen (●----●) following IPP immunization. Values represent means of triplicate cultures from 2 rats at 14 days and from 3 rats at each other time point. Vertical bars represent standard errors.

immunized PP indicating that helper cells do not migrate from immunized to nonimmunized PP.

The migration of Thα cells to non-PP effector sites in the gut, in particular the epithelium and LP, was also studied. Preparations of IEL usually yielded approximately 15-20 x 10^6 cells per rat; however, preparation of cells from LP was more difficult and usually yielded only 1-5 x 10^6 cells. Histological analysis of sections of gut after IEL preparation demonstrated that the epithelium leaves the LP substantially intact although the possibility of some cross-contamination between IEL and LPL populations cannot be excluded. Two weeks after IPP immunization Thα activity was detected in both IEL and LPL populations (Table 1). The level of help in IEL was equivalent to that observed in PP but because of difficulties in obtaining cells from the gut LP of rats data from only 1 experiment is shown for LPL in which helper activity was low. Further experiments will be required with respect to LPL isolation and the helper activity in this part of the gut. In any case, the results indicate that antigen-specific helper cells migrate to the LP and epithelium of the gut where they may assist in local proliferation of the IgA plasma cell population.

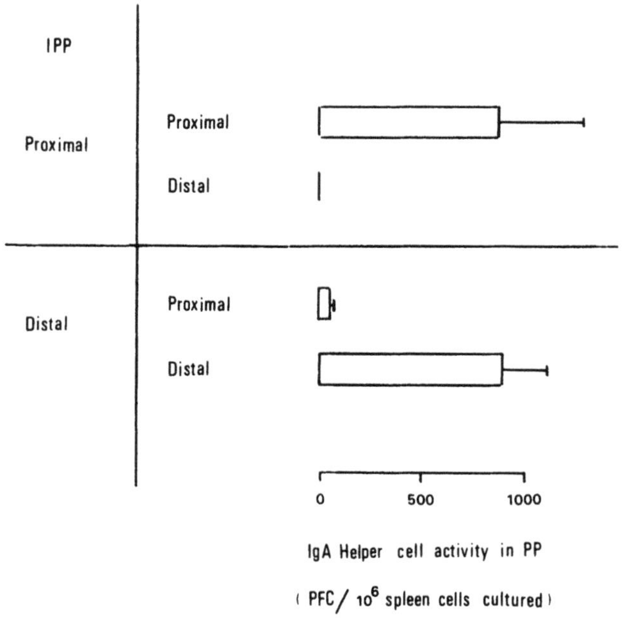

Figure 5. KLH-specific IgA helper activity among pooled proximal or distal PP cells from rats in which only the proximal half or only the distal half of the PP were immunized 2 weeks previously. Histograms represent mean IgA PFC/10^6 DNP-primed spleen cells cultured (6 experiments) and horizontal lines represent standard error.

Absence of KLH-specific suppression in the spleen after IPP immunization

There have been numerous reports of antigen-specific suppressor cells appearing in the spleen after oral immunization with soluble antigens (18-20). It was therefore considered likely that the low "net" helper activity observed in the spleen after IPP immunization (Fig. 4) may have been a reflection of the presence of suppressor cells rather than the absence of helpers. This was investigated in three ways.

In the first series of experiments OX8 antibody (1/100 ascites) was added to helper assay cultures of spleen cells. This, however, had no effect on the level of help detected in spleens from IPP immunized animals indicating that either no antigen-specific suppressor cells were present or that the OX8 receptor is not involved in suppressor function.

Secondly, spleen cells from either normal or IPP immunized rats were added to helper cultures of PP cells from IPP immunized rats. The same helper activity was observed among immunized PP cells regardless of the source of spleen cells added indicating again that antigen-specific suppressor cells were not present in spleens of immunized rats. There was,

Table 1. Helper activity in PP, gut epithelium and gut LP

	IgA PFC/10^6 spleen cells cultured
PP	2968 $\pm$ 344
IEL	2832 $\pm$ 683
LPL	267

Helper activity among PP cells, IEL and LPL from rats immunized IPP 2 wk before assay. Data represent mean of triplicate cultures from 6 rats, with the exception of IgA helper response in LPL in which data are shown from 1 rat only.

however, a reduction in helper activity compared to PP cultures with no spleen cells added but this was considered to be a crowding effect.

Thirdly, spleen cells from IPP immunized rats were panned (16) to remove $OX8^+$ cells. This would result in an increase in helper activity measured in post-panning spleen assays if $OX8^+$ cells were masking the activity of splenic helper cells. When the panned T cells were assayed for helper activity a twofold increase was observed, however, this was probably a reflection of the corresponding enrichment of $W3/25^+$ cells, as determined by flow cytometric analysis of cell aliquots after panning, and probably not due to depletion of $OX8^+$ cells.

Taken together, these observations indicate that neither helper nor suppressor cells specific for KLH appear in spleen in significant numbers following intestinal immunization with KLH by direct injection into PP.

DISCUSSION

The experiments reported here have demonstrated that antigen-specific $W3/25^+$ helper cells for IgA responses arise in PP of rats after IPP immunization with KLH. These cells appear also in MLN, thoracic duct, gut epithelium and LP. The failure of mesenteric lymphadenectomy to affect significantly the helper activity among TDL indicates that Thα cells are generated solely in PP but migrate via MLN to the thoracic duct and that the MLN are unnecessary for helper cell induction or maturation after PP immunization. The presence of helper activity among IEL and LPL suggests that Thα cells migrate, presumably via the thoracic duct and blood circulation to these effector sites. The higher Thα activity detected in IEL compared to LPL is in contrast to reports that similar numbers of $W3/25^+$ cells occur in IEL and LPL preparations (11) but that $OX8^+$ (suppressor subset) cells predominate over $W3/25^+$ (helper subset) cells in rat IEL. However, the data presented here measured "net" help and the presence of KLH-specific suppressor cells in IEL or LPL requires further investigation.

The lack of Thα activity in unimmunized PP of rats in which only half the PP received antigen suggests that Thα cells either do not migrate between PP or that antigen is essential to their retention if they do enter distant PP. The low helper activity in PLN and spleen suggests that Thα cells have a mucosally restricted distribution analogous to that described for B cells emanating from PP (21). The absence of helper activity in spleen was not due to the presence of suppressor cells and in this respect IPP immunization appears to differ from oral immunization because others have demonstrated that oral immunization results in the induction of suppressor-inducer cells in PP which migrate to the spleen to generate suppressor effector cells (18-20). The failure to generate a significant helper cell response by administration of KLH by oral or ID routes is consistent with other reports (22,23) but whether this is due to inadequate uptake of soluble antigen across the gut epithelium following lumenal presentation, insufficient concentration of antigen or stimulation of suppression is not known. The first is unlikely since in experiments with the soluble antigens ovalbumin and tetanus toxoid an ID dose of antigen was shown to elicit a strong IgA-specific B cell response in gut LP of LP primed animals (24). Antigen handling factors and the concentration and persistence of antigen in PP are probably of greater importance but in any case direct immunization of PP by subserosal injection of antigen in FCA appears not to activate the suppressor cell circuit described after oral immunization.

CONCLUSIONS

1. Immunization of PP by serosal injection of KLH in FCA generates in PP a population of antigen-specific T cells of the W3/25 phenotype which provide specific help for IgA responses (Thα cells).

2. Thα cells migrate from PP via MLN and the thoracic duct but their subsequent distribution is mucosally restricted, appearing in gut LP and epithelium but not in PLN or spleen. They do not migrate to unimmunized PP but whether they recirculate to immunized PP is not known.

3. IPP immunization with KLH in FCA does not appear to activate antigen-specific suppression in the spleen.

ACKNOWLEDGEMENTS

This work was supported by a grant from the National Health and Medical Research Council of Australia.

REFERENCES

1. Clough, J., Mims, L. and Strober, W., J. Immunol. 106, 1624, 1971.
2. Crewther, P. and Warner, N.L., Aust. J. Exp. Biol. Med. Sci. 50, 625, 1972.
3. Pritchard, H., Riddaway, J. and Micklem, H.S., Clin. Exp. Immunol. 13, 125, 1973.
4. Endoh, M., Sadai, H., Nomoto, Y., Tomino, Y. and Kaneshige, H., J. Immunol. 127, 2612, 1981.
5. McCaughan, G.W., Adams, E. and Basten, A., J. Immunol. 132, 1190, 1984.
6. Richman, L.J., Graeff, A.S., Yarchoan, R. and Strober, W., J. Immunol. 126, 2079, 1981.
7. Kawanishi, H., Saltzman, L.E. and Strober, W., J. Immunol. 129, 475, 1982.
8. Kiyono, H., Cooper, M., Kearney, J.F., Mosteller, L.M., Michalek, S.M., Koopman, W.J. and McGhee, J.R., J. Exp. Med. 159, 798, 1984.
9. Dailey, M.O., Fathman, G., Butcher, E.C., Pillemer, E. and Weissman, I., J. Immunol. 128, 2134, 1982.
10. Dunkley, M.L. and Husband, A.J., Immunology 57, 379, 1986.
11. Lyscom, N. and Brueton, M.J., Immunology 45, 775, 1982.
12. Julius, M.H., Simpson, E. and Herzenberg, L.A., Eur. J. Immunol. 3, 645, 1973.
13. Mishell, B.B. and Dutton, R.W., J. Exp. Med. 126, 423, 1967.

14. Cunningham, A.J. and Szenberg, A., Immunology 14, 599, 1968.
15. White, R.A.H., Mason, D.W., Williams, A.F., Galfre, L. and Milstein, C., J. Exp. Med. 148, 664, 1978.
16. Wysocki, L.J. and Sato, V.L., Prod. Natl. Acad. Sci. 75, 2844, 1978.
17. Webb, M., Mason, D.W. and Williams, A.F., Nature 282, 841, 1979.
18. MacDonald, T.T., Eur. J. Immunol. 12, 767, 1982.
19. Mattingly, J.A., Cell. Immunol. 86, 46, 1984.
20. Gautam, S.C. and Battisto, J.R., J. Immunol. 135, 2975, 1985.
21. Bienenstock, J. and Befus, A.D., Immunology 41, 249, 1980.
22. Arny, M., Kelly-Hatfield, P., Lamm, M.E. and Phillips-Quagliata, J.M., Cell. Immunol. 89, 95, 1984.
23. Elson, C.O. and Ealding, W., J. Immunol. 133, 2892, 1984.
24. Husband, A.J., J. Immunol. 128, 1355, 1982.

LIMITING DILUTION ANALYSIS OF FUNCTIONAL T CELLS IN THE GUT MUCOSA

T.T. MacDonald and S.B. Dillon

Department of Pediatric Gastroenterology, St. Bartholomews Hospital, London EC1A 7BE; and Department of Medicine, Duke University, Durham, North Carolina USA

INTRODUCTION

The function, nature and derivation of the lymphoid cells which are found in the gut epithelium remains controversial. In man, there is little doubt that virtually all intraepithelial lymphocytes (IEL) are of the T cell lineage because most of them are recognized by monoclonal antibodies specific for the T3 antigen complex associated with the T cell receptor (1,2). Functional data on these cells is, however, completely lacking. In rodents, the situation is much less clear because IEL have not been tested for the expression of T cell receptor related antigens and because of a body of evidence that many IEL are thymus-independent, contain granules and are Thy-1$^-$ (3-6). Indeed, we have recently shown by limiting dilution analysis that 1 in about 170 of normal mouse IEL are mast cell precursors, and that the frequency can reach as high as 1 in 60 if the mice are worm infected (7).

It is our belief that regardless of their derivation that the most important parameters to be studied in IEL are their functional capacities. In our previous work, we demonstrated for the first time that mouse IEL contain mitogen and alloantigen reactive cells (8), work which has been confirmed by others (9). More recently, we have also shown that IEL stimulated with mitogens in bulk culture produce IL-2, gamma interferon, interleukin 3 and probably granulocyte-macrophage colony stimulating factor (10). The latter 2 factors are also produced when IEL from mice recovering from a *Trichinella spiralis* infection are challenged with specific antigen *in vitro* (10). In bulk culture it is impossible to determine if the lymphokines are being secreted by many cells producing low levels or a few cells producing a lot of lymphokine. In addition, it is impossible to determine the size of the responsive population. We wish to report here our recent experiments using limiting dilution analysis to determine the numbers of IEL capable of responding to mitogen stimulation and capable of producing lymphokines.

MATERIALS AND METHODS

Animals and worm infection

Mice used were inbred BDF1 (C57BL/6 x DBA/2)F1 from Jackson Labs, Bar Harbor, Maine. Mice were infected with *Trichinella spiralis* by giving them 100 infective larvae orally by feeding tube.

Isolation of IEL

IEL were isolated as previously described by removing the small intestinal epithelium with EDTA and separating the IEL from the epithelial cells on Percoll density gradients (8). The cells were washed 3 times before any further procedure. Lyt-2^+ IEL were purified by first incubating the IEL in the undiluted supernatant of the anti-Lyt-2 hybridoma (53.6.72, ATCC) for 30 min at 4°C followed by panning on petri dishes coated with rabbit anti-rat IgG (Miles). The same procedure was used to isolate Lyt-2^+ spleen cells except that the spleen cells were first depleted of B cells by panning on anti-mouse Ig plates.

Immunofluorescence

Cells (500,000) were incubated for 30 min in the cold in either monoclonal anti-Lyt-2 (53.6.72, ATCC), monoclonal anti-IL-2 receptor (7D4, a gift from Dr. Francis Dumont), or monoclonal anti-L3T4 antibody (GK1.5, a gift from Dr. C.E. Calkins). For direct single fluorescence, the cells were washed and then incubated with a 1:50 dilution of fluorescein conjugated $F(ab')_2$ goat anti-rat IgG (Cappel) for 30 min at 4°C, washed again and examined for membrane fluorescence. For double immunofluorescence monoclonal antibody coated cells were treated next with 0.5 μg biotinylated rabbit anti-rat IgG (Vector), followed by 0.5 μg avidin-rhodamine (Becton-Dickinson). The cells were then counterstained with fluorescein conjugated anti-Lyt-2 antibody (0.5 μg, Becton-Dickinson). Fluorescence was visualized on a Zeiss Universal microscope with an epifluor 111 condenser and selective excitation and barrier filter sets for visualizing fluorescein or rhodamine conjugates. 200-500 cells per group were counted.

Cell culture

IEL were cultured in flat-bottomed microtiter wells (250,000 cells in 0.2 ml) in tissue culture medium containing 10% heat-inactivated fetal calf serum and antibiotics. The cells were stimulated with Con A (5 μg/ml), 0.5% v/v human lectin-free IL-2 (Electronucleonics, Silver Spring, MD) or a crude worm extract of Trichinella spiralis (100 μg/ml), a gift from Dr. Joan Lunney, USDA. Three days later the cell supernatants were harvested and frozen at -35°C.

Limiting dilution analysis

To determine the frequency of Con A responsive Lyt-2^+ cells, graded doses of cells in replicates of 32-48 were cultured in flat-bottomed micro-titer plates in tissue culture medium made up to contain 25% unpurified rat spleen T cell growth factor (TCGF). The TCGF contained Con A. Filler cells, T cell depleted by treatment with anti-Thy-1.2 (HO.13.4 ATCC) and complement, and irradiated (2,000 rads), were added to each well (100,000 per well). Wells were considered positive for growth if they contained clusters of proliferating lymphoblasts when examined by inverted phase contrast microscopy 14 days later.

To determine the frequency of IEL which could produce lymphokines in response to Con A, graded doses of IEL were cultured with 5 μg/ml Con A, 200,000 T cell depleted filler cells, and 0.5% human IL-2 (Electronucleonics). Eleven days later 50 μl of the supernatants were harvested from each well and frozen at -35°C.

Data from limiting dilution experiments were analysed by the chi square minimization method with a computer program written by Dr. R.A. Miller (Dept. of Pathology, Harvard University).

Lymphokine assay

Lymphokine production was measured in supernatants by their ability to support the growth of the factor dependent cell line FDC-P2. Test supernatants were added to microtiter wells and 4,000 FDC-P2 cells were added to each well. One day later, the wells were pulsed with 1 μCi tritiated thymidine and the next day the wells were harvested and incorporated radioactivity measured by liquid scintillation counting. The FDC-P2 line responds to both IL-3 and GM-CSF (10). In order to discriminate between these 2 lymphokines, supernatants were tested for their ability to support FDC-P2 proliferation in the presence of anti-IL-3 (11), a gift from Dr. J. Ihle. The human IL-2 used in this work does not support the growth of the FDC-P2 cell line.

RESULTS

As in our previous work (8), freshly isolated IEL were 50-70% Lyt-2^+ by immunofluorescence. Ten percent of the cells were L3T4^+.

The phenotype of the IEL which respond to Con A in bulk culture

To identify the IEL proliferating in response to Con A we took advantage of the fact that activated T cells express the IL-2 receptor (12) and thus we were able to detect them by double immunofluorescence using an anti-IL-2 receptor antibody and anti-Lyt-2 antibody as described in the methods. At the onset of culture no IEL showed IL-2 receptor expression. However, after 2 days in culture with Con A a substantial proportion of the cells were IL-2 receptor positive (Table 1). Interestingly, not all the cells were Lyt-2^+.

The frequency of Lyt-2^+ cells which respond to Con A

As Lyt-2^+ cells are the major cell type in the epithelium, we felt it necessary to determine the frequency of these cells which were Con A

Table 1. IL-2 receptor expression by mitogen activated IEL

	Percent Positive Cells		
	Before Culture	After culture in:-	
Surface Markers		Con A	Con A + IL-2
7D4^+, Lyt-2^+	0	38	30
7D4^+, Lyt-2^-	0	16	11

IEL were cultured at 2 x 10^5 cells per 0.2 ml with an equal number of T depleted irradiated filler cells. Two days later, cells from 10 wells were pooled and analyzed by immunofluorescence. Only large blasts were counted in the cultured cells. There were no 7D4^+ cells in the freshly isolated population or IEL cultured for 2 d in medium alone.

responsive. We have, in other studies, shown that in bulk culture IEL respond to Con A, albeit weakly. Thus, Lyt-2$^+$ cells were purified by panning which resulted in a population which was 85-95% Lyt-2$^+$. These cells were then cultured at limiting dilutions with TCGF containing Con A and the frequency of wells showing growth was determined 14 days later (Fig. 1). Using this method, it is clear that the frequency of Lyt-2$^+$ cells which respond to Con A is very low, of the order of 1 in 800 cells. This is 100 fold less than with splenic Lyt-2$^+$ cells. Immunofluorescence on cells from wells growing at limiting dilution showed that 99% of them were Lyt-2$^+$, thus confirming that it was cells from this subset which were proliferating.

Lymphokine production by mitogen and antigen activated IEL in bulk culture

Mice were infected with *Trichinella spiralis* and 21 d later their IEL were isolated and stimulated with mitogens and crude worm antigen (CWA) *in vitro*. The supernatants were harvested and tested for their ability to support the growth of the factor-dependent cell line FDC-P2 (Fig. 2). IEL from infected and control mice produced equivalent amount of factors in response to stimulation with IL-2 alone or combination of Con A and IL-2. However, only infected mice produced lymphokine in response to the CWA. Another worm antigen, an excretory/secretory product induced no lymphokine production.

Limiting dilution analysis of lymphokine secreting cells

IEL from normal or 21 d *Trichinella spiralis* infected mice were cultured at limiting dilution with Con A and IL-2. The supernatants were harvested 11 d later and individual wells tested for growth promoting activity on the FDC-P2 cell line (final dilution of the supernatant 1:4). The

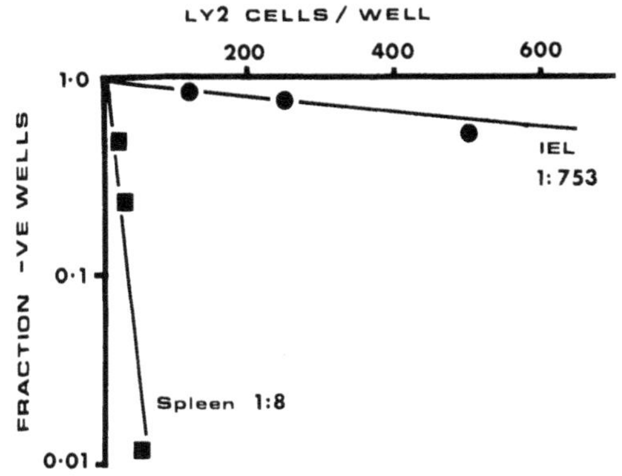

Figure 1. Limiting dilution analysis of Con A responsive Lyt-2$^+$ IEL and spleen cells.

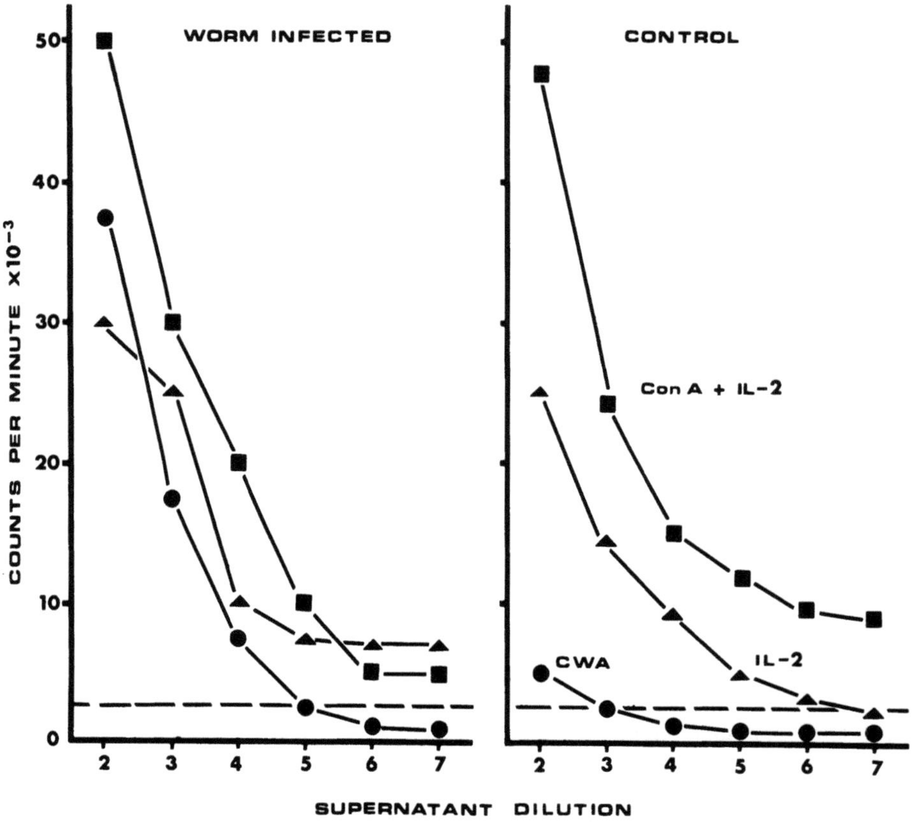

Figure 2. The ability of supernatants of IEL from worm infected mice cultured in bulk to produce FDC-P2 growth factor activity when stimulated *in vitro* with CWA or mitogen.

frequency of wells showing activity was used to determine the precursor frequency of lymphokine secreting cells in IEL. For normal mice, this was between 1:800-900 cells (Table 2). An example of the raw data used to derive these numbers is shown in Figure 3 where it can be clearly seen that this assay is sensitive enough to detect the lymphokine secreted by a single cell when the cells are plated at low numbers. Analysis of the data derived in the same way, however, from *Trichinella spiralis* infected mice was less fruitful because in both experiments the value of chi square indicated that the data did not fit that expected of single hit kinetics. In other words, the number of lymphokine secreting cells was not the only limiting factor. This could indicate regulatory cell activity in IEL from worm-infected mice.

What are the lymphokines produced by activated IEL?

The FDC-P2 cell line is a very sensitive indicator of lymphokines produced by even a single T cell, however, it does respond to both IL-3 and

Table 2. Precursor frequency of lymphokine producing cells from normal and *T. spiralis* infected mice

Expt.	Source of IEL	1/f 95% Confidence limits	$p(X^2)$	d.f.
1	Normal mice	814 (627-1161)	0.15	3
	Infected mice	1065 (814-1539)	0.001	2
2	Normal mice	868 (732-1065)	0.91	3
	Infected mice	1815 (1544-2202)	<0.001	3

1/f equals the reciprocal of the number of IEL containing 1 factor producing precursor cell. To determine 1/f, IEL were cultured at limiting dilutions with T cell depleted, irradiated splenic filler cells, 5 µg/ml Con A and 0.5% (vol/vol) human IL-2. On d 11 of culture, when proliferating cells were visible in the wells, supernatants from individual wells were tested at a 1:4 final dilution for factor activity on FDC-P2 cells. $p(X^2)$, the probability of chi-square, measures the goodness of fit to the hypothesis of a single precursor cell. This must be greater than 0.1. d.f. is the number of cell doses tested minus 1.

GM-CSF (10). To distinguish between these 2 factors, we used a specific anti-IL-3 rabbit antiserum to neutralize any IL-3 in our supernatants. Thus, the failure to neutralize FDC-P2 growth activity with anti-IL-3 indicates that the factor in the supernatant with FDC-P2 growth factor activity is probably GM-CSF. The anti-IL-3 neutralized most of the activity of a WEHI-3B supernatant which is known to contain significant levels of IL-3 (Table 3). In contrast, it had little effect on lung conditioned medium (a standard source of GM-CSF) or a mouse spleen Con A supernatant. It also failed to inhibit the activity of any of the IEL supernatants tested regardless of whether they were mitogen or antigen-induced. So that sufficient material was available for analysis the supernatants were harvested from IEL cultured in bulk. Thus, it appears that the factors produced by IEL contain GM-CSF.

DISCUSSION

Lyt-2 cells make up the majority of murine IEL. When unseparated IEL are stimulated with Con A *in vitro*, they make a weak proliferative response

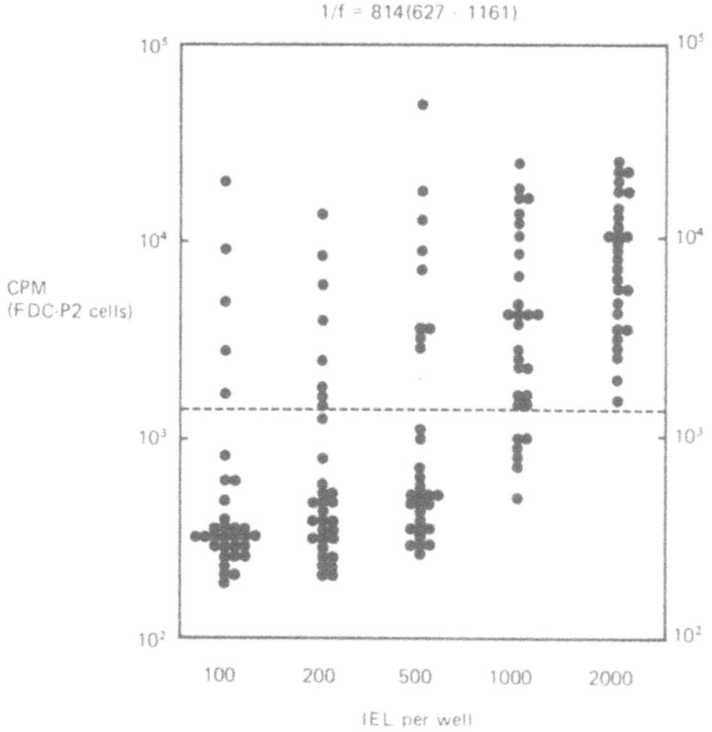

Figure 3. The ability of the supernatants from cultures of IEL stimulated with Con A at limiting dilution to support the proliferation of the FDC-P2 cell line. Each point is the amount of proliferation induced by the supernatant of a single well. Counts were considered significant if they were greater than 3 standard deviations above the proliferation of FDC-P2 cells in medium alone (-----).

(8). In this work we now directly show that some Lyt-2$^+$ IEL respond to Con A. This was demonstrated by the fact that whole Con A stimulated IEL contain large Lyt-2$^+$ positive blasts which simultaneously express the IL-2 receptor. In fact, these make up two-thirds of the IL-2 receptor bearing cells in stimulated cultures. We did not attempt to identify the phenotype of the other one-third of the activated cells. Limiting dilution analysis experiments confirmed this observation but yielded the surprising result that only 1 in 800 Lyt-2$^+$ IEL were capable of responding to Con A, 100-fold less than splenic Lyt-2$^+$ cells. This explains the weak proliferative responses of IEL to mitogens. IEL are also characterized by a unique population of cells which are Thy-1$^-$, Lyt-2$^+$ (6,13). These make up about 50% of the total IEL. Elsewhere we have shown that after mitogen stimulation most of the Lyt-2$^+$ cells which respond are Thy-1$^+$, Lyt-2$^+$ which are only

Table 3. Neutralization of FDC-P2 growth factor activity with anti-IL-3

Standards	% Inhibition	Test Supernatants	% Inhibition
WEHI-3B	70-75%	IEL (Con A + IL-2)	< 10%
Lung CM	20%	Trich IEL (Con A + IL-2)	10-30%
Spleen CM	10%	Trich IEL (CWA)	10%

Details of the supernatants are as follows: WEHI-3B, the supernatant taken after 4 d of culture of WEHI-3B cells at 250,000 per ml. Lung conditioned medium, the 7 d supernatant of teased apart lungs from mice treated previously with LPS. Spleen CM, the 48 h supernatant of mouse spleen cells cultured with 5 μg/ml Con A. The IEL supernatants were harvested 72 h after culture of the cells at 250,000 per 0.2 ml with mitogen or antigen as described in the methods. Rabbit anti-IL-3 (1 mg - 10 μg/ml) was incubated with the test supernatants for 3 h prior to testing the activity on the FDC-P2 cells. Results are expressed as the maximal percent inhibition of activity induced by the anti-IL-3 compared to the effects of normal rabbit IgG.

20% of the starting population (13). The major cell population of $Thy\text{-}1^-$, $Lyt\text{-}2^+$ cells do not appear to be mitogen responsive and thus their function remains obscure.

We and others have used LDA to identify the precursor frequency of cells in the gut epithelium. Ernst et al. (9) have recently shown that 1 in 500 IEL can develop into allogeneic cytotoxic effector cells. These cells are of the $Thy\text{-}1^+$, $Lyt\text{-}1^+$, $Lyt\text{-}2^+$ phenotype which is a minority of IEL. We have recently shown that 1 in 200-300 IEL are mast cell precursors (6).

Another major observation made in this work is on the frequency of IEL which can produce factors which promote the growth of FDC-P2 cell line. Despite the fact that this cell line responds to more than 1 lymphokine it is an excellent tool to study factor production by IEL because of it's high level of responsiveness to low levels of lymphokines. This makes it superior to some other cell lines such as the DA-1 cell line which is strictly IL-3 dependent (14) but which proliferates poorly even in large amounts of IL-3 (13). Our results indicated that only 1 in 800 IEL produce factors when stimulated with Con A. Because this frequency was so low we did not consider it worthwhile to determine the phenotype of the cells producing these factors.

When IEL from mice recovering from Trichinella spiralis infection were stimulated with crude worm antigen (CWA) or mitogens in bulk culture, lymphokines were produced. Attempts were made to determine if the frequency of mitogen inducible lymphokine secreting cells was increased in the epithelium of worm infected mice but unfortunately this could not be done, the LDA indicating that more than 1 cell type was limiting. This could be due to regulatory cell activity but this requires experimental verification. Experiments are also planned to determine the frequency of the IEL from worm infected which produce lymphokines to CWA.

The nature of the lymphokines produced by IEL was of special interest because it has long been speculated that lymphokines are involved in some enteropathies (15,16). Antigen specific IL-3 release by mucosal lymphocytes from Nippostrongylus infected mice has also been recently demonstrated (17). Cell lines with defined factor dependencies have proved very useful in the identification of specific lymphokines and so we used the cell line FDC-P2 to detect lymphokine in our test supernatants. This cell line was originally strictly IL-3 dependent (18) but we have shown that it now responds to recombinant GM-CSF (10). Thus, a specific anti-IL-3 antiserum was used to determine whether it was IL-3 or GM-CSF which was inducing the FDC-P2 cells to proliferate. To our surprise the anti-IL-3 did not neutralize the activity and so we can conclude that activated IEL probably produce GM-CSF. We have also shown elsewhere, however, that the supernatants of activated IEL contain growth factor activity for the DA-1 cell line (10) which is reportedly strictly IL-3 dependent. Thus, it is probable that IEL, like most activated T cells produce multiple lymphokines.

CONCLUSIONS

We have shown that the number of Lyt-2^+ IEL which can respond to mitogens is very low, thus explaining their low proliferative responses. The number of IEL capable of producing lymphokines in response to mitogens is also very low. IEL also produce lymphokines in response to specific antigen but the precursor frequency has not yet been established. Evidence is presented that at least one of the lymphokines IEL produce is GM-CSF.

REFERENCES

1. Selby, W.S., Janossy, G., Bofill, M. and Jewell, D.P., Clin. Exp. Immunol. 52, 219, 1983.
2. Meuer S.C., Acuto, O., Hussey, R.E., Hodgdon, J.C., Fitzgerald, K.A., Schlossman, S.F. and Reinherz, E.L., Nature 303, 808, 1983.
3. Mayrhofer, G., Blood 55, 532, 1980.
4. Mayrhofer, G. and Whately, R.J., Int. Arch. Allergy Appl. Immunol. 71, 317, 1983.
5. Ferguson, A. and Parrott, D.M.V., Clin. Exp. Immunol. 12, 477, 1982.
6. Parrott, D.M.V., Tait, C., MacKenzie, S., Mowat, A.McI., Davies, M.D.J. and Micklem, H.S., Ann. N.Y. Acad. Sci. 409, 307, 1983.
7. Dillon, S.B. and MacDonald, T.T., Parasite Immunology, 8, 503, 1986.
8. Dillon, S.B. and MacDonald, T.T., Immunology 52, 501, 1984.
9. Ernst, P.B., Clark, D.A., Rosenthal, K.A., Befus, A.D. and Bienenstock, J., J. Immunol. 136, 2121, 1986.
10. Dillon, S.B., Dalton, B.J. and MacDonald, T.T., Cell. Immunol., 103, 326, 1986.
11. Bowlin, T.L., Scott, A.N. and Ihle, J.N., J. Immunol. 133, 2001, 1984.
12. Robb, R.J. and Greene, W.C., J. Exp. Med. 158, 1332, 1983.
13. Dillon, S.B. and MacDonald, T.T., Immunology, 59, 389, 1986.
14. Ihle, J.N., Contemp. Topics in Molec. Biol. 10, 93, 1985.
15. Ferguson, A., MacDonald, T.T., McClure, J.P. and Holden, R.J., Lancet 1, 895, 1975.
16. Ferguson, A. and MacDonald, T.T., Ciba. Fdn. Symp. 46, 305, 1977.
17. Guy-Grand, D., Dy M., Luffau, G. and Vassalli, P., J. Exp. Med. 160, 12, 1984.
18. Dexter, T.M., Garland, J., Scott, D., Scolnick, E. and Metcalf, D., J. Exp. Med. 152, 1036, 1980.

ISOTYPE-SPECIFIC IMMUNOREGULATION: T CONTRASUPPRESSOR CELLS PROTECT IgA RESPONSES IN ORAL TOLERANCE

K. Kitamura, I. Suzuki, H. Kiyono*, T. Kurita, A.K. Berry, D.R. Green** and J.R. McGhee

Departments of Microbiology, *Oral Biology and Preventive Dentistry, The Institute of Dental Research, University of Alabama at Birmingham, University Station, Birmingham, Alabama USA; and **Department of Immunology, Faculty of Medicine, University of Alberta, Edmonton, Alberta, Canada T6G 2H7

INTRODUCTION

Murine Peyer's patches (PP) are enriched in T cell subsets with helper amplifier and contrasuppressor (Tcs) activity (1), and the Tcs cells may play a role in allowing IgA response induction in the presence of T suppressor (Ts) cells which mediate systemic unresponsiveness (1). Continuous oral exposure to thymus-dependent (TD) antigen results in two seemingly-opposite responses, the induction of IgA responses at mucosal sites and systemic unresponsiveness, termed oral tolerance (2,3). C3H/HeJ mice, which are genetically resistant to oral tolerance induction with sheep erythrocytes (SRBC), possess a splenic Tcs cell subset which abolishes oral tolerance when adoptively transferred to syngeneic, C3H/HeN mice. In this study, we summarize recent studies which show that C3H/HeJ PP contain abundant Tcs cell activity which may account for their lack of oral tolerance, and the existence of a Tcs cell subset which preferentially enhances Th cell-mediated IgA responses.

MATERIALS AND METHODS

Groups of C3H/HeN and C3H/HeJ mice ($H-2^{k}$) were intubated with SRBC for 28 consecutive days and splenic and PP T cells were prepared from C3H/HeJ mice for adoptive transfer to the orally tolerant C3H/HeN strain. Purified T cells from SRBC-orally fed C3H/HeJ mice were enriched by adherence to Vicia villosa lectin and adoptively transferred to orally tolerant, C3H/HeN mice. V. villosa adherent T cells allowed the development of IgM, IgG and especially IgA responses, a pattern similar to that seen in C3H/HeJ mice given oral SRBC and systemically challenged with antigen (4). The nonadherent fraction, which was enriched in Th cells, did not reverse oral tolerance. This suggests that C3H/HeJ mice given oral SRBC develop a PP T cell subset which reverses oral tolerance when small numbers are adoptively transferred, and shares the property of V. villosa binding with previously described Tcs cells (4-6).

The T cell subset responsible for oral tolerance reversal is Lyt-1$^+$, since enrichment of V. villosa adherent PP T cells by treatment with anti-Lyt-2 and rabbit complement (C), gave a cell fraction which abrogated oral tolerance when adoptively transferred to C3H/HeN mice (Fig. 1). However, reversal was not due to mature Th cells, since treatment of V. villosa adherent PP T cells with monoclonal anti-L3T4 and C, did not affect the ability of transferred T cells to abrogate tolerance (Fig. 1). Furthermore, treatment of Lyt-1$^+$, V. villosa adherent PP T cells with anti-L3T4 and C, did not alter their ability to reverse oral tolerance in the C3H/HeN strain (Fig. 1). However, treatment of this fraction with anti-Lyt-1 and C completely removed this activity.

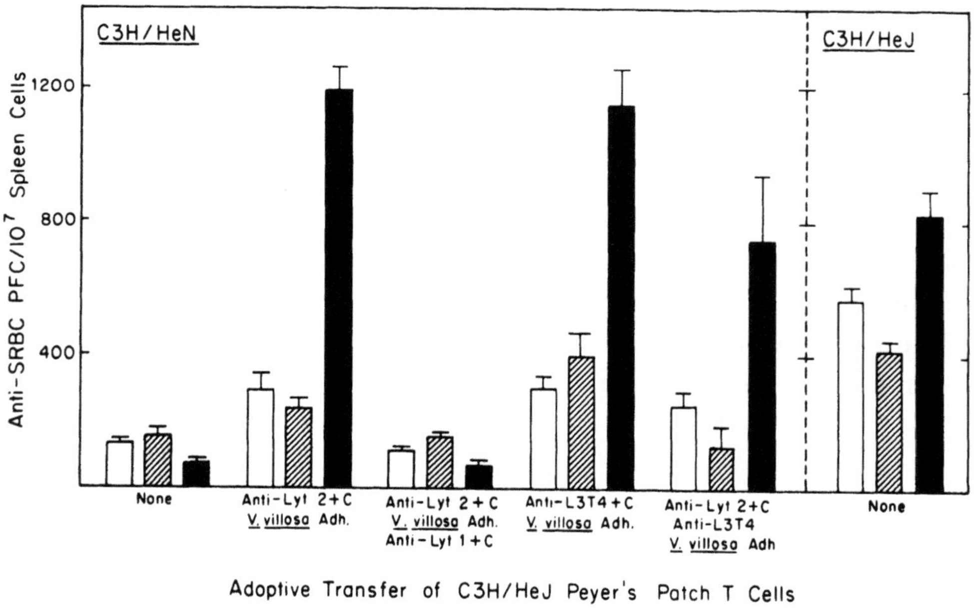

Figure 1. Reversal of oral tolerance in C3H/HeN mice by adoptive transfer of C3H/HeJ PP V. villosa-adherent cells. After transfer, mice were challenged i.p. with SRBC and splenic anti-SRBC PFC of the IgM (□), IgG (▨) and IgA (■) isotype were determined 4 d later.

Tcs cells share the important property of expression of the I-J determinant and Tcs cell-derived factors which mediate contrasuppression also express this molecule (7,8). When C3H/HeJ PP Lyt-1^+ T cell enriched fractions were treated with either polyclonal anti-I-J^K or monoclonal anti-I-^{K} antibodies and C, complete removal of Tcs activity was achieved. The Tcs cell fractions prepared by various treatments were also effective in restoring tolerant C3H/HeN spleen cell cultures to IgM, IgG and IgA anti-SRBC PFC responses _in vitro_. Lyt-1^+, _V. villosa_ adherent T cells supported _in vitro_ PFC responses of all isotypes, while the nonadherent, Th cell enriched fraction was ineffective. Additional treatment of Lyt-1^+ T cells with anti-I-J^K and C, or with anti-Lyt-1 and C completely blocked Tcs cell activity. As predicted from the _in vivo_ studies, anti-L3T4 and C treatment did not affect Tcs cell function _in vitro_. We conclude from these results that C3H/HeJ mice given oral SRBC possess a PP Tcs cell subset which is Lyt-1^+, 2^-, _V. villosa_ adherent, I-J^{K+} and L3T4^-. It is suggested that this activity in murine PP is due to a mature, effector Tcs cell population (4-6,9).

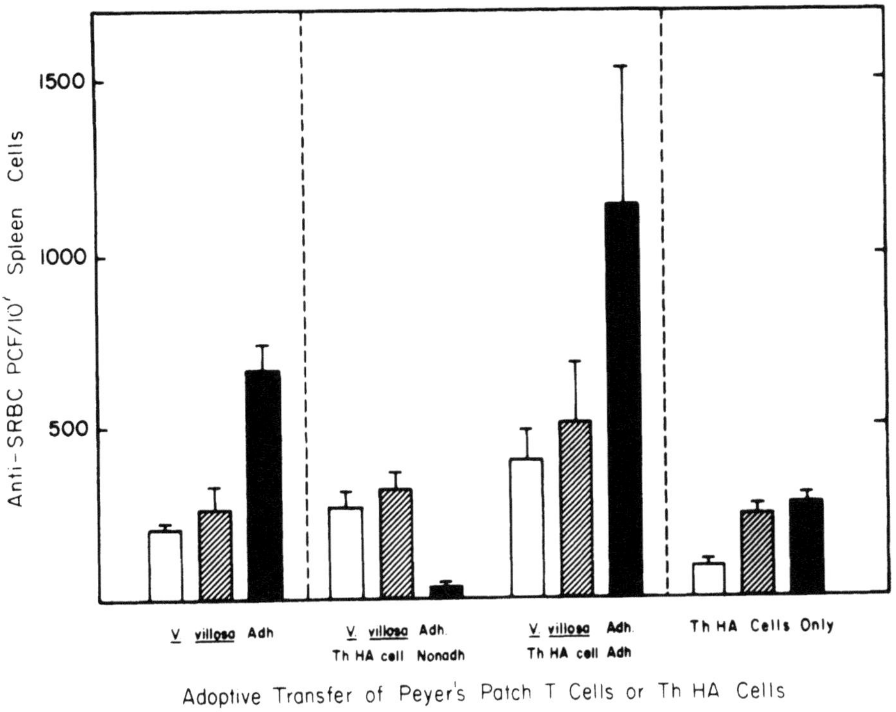

Figure 2. Tcs cells are isotype specific. C3H/HeJ PP _V. villosa_ adherent Tcs cells were added to wells containing fixed Th HA_1 #9 cells and adherent and nonadherent cell fractions were adoptively transferred. See Fig. 1 legend.

Our previous studies have shown that PP possess IgA specific Th cells which collaborate with IgA-committed B cells through an apparent FcαR-mediated mechanism (10,11). If FcαR$^+$ PP Th cells are the major helper population involved in the IgA response, then one could postulate that isotype-specific Tcs cells potentiate IgA responses by an effect on this cell type. To test this assumption, C3H/HeJ PP T cells were enriched on V. villosa plates and further fractionated by adherence to solid-phase absorbents of the Th HA_1 #9 cell line. PP T cells failed to adhere to FcαR$^+$ Th HA cells, when adoptively transferred to C3H/HeN mice, supported only IgM and IgG anti-SRBC PFC responses (Fig. 2). On the other hand, V. villosa$^+$, Th HA$^+$ Tcs cells supported all 3 isotypes when adoptively transferred (Fig. 2). However, the IgA response was clearly favored. Since fractionation on solid-phase Th HA cells resulted in two populations of Tcs cells, one which supported good IgA responses while a second, non-adherent Tcs cell did not, we conclude that isotype-specific Tcs cells occur. Furthermore, IgA-specific Tcs cells are enriched at IgA inductive sites, e.g., the PP.

DISCUSSION

The LPS unresponsive C3H/HeJ mouse offered a unique opportunity to study GALT contrasuppression, since this strain exhibits elevated Th cell activity in PP an enhanced IgA responses to oral TD antigen (12), and failed to elicit oral tolerance to SRBC (13,14). The syngeneic, LPS responsive C3H/HeN strain, however, is easily tolerized by feeding SRBC (13,14). Adoptive transfer of C3H/HeJ PP V. villosa adherent T cells in small numbers, readily reversed oral tolerance in the C3H/HeN mouse strain. This was not due to an active population of Th cells in this fraction, since treatment of anti-L3T4 antibody and C had no effect on the ability of Tcs cells to abrogate oral tolerance (Fig. 1). Our recent studies with FACS-separated cells shows that the effector Tcs cells which abrogate oral tolerance are distinct from T helper (L3T4$^+$) and T suppressor (Lyt-2$^+$) cells, since the active Tcs cell does not express either L3T4 or Lyt-2 antigens. The active Tcs cell in C3H/HeJ PP exhibited the characteristics associated with contrasuppressor-effector cells and was Lyt-1$^+$,2$^-$, L3T4$^-$, I-J^{k+} and adherent to V. villosa lectin.

The fact that active Tcs effector cells from non-tolerant C3H/HeJ PP convert tolerant C3H/HeN mice to responsiveness, clearly indicates that oral tolerance to SRBC is mediated by Ts cells. Since effector Tcs cells were adoptively transferred, it also suggests that Th cells already occur in tolerant mice, and are not induced in a protected environment of a complete contrasuppressor circuit. The absence of Th cell function indicates that Ts cells override their activity and systemic unresponsiveness ensues. However, Tcs effector cells, together with Th cells, can overcome Ts cell-mediated tolerance and result in anamnestic-type responses to systemic antigen.

Enrichment of C3H/HeJ PP Tcs cells by sequential adherence to V. villosa and Th HA_1 #9 cells, gave a population which enhanced IgM, IgG and especially IgA responses upon adoptive transfer (Fig. 2). Due to the low cell yields obtained by this procedure, it has been difficult to further characterize this Tcs cell fraction. We cannot, at present, discern whether one Tcs cell type is responsible for all 3 isotypes with preference for IgA, or whether Tcs cells which support IgM and IgG contaminate the Tcs cell fraction which supports IgA responses. In our current studies, we are using various competitive inhibitors such as purified IgA, monoclonal anti-FcαR and antibodies to other T cell antigens to selectively elute Th HA cell bound Tcs cells. This should provide additional information regarding the mechanisms of Tcs-Th cell interactions and allow further characterization of isotype-specific Tcs cells.

ACKNOWLEDGEMENTS

This work was supported by U.S.P.H.S. grants AI 19674, AI 18958, DE 04217, New Investigator Research Award 21032 (to H.K.) and The Alberta Heritage Foundation (to D.R.G.).

REFERNCES

1. Green, D.R., Gold, J., St. Martin, S., Gershon, R. and Gershon, R.K., Proc. Natl. Acad. Sci. USA 79, 889, 1982.
2. Tomasi, T.B., Jr., Transplantation (Baltimore) 29, 353, 1980.
3. Challacombe, S.J. and Tomasi, T.B., Jr., J. Exp. Med. 152, 1459, 1980.
4. Suzuki, I., Kiyono, H., Kitamura, K., Green, D.R. and McGhee, J.R., Nature 320, 451, 1986.
5. Iverson, M., Ptak, W., Green, D.R. and Gershon, R.K., J. Exp. Med. 158, 982, 1983.

6. Green, D.R., Eardley, D.D., Kimura, A., Murphy, D.B., Yamauchi, K. and Gershon, R.K., Eur. J. Immunol. 11, 973, 1981.
7. Green, D.R., Flood, P.M. and Gershon, R.K., Ann. Rev. Immunol. 1, 439, 1983.
8. Yamauchi, K., Green, D.R., Eardley, D.D., Murphy, D.B. and Gershon, R.K., J. Exp. Med. 153, 1547, 1981.
9. Gershon, R.K., Eardley, D.D., Durum, S., Green, D.R., Shen, F.W., Yamauchi, K., Cantor, H. and Murphy, D.E., J. Exp. Med. 153, 1533, 1981.
10. Kiyono, H., Cooper, M.D., Kearney, J.F., Mosteller, L.M., Michalek, S.M., Koopman, W.J. and McGhee, J.R., J. Exp. Med. 159, 798, 1984.
11. Kiyono, H., Phillips, J.O., Colwell, D.E., Michalek, S.M., Koopman, W.J. and McGhee, J.R., J. Immunol. 133, 1087, 1984.
12. Kiyono, H., Babb, J.L., Michalek, S.M. and McGhee, J.R., J. Immunol. 125, 732, 1980.
13. Kiyono, H., McGhee, J.R., Wannemuehler, M.J. and Michalek, S.M., J. Exp. Med. 155, 605, 1982.
14. Michalek, S.M., Kiyono, H., Wannemuehler, M.J., Mosteller, L.M. and McGhee, J.R., J. Immunol. 128, 1992, 1982.

REGULATORY T CELLS IN THE GALT

G.A. Enders

Institute for Surgical Research
Marchioninistr. 15, D-8000 München 70
West Germany

INTRODUCTION

The discussion about the importance of regulatory T cells for the differentiation of B cell precursors into IgA producing cells is controversial. Whereas the antigen driven differentiation of precursor cells is the central point of the B cell centered theories (1), others have suggested a crucial influence of T cells for the end stage differentiation of bone marrow derived cells into IgA secreting cells (2). Our own experiments with PP-deprived rats and mice show that these animals have lower IgA-positive cells in the lamina propria (LP) of the small intestine. This result points to the fact that the antigenic load, which due to gut motility should induce a more intense contact with the GALT, was not the ultimate inducer for an IgA response in the intestine. These findings made us consider the role of regulatory T cells for the IgA secretion in the LP. As a source of T cells we used phytahemagglutinin (PHA)-driven PP T cells and investigated their influence on bone marrow cells and as a source of precursor B cells PNA separated bone marrow cells. In another experiment we looked for the role of PHA directly on unseparated Peyer's patch, spleen and LP cells.

MATERIALS AND METHODS

Animals. BALB/c mice were purchased from Charles River (Sulzfeld, FRG) and were kept under routine conditions.

Medium and mitogens. Culture medium was Dulbecco's modified eagle (Gibco Laboratories) supplemented with L-glutamine (2 mM), sodium pyruvate (1 mM), MEM non-essential amino acids (1% solution, Gibco), L-asparagine (0.2 mM) and antibiotics (100 U/ml penicillin and 100 μg/ml Streptomycin). Fetal calf serum was obtained from Boehringer (Mannheim, FRG), heat-inactivated and used as 5% solution.

Lymphocyte separation. Single cell suspensions from PP and spleen were prepared by dissociation of the organs in a loosely fitting tissue homogenizer. Cells were washed twice and used in the culture system. LP lymphocytes were separated by filling everted intestinal gut segments with pronase (7 mg/ml) (Merck, Darmstadt, FRG) and incubation of the segments in Ca^{++} Mg^{++} free HBSS containing EDTA 2 mM for 3 x 30 min. The 4th incubation step was in HBSS with 20 mg % BSA under mild agitation. All incubation steps were performed at 37°C. The cells of the fourth step were then cleared by centrifugation through FCS and washed. Bone marrow cells were isolated by flushing the femur with HBSS. The cells were Ficoll-separated. PNA (Vector Laboratories, Burlingame, CA) positive cells were isolated as described (3).

Activation of T cells. Peyer's patch lymphocytes were separated as described and cultured in DME plus 1% autologous serum at a cell density of 1 x 10^6/ml in 10 ml Petri dishes (Falcon). PHA was added at a concentration of 2.5 μg/ml. After 3-4 days the PHA blasts were Ficoll-separated and expanded in medium containing 15% IL 2 supernatant (from C3H spleen cells cultured for 24 hr together with 5 μg/ml Con A). Medium was changed every 3 to 4 d. Cells were cultured for up to 2 wk before use in the coculture experiment.

Culture conditions for immunoglobulin production. Cells were cultured in DME supplemented with 5% FCS at a cell density of 2 x 10^5/ml bone marrow cells over 5 to 7 d. PWM (Seromed, Berlin, FRG) was added at a concentration of 2.5 μg/ml. Different numbers of PHA activated PP T cells were added. In the second experiment single cell suspensions of PP, spleen and LP lymphocytes were cultured with PHA at a cell density of 1 x 10^6/ml over 5 days. The final volume was 2 ml. All cultures were set up in triplicate. The vials were incubated in a humidified atmosphere containing 10% CO_2. After centrifugation, supernatants were removed and stored at -20°C prior to analysis by ELISA.

ELISA. Culture supernatants were used for the immunoglobulin determination using standard ELISA procedure. Immunoglobulin references were class specific myeloma proteins.

Statistics. Student's *t*-test.

RESULTS

The cocultivation of PHA driven, IL 2 expanded PP T cells (Thy 1.2^+, $Ly\text{-}2^-$) together with isolated PWM driven bone marrow cells from BALB/c mice resulted in an increase of the IgA concentration from 140 ± 30 ng/ml to 789 ± 140 ng/ml. However, the elevation of the IgM and IgG concentration was even more marked. The IgM production of bone marrow cells in the presence of PWM was 461 + 110, and in culture substituted with PP T cells 8140 + 520 ng/ml, the IgG concentration 331 + 65 and 2932 + 320 ng/ml, respectively (Fig. 1).

In cultures where PNA separated bone marrow cells were used as indicator cells the PWM induced immunoglobulin production was 498 + 50 ng/ml IgA, 200 + 30 IgM and 706 + 45 IgG. In this system the addition of PP

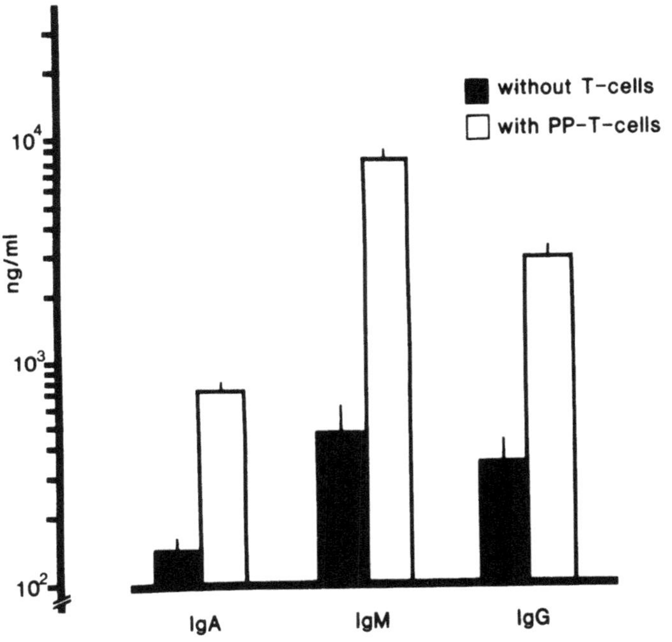

Figure 1. Ig-secretion of BALB/c BM-cells (2×10^5) in the presence of PWM (2.5 μg/ml). Black bars represent BM-cells without T cells; open bars, with PP-derived T cells.

derived, PHA driven IL 2 prolonged T cells led to an IgA concentration of 1240 + 35, IgM 1545 + 70 and IgG 1730 + 20 ng/ml (Fig. 2).

The highest IgA concentrations could be obtained in a culture system, where pronase treated LP lymphocytes were cultured in the presence of PHA over 5 d. Here the IgA concentration was 6375 + 710, IgM 330 + 160 and IgG 581 + 50 ng/ml. These IgA concentrations exceeded by far PHA induced IgA secretion by spleen (155 ng/ml) and PP lymphocytes (195 ng/ml). In contrast, spleen cells produced considerable amounts of IgM (3547 ng/ml), whereas the IgG secretion of spleen and PP lymphocytes and IgM of PP was very low (Fig. 3).

DISCUSSION

Recent reports have pointed out that PP contain helper T cells which influence the IgA differentiation/secretion. In all these studies spleen cells (4) or PP T cells (5-7) were used as indicator cells. Despite separation processes these cells might have a background IgA secretion. We, therefore, used bone marrow cells and, as a source of precursor B cells, PNA-separated BM cells (8) as indicator cells. In these two systems

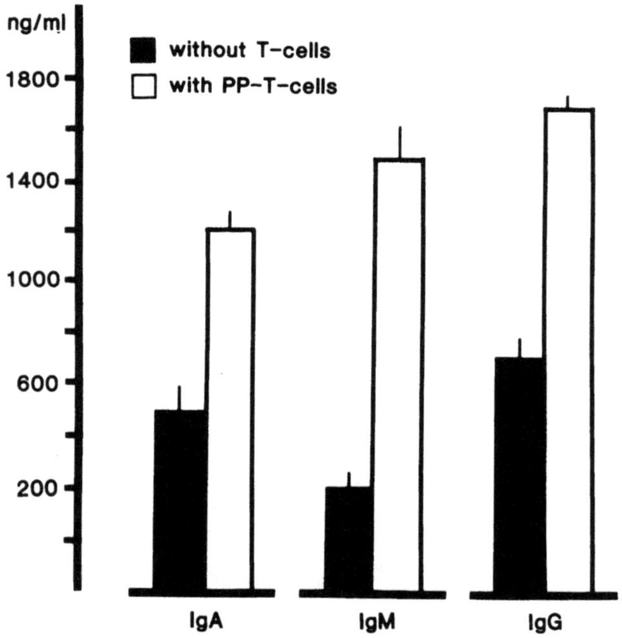

Figure 2. Ig secretion of BALB/c PNA separated BM cells (2 x 10^5) in the presence of PWM (2.5 μg/ml). Black bars represent PNA separated BM cells without T cells; open bars, with PP derived T cells.

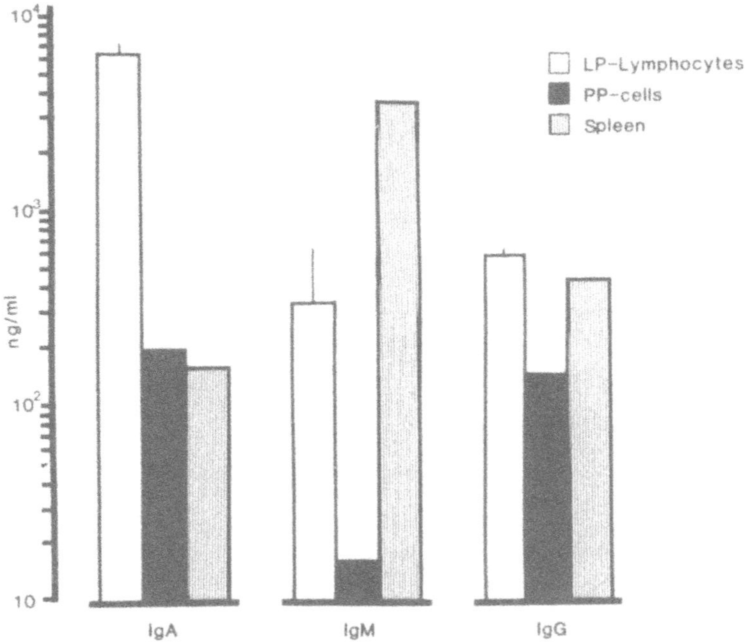

Figure 3. Ig secretion of PHA driven LP lymphocytes, PP lymphocytes and spleen cells (2 x 10^6). The Ig concentrations are given in a log scale.

PP derived PHA driven and IL 2 expanded T cells influence the immunoglobulin production. But in contrast to reports from the literature this influence was not restricted to the IgA production but intense changes in IgG and IgM secretion could be measured. From these results we must conclude that PP T cells may cooperate with pre-switched B cells (probably in the PP follicles), but not with B cell precursors immigrating from the bone marrow into the PP. Using immunohistology, in the neighborhood of differentiated IgA producing plasma cells in the lamina propria many T helper cells can be found. To test the inductive role of these T cells, we cultured LP lymphocyte preparations in the presence of PHA, a T cell mitogen. This culture resulted in very high IgA concentrations, compared with PP lymphocytes and spleen cells. We, therefore, suggest the importance of local regulatory T cells for IgA production. Their influence on the differentiation of B cell precursors, on the other hand, is the object of current experiments.

REFERENCES

1. Cebra, J.J., Cebra, E.R., Clough, E.R., Fuhrman, J.A., Komisar, J.L., Schweitzer, P.A. and Shahin, R.D., Ann. N.Y. Acad. Sci. 409, 25, 1983.
2. Strober, W. and Jacobs, D., in Advances in Host Defense Mechanisms, (Edited by Gallin, J.I. and Fauci, A.S.), p. 1, Raven Press, 1985.
3. Reisner, Y.M., Israeli, L. and Sharon, N., Cell. Immunol. 25, 129, 1976.
4. Campbell, D. and Vose, B.M., Immunology 56, 81, 1985.
5. Kiyono, H., Mosteller-Barnum, L.M., Pitts, A.M., Williamson, S.I., Michalek, S.M. and McGhee, J.R., J. Exp. Med. 161, 731, 1985.
6. Spalding, D.M., Williamson, S.I., Koopman, W.J. and McGhee, J.R., J. Exp. Med. 160, 941, 1984.
7. Kawanishi, H., Saltzman, L. and Strober, W., J. Exp. Med. 158, 649, 1983.
8. Osmond, W., Melchers, F. and Paige, C.H., J. Immunol. 133, 86, 1984.

T DEPENDENT INDUCTION OF AN IgA AND IgM ANTI-POLYSACCHARIDE RESPONSE

M.F. Kagnoff and P.D. Murray

Laboratory of Mucosal Immunology
Department of Medicine, M-023-D
University of California
San Diego, La Jolla, CA USA

INTRODUCTION

The intestinal mucosa is the first site of interaction between the immune system and many foreign antigens and pathogens (1). Major interactions with polysaccharide antigens take place in the gut, and immune responses to bacterial polysaccharides are important in host defenses at mucosal surfaces. Morbidity and mortality from infections with encapsulated bacteria is high in neonates and the elderly. Information regarding how anti-polysaccharide immunity is regulated at mucosal surfaces and changes in that regulation during aging could be of substantial value for strategies to alter anti-polysaccharide immunity and for the design of immunization programs.

The induction and regulation of antibody responses to polymeric polysaccharides like the dextrans or levans differs in several respects from that to proteins or polysaccharides coupled to proteins (2-8). For example, responses to bacterial polysaccharides are largely of the IgM and IgA class, and the IgG3 subclass in mice (2,9-12). Such molecules have a limited number of antigenic determinants and elicit antibodies of restricted heterogeneity (13,14). B cell precursors for polysaccharides can be detected a few days after birth (15). Nonetheless, compared to proteins, antibody responses to polysaccharides may be delayed in ontogeny after *in vivo* immunization (2,4,15,16). Delays in the age of onset of antipolysaccharide immunity are seen also in humans (17).

Dextran B1355S is a water soluble dextran derived from *Leuconostoc mesenteroides*. Responses to this type II antigen in BALB/c mice are predominantly of the IgA and IgM class and are directed to α(1,3) glycosidic linkages (2,18). Immune responses to polysaccharide antigens like the dextrans generally have been regarded as thymus-independent (i.e., not requiring T cell help) (19-22). However, previous studies from this laboratory challenged that notion and demonstrated that anti-dextran responses are T dependent *in vivo* and *in vitro* (2,12). In the present studies, we have used the response to dextran B1355S to define the requirement for T cells and T cell lymphokines in the induction and regulation of an IgA and IgM anti-polysaccharide response.

MATERIALS AND METHODS

Mice

BALB/c mice, 2 to 14 months old, were bred in our laboratories.

Antigens

Dextran B1355 (NRRL Dextran, fraction S) from *Leuconostoc mesenteroides* and dextran B512 (fraction S) were provided by Dr. M.E. Slodki, Northern Regional Research Center, Peoria, IL. The α-D-glucopyranosidic linkages of dextran B1355 are 43% α(1,3) and 57% α(1,6), whereas those of dextran B512 are 95% α(1,6) and 5% α(1,3) (23).

Lymphocytes and cell culture

Single cell suspensions of spleen and Peyer's patch lymphocytes were prepared as described before (24-26). To obtain B cells, mice were pretreated *in vivo* with antithymocyte serum (24,25). Cell suspensions were treated before use *in vitro* with a cocktail of monoclonal anti-Thy-1 (HO.13.4) (27) and anti-Lyt 2.2 antibody (AD 4.15) (28) plus complement. Subsequently, antibody secreting and accessory cells were removed on Sephadex G-10 columns (29). T cells were enriched by depleting spleen or Peyer's patch cells of surface immunoglobulin bearing cells by panning on $F(ab')_2$ rabbit anti-mouse immunoglobulin coated plates, or by passage over nylon wool columns followed by treatment with anti-Lyt-2.2, anti-Ia^d and J11d monoclonal antibodies and complement to further deplete B cells and Ia bearing accessory cells (30,31). Lymphocytes were cultured in 24 or 96 well tissue culture plates in RPMI 1640 supplemented with 10% fetal calf serum, 2-mercaptoethanol (5×10^{-5}M), penicillin (40 U/ml), streptomycin (40 μg/ml), 2.4 mM glutamine and 12% nutritional cocktail (12,25,32).

Lymphokines

Recombinant human interleukin 2 (IL 2) was provided by Cetus Corp. E. coli derived murine recombinant gamma interferon (IFN-γ) was provided by Genentech Inc. BCGF II was obtained from EL-4 supernatants or the rat AT-2 hybridoma as described before (25). Supernatant from the Id-1 T helper cell line stimulated with Con A (3 μg/ml) contains BCGF II and IL-2 (26).

Plaque forming cell (PFC) assay

IgM and IgA anti-dextran PFC were assayed as described before (2). Specificity of the anti-dextran B1355 response for α(1,3) glucan determinants was determined by adding titrated concentrations of dextran B1355 or dextran B512 to the PFC assay and measuring PFC inhibition (2).

Limiting dilution cultures

Spleen cells were seeded in limiting cell concentrations in microwells in the presence of rat thymocytes (6×10^5/well) and LPS (25 μg/ml; E. coli 0111:B4) (33), with 36 replicate cultures for each responder cell concentration. Supernatants were harvested after 7 days of culture and assayed for anti-dextran antibodies in a micro-ELISA assay.

RESULTS

The T cell dependence of the anti-dextran response reflects a requirement for T cell lymphokines

We showed before that supernatants from long-term alloreactive T cell lines and T cell hybridomas contain non-specific helper factors which can substitute for T cells in the antigen specific activation of IgA and IgM anti-dextran responses in vitro (34). The experiments below define the specific T cell lymphokines in those supernatants that are important for the induction of the anti-dextran response.

Three different T cell lymphokines that affect B cell growth and differentiation can substitute for T cells in the induction of the IgM and IgA anti-α(1,3) dextran response. These are a) IFN-γ, (b) a late acting

B cell growth and differentiation factor known as BCGF II, and (c) IL 2. Of note, when tested alone, recombinant IFN-γ, BCGF II or IL 2 had little affect on the induction of the anti-α(1,3) dextran response, although BCGF II or IL 2 could stimulate low level IgM and IgA responses and IFN-γ variably could stimulate low level IgA responses (Fig. 1A-C).

The striking finding of these studies was that dextran stimulated murine spleen B cell cultures supplemented with a combination of murine recombinant IFN-γ and BCGF II produced substantial IgA and IgM anti-dextran responses (Figs. 1 and 2). IL 2 was not required for those responses (Fig. 1). In contrast, recombinant IFN-γ and recombinant IL-2 in combination supported the induction of IgA but not IgM anti-α(1,3) dextran PFC (Figs. 1 and 3). The B cells responding to those lymphokines were committed already to IgA expression. Thus, depletion of surface IgA (sIgA) bearing B cells significantly decreased the IgA response in lymphokine supplemented cultures (Table 1).

In contrast to the above studies, which tested lymphokines and spleen cells from 10-14 month old mice, spleen B cells from young (2 month old) mice did not produce an <u>in vitro</u> anti-α(1,3) dextran response (Table 2). This was the case regardless of whether BCGF II, IL 2 or IFN-γ alone or in combination were added to culture. We have investigated the mechanisms responsible for the failure of spleen B cells from young mice to produce an anti-dextran response. Suppressor cells did not appear to be responsible

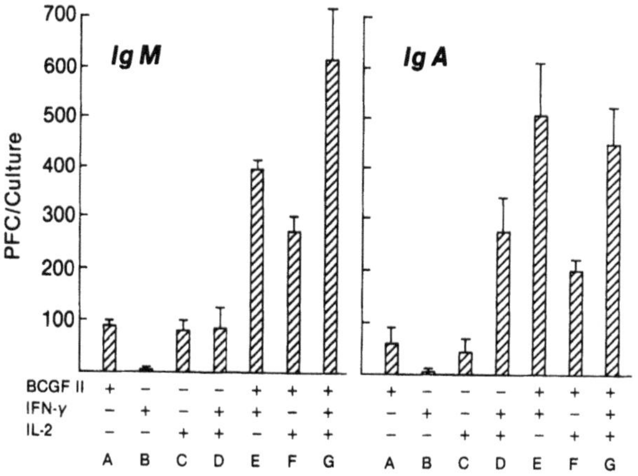

Figure 1. Anti-dextran PFC responses in B cell cultures stimulated with purified (AT.2)BCGF II, recombinant IFN-γ, and/or recombinant IL 2. B cells (5 x 10^5) were stimulated with dextran (0.1 ng/culture) and IFN-γ (1 U/culture) on day 0, and (AT.2)BCGF II (15 U/culture) and IL 2 (200 U/culture) were added on day 1. PFC were assayed on day 5. Results represent the mean (±SEM) of three repeated experiments.

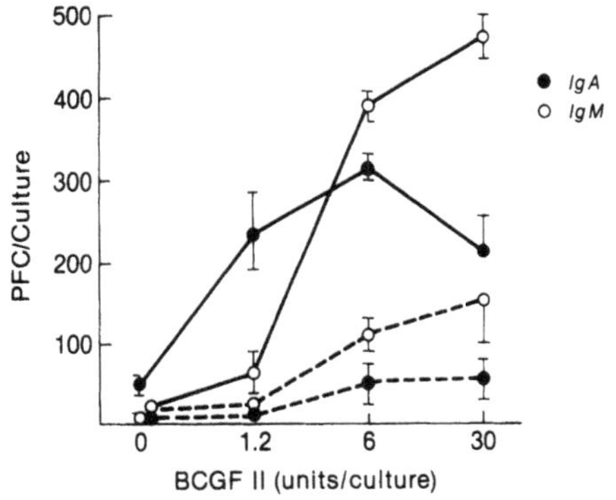

Figure 2. Anti-α (1,3) dextran responses in B cell cultures supplemented with BCGF II (---) or BCGF II + IFN-γ (——). Spleen B cells (5 x 10^5) were stimulated with dextran (0.1 ng/culture), recombinant IFN-γ (1 U/culture), and titrated concentrations of BCGF II. Lymphokines and antigen were added at the initiation of culture and PFC were assayed on day 5. Results represent the mean (±SEM) of four repeated experiments. PFC obtained from cultures stimulated with dextran alone ranged from 0 to 10 for IgM and 0 to 3 for IgA and have been subtracted from the data. Cultures supplemented with BCGF II (30 U/culture) and IFN-γ but no antigen yielded 41 ± 11 IgM and 17 ± 8 IgA PFC, respectively.

in that, in cell mixing experiments, spleens of young mice did not suppress the induction of the anti-dextran response by spleen cells from old mice (12). Further, the lack of anti-dextran PFC in spleen cell cultures from young mice is not due to a lack of anti-α(1,3) dextran B cell precursors in the spleens of these mice (26). Thus, using limiting dilution analysis with LPS to reveal the B cell repertoire (33), we found the spleens of young (2 month old) mice to contain twice as many LPS inducible α(1,3) dextran specific B cell precursors as the spleens of older (14 month old) mice (26). However, when neonatal mice were primed with dextran and their splenic B cells obtained at 2 months of age, IgM anti-dextran responses could be stimulated in cultures supplemented with BCGF II and IL 2; IFN-γ synergized with those lymphokines in the production of that response (Table 3). This suggests that the difference in the B cell response between young and old mice reflects the ability of primed or memory B cells as compared to unprimed B cells to respond to dextran in the presence of lymphokines.

Requirement for T cells in the induction of the anti-dextran response

Peyer's patches are the initial site of interaction between the host and many environmental antigens. However, the response of lymphocytes from Peyer's patches to polysaccharide antigens had not been investigated.

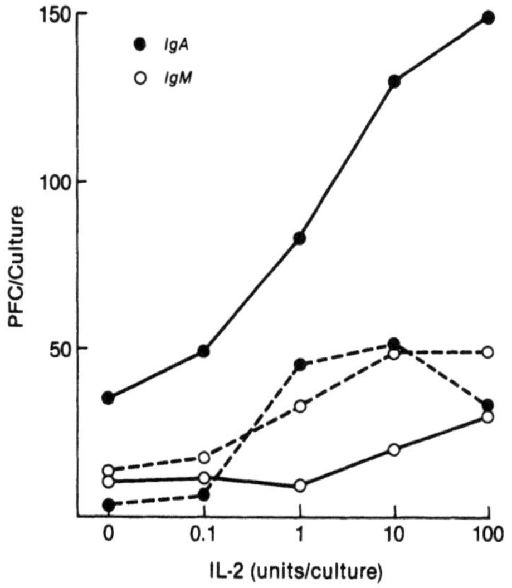

Figure 3. Anti-α(1,3) dextran responses in cultures supplemented with recombinant IL-2 (---) or recombinant IL-2 + IFN-γ (——). Splenic B cells were stimulated with dextran B1355 (0.1 ng/culture). IFN-γ (4 units/culture) and titrated concentrations of IL-2 were added at the initiation of culture and PFC was assayed on day 5. Concentrations of IL-2 greater than 100 units/culture did not result in incremental increases in IgM or IgA responses.

We noted that dextran stimulated Peyer's patch cells from 2 month old mice could generate anti-α(1,3) dextran PFC, whereas spleen cells from the same mice could not (Table 4). This observation, and the fact that young spleens do contain anti-α(1,3) dextran B cell precursors, suggested that T cells and/or accessory cells in Peyer's patches may be important in the initiation of the anti-dextran response. To assess this possibility, T cells from Peyer's patches were tested for their ability to help in the induction of the anti-dextran response of young spleen B cells. As shown in Table 5, freshly isolated Peyer's patch T cells, but not spleen T cells from the same mice, supported the induction of spleen B cells to anti-dextran PFC. Thus, Peyer's patches appear to contain a T helper population that either is not present or is not active functionally in the spleens of young mice. Other data confirmed that the cell active in the induction of the anti-dextran response by young spleen B cells is, in fact, a T cell. Thus, PT-1 (a $L3T4^+$ long-term Peyer's patch T cell line generated in our laboratory by stimulation of Peyer's patch cells with syngeneic B cells), but not supernatants of PT-1, supported the induction of young spleen B cells to anti-α(1,3) dextran antibody forming cells.

Table 1. Anti-α(1,3) dextran responses in splenic B cell cultures depleted of sIgA bearing cells[a]

Factor	B Cells	PFC/Culture	
		IgM	IgA
BCGF II + IFN-γ	Unfractionated	305	275
	sIgA[-b]	375	20
IL-2 + IFN-γ	Unfractionated	25	150
	sIgA[-]	16	1

[a]Splenic B cells from 14 month old mice were stimulated with dextran (0.1 ng/culture) and either BCGF II and IFN-γ or IL 2 and IFN-γ.

[b]Nonadherent cells obtained after panning of spleen B cells on goat anti-mouse IgA plates.

Table 2. Comparison of the response of spleen B cells from 2 and 14 month old mice to T cell lymphokine-mediated help

Source of B cells[a]	Age of Mice	Lymphokines[b]	Anti-dextran PFC/culture[c]	
			IgM	IgA
		None	2	4
Spleen	14 month	BCGF II-IL-2	50	59
		BCGF II-IL-2+IFN-γ	356	317
		None	5	14
Spleen	2 month	BCGF II+IL-2	28	3
		BCGF II+IL-2+IFN-γ	10	3

[a]After T cell depletion as described in Materials and Methods, spleens were twice Sephadex G-10 passed to deplete antibody secreting cells and accessory cells. 5×10^5 B cells were cultured in 0.1 ml in microwells with dextran B1355S (0.1 ng/culture).

[b]Supernatant from the T cell line Id-1 was added on day 1 culture as a source of BCGF II and IL-2. Supernatants were titrated in culture over a dose range of 0.2 to 20% final concentration and doses yielding maximum PFC responses are shown. Maximum responses correspond to 3-15 units BCGF II/culture and 50-250 units IL-2/culture. IFN-γ (1 unit/culture) was added at the initiation of culture. PFC responses with lymphokines but no antigen ranged from 0-22 and 0-18 for IgM and IgA PFC, respectively.

[c]PFC were assayed on day 5 of culture. Data represents the geometric mean from triplicate cultures.

Table 3. Anti-dextran response in spleen B cell cultures from 2 month old unprimed or neonatally dextran primed mice[a]

Lymphokine added to culture	IgM anti-dextran PFC/culture[b] Not primed with dextran[c]	Neonatally primed with dextran[d]
None	5	0
BCGF II + IL 2	28	109
BCGF II + IL 2 + IFN-γ[e]	10	286

[a]B cells were prepared as described in Table 2.

[b]PFC were assayed on day 5 of culture. Data represent the geometric means from triplicate cultures.

[c]Spleens were removed at 2 months of age.

[d]Mice were primed at 3 days of age with 5 μg dextran B1355 i.p. Spleen cells were obtained at 2 months of age.

[e]Lymphokines were added as described in Table 2.

Table 4. Comparison of anti-dextran responses in cultures of spleen and Peyer's patch cells from 2 month old mice[a]

Expt.	Source of Lymphocytes	Age of mice (mo)	Anti-dextran PFC/culture IgM	IgA
1	Spleen	2	32	0
	Peyer's patch	2	588	2500
2	Spleen	2	40	0
	Peyer's patch	2	420	1600
3	Spleen	2	68	0
	Peyer's patch	2	388	840

[a]Spleen and PP cells (2.5×10^6/0.5 ml) from 2 month old BALB/c mice were stimulated in culture with 0.5 ng dextran B1355. On day 5, triplicate cultures were pooled and IgM and IgA PFC were enumerated. Background responses in cultures not stimulated with dextran ranged from 0-18 PFC.

Table 5. Peyer's patch T cells help in the induction of young spleen B cells[a]

Source of T cells[b]	Source of B cells	Dextran	IgA anti-dextran PFC/culture IgM
-	Spleen	+	60
PP	Spleen	+	764
PP	Spleen	-	98
PP	-	+	0
Spleen	Spleen	+	24
PP + Spleen	Spleen	+	650

[a]Spleen and Peyer's patch cells were obtained from 9-11 wk old mice. 1.25 x 10^6 T cells from spleen or PP were cultured with 1.25 x 10^6 spleen B cells in 0.5 ml volumes. Dextran (1 ng/ml) was added at the initiation of culture and PFC were determined on day 5.

[b]Similar findings were seen when Peyer's patch and spleen cells used as a source of T cells were added at various T cell:B cell ratios varying from 1:1 to 4:1.

DISCUSSION

Three B cell growth and differentiation factors have been identified that, in combination, are required for the induction of splenic B cells to IgA and IgM anti-α(1,3) dextran antibody forming cells. IFN-γ and IL 2 in combination were required for the induction of IgA anti-dextran responses, but did not support IgM anti-dextran responses. IFN-γ and BCGF II in combination supported the induction of both IgM and IgA responses. Alone, such lymphokines support little or no anti-dextran response. In combination, these lymphokines had synergistic and not simply additive activities.

BCGF II and IL 2 are known to stimulate B cell proliferation and differentiation (35-40). The enhanced anti-dextran response in cultures containing IFN-γ and BCGF II may reflect an anti-proliferative effect of IFN-γ on B cells (41-43). Such an anti-proliferative effect may permit the differentiation properties of BCGF II on B cells to be revealed preferentially. In this regard, we have noted proliferative responses of B cell cultures stimulated with BCGF II containing supernatants to be reduced significantly by the addition of IFN-γ to culture. Alternatively, IFN-γ may directly influence B cell differentiation.

Others have suggested that IL 2 is the important lymphokine in T cell supernatants that can substitute for T cells in the response of B cells to thymus-dependent antigens (44,45). Our results clearly indicate that IL 2 is not required for the IgA and IgM anti-dextran PFC response in B cell cultures supplemented with BCGF II and IFN-γ. However, high concentrations of IL 2 (> 100 U/culture), corresponding to those required to induce B cell differentiation, increased PFC responses in cultures containing suboptimal BCGF II concentrations (25).

In striking contrast to spleen B cells from older mice, dextran stimulated spleen B cells from young mice did not produce an anti-dextran response when cultures were supplemented with IFN-γ, BCGF II, or IL 2 alone or in combination. This was not due to a lack of dextran specific precursors in the spleen of young mice, since anti-α(1,3) dextran B cells were, in fact, more prevalent in the spleens of young compared to aged mice. Further, other experiments indicated that spleen B cells from young mice primed to dextran were capable of responding to dextran and lymphokines. Thus, differences in the splenic B cell response to dextran and lymphokines between the young and old mice appears to reflect a difference in the ability of primed or memory B cells compared to unprimed B cells to respond to T cell lymphokines.

The induction of antibody responses to polysaccharide antigens traditionally has been considered as thymus-independent. Initially, it was thought that T cell help was not required for such responses, and more recently, that non-specific T cell lymphokines, as reported above, but not a direct T cell interaction was required. However, as demonstrated herein, dextran stimulated spleen B cells from young mice required the physical presence of a T helper cell for their induction. Whereas, the T cells necessary for such responses are not present or are functionally less active in young spleen, they are present in Peyer's patches freshly isolated from young mice. Further support for the fact that a T cell is required for the initial induction of dextran specific B cells was derived from experiments using the Peyer's patch T cell line, PT-1. This $L3T4^+$ line, generated in our laboratory in response to stimulation with syngeneic B cells, was sufficient to provide T help to young spleen B cells in the induction of the anti-dextran response. Further, we note that, in the absence of added T cells, supernatants from freshly isolated Peyer's patch

T cells and Peyer's patch T cell lines have consistently failed to support anti-α(1,3) dextran responses among young spleen B cells.

We propose that before becoming responsive to T cell lymphokines like BCGF II, IL 2 and IFN-γ, dextran specific B cells require a signal provided by a T cell. In this regard, it has not been possible to demonstrate MHC restricted T helper cells that recognize epitopes on dextran, despite repeated attempts to identify such cells (8,12). It may be that the T cell repertoire does not contain T cells that recognize α(1,3) glucan determinants. We suggest that a critical step in the induction of B cells to become responsive to polysacchride antigens and lymphokines involves an interaction between a B cell precursor and a T cell that recognizes self class II molecules (46), either alone or in combination with another B cell surface marker. Such T cells may be particularly abundant in Peyer's patches, a site where the immune system first encounters many environmental antigens, including bacterial polysaccharides (47).

One final point warrants comment. Among lymphokine responsive B cells, we noted a differential effect of IFN-γ and IL 2 on the induction of the IgA, compared to the IgM anti-α(1,3) dextran response. It is possible that the IgA and IgM B cells were at different stages of differentiation, and therefore, exhibited different lymphokine requirements for their induction. Alternatively, B cells destined to produce varying isotypes may differ in the expression of receptors for different lymphokines. Further, B cells at different stages of activation may exhibit different responses to identical lymphokines. We suggest that quantitative or qualitative differences in the production of B cell growth and differentiation factors in different lymphoid compartments could be important in the selective regulation of B cell proliferation and differentiation in different sites, and may influence the distribution of immunoglobulin isotypes produced in a response. Such mechanisms may be particularly relevant for B cell development in Peyer's patches and for the selective expression of IgA responses in the microenvironment of the intestinal tract.

ACKNOWLEDGEMENTS

The authors wish to thank Ms. Debby Sagal for the preparation of this manuscript. These studies were supported by NIH grant AM 35108.

REFERENCES

1. Kagnoff, M.F., in Physiology of the Gastrointestinal Tract, Second Edition, (Edited by L. Johnson), Raven Press, 1987 (in press).
2. Kagnoff, M.F., J. Immunol. 122, 866, 1979.
3. Ivars, F., Nyberg, G., Holmberg, D. and Coutinho, A., J. Exp. Med. 158, 1498, 1983.
4. Bona, C., Mond, J.J., Stein, K.E., House, S., Lieberman, R. and Paul, W.E., J. Immunol. 123, 1484, 1979.
5. Ward, RE. and Kohler, H., J. Immunol. 126, 146, 1981.
6. Ward, R.E. and Kohler, H., J. Immunol. 134, 1430, 1985.
7. Froscher, B.G and Klinman, N.R., J. Exp. Med. 162, 1620, 1985.
8. Tittle, T.V., Mawle, A. and Cohn, M., J. Immunol. 135, 2582, 1985.
9. Mayers, G.L., Bankert, R.B. and Pressman, D., J. Immunol. 120, 1143, 1978.
10. Slack, J., Der-Balian, G.P., Nahm, M. and Davie, J.M., J. Exp. Med. 151, 853, 1980.
11. Perlmutter, R.M., Hansburg, D., Briles, D.E., Nicolotti, R.A. and Davie, J.M., J. Immunol. 121, 566, 1978.
12. Trefts, P.E., Rivier, D.A. and Kagnoff, M.F., Nature 292, 163, 1981.
13. Hansburg, D., Briles, D.E. and Davie, J.M., J. Immunol. 117, 569, 1977.
14. Briles, D.E. and Davie, J.M., J. Exp. Med. 141, 1291, 1975.
15. Stohrer, R. and Kearney, J.F., J. Immunol. 133, 2323, 1984.
16. Rivier, D.A., Trefts, P.E. and Kagnoff, M.F., Scand. J. Immunol. 17, 115, 1983.
17. Ambrosino, D.M., Schiffman, G., Gotschlich, E.C., Schur, P.H., Rosenberg, G.A., DeLange, G.G., van Loghem, E. and Siber, G.R., J. Clin. Invest. 75, 1935, 1985.
18. Blomberg, B., Geckeler, W.R. and Weigert, M., Science 177, 178, 1972.
19. Howard, J.G., Christie, G.H., Courtenay, B.M., Leuchars, E. and Davies, A.J.S., Cell. Immunol. 2, 614, 1971.
20. Howard, J.G. and Courtenay, B.M., Immunology 29, 599, 1975.
21. Fernandez, C. and Moller, G., Scand. J. Immunol. 7, 331, 1978.
22. Mitchison, N.A., Eur. J. Immunol. 1, 18, 1971.
23. Misaki, A., Torii, M., Jr., Sawai, T. and Goldstein, I.J., Carbohydr. Res. 84, 273, 1980.
24. Murray, P.D. and Kagnoff, M.F., Cell. Immunol. 95, 437, 1985.
25. Murray, P.D., Swain, S.L. and Kagnoff, M.F., J. Immunol. 135, 4015, 1985.
26. Murray, P.D. and Kagnoff, M.F., J. Immunol. 1986 (in press).

27. Marshak-Rothstein, A., Fink, P., Gridley, I., Raulet, D.H., Bevan, M.J. and Gefter, M.L., J. Immunol. 122, 2491, 1979.
28. Raulet, D.H., Gottlieb, P.D. and Bevan, M.J., J. Immunol. 125, 1136, 1980.
29. Ly, I. and Misehll, R., J. Immunol. Meth. 5, 239, 1974.
30. Wysocki, L.J. and Sato, V.L., Proc. Natl. Acad. Sci. USA 75, 2844, 1978.
31. Bruce, J., Symington, F.W., McKearn, T.J. and Sprent, J., J. Immunol. 1127, 2496, 1981.
32. Mishell, R.I. and Dutton, R.W., J. Exp. Med. 126, 423, 1967.
33. Andersson, J., Coutinho, A. and Melchers, F., J. Exp. Med. 145, 1511, 1977.
34. Kagnoff, M.F., Arner, L.S. and Swain, S.L., J. Immunol. 131, 2210, 1983.
35. Ralph, P., Deong, G., Welte, K., Mertelsmann, R., Rabin, H., Henderson, L.E., Souza, L.M., Boone, T.C. and Robb, R.J., J. Immunol. 133, 2442, 1984.
36. Mingara, M.C., Gerosa, F., Carra, G., Accola, R.S., Moretta, A., Zubler, R.H., Waldman, T.A. and Moretta, L., Nature 312, 641, 1984.
37. Nakanishi, K., Malek, T.R., Sith, K.A., Hamaoka, T., Shevach, E. and Paul, W.E., J. Exp. Med. 160, 1605, 1984.
38. Muraguchi, A., Kehrl, J.H., Longo, D.L., Volkman, D.J., Smith, K.A. and Fauci, A.S., J. Exp. Med. 161, 181, 1985.
39. Swain, S.L. and Dutton, R.W., J. Exp. Med. 156, 1821, 1982.
40. Swain, S.L., J. Immunol. 134, 3934, 1985.
41. Rubin, B.Y. and Gupta, S.L., Proc. Natl. Acad. Sci. USA 77, 5928, 1980.
42. Gewert, D.R., Shah, S. and Clemens, M.J., Eur. J. Biochem. 116, 487, 1981.
43. Mond, J.J., Sarma, C., Ohara, J., Finkelman, F.D. and Seratti, S., Fed. Proc. 44, 1296, 1985.
44. Mond, J.J., Mongini, P.K., Sieckmann, D. and Paul., W.E., J. Immunol. 125, 1066, 1980.
45. Mond, J.J., Farrar, J., Paul, W.E., Fuller-Farrar, J., Schaefer, M. and Howard, M., J. Immunol. 131, 633, 1983.
46. Kawanishi, H., Ozato, K. and Strober, W., J. Immunol. 134, 3586, 1985.
47. Kearney, J.F., McCarthy, M.T.M., Stohrer, R., Benjamin, W.H., Jr., and Briles, D.E., J. Immunol. 135, 3468, 1985.

A PREDOMINANT IDIOTYPE IN THE GUT ASSOCIATED LYMPHOID TISSUE

P.M. Andre and T.B. Tomasi

Laboratoire de Microbiology, Faculte de Medecine, Rennes, France and Department of Cell Biology, University of New Mexico, Albuquerque, New Mexico; and Roswell Park Memorial Institute, Buffalo, New York USA

INTRODUCTION

A high percentage of gut lamina propria plasma cells in tissue sections were stained by three fluoresceinated rabbit anti mouse IgG3 antisera. Similar cytoplasmic staining was found in several mouse strains including CBA/N mice. To further extend these data, northern hybridization experiments with a cDNA probe specific for IgG3 was performed with total RNA isolated from the small intestine or from cell preparations enriched for lamina propria plasma cells (data not shown). In contrast to the fluorescent studies, little or no mRNA for IgG3 was found. In all cases the antigen used in producing the anti-mouse IgG3 serum was the J 606 (IgG3) myeloma protein, which reacts with certain polysaccharides such as inulin [β(2-1) poly fructosan] and bacterial levan [β(2-6) polyfructosan].

The possibility that the anti IgG3 sera were reacting with idiotypic determinants of J 606 was investigated using ABPC 4, an IgA myeloma protein which has the same antigen specificity as J 606 and shares cross reactive idiotypes (1). All of the antisera reacted strongly with ABPC 4. The idiotypes associated with levan specificity were present in a high proportion of plasma cells of the gut associated lymphoid tissues (GALT) of several mouse strains, including CBA/N mice which have an X-linked immune defect (Xid) and do not respond to thymus independent class 2 (TI-2) antigens such as levan (1). It was, therefore, of interest to further characterize the specificity of the antisera and to quantify the expression of these idiotypes in the gut lymphoid tissues (GLT).

MATERIALS AND METHODS

Mice

CBA/N were obtained from Bommice, Netherlands. CBA/J and (C57BLxDBA2) F1 were bred in our animal facility. All mice were between 8 and 12 weeks of age.

Myeloma proteins

Myeloma proteins were purified from ascitic fluid either by chromatography on a Mono Q column (Pharmacia, Piscataway, NJ) for ABPC 4 (IgA, κ), by low salt precipitation followed by a pH gradient elution from a protein-A column for J 606 and FLOPC 21 (IgG3, κ), or by affinity chromatography for TEPC 15 (IgA, κ). Other myeloma proteins were purchased from Litton Bionetic (Charleston, SC). The purity of the proteins was tested by SDS polyacrylamide gel electrophoresis and immunoelectrophoresis.

Antigens

β(2-1) and β(2-6) poly fructosans were provided by Dr. P. Legrain, Pasteur Institut, France. Inulin was obtained from Sigma (St. Louis, MO).

Anti-Id J 606 serum

White New Zealand rabbits were immunized with J 606 emulsified in complete Freund's adjuvant. Following immunization, anti Id J 606 antibodies were purified by affinity chromatography on J 606 conjugated to Sepharose, followed by thorough absorption of the anti J 606 antibodies with FLOPC 21-Sepharose.

ELISA

Microtiter plates were coated with 2 μg/ml of the relevant protein (J 606 or ABPC 4). Binding of the anti-Id J 606 serum was inhibited with myeloma proteins or levans. Bound anti-Id J 606 was detected using alkaline phosphatase conjugated goat anti rabbit IgG (Cappel/Worthington, Malvern, PA).

Immunofluorescence

Sections of frozen small intestine were fixed in 95% alcohol at room temperature. A two step procedure was performed for staining gut plasma cells. The first step reagent was the anti-IgG3 (anti-Id) followed by an FITC-goat anti-rabbit IgG (Cappel/Worthington) as the second step antibody. For inhibition experiments, myeloma proteins were added at 5 μg/ml and levans at 100 μg/ml. For double staining, plasma cells were also stained with TRITC-goat anti mouse-kappa, -IgG, -IgA or -IgM (Cappel/Worthington).

RESULTS

Characterization of the anti-Id J 606 serum

The specificity of the anti-Id J 606 was tested by an enzyme linked immunoassay (ELISA) as shown in Table 1. The data show that 0.09 μg/ml of J 606 inhibits 50% binding while more than 100 μg/ml of FLOPC 21 failed to inhibit. Except for ABPC 4, the other isotypes do not inhibit the binding at a concentration of >100 μg/ml. The anti-Id J 606 reacts strongly with ABPC 4 (IgA) which has the same antigen specificity as J 606 (IgG3) and which differs by only one amino acid in the V_H region. The V_L of J 606 and ABPC 4 are also closely related (2). Figures 1A, 1B and 1C show staining of GLT with anti-J 606 and inhibition with the J 606 and ABPC-4 proteins, respectively.

Anti-Id J 606 does not bind UPC 10 (IgG2a) which recognizes β(2-6) poly fructosan and shares an idiotype with ABPC 4 but not with J 606 (3).

Figure 2 shows only slight inhibition of anti-Id J 606 binding to J 606 by β(2-1) and β(2-6) poly fructosans. Using ABPC 4 instead of J 606, there is no inhibition by these haptens (data not shown).

Table 1. ELISA assay of anti-Id J 606 binding to different myeloma proteins

Myeloma	Ig class	50% inhibition (μg/ml)
J 606	IgG3	0.09
FLOPC 21	IgG3	>100
ABPC 4	IgA	1.0
TEPC 15	IgA	>100
MOPC 21	IgG1	>100
UPC 10	IgG2a	>100
MOPC 195	IgG2b	>100
MOPC 104E	IgM	>100

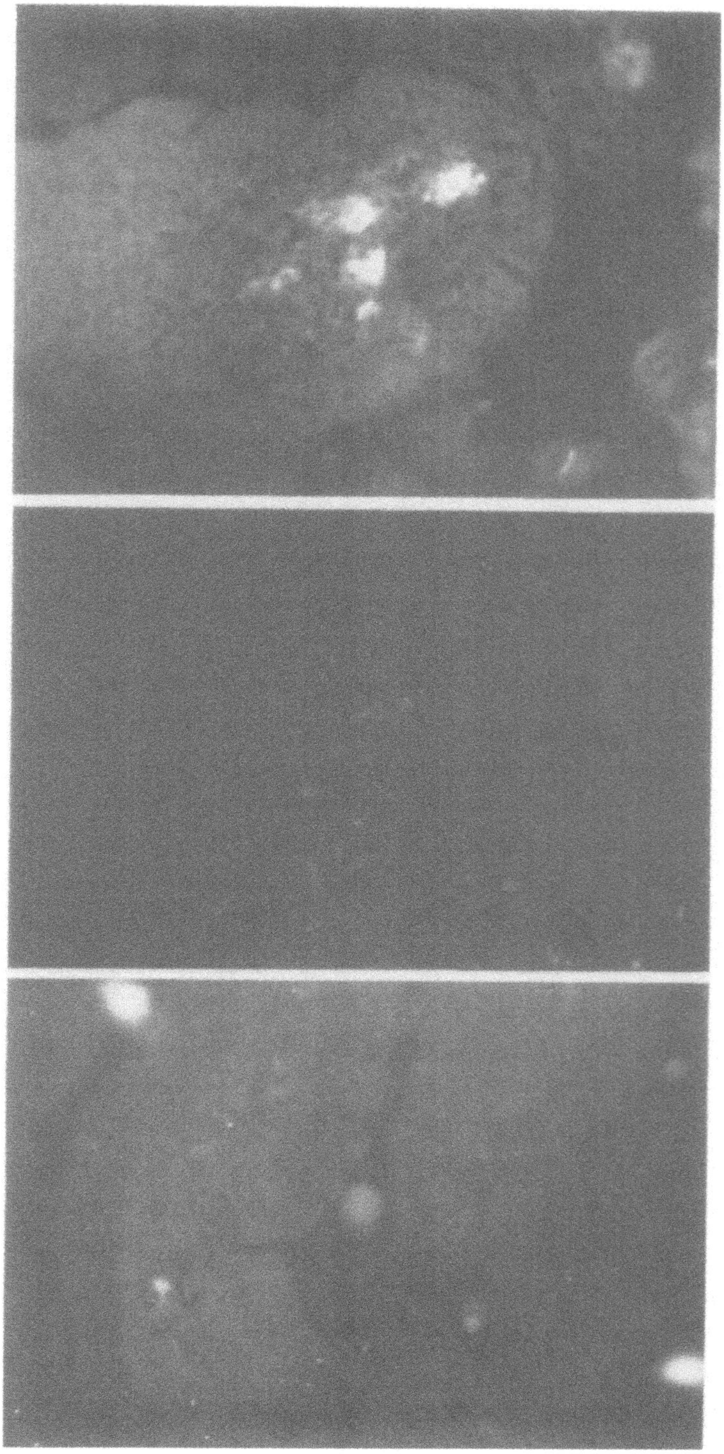

Figure 1. (A) Frozen gut section stained with anti-Id J 606; (B) Frozen gut section stained with anti-Id J 606 in the presence of J 606; and (C) Frozen gut section stained with anti-Id J 606 in the presence of ABPC 4.

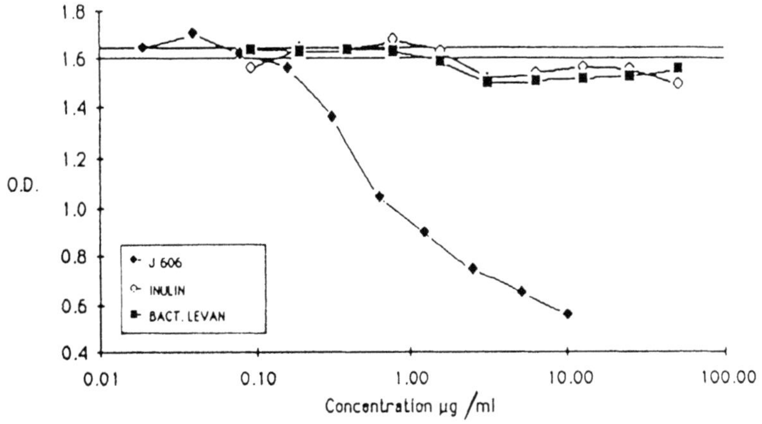

Figure 2. Inhibition of anti-Id J 606 binding to J 606 by levans and J 606.

Taken together, the data suggest that the anti-Id J 606 recognizes predominantly the V-region framework of J 606 and ABPC 4 and not the idiotypes involved in the antigen binding site.

Quantification of Id J 606 positive plasma cells in the intestinal lamina propria by immunofluorescence

Plasma cells of the small intestine of CBA/J, CBA/N and F1 (C57BLxDBA2) mice which stained with anti-Id J 606 and anti-mouse kappa were enumerated. All cells stained by anti-Id J 606 were also stained by anti-mouse kappa chain. As shown in Table 2, betwen 17 and 23% of intestinal plasma cells are Id J 606 positive. The anti-Id sera detcted both V_H and V_L of J 606, and thus these percentages include cells bearing either V_H and/or V_L related to J 606.

Table 2. Id J 606 plasma cells in gut lamina propria

Strain	Ig^+ cells	Id 606^+ cells	%
CBA/J	1862	434	23.3
CBA/N	2084	379	18.2
C57BL/DBA2	1319	225	17.1

DISCUSSION

The rabbit anti-Id J 606 employed in this study is specific for the V_L and V_H regions of J 606, and the idiotypes are likely to be in the framework and not in the hypervariable regions. The antisera has little, if any reactivity with idiotypic determinants involved in the antigen binding site, at least as measured by levan inhibition studies. The slight inhibition of the anti-Id J 606 by haptens probably represents a private idiotype of J 606 since an assay employing ABPC 4 showed no inhibition, and ABPC 4 has the same specificity as J 606 and very closely related V_H and V_L chains (2). Thus, although it is not possible to completely rule out activity of anti-Id J 606 for the D and J segments this seems unlikely.

The anti-Id J 606 stained 23% of GALT plasma cells in CBA/J mice and 17-18% in CBA/N and F1 (C57BLxDBA2) mice. There is a preferential isotype-idiotype association for the response to T-2 antigens (such as inulin and levan) in the spleen, where IgG3 is the preferred isotype (1). As there is little IgG3 Fc staining and mRNA for the heavy chain of IgG3 in the GALT, our findings show that the preferential association noted between the J 606 idiotype and TI-2 antigens is probably a manifestation of regulatory mechanisms that act on B cells rather than a preferential paring of specific V_H regions with the C_H of IgG3.

Moreover, the presence of approximately 18% Id J 606 bearing IgA plasma cells in CBA/N mice indicates that this is a predominant system in the selection among the available V_H and V_L. This data confirms those of other investigators who found that J 606 V_H is expressed in 5-10% of splenic B cells of different strains (4), and argues against the hypothesis that B cells in CBA/N mice use different V-region repertoire (5).

It would be of interest to determine if Id J 606 positive cells can also be stained by labeled levans. If so, that would imply that CBA/N B cells can be primed by TI-2 antigens and proliferate, but have blocked immunoglobulin secretion, as suggested by other investigators (6,7). Another possibility is that B cells can mature and secrete immunoglobulin only in the gut environment (8). If labeling of cells with antigen does not occur either in CBA/N or in normal mice, it would indicate that the same V_H (or a family of closely related V_H) results in different specificities as a consequence of somatic mutations, and these are of prime importance for the diversity of the repertoire. Experiments to test this hypothesis are in progress.

CONCLUSIONS

Plasma cells recognized by an anti-Id J 606 serum are dominant in the mouse GALT (23% of the kappa bearing cells). Myeloma proteins included in the J 606 V_H family have specificity for TI-2 antigens. The preferential isotype of the serum response to certain TI-2 antigens such as inulin and levan is IgG3, while the same antigens elicit predominantly an IgA response in the gut. The predominance of Id J 606 in IgA bearing plasma cells in the GLT, while the Id J 606 is mainly associated with IgG3 in other sites, demonstrates that there is no preferential V_H-C_H pairing. CBA/N mice which do not manifest a serum response to TI-2 antigens have similar numbers of Id J 606 IgA positive cells in the gut lamina propria. This suggests that CBA/N B lymphocytes use the same V_H repertoire as other mouse strains. More work is needed to determine whether the Id J 606 expression is related only to TI-2 antigens, and whether the J 606 Id positive cells in the gut of CBA/N and other strains of mice bind the corresponding antigen.

REFERENCES

1. Mosier, D.E. and Subbarao, B., Immunol. Today 3, 217, 1982.
2. Johnson, N., Slankard, H., Paul, L. and Hood, L., J. Immunol 128, 302, 1982.
3. Lieberman, R., Potter, M., Humphrey, W., Mushinski, E.B. and Vrana, M., J. Exp. Med. 142, 106, 1975.
4. Basta, P., Kubagawa, H., Kearney, J.F. and Briles, D.E., J. Immunol. 130, 2423, 1983.
5. Slack, J., Der Balian, G., Nahm, M. and Davie, J.M., J. Exp. Med. 151, 853, 1980.
6. Ohriner, W.D. and Cebra, J.J., Eur. J. Immunol. 15, 906, 1985.
7. Teale, J.M., J. Immunol. 130, 72, 1983.
8. Eldridge, J.H., Kiyono, H., Michalek, S.M. and McGhee, J.R., J. Exp. Med. 157, 789, 1983.
9. Brodeur, P.H. and Riblet, R., Eur. J. Immunol. 14, 92, 1984.

ISOLATION OF PEYER'S PATCH T CELL SUBSETS INVOLVED IN ISOTYPE SPECIFIC IMMUNOREGULATION

K.W. Beagley, H. Kiyono*, C.D. Alley**, J.H. Eldridge and J.R. McGhee

Departments of of Microbiology, *Oral Biology and **Cell Biology and Anatomy, University of Alabama at Birmingham, Birmingham, AL USA

INTRODUCTION

Antigenic stimulation of the gut-associated lymphoreticular tissue (GALT) in the mouse results in an immune response at mucosal sites distant from the gut which is dominated by antibody of the IgA isotype. The morphology of murine Peyer's patch and the composition of the resident lymphoid and accessory cells is now well established. T and B lymphocytes are found in distinct zones beneath a specialized epithelial tissue. The B cell areas contain numerous IgA precursor B cells and within the T cell zone all T cell subsets are present (Lyt 1^+/L3T4$^+$, Lyt 2^+ and T contrasuppressor cells). Contrary to earlier reports, Peyer's patch cells prepared by enzymatic digestion also contain accessory cells, e.g., both macrophages and dendritic cells.

To date little is known of the regulatory mechanisms involved in promoting the IgA isotype, including specific response to orally-administered antigens. To address this we have made use of the oxidative mitogen, sodium periodate ($NaIO_4$), to enrich for PP T cell and accessory cell populations which enhance IgA responses. Coculture of periodate induced dendritic cell-T cell clusters with either PP B lymphocytes or bone marrow mononuclear cells resulted in a significant enhancement of IgA production over control cultures.

MATERIALS AND METHODS

Preparation of Peyer's patch cell suspensions

Peyer's patches from C3H/HeJ mice were dissociated using the neutral protease Dispase® according to published methods (1).

Isolation of periodate induced dendritic cell-T cell (DC-T) clusters

Peyer's patch cell suspensions obtained by enzymatic disaggregation were treated with the oxidative mitogen sodium periodate (2) and incubated overnight in complete RPMI-1640 supplemented with 10% fetal calf serum (FCS) at 10×10^6 cells per well in 24 well plates. The resulting cell clusters were isolated on a continuous density gradient of BSA (p 1.008-1.030) (2).

Purification of Peyer's patch B lymphocytes

C3H/HeN Peyer's patch cell suspensions obtained by enzymatic disaggregation were "panned" on petri dishes coated with the IgG fraction of goat anti-mouse immunoglobulin antisera (3), followed by treatment with anti-Thy 1.2 plus complement.

Purification of bone marrow cells

Femurs and tibiae were removed and the marrow cavities flushed with RPMI-1640 without FCS and 2 ME after removal of the epiphyses. The cells were aspirated off the spicules and further separated over Ficoll-hypaque, washed twice and suspended in complete RPMI 1640 plus 10% FCS (4).

Co-culture experiments

Peyer's patch B cells or bone marrow mononuclear cells, purified as described above, were suspended in complete RPMI-1640 supplemented with 10% FCS and 1×10^6 cells in 500 µl was dispensed to wells in 24 well plates. Peyer's patch DC-T cluster cells were treated with anti-Ig plus complement to remove residual B cells and added to PP B cells or bone marrow mononuclear cells and the cultures incubated at 37°C in Mishell-Dutton gas mixture for 7 days. After 7 days, immunoglobulin in the culture supernatants was assayed by isotype-specific radioimmunoassay (1).

Production of T cell hybridomas from DC-T cluster T cells

Peyer's patch DC-T clusters were treated with anti-Ig plus complement and then incubated for 3 days in complete RPMI 1640 plus 10% FCS. Activated T cells from the clusters were isolated by flotation on a BSA cushion (d 1.078). These cells were fused with the HAT sensitive T lymphoma R1.1 at a 1:1 ratio. Positive wells were cloned by limiting dilution and supernatants from the resulting hybridomas were assayed for the ability to enhance polyclonal IgA production in C3H/HeJ Peyer's patch cultures.

RESULTS

Cell clusters isolated from sodium periodate treated Peyer's patch cells comprise 12% of the starting cell population (range 8%-15%). Table 1 shows the surface phenotypes of whole Peyer's patch and periodate induced cluster cells as determined by FACS analysis. Cells in the cluster population are enriched 3-4 fold in cells of the L3T4$^+$ phenotype (T helper) compared to whole Peyer's patch cells.

Because the cluster populations contained residual B cells which could contribute to immunoglobulin production in co-culture experiments, these populations were treated twice with anti-Ig plus complement before addition to PP B cells or bone marrow mononuclear cells. This resulted in a 95% reduction in background IgA production by cluster populations (data not shown). In some experiments cluster populations were cultured for 3 days and the activated T cells isolated by further centrifugation on BSA (d 1.078).

Figures 1 and 2 show the effects of coculturing periodate induced cluster cells with PP B cells and bone marrow mononuclear cells. In all experiments addition of DC-T clusters to the cultures resulted in marked enhancement of polyclonal IgA production, with little enhancement seen in IgM or IgG production.

To further investigate a possible role of T cell derived isotype specific helper factor(s) in the control of immunoglobulin production, activated T cells from cluster populations were fused with the T lymphoma R1.1. T cell hybridomas were cloned by limiting dilution and supernatants from the hybridoma lines were added to whole Peyer's patch cell cultures to screen for IgA isotype-specific enhancing activity. Immunoglobulin levels in culture supernatants were measured by isotype specific radioimmunoassay. Table 2 shows the surface phenotypes of 3 T cell hybridomas which produced factors that enhanced IgA isotype production in Peyer's patch cultures.

Table 1. Surface phenotypes of Peyer's patch lymphocytes (FACS analysis)

(A) Whole PP Population		
Lyt 1^+ 37% (33-40)	sIg^+ 58% (58-59)	Ia^{k+} 63% (55-70)
Lyt 2^+ 6.5% (2-11)	$B220^+$ 48% (45-53)	Mac 1^+ 8% (6-10)
$L3T4^+$ 12% (5-19)	$sIgA^+$ 11% (6-17)	
(b) $NaIO_4$ Induced Clusters		
Lyt 1^+ 45% (42-49)	sIg^+ 44% (37-51)	Ia^{k^+} 44.2% (43-45)
Lyt 2^+ 10% (7-14)	$B220^+$ 32% (27-37)	Mac 1^+ 9% (4-24)
$L3T4^+$ 41% (37-47)	$sIgA^+$ 7.5% (4-10)	

Table 2. Hybridoma supernatants enhancing IgA synthesis in PP lymphocyte cultures

	Hybridoma	Enhancement over control values
Experiment 1	1J	>3X
	3U	>3X
	5K	>3X
	4C	>3X
	12B	>3X
	12D	>3X
Experiment 2	1J	2.5X
	3U	6X
	4C	3.2X

Surface phenotype of hybridomas

	Thy 1.2	Lyt 1	Lyt 2	L3T4	Ia^k	Fcμ	Fcγ	Fcα
1J	++	±	±	++	-	-	-	-
3U	++	-	++	±	-	-	-	-
4C	++	-	++	+	-	-	-	-

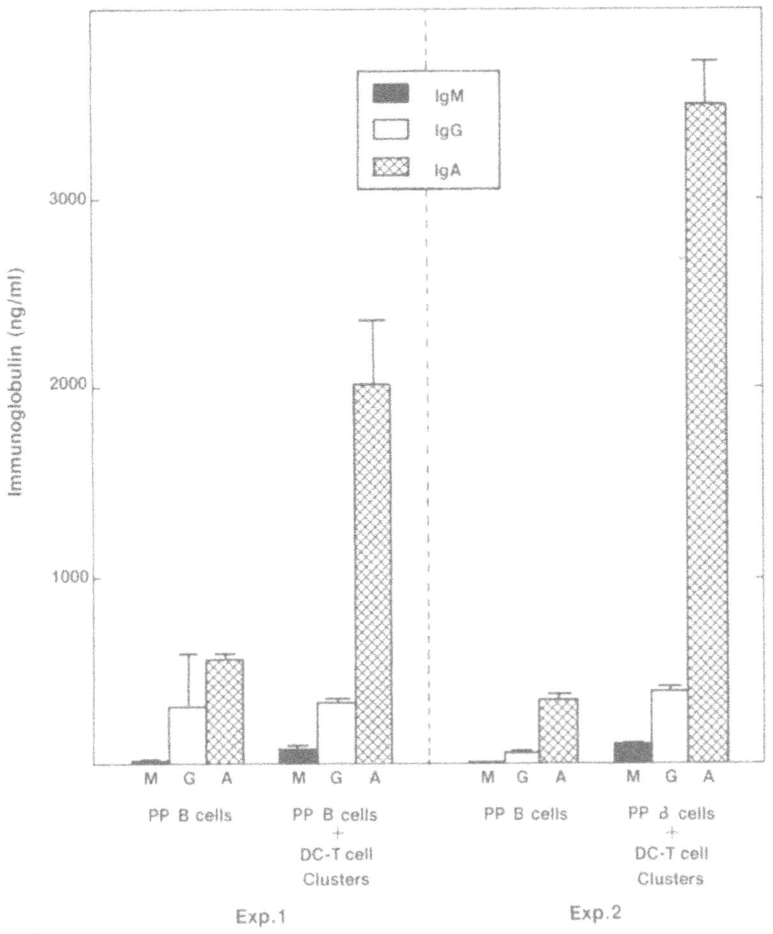

Figure 1. Sodium periodate induced PP cluster cells enhance IgA synthesis in Peyer's patch B lymphocyte cultures. 2.5×10^5 B cell-depleted cluster cells were co-cultured with 1×10^6 PP B lymphocytes for 7 days in complete medium. Supernatants were assayed for immunoglobulin by radioimmunoassay.

All 3 hybridomas stained strongly for Thy 1.2 and were also positive for L3T4 although staining for this marker appeared to be cell cycle dependent, especially in the case of hybridoma 3U. Hybridomas 3U and 4C stained strongly with anti-Lyt 2 antibody. Little staining with anti-Lyt 1 was seen with any of the 3 lines. In contrast to antigen-specific T helper hybridomas reported previously by this laboratory none of the hybridomas reported here demonstrated membrane Fc receptors for any isotype.

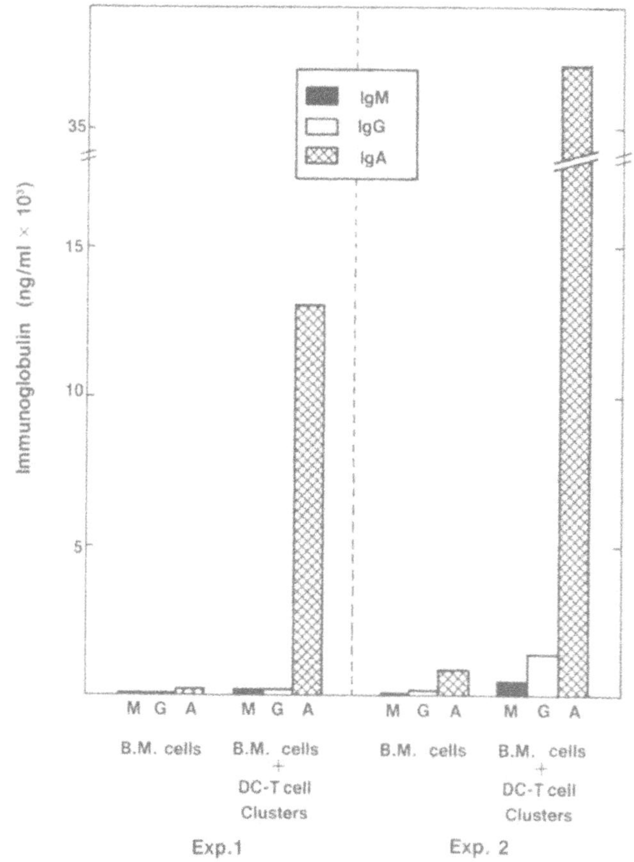

Figure 2. Sodium periodate induced PP cluster cells enhance IgA synthesis in bone marrow mononuclear cells. 1 x 10^6 cell-depleted cluster cells were co-cultured with 1 x 10^6 bone marrow mononuclear cells for 7 days in complete medium. Supernatants were assayed for immunoglobulin by radioimmunoassay.

DISCUSSION

Treatment of whole Peyer's patch cell populations with the oxidative mitogen sodium periodate resulted in the formation of cell clusters which were enriched approximately four-fold in cells of the L3T4 phenotype (T helper/inducer) and contained numerous Ia positive dendritic cells. When residual B lymphocytes were removed from this cluster population the remaining cells significantly enhanced immunoglobulin synthesis by Peyer's patch B lymphocytes and bone marrow mononuclear cells. The greatest enhancement was seen in the IgA isotype. Preliminary experiments with periodate induced clusters from murine splenic lymphocytes indicated that these cells do not enhance IgA synthesis in co-culture experiments.

T cell hybridomas derived from cluster T cells have been shown to produce factor(s) which enhance IgA production in Peyer's patch cultures. Of particular interest was the finding that none of the hybridomas described here expressed membrane Fc receptors, in contrast to our earlier findings with antigen specific T helper hybridomas. Detailed analysis of these hybridoma products will yield further information on the role of T cell factors involved in isotype-specific immunoregulation.

ACKNOWLEDGEMENTS

The results discussed in this paper were supported by U.S. P.H.S. grants AI 18958, AI 19674, DE 04217, AI 21032 and AI 21774.

REFERENCES

1. Frangakis, M.V., Koopman, W.J., Kiyono, H., Michalek, S.M. and McGhee, J.R., J. Immunol. Meth. 48, 33, 1981.
2. Spalding, D.M., Koopman, W.J., Eldridge, J.H., McGhee, J.R., Steinman, R.M., J. Exp. Med. 157, 1646, 1983.
3. Wysocki, L.J. and Sato, V.L., Proc. Natl. Acad. Sci. (USA) 75, 2844, 1978.
4. Alley, C.D., Kiyono, H. and McGhee, J.R., J. Immunol. 136, 4414, 1986.

EXPRESSION OF SUBSTANCE P AND SOMATOSTATIN RECEPTORS ON A T HELPER CELL LINE

R. Scicchitano, A.M. Stanisz, D.G. Payan, H. Kiyono,
J.R. McGhee and J. Bienenstock

The Department of Pathology, Intestinal Diseases Research
Unit and Host Resistance Program, McMaster University,
Hamilton, Ontario, Canada; the Department of Medicine,
Howard Hughes Medical Institute, University of California,
San Francisco, CA USA; and the Department of Microbiology,
University of Alabama at Birmingham, Birmingham, AL USA

INTRODUCTION

Recent evidence has demonstrated the involvement of the neuroendocrine system in immunoregulation (1,2). Several in vitro studies have shown that the function of immune cells can be altered by hormones (3) and neurotransmitters including peptides, polypeptides and biogenic amines (4,5).

Stanisz et al. (6) showed that the neuropeptides (NP) substance P (SP) and somatostatin (SOM) effect mitogen-induced cell proliferation and immunoglobulin synthesis by murine Peyer's patch (PP) and splenic lymphocytes. Somatostatin acted generally as an inhibitory peptide but SP had profound enhancing effects especially on IgA synthesis by PP.

Several studies have now shown the presence of T cells which promote IgA responses in PP (7,8). Kiyono et al. (9) have cloned T cells from murine PP which provide antigen-specific help for IgA and to a lesser extent IgM and IgG responses (Th A cells) (9). These Th A cells have been fused with the murine T lymphoma R 1.1 to produce T-T hybridoma cells which have many of the properties of the Th A clones: they bear surface receptors for IgA ($RFc\alpha^{+}$) and secrete IgA-binding factor(s) which provide antigen-specific help for IgA responses in vitro (Th HA cells) (10). None of these properties are demonstrated by the fusion partner, R 1.1.

To further study the role of neuropeptides in IgA immunoregulation we investigated the presence and properties of NP receptors on these Th HA cells.

METHODS AND RESULTS

Cytofluorimetric and radioligand analysis of NP receptors on Th HA cells

Cells were stained with fluorescein-SP (*SP) or -SOM (*SOM) and the proportion of cells which bound NP determined by flow cytometry. Th HA cells bound both *SP and *SOM (54.3 ± 6.5% and 30.6 ± 0.9%, respectively). Dual parameter analysis showed that binding was solely to the small cell population. ^{125}I-NP binding experiments confirmed that there was specific binding for both NP (Table 1). This binding was temperature-dependent, reached a plateau by 30 min incubation at 4°C and was inhibitable by incubation with excess (10^{-5}M) unlabeled NP.

Cell proliferation and RFcα expression

Incubation of Th HA cells with SOM or SP (10^{-7}M) for 6 h increased cell proliferation as determined by ^{3}H-thymidine uptake (Fig. 1). When cells were incubated with NP for 72 h, SOM decreased, while SP had no significant effect on cell proliferation.

Table 1. (^{125}I)-SP and (^{125}I)-SOM binding

	Total CPM Bound	*Specific CPM Bound	Percent Specific Binding
SP	3878 ± 2620	993 ± 258	35.8 ± 4.4
SOM	10865 ± 1003	4544 ± 117	42.3 ± 3.2

Values are mean ± SE of 3 experiments performed in duplicate. Cells (5 x 10^6/0.2 ml) were incubated with (^{125}I)-NP (10^{-9} M) for 45 min at 4°C.
*Specific binding =

$$\frac{[\text{CPM bound in absence cold NP}] - [\text{CPM bound in presence cold NP } (10^{-5}\text{M})]}{\text{CPM bound in absence cold NP}} \times 100$$

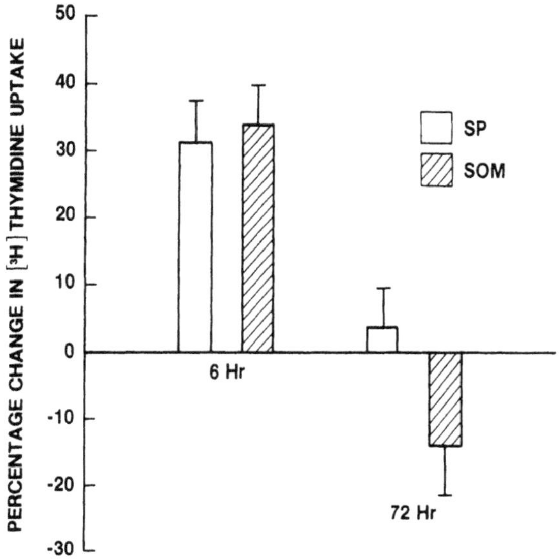

Figure 1. Values are mean ± SD of 3 experiments (12 wells per experiment). Cells (2.5×10^5/0.2 ml) were incubated in 96 well plates in absence or presence of neuropeptides (10^{-7}M) for 6 or 72 h. ^{3}H-thymidine was added for 6 and 24 h, respectively.

The proportion of cells which expressed RFcα was determined by flow cytometry. Cells were cultured for 18-24 h in the presence or absence of NP (10^{-7}M). In all experiments, SOM significantly decreased the percentage of cells which expressed RFcα ($p < .05$) while SP had no significant effect (Table 2).

Antigen specific splenic plaque forming cell responses

The HA cells were cultured in the absence or presence of NP (10^{-7} M) for 72 h. Culture supernatants were extensively dialyzed to remove NP and then tested in vivo for their ability to promote anti-sheep red blood cell plaque forming cell responses (PFC) (Table 3).

Control Th HA supernatants enhanced the IgA, IgG and IgM PFC response to SRBC. Incubation of cells with SP did not significantly alter this effect. However, prior treatment of Th HA with SOM abolished the enhancing effect of the culture supernatant.

Table 2. Effect of neuropeptides on RFα expression

		% RFcα$^+$	
A (5)	Control	69.2 ± 1.6	p < .05
	SOM	54.0 ± 12.3	
B (4)	Control	46.6 ± 9.7	NS
	SP	42.8 ± 9.9	

Values are means ± S.E. of number experiments indicated (n). Cells (10^6/ 0.1 ml) incubated with IgA (45 μg) followed by FITC-rabbit anti-mouse IgA. Cells were incubated (18-24 h) in absence or presence of neuropeptide (10^{-7} M).

Table 3. Effect of neuropeptides on immunoglobulin synthesis

Culture Supernatant	Anti-SRBC plaques/10^6 spleen cells IgA	IgG	IgM
NIL	295	480	290
THCS*	1655	2285	1555
SP treated THCS	1230	1885	1260
SOM treated THCS	421	980	435

Values are means of two experiments performed in triplicate. Cells were cultured in absence or presence of neuropeptides (10^{-7}M) for 72 h. *Th HA culture supernatants (THCS) were extensively dialyzed to remove neuropeptides. Mice were immunized with SRBC intravenously on day 0, and given 0.2 ml of culture supernatant intravenously on day 3. Splenic anti-SRBC plaques were assessed on day 5.

CONCLUSIONS

1. Murine T-T hybridoma cells (Th HA) produced by fusion between R 1.1 T lymphoma and cloned Peyer's patch T helper cells that promote IgA responses (Th A cells), express specific receptors for substance P and somatostatin.

2. Substance P enhanced cell proliferation. Somatostatin initially enhanced (6 h) then decreased cell proliferation (72 h).

3. Somatostatin decreased RFcα expression. Substance P had no significant effect on RFcα expression.

4. Somatostatin abolished and SP had no significant effect on the enhancing effect of in vivo administration of culture supernatants on the splenic PFC responses to SRBC. This effect was not isotype specific. We concluded that the profound in vitro effect of SP on IgA synthesis may not relate to the exclusive effect of SP on T helper subpopulations in PP.

5. Both the flow cytometry data showing binding of *NP to a subpopulation of small Th HA cells, and the differential effect with time on cell proliferation, suggest that the effects of SP and SO may be cell cycle dependent.

6. Experiments such as these with cloned cell populations may provide a suitable in vitro model to study the role of neuropeptides in immunoregulation.

REFERENCES

1. Ader, R., Psychoneuroimmunology, Academic Press, New York, 1981.
2. Besedovsky, H.O., del Rey, A.E. and Sorkin, E., Immunol. Today 4, 342, 1983.
3. Comsa, J., Leonhardt, H. and Wekerle, H., Rev. Physiol. Pharmacol. 92, 169, 1982.
4. Johnson, H.M., Smith, E.M., Torres, B.A. and Blalock, J.E., Proc. Natl. Acad. Sci. USA 79, 4171, 1982.
5. Plotnikoff, N.P. and Miller, G.C., Int. J. Immunopharmacol. 5, 437, 1983.
6. Stanisz, A.M., Befus, D. and Bienenstock, J., J. Immunol. 136, 152, 1986.
7. Elson, C.O., Heck, J.A. and Strober, W., J. Exp. Med. 149, 632, 1979.
8. Richman, L.K., Graeff, A.S., Yarchoan, R. and Strober, W., J. Immunol. 126, 2079, 1981.

9. Kiyono, H., Cooper, M.D., Kearney, J.F., Mosteller, L.M., Michalek, S.M., Koopman, W.J. and McGhee, J.R., J. Exp. Med. 159, 798, 1984.
10. Kiyono, H., Mosteller-Barnum, L., Pitts, A.M., Williamson, S.I., Michalek, S.M. and McGhee, J.R., J. Exp. Med. 161, 731, 1985.

N-TERMINAL TEN AMINO ACID SEQUENCE DETERMINED FOR B-CELL DIFFERENTIATION FACTOR DERIVED FROM RABBIT BREAST MILK CELL SUPERNATANT

R.H. Reid, D.A. Axelrod, L.Y. Tseng, W.T. McCarthy, C.A. Hooper, R.C. Chung* and R.C. Seid*

Departments of Gastroenterology and *Bacterial Diseases
Walter Reed Army Institute of Research
Washington, DC USA

INTRODUCTION

The rabbit has provided a useful model for the study of mucosal immunity (1). Indeed, the bulk of the rabbit immune system lies within the gut associated lymphoid tissue. At birth, these tissues are poorly developed; however, shortly after birth, these gut associated lymphoid tissues enlarge and become capable of mounting an immune response (2). Temporally, these changes occur during breast feeding. Breast milk contains a variety of cellular elements, including T cells and B cells, as well as a predominance of macrophages, all capable of responding to polyclonal activation and antigen (3). This study defines the N-terminal 1-10 AA sequence for a naturally occurring B-cell differentiation factor arising from rabbit breast milk cells.

MATERIALS AND METHODS

Rabbit breast milk was obtained by gentle suction from lactating, 14 day post-partum, New Zealand White rabbits. The milk was spun at 1200 rpm for ten minutes. The cellular pellet was resuspended and washed twice in RPMI 1640 with 20% heat inactivated fetal calf serum, penicillin (100 units/ml), streptomycin (100 μg/ml), gentamicin (40 μg/ml), 5-flurocytosine (10 μg/ml) and L-glutamine (4 mM) (pH 7.4). 1 ml cultures containing 2 x 10^6 cells were added to Falcon 2058 tubes and incubated at 37°C and 5% CO_2 in air. After seven days of culture, supernatants were collected and pooled (for each animal used) and frozen at -20°C until used.

Rabbit Peyer's patches were aseptically removed from adult (12-16 wk old) New Zealand White rabbits and placed into Dulbecco's Modified Eagles Medium (DMEM). Peyer's patch lymphoid cells were collected by flushing the aseptically severed organs with DMEM. All final cell concentrations were made in DMEM with 10% heat inactivated fetal calf serum, penicillin (100 units/ml), streptomycin (100 μg/l) and L-glutamine (2 mM). Maximal immunoglobulin responses were obtained at a final cell density of 3×10^5 cells/ml (total volume 0.2 ml) in round-bottom microculture plates for 48 h.

Supernatant immunoglobulin concentrations were determined by enzyme-linked immunosorbent assay (ELISA) (4). Soft, 96-well round bottom microtiter plates were sensitized overnight with isotype-specific goat anti-rabbit immunoglobulin (Fc specific) in a 0.1 M carbonate buffer (pH 9.8). Plates were washed with a phosphate buffered saline solution (pH 7.4), containing 0.1% bovine serum albumin. Culture supernatants and rabbit immunoglobulin controls (IgG, IgA and IgM) were added to the plates. After 90 minutes incubation and washing, isotype specific, anti-rabbit immunoglobulins, antibodies conjugated to peroxidase were added and incubated for 60 min. The enzyme reaction was developed using an ELISA substrate (ABTS, Kikegaard-Perry, Gaithersberg, MD). "Developed" ELISA plates were read by a Dynatech MR580 ELISA reader. Experimental values were quantitated by comparison to known controls on each plate.

BMS was passed over a Biogel P300 sizing column (102 cm x 2.5 cm) in a phosphate buffered saline solution (pH 7.4). Two ml aliquots were collected and tested as above for <u>in vitro</u> induction of immunoglobulin generation. Aliquots having activity and containing protein were subjected to gel electrophoresis to determined the molecular weight of the protein.

To determine the presence of one or more proteins which induce immunoglobulin production and their molecular weights in the aliquots from the P300 column, 10 μg of protein from positive aliquots #51-60 were subjected to sodium dodecyl sulfate 8% polyacrylamide gel electrophoresis (SDS PAGE) (5).

To determine the N-terminal amino acid sequence of the major protein in aliquots having a single protein band and positive for immunoglobulin production, a 65 ng sample of protein from aliquots #56-60 was subjected to N-terminal amino acid sequence analysis by Edman degradation using a gas phase protein sequenator (6).

Peyer's patch lymphoid cells were cultured in 96 well flat-bottom microtiter plates with and without BMS and pokeweed mitogen (PWM). After 48 h of culture at 37°C, and 5% CO_2 in air, 0.1 µCi ^{3}H-thymidine (tritiated thymidine) (S.A. = 25 Ci/mmole) was added to each well and six hours later, cells were harvested on a Mash II cell harvester to 934 AH glass fiber filter. Samples were placed in glass counting vials in Scintiverse and radioactivity was counted in a Mark II liquid scintillation counter. Radioactivity was expressed as counts per minute.

RESULTS

To determine the effect of the rabbit breast milk cell supernatant (BMS) upon rabbit Peyer's patch and spleen lymphoid cells, pooled breast milk cell supernatant was added to lymphoid cell cultures at varying dilutions. Preliminary results suggested that 48 h of culture provided maximal immunoglobulin generation with the BMS at a 1:30 dilution. As can be seen in Table 1, exposure of rabbit Peyer's patch lymphoid cultures to BMS (1:30 dilution) resulted in the generation of immunoglobulins of all isotypes tested (IgG, IgA and IgM).

BMS passed over a Biogel P300 column revealed a single protein peak in sequential samples 51-60 containing 2 ml aliquots. These fractions were further analyzed by SDS PAGE and found to contain a single major protein peak at approximately 66 KD. Silver staining of similarly prepared gels did not reveal any additional protein bands (data not shown). Also, to determine if there were more than one protein present in the 66KD protein band, a 65 ng protein sample was found by amino acid sequential analysis to have the following N-terminal 1-10 AA sequence: ILE-PRO-LEU-LYS-PRO-VAL-ALA-GLY-TYR-LYS as the major protein and a minor protein contaminant with the sequence expected for bovine serum albumin. The 66 KD protein from pooled aliquots samples 56-60, at the same concentration as the BMS (1:30) was assayed using Peyer's patch cells from 3 rabbits. All three immunoglobulin isotypes (IgG, IgA and IgM) were produced by the 66KD protein as seen in Table 1. Also, individual aliquot samples 51-60 contained the polyclonal activating factor (data not shown).

Table 1. Immunoglobulin generation from rabbit Peyer's patch lymphoid cell cultures by rabbit breast milk supernatant (BMS) and BMS 66KD Protein, N[a]=3

	Immunoglobulin Generation (Mean Ig ng/ml ± 1 S.D.)		
	IgG	IgA	IgM
BMS 1:30	1138 ± 110[b]	1201 ± 101	1620 ± 98
BMS 66K Protein	960 ± 100	1120 ± 103	1490 ± 99
Media Control	10 ± 1	10 ± 2	10 ± 1

[a]N = number of animals.

[b]Mean results in ng/ml ± 1 standard deviation (S.D.) (individual rabbits tested with triplicate cultures).

To determine whether B cell activation by BMS results in blast transformation or whether BMS behaves like a B cell differentiation factor not producing blast transformation, Peyer's patch cell cultures were exposed to BMS and pokeweed mitogen (PWM) followed by ^{3}H-thymidine. ^{3}H-thymidine incorporation was measured in counts per minute. As can be seen in Table 2, PWM induced substantial ^{3}H-thymidine uptake. In contrast, BMS at three different dilutions which stimulated IgG, IgA and IgM immunoglobulin production did not stimulate ^{3}H-thymidine uptake indicating a lack of blast transformation.

DISCUSSION

This study describes the N-terminal AA sequence (ILE-PRO-LEU-LYS-PRO-VAL-ALA-GLY-TYR-LYS) for a protein factor of approximately 66 kilodaltons molecular weight which was derived from rabbit breast milk cells and induces the polyclonal B cell generation of immunoglobulins from rabbit Peyer' patch lymphoid cells. The typical polyclonal activator causes cellular proliferation; however, immunoglobulin generation to BMS is associated with only minimal ^{3}H-thymidine uptake as compared to PWM suggesting that this

Table 2. Lack of blast transformation of rabbit Peyer's patch lymphocytes by rabbit breast milk cell supernatant (BMS) compared to pokeweed mitogen (PWM)

	^{3}H-Thymidine Incorporation (Mean CPM ± S.D.[a])	
	Exp. #1	Exp. #2
Media control	168 ± 17[b]	183 ± 17
BMS 1:10	150 ± 12	120 ± 8
BMS 1:100	140 ± 11	113 ± 12
PWM 1:100	12,000 ± 800	5,040 ± 600

[a]Mean counts per minute (CPM) ± 1 standard deviation (S.D.).

[b]Mean CPM ± 1 S.D. of triplicate counts.

breast milk cell derived factor is not a growth factor. Indeed, by virtue of its polyclonal activation of the B cells tested, this factor probably represents a naturally occurring rabbit B cell differentiation factor (BCDF).

The BCDF described in the current study is different from previously described BCDF's (7-10) in that prior activation of normal B cells is not a requirement and it has a large molecular weight, 66,000 compared to 19-21,000 (11). Since T cells have been the source of other BCDF's the T cells in the milk are the most likely source of this rabbit BCDF; however, the predominant cell in milk is the macrophage (3). This BCDF may be unique to the rabbit or similar BCDF's may be found in the milk cell supernatants of other mammalian species such as human and mouse.

CONCLUSIONS

1. Rabbit breast milk cell supernatant contains a protein factor which induces polyclonal B cell immunoglobulin production from Peyer's patch lymphoid cells.

2. The factor functions without B cell activation and proliferation.

3. This 66 KD molecular weight B cell differentiation factor has the following N-terminal 1-10 AA sequence: ILE-PRO-LEU-LYS-PRO-VAL-ALA-GLY-TYR-LYS.

REFERENCES

1. Befus, A.D. and Bienenstock, J., in Animal Models of Immunological Processes, (Edited by Hay, J.B.), p, 167, Academic Press, New York, 1982.
2. Henry, C., Faulk, W.P., Kuhn, L., Yoffee, J.M. and Fudenberg, H.H., J. Exp. Med. 131, 1200, 1970.
3. Parmely, M.J., Beer, A.E. and Billingham, R.E., J. Exp. Med. 144, 58, 1976.
4. Engvall, E. and Perlmann, P., Immunochemistry 8, 871, 1971.
5. Laemmli, U.K., Nature (London) 277, 680, 1970.
6. Hewick, R.A., Hunkapiller, M.W., Hood, L.E. and Dreyer, W.J., J. Biol. Chem. 56, 790, 1981.
7. Okada, M., Sakaguchi, N., Yoshimura, N., Hara, H., Yamamura, Y. and Kishimoto, T., J. Exp. Med. 583, 590, 1983.
8. Yoshizaki, K., Nakaguwa, T., Kaieda, T., Muraguchi, A., Yamamura, Y., and Kishimoto, T., J. Immunol. 128, 1296, 1982.
9. Hirano, T., Teranishi, T., Lin, B.H. and Onoue, K., J. Immunol. 133, 798, 1984.
10. Teranishi, T., Hirano, T., Lin, B.H. and Onoue, K., J. Immunol. 133, 3062, 1984.
11. Hirano, T., Taga, T., Nakano, N., Yasukawa, K., Kashiwimura, S., Shimiza, K., Nakajima, K., Pyun., K.H. and Kishimoto, T., Proc. Natl. Acad. Sci. USA 82, 5490, 1985.

A NOVEL PRE-B CELL PRECURSOR: PHENOTYPIC CHARACTERIZATION AND DIFFERENTIATION INDUCTION BY DENDRITIC CELL-T CELL MIXTURES

D.M. Spalding and J.A. Griffin

Division of Clinical Immunology and Rheumatology, and
Departments of Medicine, Microbiology and Biochemistry,
University of Alabama at Birmingham and the Birmingham
Veterans Administration Hospital, Birmingham, Alabama USA

INTRODUCTION

Recently, culture systems have been developed which support the growth of multipotential stem cells (1), pro-B cells (2), pre-B cells (3) or mixtures of several early stages (4,5), and these have begun to improve our understanding of very early stages of B lymphocyte differentiation. In some of these systems, differentiation to a subsequent developmental stage can be induced, but multiple levels of differentiation have not been observed under conditions suitable for detailed analysis of phenotypic and genotypic events during these maturation processes.

We have previously described the establishment of cultures of non-transformed cell populations that have a pre-B cell phenotype and can be induced to differentiate *in vitro* in response to a stimulus provided by mixtures of dendritic cells and activated T cells (DC-T) (6). After induction, these pre-B cells increase their transcription of all light and heavy chain genes, begin to synthesize heavy and light chain polypeptides, and finally secrete immunoglobulin. The pattern of isotypes secreted by these cells varies depending upon the source of the inducing DC-T population, with exclusive secretion of IgM when induced by spleen DC-T and preferential secretion of IgG and IgA isotypes after induction by Peyer's patches (PP) DC-T populations. We now report the identification of B lineage cells with unique morphologic and phenotypic features compatible with the pre-pre-B cell stage as described by Muller-Sieburg, et al. (5). Even this very early B lineage cell can be induced by mixtures of DC and T cells to enter the B cell differentiation pathway to the ultimate secretions of antibody.

METHODS

Preparation and maintenance of pre-B precursor cell lines

Cell lines were prepared as previously described (6) from spleens of 4-6 week old nude mice, except that surface immunoglobulin-bearing B cells were depleted by panning the spleen cell suspension on anti-mouse light chain coated petri dishes. The non-B cell population was cultured at 1 x 10^6 cells/ml in WEHI-Conditioned Media (WEHI-CM) which included RPMI 1640 media containing 10% FCS, 50 μg/ml gentamicin, 2 mM L-glutamine and 10% (vol/vol) WEHI supernatants prepared as described (3). After 3-4 days in culture, non-adherent cells were removed and replated in fresh WEHI-CM at 2.5 x 10^5 cells/ml, 1.5 ml well. Cells were passed in this fashion every three days and were generally used in experients between the 10th and 20th passages.

Preparation of mixtures of DC and activated Ly-1 T cells (DC-T)

Methods for the preparation of the various mixtures of DC-T used in these studies was identical to those described in detail previously (6,7). Briefly, DC-T were prepared either from $NaIO_4$-treated, B cell depleted spleen or PP cell suspensions or from populations of DC prepared by previously described methods (8,9) and $NaIO_4$-treated T cells prepared by nylon wool column purification or by panning on either Thy 1.2 or Ly-1 (Becton Dickinson, Sunnyvale, CA) coated petri dishes.

Culture conditions

WEHI-CM-maintained cell lines were harvested, washed twice in 50 ml of RPMI 1640 and cultured at 1.5 x 10^5 cells/ml/well in 24 well plates with varying concentrations of different DC-T populations in RPMI 1640 containing 10% FCS, 2 mM L-glutamine, 50 μg/ml gentamicin and 2 μg/ml Concanavalin A. After varying intervals of time cultures were harvested, cells and supernatants separated by centrifugation, and cells were processed for immunofluorescence, while supernatants were assayed for IgM, IgG and IgA by isotype-specific RIA previously described in detail (8,10).

Immunofluorescence studies

Surface and cytoplasmic staining for IgM, IgG and IgA were performed as previously described (6). In addition, surface and cytoplasmic staining for B220 antigen were performed using 14.8 (11) kindly provided by Dr. M.D. Cooper as the first layer antibody and a fluorescein-labeled, rat anti-mouse antibody (Cappel Labs) as the second antibody. Surface staining was also performed with fluorescein-labeled anti-Thy 1.2 (Becton Dickinson) and anti-Ia^d (Becton-Dickinson) with a second layer of fluorscein-labeled goat anti-mouse immunoglobulin (Southern Biotechnological Associates, Birmingham, AL).

RESULTS

Characterization of pre-pre-B cell lines

The culture conditions established as described in Methods resulted in cultures with reproducible growth patterns. The majority of cells died during the first five days of culture after which residual cells proliferated. During the first two-four weeks in culture cell counts rose steadily, and the morphology of the population became progressively more homogeneous, such that by 32 days in culture most cells had a large nuclei and a granular cytoplasm (Fig. 1A). When the cell lines had been in culture for one to two months, cell numbers plateaued and proliferation matched cell death. By four months most cultures had begun to decline and could not be maintained in WEHI-CM.

Surface and cytoplasmic staining of three different cell lines were completely negative for μ, γ and α heavy chain, and k and λ light chain. B220 surface staining was also negative. However, 60-70% of cells from different cell lines (Fig. 1B) were positive for cytoplasmic B220. These cells also had undetectable surface staining for Thy 1.2 and Ia^d. Therefore, this population of large cells with phenotype cIg^-, sIg^-, $sB220^-$, $cB220^+$, Thy 1.2^- and Ia^- cells represent a pre-pre-B cell stage similar to one described by Muller-Sieburg et al. (5).

Southern blot analysis of pre-pre-B cell DNA exhibited no rearrangement compared with germline sequences of the immunoglobulin Cμ heavy chain. By Northern blot analysis uninduced pre-pre-B cells showed no Cμ RNA, but after 24 hours induction with spleen DC-T cells Cμ RNA appeared (manuscript in preparation).

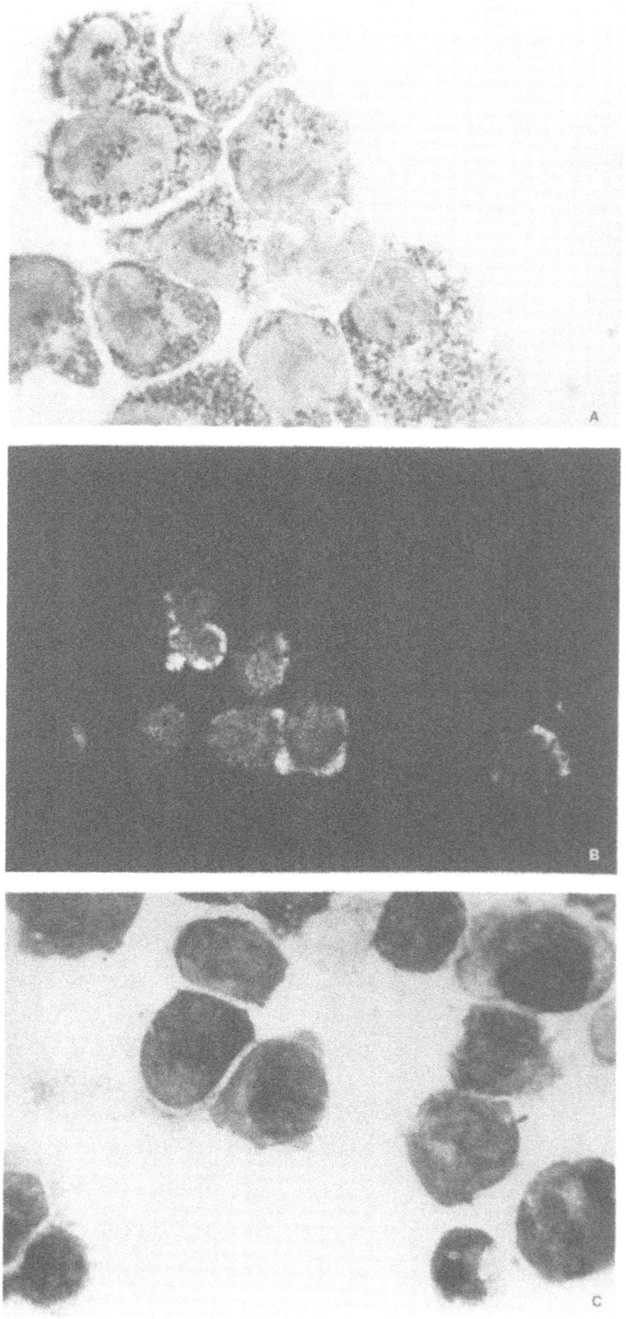

Figure 1. (A) Wright stain of a cytocentrifuge preparation of PF16 cells after 32 d in culture (7th passage). Note one residual myeloid cell. By 10th passage all cells had a granular cytoplasm. (B) Cytoplasmic stain of a cytocentrifuge preparation of PF16 cells. First antibody was 14.8 (a monoclonal anti-B220 antibody) with a second antibody of fluoresceinated rat anti-mouse antibody. Control slide with labeled antibody alone was completely negative. Note perinuclear positivity in the majority of the cells. (C) Wright stain of a cytocentrifuge preparation of cells taken from a co-cultivation of PF16 with PP DC-T. PP DC-T control had inadequate numbers of cells to visualize. Note dramatic change in morphology after induction.

Induction of pre-pre-B cells by DC-T

Since we had recently demonstrated that non-transformed pre-B cells could be induced to differentiate by mixtures of DC and T cells (6), we next determined whether or not an earlier B lineage cell could also respond to signals delivered by DC-T. Initially, we monitored cell surface expression of B220 after intervals of co-cultivation of pre-pre-B cells with DC-T. We cultured 1.5×10^5 pre-pre-B cells (PF16 line) with 5×10^4 PP DC-T for 0, 4 , 22 and 46 hours. A rapid increase occurred in the percentage of cells expressing B220 on the surface: 0% at 0 h to 6.6% at 4 h, 40% at 22 h and 49% at 46 h. The rapid increase in expression from 0-22 h occurred in the absence of cell proliferation.

There was a distinct change in the morphology of cells in induced cultures. We performed Wright stains before and after four days of co-cultivation of PF16 with PP DC-T culture. During that time the numbers of induced cells more than doubled, while the non-induced PF16 decreased to <15% of starting numbers. PP DC-T cultured alone decreased to < 20% of starting numbers. Approximtely 75% of the cells acquired lymphoid or lymphoblastoid morphology during four days of induction (Fig. 1C). Experiments with spleen DC-T and PF16 gave a similar result.

Finally, we examined changes in immunoglobulin synthesis after induction. In the PF16 cells induced with PP DC-T cytoplasmic staining for μ chain first appeared at 46 hours, a time at which γ, α, and light chain were essentially undetectable. After 69 hr in culture staining for all isotypes in the cytoplasm was weakly positive (Fig. 2). In addition to synthesis of immunoglobulin we assayed for secreted immunoglobulin at varying time intervals after initiation of co-cultivation (Table 1). Terminal differentiation, as reflected by secretion, followed the initial appearance of immunoglobulin synthesis by 3-4 days.

Differential capacity of PP DC-T versus spleen DC-T to induce differentiation in pre-pre-B cells

In our previous studies of pre-B cell differentiation, DC-T from PP had a broader range of inductive potential than did spleen DC-T. We undertook similar studies with these pre-pre-B cell populations. Both spleen and PP DC-T could induce differentiation to IgM secretion, but IgG and IgA secretion required PP DC-T be the source of the inducing stimulus (Table 2). However, the pattern of isotype secretion was predominantly IgM

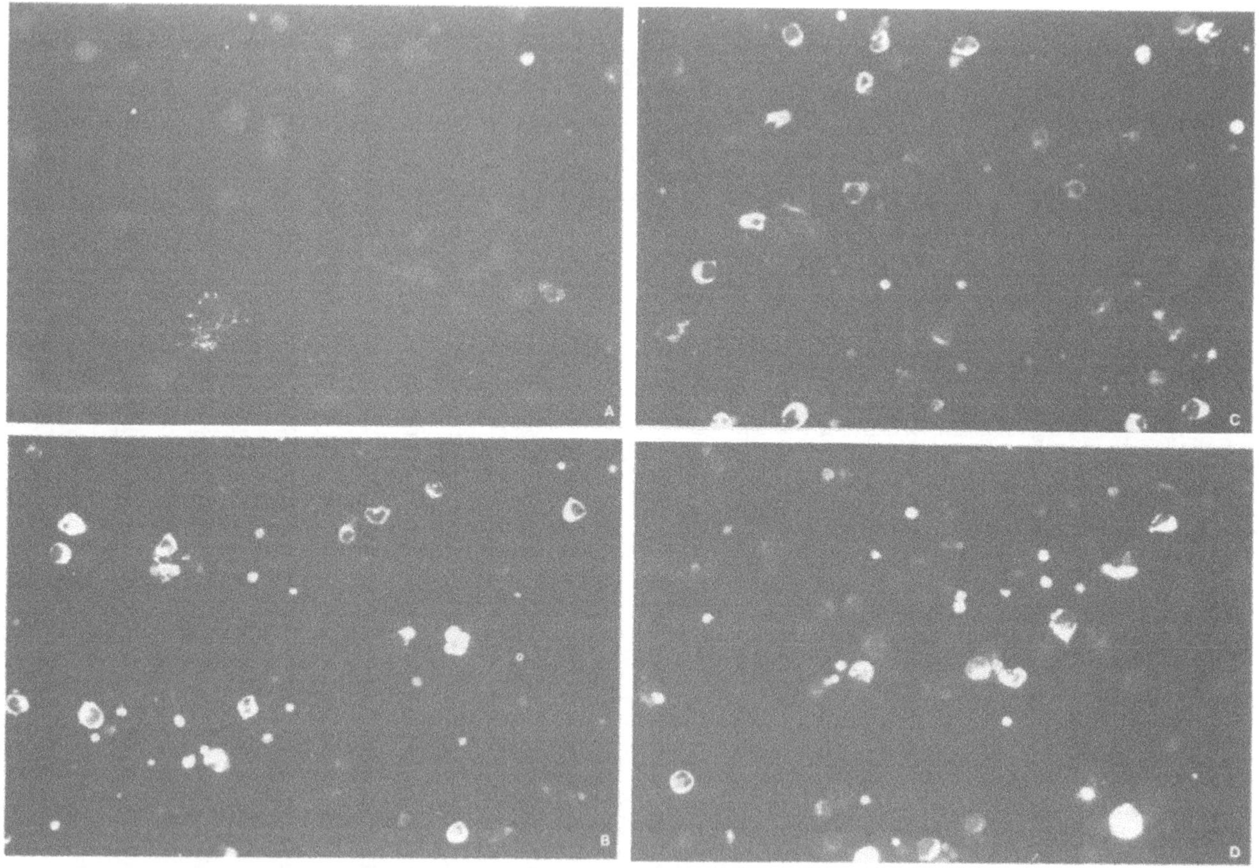

Figure 2. Cytoplasmic immunofluorescence of PF16 cells after induction with PP DC-T. (A) IgM after 12 h of co-cultivation (note complete absence of cytoplasmic staining; staining for IgG and IgA were also completely negative at 22 h). (B-D) After 69 h of co-cultivation (note positive staining for IgM in 35% of cells (2B), IgG in 25% of cells (2C) and IgA in 14% of cells (2D) for a total of 74% of all cells with positive immunofluorescence (essentially no double staining cells were seen when two-color immunofluorescence with different isotypes were performed).

Table 1. Time course of antibody secretion by pre-pre-B cells after induction by DC-T*

	IgM (ng/ml)	IgG (ng/ml)	IgA (ng/ml)
PF16 + PP DC-T			
4 hr	< 125	< 12.5	< 12.5
23 hr	< 125	< 12.5	< 16.3
46 hr	< 125	16.7	63.4
69 hr	436	120	172
6 day	2212	700	277
7 day	5234	1197	477
PF16 Alone			
4 hr	< 125	< 12.5	< 12.5
46 hr	< 125	< 12.5	< 12.5
69 hr	< 125	< 12.5	< 12.5
PP DC-T Alone			
4 hr	< 125	< 12.5	< 12.5
46 hr	< 125	< 12.5	< 12.5

* PF16 cells, 1.5×10^5 cells/ml/well, were cultured with PP DC-T, 5×10^4 cells/ml/well, in complete media for varying time intervals. Supernatants were harvested and assayed for IgM, IgG and IgA.

with significantly less IgG and IgA than that seen previously with pre-B cell lines (Table 3).

We also assessed secretion patterns of cells which came into physical contact with the inducing DC-T mixtures. We had previously reported enhanced differentiation in pre-B cells that formed clusters with DC-T verus those that did not cluster. This was true for pre-pre-B cells as well (Table 4). Almost 10-fold more immunoglobulin was secreted by cells that were incorporated into clusters within the first day of co-cultivation of pre-pre-B cells with DC-T. With additional time, the single cell population was progressively more competent to complete differentiation to the stage of secretion of immunoglobulin, indicating that continual contact between B cells and DC-T was not required.

Table 2. Spleen and PP DC-T induce different differentiation pathways[a]

DC-T	IgM (ng/ml)	IgG (ng/ml)	IgA (ng/ml)
PF16 + SP DC-T (5×10^4)	30000	334	328
PF16 + PP DC-T (5×10^4)	32175	4525	1835

[a]PF16 cells, 1.5×10^5, were cultured with spleen or PP DC-T for 7 days followed by collection of supernatants and RIA for IgM, IgG and IgA. Background secretion of immunoglobulin, by DC-T alone was < 5% of induced cultures for spleen and < 25% of induced cultures for PP. Note that although quantities of total immunoglobulin secreted varied between experiments on different days the same pattern of isotype profile was seen throughout all experiments.

Table 3. Induction of PF16 cells by different mixtures of DC and T cells[a]

	IgM (ng/ml)	IgG (ng/ml)	IgA (ng/ml)
PPDC-PP Lyl T			
5×10^4	13,630	2,007	1,207
2.5×10^4	10,611	1,264	571
1.25×10^4	4,418	340	--
PPDC-Sp Lyl T			
5×10^4	5,525	443	548
2.5×10^4	3,884	228	170
1.25×10^4	2,505	169	87
Sp DC-Sp Lyl T			
5×10^4	1,581	96	21
2.5×10^4	1,594	111	13
1.25×10^4	470	16	<12.5

[a]PF16 cells, 1.5×10^5 cells/ml/well, cultured with DC-T prepared from enriched DC populations from SP or PP and T cells from SP or PP prepared by panning on Lyl-coated petri dishes. Background secretion by DC-T alone was generally < 5% of that from induced cultures.

Table 4. Immunoglobulin secretion by clustered vs. single PF16 cells[a]

PF16 + PPDCT	IgM (ng/ml)	IgG (ng/ml)	IgA (ng/ml)
day 1			
clusters 5×10^4	1986	172	168
singles 5×10^4	263 (13%)[b]	<12.5 (<7%)	17 (10%)
day 2			
clusters 5×10^4	1242	95	162
singles 5×10^4	235 (19%)	18 (19%)	33 (20%)
day 3			
clusters 5×10^4	1509	93	164
singles 5×10^4	606 (40%)	55 (59%)	44 (21%)

[a]PF16 cells, 1.5×10^5 cells/ml/well, were cultured with 5×10^4 PP DC-T cells/ml/well. At various intervals after initiation of culture (day 1, 2 or 3), clustered cells were separated from single cells on a continuous density BSA gradient and recultured at 5×10^4 cells/ml/well in fresh complete media. Supernatants were harvested from all cultures after 7 days total culture and assayed by RIA.

[b]Represents % immunoglobulin secreted by single versus clustered cells.

DISCUSSION

In these studies, we have stably maintained in cultures a previously undefined early stage of B cell differentiation characterized by large granular cells that are genotypically characterized by unrearranged immunoglobulin genes, also lack detectable immunoglobulin RNA and are phenotypically cIg^-, sIg^-, Thy 1^-, Ia^-, $sB220^-$ but $cB220^+$. These very early B lineage cells can be induced *in vitro* to differentiate through the B cell lineage to immunoglobulin secretion. The cell lines we have described are heterogeneous; approximately 60-70% stain for B220 in the cytoplasm. In the bone marrow culture system described by Muller-Sieburg et al. (5), the population identified as Thy $1^-B^-G^-M^-$ had a limited life span in culture. Although these cells survived longer than the granulocytic and monocytic precursors, which survived only three-five days, their cell numbers had decreased by 99% in two weeks. This appeared to be due to *in vitro* differentiation of cells to $B220^+$, since 80% of the cells expressed B220 within that time. There are at least two reasons that our cultures can be maintained longer as proliferating $B220^-$ cells: (1) our nude spleen cultures lack bone marrow stroma that contains cells capable of initiating the $B220^-$ to $B220^+$ differentiation step, and (2) our $B220^-$ cultures are supported by some factor in WEHI-3B supernatant, without which they die within three days. Although this factor may be IL-3, a known product of WEHI-3B, the growth requirements may be more complex. These culture conditions select for a very immature B cell stage in spleens of athymic mice which may be too small a pool to be detected in spleens of normal mice. This stage closely resembles that of the pre-pre-B cells described by Muller-Sieburg et al. (5). Although they did not report the presence or absence of cytoplasmic B220 when defining their pre-pre-B cell stage that was Thy 1^-, our cell could be identical to or somewhat more mature than theirs. A continuum of differentiation probably exists and can be blocked at selected stages under the correct culture conditions (1,2,6,7) or by viral transformation or cell fusion.

Even though these pre-pre-B cells can be maintained at a blocked level of differentiation, they remain susceptible to differentiaton-inducing stimuli. Therefore, this system represents an ideal tool for studying *in vitro* the events that occur during B lymphcyte differentiation. The earliest definable change appears to be the expression of B220 on the surface of the pre-pre-B cells, and this occurs without cell division during the time that pre-pre-B cells and DC-T begin to physically interact through the formation of cell aggregates. During the physical interaction of cells in the induced cultures there is initiation of synthesis of μ heavy chain. The data in Table 4 suggest that induced cells leave clusters and complete differentiation to secretion of immunoglobulin as single cells.

These data, combined with our earlier findings that DC-T could induce terminal differentiation of both cytoplasmic $C\mu^+$ pre-B cells (6) and mature, surface immunoglobulin-bearing B cells (7), demonstrate that DC-T can interact with cells at several stages of maturation to initiate B cell differentiation. The isotype pattern of secreted immunoglobulin is different in cultures of cells that represent different stages of maturation, and we suspect that the level of differentiation of the B cell at that time it encounters the DC-T must be critical in determining the pathway of terminal differentiation. Additional data with three pre-B cell lines support this notion (Griffin and Spalding, manuscript in preparation).

SUMMARY

We have derived from spleens of nude mice early B lineage cell lines that are dependent upon factor(s) in supernatants of the WEHI-3B cell line. The cells are phenotypically at the pre-pre-B cell stage of differentiation. These cells are large and have basophilic granules in the cytoplasm. They are negative for cytoplasmic and surface immunoglobulin heavy or light chain, surface B220, surface Thy 1.2 and surface Ia but are positive for cytoplasmic B220. These cells at this early stage of maturation can be induced by mixtures of DC-T cells to express B220 on their surfaces and later to synthesize and ultimately to secrete immunoglobulin. These events are associated with morphologic changes in the cells to a lymphoblastoid appearance. Different pattern of immunoglobulin secretion were induced by DC-T from different tissues. The inductive event appears to occur during cell contact of pre-pre-B cells with the inducing DC-T cell mixture, but it does not appear to require IL-3. These data indicate that DC-T cell mixtures can provide signals for B cell differentiation at pre-pre-B cell stage as well as pre-B and mature B cell stage.

ACKNOWLEDGEMENTS

The authors would like to thank S. Tice, S. Johnson and J. Morgan for their expert technical assistance, M. Mullican and S. Reid for preparation of the manuscript, and VA Medical Media Service for photographs. Support for these studies was provided by a Veteran's Administration Merit Review Award (DMS), Arthritis Foundation Investigator Award (DMS), NIH AI 18958 (DMS) and NIH GM 31883 (JAG).

REFERENCES

1. McKearn, J.P., McCubrey, J. and Fagg, B., Proc. Natl. Acad. Sci. USA 82, 7414, 1985.
2. Palacios, R. and Steinmetz, M., Cell 41, 727, 1985.
3. Palacios, R., Henson, G., Steinmetz, M. and McKearn, J.P., Nature 309, 1984.
4. Denis, K.A. and Witte, O.N., Proc. Natl. Acad. Sci. USA 83, 441, 1986.

5. Muller-Sieburg, C.E., Whitlock, C.A. and Weissman, I.L., Cell 44, 653, 1986.
6. Spalding, D.M. and Griffin, J.A., Cell 44, 507, 1986.
7. Spalding, D.M., Williamson, S.I., Koopman, W.J. and McGhee, J.R., J. Exp. Med. 160, 941, 1984.
8. Spalding, D.M., Koopman, W.J., Eldridge, J.H., McGhee, J.R. and Steinman, R.M., J. Exp. Med. 157, 1646, 1983.
9. Steinman, R.M., Van Voorhis, W.C. and Spalding, D.M., in Handbook of Experimental Immunology, 4th Edition, (Edited by Weir, D.M., Herzenberg, L.A., Blackwell, C.C. and Herzenberg, L.A.), Blackwell Scientific Publications, Ltd., Edinburg (in press).
10. Spalding, D.M. and Koopman, W.J., Meth. Enzymol. 116, 146, 1985.
11. Scheid, M.P., Landreth, K.S., Tung, J.-S. and Kincade, P.W., Immunol. Rev. 69, 141, 1983.

THE ROLE OF EPITHELIAL CELLS AS ACCESSORY CELLS

L. Mayer

Division of Clinical Immunology, The Mount Sinai
School of Medicine of the University of
New York, New York, NY USA

INTRODUCTION

Mucosal immunity is characterized by poor or absent responses to most orally administered antigens (1,2). Antigens access into gut-associated lymphoid tissues (GALT) is partially inhibited by a mucous coat containing glycoproteins and secretory IgA (3). Those antigens which do gain access to GALT are thought to enter through specialized epithelial cells overlying Peyer's patches, the so-called M cell (M). Although it has been suggested that these cells bear receptors for a number of bacterial and viral antigens (4), the relative numbers of these cells are small and therefore antigen processing via such a mechanism may not be very efficient.

There have been several recent reports of the presence of Class II antigens on the surface of intestinal epithelial cells in rat (5) and human (6,7). Although the distribution of molecules appears to be polar and luminal, redistribution can be demonstrated in actively inflamed states (7). The presence of such molecules raises questions as to their role in local mucosal immune responses. Class II antigens have been described on other epithelial/endothelial cells, keratinocytes (8), endothelial cells (9), etc. with evidence for their function as accessory cells (9). Gut epithelial cells have a known function in mucosal immune responses, that being production of secretory component and transport of secretory IgA to the lumen. However, it is possible that, in view of the presence of class II antigens, these cells can serve other functions in the mucosal immune response. In this paper, we demonstrate that not only can epithelial cells function as effective accessory cells, processing and presenting antigens, but that they appear to selectively stimulate functional suppressor T cells.

MATERIALS AND METHODS

Isolation of gut epithelial cells

Surgically resected intestinal specimens were obtained sterilely from the operating room and transported in Hanks' balanced salt solution (HBSS) (Gibco, Grand Island, NY) containing penicillin/streptomycin 100 μg/ml (Gibco), gentamicin 50 μg/ml and fungizone 1%. The mucosa was carefully dissected free of submucosa, washed and minced into small 1-3 mm pieces. These pieces were incubated for 5' in 1 mM dithiothreitol (Sigma) in HBSS. After washing, mucosal pieces were incubated at 37°C in CMF-HBSS containing 100 mM EDTA (Fisher, Springfield, NJ) on a platform rotator in a siliconized flask. After 60', epithelial cells were isolated by straining mucosal pieces through a metal sieve. The flow through, containing epithelial cells and contaminating mononuclear cells, was centrifuged at 1400 RPM for 8' and the pellet resuspended in HBSS. This cell suspension was separated on a Percoll density gradient (Pharmacia Fine Chemicals - 0, 10%, 30%, 100%) to improve viability (>90%) and reduce mononuclear cell contamination (<0.1% $M1^+$, <0.1% sIg^+, <0.1% $T6^+$, 2-3% $T3^+$). In most experiments, epithelial cells were fixed with paraformaldehyde or irradiated 3000 R using a cesium source. In experiments involving antigen processing, cells were fixed only after antigen pulsing for 30-60' in culture medium (CM) (RPMI 1640, 5% human a γ serum, antibiotics) at 37°C.

Mixed lymphocyte responses (MLR)

Autologous and allogeneic MLRs were performed as previously described (10) using 1 x 10^5 peripheral blood T cells as responder cells and either irradiated epithelial cells, peripheral blood adherent cells or peripheral blood non T cells as stimulators in varying concentrations. Cultures were maintained for 120 hours at 37°C in CM. ^{3}H thymidine (2uCi) was added during the last 18 hours of culture.

Cell surface staining - immunofluorescence

Monoclonal antibodies OKT3, T4, T8, M1, T6 were obtained from Ortho

Diagnostics, Raritan, NJ. Fluorescein conjugated T4 and RD-1 conjugated T8 were obtained from Coulter, Hialeah, FL. Monoclonal antibody 9.3 recognizing cytotoxic T cells was a kind gift of Dr. John Hansen. VG2, an anti-framework DR monoclonal antibody, was generously provided by Dr. Shu Man Fu (Oklahoma Medical Research Foundation, Oklahoma City, OK). Leu 7 was obtained from Becton Dickinson. Fluorescein conjugated $F(ab')_2$ goat anti-mouse Ig was obtained from Cappel Laboratories (Cochranville, PA). Immunofluorescence staining was performed as previously described (11). At least 5000 stained cells were counted on a Epics C cytofluorograph (Coulter) gating for live cells.

Isolation of activated T cells

MLRs were set up in T25 flasks (Falcon, Oxnard, CA) with 5×10^6 T cells and 5×10^6 irradiated or fixed stimulator cells (epithelial, adherent or non-T cells). After 48-72 hours in culture, cells were layered over Ficoll Hypaque (Pharmacia) and T cell blasts were collected from the interface. T cell blasts were either stained as described above or used in functional assays as detailed in the results section.

RESULTS AND DISCUSSION

Gut epithelial cells function as stimulator cells in MLR

Since we and others have previously demonstrated the presence of class II antigens on epithelial cells in the GI tract, we initiated studies to determine whether these cells could function in a manner analogous to other class II antigen positive accessory cells. Epithelial cells, peripheral blood adherent cells and T cells were obtained from patients undergoing bowel resections for non-inflammatory conditions (cancer, colonic inertia, familial polyposis, etc.). Both autologous and allogeneic MLR cultures were established. As seen in Figure 1, both allogeneic adherent cells and epithelial cells were simulatory in MLR although, in general, adherent cells were more potent stimulators (possibly due to greater Ia density on adherent cells - 10-100 fold greater). Similarly, both cell populations were capable of stimulating autologous T cells in an autologous MLR. These responses could be blocked by the addition of a rabbit anti-human Ia heteroantiserum, 962 (Fig. 2) (developed by C.Y. Wang, Rockefeller

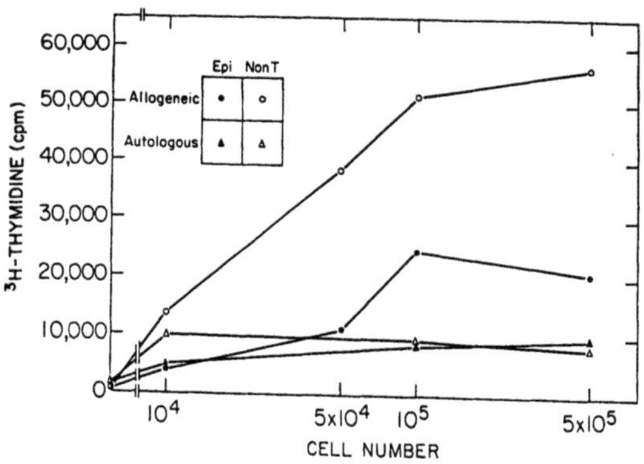

Figure 1. Graded numbers of irradiated epithelial (closed symbols) or non-T cells (open symbols) are added to 1×10^5 autologous (triangles) or allogeneic (circles) T cells for 5 days. After 120 h, 2μCi ^{3}H thymidine are added and cells are harvested and counted after an additional 18 h incubation. Results are expressed as mean counts per minute (cpm).

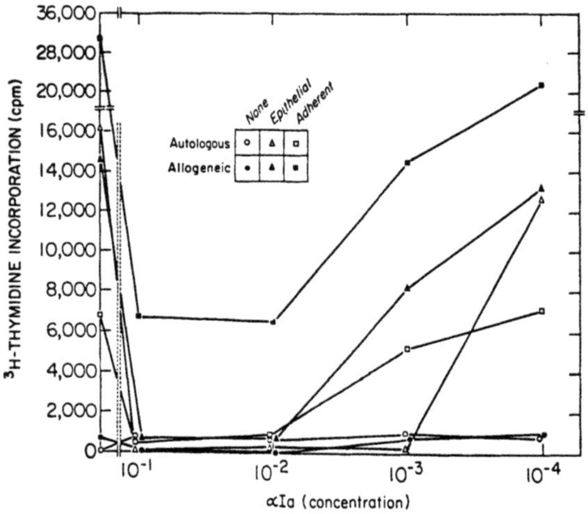

Figure 2. Graded doses of rabbit hetero-anti-Ia antibody 962 are added to cultures of 1×10^5 autologous (closed symbols) or allogeneic (open symbols) T cells with or without irradiated 1×10^5 epithelial cells (triangles) or 1×10^5 adherent cells (squares). Cultures are pulsed, harvested and counted as in Figure 1.

University, NYC). Since the stimulation by isolated epithelial cells could conceivably be due to cells contaminating this preparation (dendritic cells, macrophages, B cells), these studies were repeated using the human colonic epithelial cell line T84 (kindly provided by Dr. K. Dharmasathaphorn, UCSD, San Diego, CA). As seen in Table 1, this cell line is faintly Ia^+ in culture but can be induced to express significant HLA DR after induction with 50-500 U of recombinant γ IFN (Interferon Sciences, New Brunswick, NJ). These induced Ia^+ epithelial cells were now capable of stimulating allogeneic T cells in MLR in a manner comparable to that seen with freshly isolated epithelial cells (Table 2). Thus, it appears that Ia^+ epithelial cells can present foreign Ia to alloreactive T cells and autologous Ia to autoreactive cells.

Antigen processing

Although epithelial cells are capable of macromolecular uptake as part of the normal transport and absorptive function of these cells, it is not known whether antigens can be taken up, processed and re-expressed on the cell surface in association with Ia. To assess this possibility, epithelial cells, adherent cells and T cells were isolated from patients recently boosted with tetanus toxoid (TT). Epithelial cells or adherent cells were pulsed with TT (40 μg/ml), subsequently fixed with paraformaldehyde (0.1%) and co-cultured with macrophage depleted T cells (plastic adherence and carbonyl iron treated). In the absence of accessory cells, no response to TT was noted (Fig. 3). However, restoration of the proliferative response was noted with the addition of either antigen pulsed adherent cells or epithelial cells. Thus, it appears that gut epithelial cells can function appropriately as accessory cells, processing and presenting antigen to immunocompetent T cells. As previously demonstrated for monocytes and B cells, antigen processing by epithelial cells could be blocked by pretreatment with chloroquine (0.1 mM) or paraformaldehyde (data not shown).

Preferential induction of suppressor T cells

In order to determine the type of immune response generated using epithelial cells as accessory cells, T cell blasts were isolated after 48 hours from allogeneic MLR combinations. As seen in Figure 4, without stimulator cells (4a), $T4^+$ cells were roughly 2 fold greater than $T8^+$ (suppressor/cytotoxic) T cells. Addition of allogeneic macrophages as stimulators in MLR (4b) did not appreciably alter these ratios. However, use of epithelial cells as stimulators resulted in a significant increase in $T8^+$ cells (4c)

Table 1. γ-IFN induces Ia on T84 cell line

γ-IFN (U/ml)	α- γ IFN (Neutralizing U/ml)	T84 Cells % Staining	Fluorescence Intensity
-	-	2.1	tr-1$^+$
5000	-	88.6	3-4$^+$
500	-	81.4	3-4$^+$
50	-	32.6	2$^+$
5	-	4.8	1$^+$
5000	5000	1.6	tr-1$^+$
500	5000	1.5	tr-1$^+$

One million T84 cells were cultured on coverslips in 6 well plates. Recombinant γ-IFN was added for 24-48 hours after which cells were washed and stained with anti-Ia monoclonal VG2. Anti-γ-IFN was added at the onset of some cultures at the concentrations noted.

Table 2. γ-IFN induced T84 cells stimulate in MLR

T cells	γ-IFN U/ml	T84 cells 0	10^5	10^4 cpm	10^3
10^5	-	216	6123	3144	1610
10^5	50	-	22177	18164	12651
10^5	500	-	23143	26128	14564

T84 cells were plated at the cell concentrations noted above in triplicate microwell plates. γ-IFN was added in varying concentations for 24-48 h to these cultures. After this time period, wells were washed free of contaminating γ-IFN and 1 x 10^5 T cells were added to the treated and untreated cells. ^{3}H-thymidine incorporation was measured on day 5 of culture.

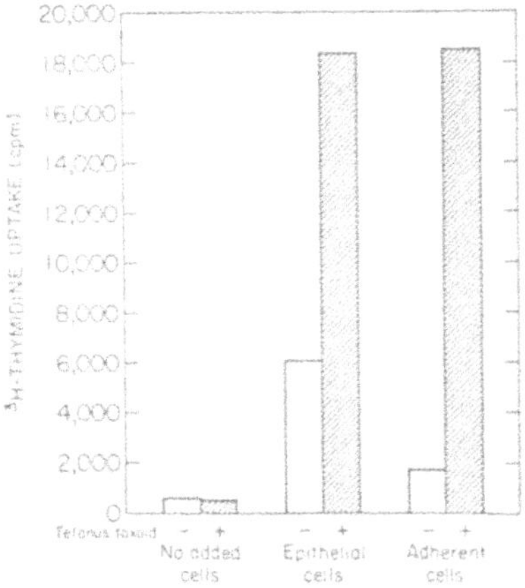

Figure 3. 1 x 10^5 severely monocyte/dendritic cell depleted tetanus primed T cells are cultured with or without tetanus toxoid (40 μg/ml) in the presence or absence of 1 x 10^5 autologous epithelial or adherent cells. Cultures are pulsed, harvested and counted as described in Figure 1.

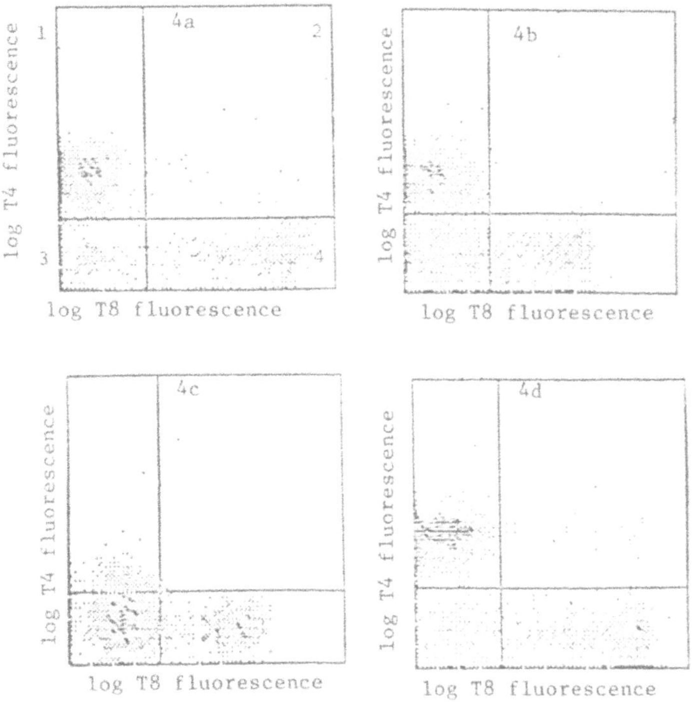

Figure 4. (a) T cells (medium control). Control T cells are cultured in CM alone for 48 h, and harvested as described in MATERIALS AND METHODS. Cells are stained with rhodamine conjugated T4 (helper/inducer T cells) and fluorescein conjugated T8 (suppressor/cytotoxic T cells) and analyzed by cytofluorograph. Control staining with rhodamine and fluorescein conjugated mouse IgG was negative. (b) T x allogeneic monocytes. Normal control T cells stimulated with equal numbers of fixed or irradiated adherent cells and stained as above. (c) T x allogeneic normal epithelial cells. Control T cells stimulated with equal numbers of fixed or irradiated isolated epithelial cells from the same donor as the adherent cells, harvested and stained as described above. (d) T x allogeneic Crohn's epithelial cells.

and a dramatic decrease in T4^{+} cells. These T8^{+} cells did not bear the surface antigen 9.3, a marker of cytotoxic T cells (Fig. 5c), in contrast to T8^{+} cells stimulated by adherent cells (Fig. 5b). Therefore, by staining, epithelial cells appear to preferentially stimulate T8^{+} suppressor T cells. To determine whether these cells were functional suppressor cells, T cell blasts from primary MLRs (adherent cell or epithelial cell stimulated) were added back to MLRs of DR matched (epithelial cell or adherent cell DR) or mismatched cells. In contrast to adherent cell stimulated T blasts which preferentially suppressed DR matched MLRs (Table 3) epithelial

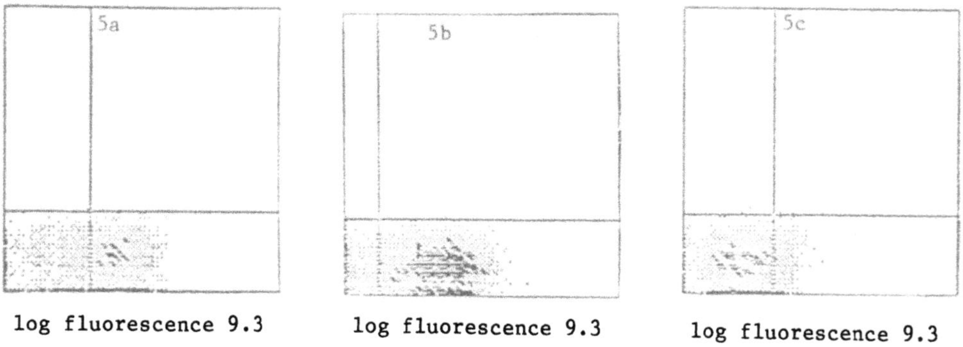

Figure 5. (a) T cells (medium control). Control T cells cultured in CM alone for 48 h as in Figure 4. Here, cells are stained indirectly with monoclonal 9.3 (cytotoxic T cells) followed by fluorescein conjugated F(ab)'$_2$ goat anti-mouse IgG. Control staining using second antibody alone was negative. (b) T x allogeneic monocytes. Same population as 4b stained with monoclonal 9.3. (c) T x allogeneic normal epithelial cells. Same population as 4c stained with monoclonal 9.3.

Table 3. Epithelial cell stimulated T cells mediate nonspecific suppression

		^{3}H-thymidine incorp. CPM added T cells	
MLR	0	Tx Epi[a]	Tx adh cells[b]
FR "T" x Mc EPI	23164	463	6388
FR "T" x Mc non-T	44321	324	29244
FR "T" x LA non-T	68129	1625	61683
FR "T" x FR non-T	11324	902	10443

(a) Derived from FR "T" x MC EPI MLR. (b) Derived from FR "T" x Mc non-T MLR. Mixed lymphocyte cultures were performed using either allogeneic or autologous epithelial cells or adherent monocytes/dendritic cells in tissue culture flasks for 48-72 hours. After this culture period, T cell blasts were isolated by Ficoll-Hypaque density gradient and either added back to a mixed lymphocyte culture involving the original pairing or to an irrelevant MLR. Inhibition of ^{3}H thymidine incorporation was detected at day 5 of culture for T cells induced by epithelial cells (regardless of the MLR combination) whereas the T cells induced by adherent cells suppressed only MLRs involving the original pairing.

cell stimulated T blasts suppressed in an antigen nonspecific fashion. In fact, these cells functioned as potent antigen nonspecific suppressor cells of T cell mitogenesis and B cell differentiation as well (data not shown).

CONCLUSIONS

These data suggest that gut epithelial cells may have a significant role in mucosal immune responses, in that they are capable of processing and presenting antigens to immunocompetent T cells. The finding of selective induction of antigen nonspecific suppressor T cells may help explain the immunologic nonresponsiveness of the gut and aid in our understanding of the concept of oral tolerance. More careful dissection of these processes will allow us to develop methods to selectively bypass this barrier and enhance our future capabilities with oral vaccination.

ACKNOWLEDGEMENTS

This work is supported, in part, by the National Foundation of Ileitis and Colitis, the Burrill Crohn Research Foundation and by grants CA 41583 from the NIH. Dr. Mayer is the recipient of the Irma T. Hirschl Trust Career Development Award.

The authors wish to thank Chris Thompson and David Eisenhardt for their technical expertise and Mrs. Hyacinth Fyffe for preparation of this manuscript.

REFERENCES

1. Challacombe, S.J., Tomasi, T.B., J. Exp. Med. 152, 1459, 1980.
2. Chase, M.W., Proc. Soc. Exp. Biol. 61, 257, 1946.
3. Hanson, L.A., Ahlstedt, S., Andersson, B., Carlson, B., Cole, M.F., Ann. N.Y. Acad. Sci. 409, 1, 1983.
4. Wolf, J.L., Rubin, D.H., Finberg, R., Kauffman, R.S., Sharpe, A.H., Trier, J.S., Fields, B.N., Science 212, 471, 1981.

5. Mason, D.W., Dallman, M., Barclay, A.N., Nature 293, 150, 1981.
6. Natali, P.G., DeMartinio, C., Quaranta, V., Nicotra, M.R., Frezza, F., Pellegrino, M.A., Ferrone, S., Transplantation 31, 75, 1981.
7. Selby, W.S., Janossy, G., Mason, D.Y., Jewell, D.P., Clin. Exp. Immunol. 53, 614, 1983.
8. Volc-Platzer, B., Majdic, O., Knapp, W., Wolff, K., Minter Berger, W., Lechner, K., Stingl, G., J. Exp. Med. 159, 1784, 1984.
9. Geppert, T.D., Lipsky, P.E., J. Immunol. 135, 3750, 1985.
10. Gottleib, A.B., Fu, S.M., Yu, D.T.Y., Wang, C.Y., Halper, J.P., Kunkel, H.G., J. Immunol. 123, 1497, 1979.
11. Mayer, L., Fu, S.M., Cunningham-Rundles, C., Kunkel, H.G., J. Clin. Invest. 74, 2115, 1984.

ANTIGEN PRESENTATION BY GUT EPITHELIAL CELLS: SECRETION BY RAT ENTEROCYTES OF A FACTOR WITH IL-1-LIKE ACTIVITY

P.W. Bland

Department of Veterinary Medicine, University of Bristol
Langford House, Langford, Bristol BS18 7DU, U.K.

INTRODUCTION

Evidence is emerging that the epithelial interface of the gut may play an important role in directing the type of immune response initiated towards enteric antigens. Soluble protein antigens are processed to constituent antigenic peptides during absorption from the lumen (1) and such processing may give rise to circulating fragments with greater tolerogenicity than the native protein (2). In addition to its antigen processing function, the epithelium may be directly involved in the presentation of absorbed antigen, and the local induction of immunoregulatory lymphocytes. Thus, fully differentiated absorptive epithelial cells (EC) isolated from the rat small intestine can present soluble protein antigens to immune lymph node T cells *in vivo* (3), causing them to proliferate and differentiate into antigen-specific suppressor cells (4).

A series of initiating and enhancing signals are required to effect T cell activation by polypeptide antigens. A degree of antigen processing by the antigen-presenting cell (APC), to reveal epitopes reactive with the T cell receptor, is usually required (5); interaction of processed antigen with the T cell receptor is regulated by products of the major histocompatibility complex residing in the APC surface membrane (6); and release by the APC of the cytokine, interleukin 1 (IL-1) is required to induce the synthesis of receptors for interleukin 2 (IL-2) on the T cell (7). A role for soluble mediators in antigen presentation by EC has not been previously investigated and evidence is presented here for a factor, secreted during short-term culture of EC (ECF), which is reactive in the thymocyte co-stimulation assay for IL-1.

METHODS

Male WF rats were used at seven to ten weeks of age. Proliferation assays were carried out in RPMI-1640 supplemented with 10% heat-inactivated fetal calf serum (FCS), 2 mM L-glutamine, 1 mM sodium pyruvate, 50 μM 2-ME, 100 u/ml penicillin, 100 μg/ml streptomycin, 40 μg/ml gentamicin and 20 mM HEPES. ECF supernatants were prepared in serum-free medium. IL-1 was prepared as the supernatant from splenic MØ (10^6/ml) incubated at 37°C with 1 μg/ml muramyl dipeptide (N-acetylmuramyl-L-alanyl-D-isoglutamine) for 24 h. IL-2 was prepared by incubation of unfractionated spleen cells (5×10^6/ml) in medium containing 2 μg/ml concanavalin A (Con A) for 24 h at 37°C and was subsequently delectinized using Sephadex G-50. IL-1 and IL-2 containing supernatants were dialyzed and filter sterilized before use. Cell preparation and purity was as previously described (3). Briefly, EC were released from everted duodenal/jejunal sacs by brief stirring in 0.5 mM EDTA. T cells were derived from two successive nylon wool column treatments of draining lymph node cells from rats immunized in the footpads with 100 μg OVA in FCA 8 - 15 days previously. Pooled EC, freshly isolated from four unimmunized rats were used for each preparation of ECF. EC were incubated at 2×10^6 cells/ml for the time periods shown at 37°C. The supernatant was clarified by centrifugation and dialyzed against RPMI 1640. RPMI 1640 incubated alone for the corresponding time periods and dialyzed was used as a control. Proliferation assays were carried out in flat-bottomed microtiter wells and all cultures were pulsed with 1 μCi ^{3}H-TdR 4 h before harvesting.

RESULTS

Initial experiments to detect in vitro presentation of antigen by EC involved continuous co-culture of EC with antigen and immune T cells for 96 h. As seen in Table 1, under these conditions, splenic MØ successfully presented OVA to T cells, causing them to proliferate. T cells, however, did not proliferate in the presence of EC APC. In fact, in many cases uptake of ^{3}H-TdR in the presence of EC was less than that seen in T cells cultured with antigen alone. It is well known that the expression of antigen presentation in vitro represents a balance between induction of T cell proliferation and suppression of proliferation by non-specific factors secreted by APC. Even MØ in our experiments were suppressive at high concentrations (not shown). To overcome a possible dominant suppressive influence of EC in long-term co-cultures, the co-culture induction period

Table 1. Presentation of OVA to sensitized T cells by macrophages or epithelial cells (96 h co-culture)

Antigen	Accessory Cell	Proliferative Response (cpm)
-	-	586
+	-	808
-	MØ	4,839
-	EC	175
+	MØ	60,305
+	EC	299

allowing antigen presentation to take place was reduced to 18 h. Thus, T cells and EC were co-cultured with and without OVA for 18 h and were then separated on Ficoll-Hypaque gradients. Following washing, the T cells were then re-plated and cultured for a further 96 h. Figure 1 shows that under these conditions, T cells which had experienced antigen in the context of EC APC showed significant proliferation, whereas control groups did not. This was considered to be further evidence for a suppressive, anti-proliferative factor secreted by EC in long-term culture. Increasing the EC-T cell ratio above an optimum of 1:5 again swung the balance in favor of suppression which was not due to simple cell crowding (not shown). In subsequent time-course experiments, an 18 h induction culture period was found to be optimum with significant suppression of proliferation evident following a 48 h induction culture (Fig. 2).

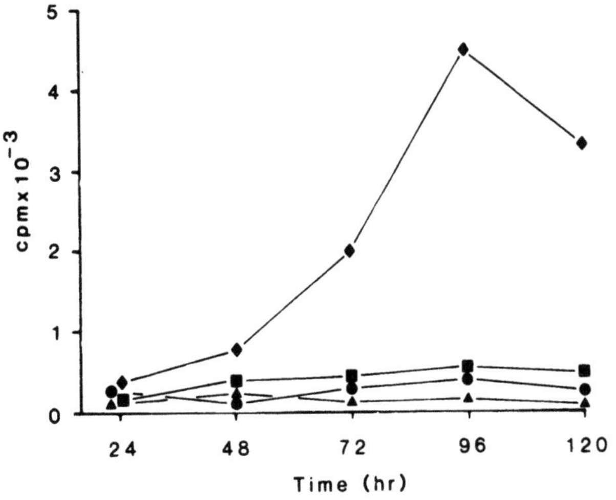

Figure 1. Proliferation of OVA-immune T cells induced following antigen presentation by epithelial cells. T cells were cultured alone (▲); with EC only (●); with OVA only (■); or with EC + OVA (◆) for 18 h, isolated over Ficoll-Hypaque and allowed to proliferate for the times indicated.

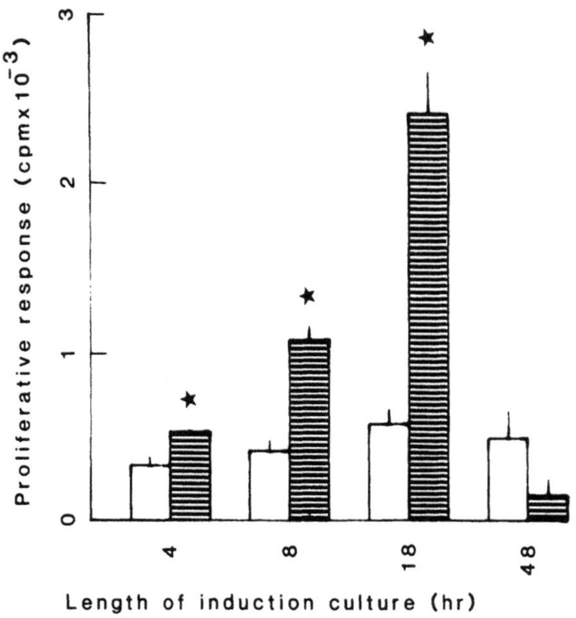

Figure 2. Optimum period of co-culture to demonstrate antigen presentation by epithelial cells. T cells were cultured with OVA alone (□) or with EC + OVA (▥) for the times indicated, isolated over Ficoll-Hypaque and allowed to proliferate for 96 h.

To determine the role of EC-secreted factors in antigen presentation, ECF was prepared from normal, unstimulated EC cultured for a range of time periods and was tested for its effect on the proliferative response of spleen cells to Con A. The results are shown in Figure 3. It is clear from these experiments that at least two factors with conflicting effects on T cell proliferation are synthesized by isolated EC in culture. Thus, ECF from EC cultured for 24 h or less enhanced lymphocyte proliferation, but in ECF prepared from longer cultures a suppressive effects was dominant. The inhibitory effect of 48 h ECF indicated either the rèlease of a toxic or anti-proliferative factor and/or the accumulation of an inhibitory factor competing with the early synthesized enhancing factor.

Finally, the enhancing effect of $\leq$ 24 h ECF was investigated to determine its functional similarity to IL-1. Figure 4a shows that 6 h ECF, but not 48 h ECF, enhanced the proliferative response of thymocytes to PHA in a dose-dependent manner. However, this assay is not specific for IL-1 as IL-2 also induces thymocyte proliferation. Maintenance of the murine cytotoxic T cell line, CTLL, is specifically IL-2 dependent. Figure 4b shows that neither 6 h ECF nor 24 h ECF was capable of supporting CTLL proliferation, confirming that IL-2 did not account for the enhancement of proliferation induced by early ECF.

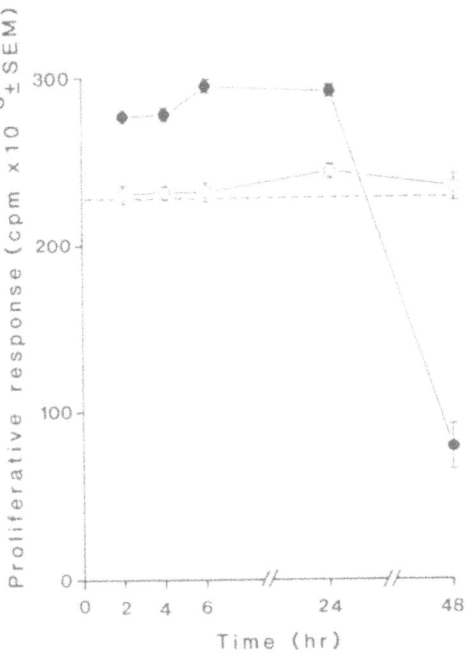

Figure 3. Effect of ECF on concanavalin A-induced spleen cell proliferation. Unfractionated spleen cells were cultured with Con A for 72 h at 37°C: alone (-----); with the dialyzed supernatant from EC cultured for the time periods shown (●); or with RPMI cultured alone for the same time periods (○). Additions were made at a final dilution of 1 in 4.

DISCUSSION

The results suggest that unstimulated EC secrete a factor with properties similar to IL-1. Biochemical analysis is currently underway to analyze the molecular relationship between ECF and IL-1. Although, immunologically, IL-1 is usually thought of as a macrophage/monocyte-secreted factor, there are now reports of IL-1-like activity in the secretions of many cell types: keratinocytes (8), astrocytes (9), glomerular mesangial cells (10), endothelial cells (11), and normal and virus-infected B cells (12). The *in vivo* immunological significance of many of these factors, however is questionable. On the other hand, we have shown that rat intestinal EC can act as antigen-presenting cells (3), suggesting that an EC-synthesized IL-1-like molecule may play an important role. Factors with IL-1-like activity from other cell types are usually undetectable unless the cell is stimulated *in vitro* with lipopolysaccharide (LPS) or a phorbol ester. The release of detectable amounts of an IL-1-like factor by EC without *in vitro* stimulation

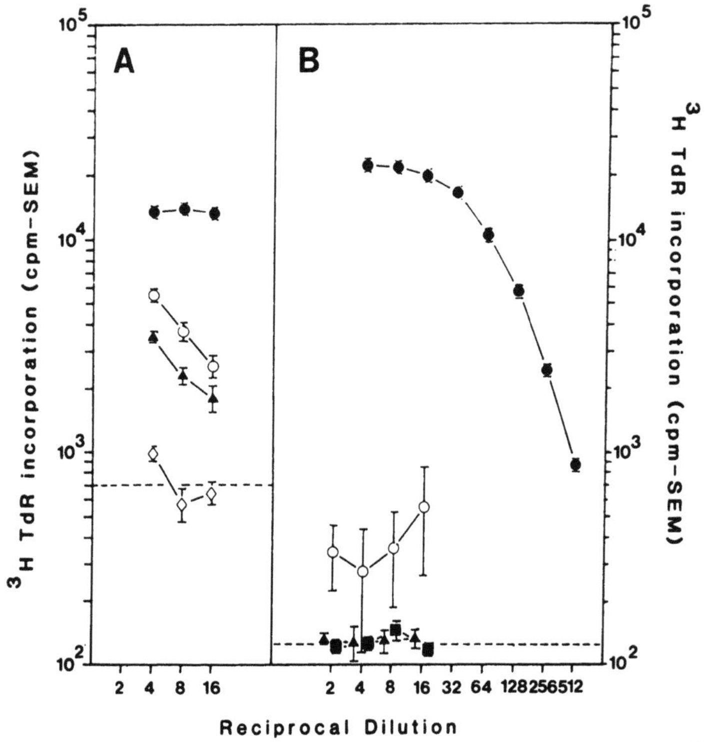

Figure 4. Effect of IL-1, IL-2 and ECF on thymocyte (A) and CTLL (B) proliferation. Cultures were treated with IL-1 (○), IL-2 (●), 6 h ECF (▲), 24 h ECF (■), or 48 h ECF (◇) at the final dilutions shown. Thymocytes were cultured with PHA for 72 h at 37°C; CTLL were cultured for 24 h at 37°C. (-----), response of thymocytes to PHA alone and CTLL to medium control.

however, may reflect the unique location of this antigen-presenting cell at the antigen-sampling interface of the gut lumen. In this location, EC are constantly exposed to LPS and other bacterial cell wall products. Indeed, fluctuations in the levels of these endotoxins could conceivably exert control over the synthesis by the epithelium of factors with IL-1-like activity and, in turn, modulate the presentation of luminal antigens by the epithelium.

CONCLUSIONS

A factor released from rat intestinal epithelial cells (EC) in short term culture ($\leq$ 24 h) has an activity profile resembling IL-1, but is not reactive in a specific IL-2 assay. This co-stimulatory activity is inhibited or obscured in supernatants from prolonged EC cultures. It is suggested that this factor may participate in the regulation of antigen presentation in the gut.

ACKNOWLEDGEMENTS

This work was supported by a grant from The National Foundation for Ileitis and Colitis.

REFERENCES

1. Stern, M. and Walker, W.A., Am. J. Physiol. 246, G556, 1984.
2. Bruce, M.G. and Ferguson, A., Immunology 57, 627, 1986.
3. Bland, P.W. and Warren, L.G., Immunology 58, 1, 1986.
4. Bland, P.W. and Warren, L.G., Immunology 58, 9, 1986.
5. Ziegler, K. and Unanue, E., J. Immunol. 127, 1869, 1981.
6. Lee, K.C., Wilkinson, A. and Wong, M., Cell. Immunol. 48, 79, 1979.
7. Kaye, J., Gillis, S., Mizel, S.B., Shevach, E.M., Males, T.R., Dinarello, C.A., Lachman, L.B. and Janeway, C.A., J. Immunol. 133, 1339, 1984.
8. Luger, T.A., Stadler, B.M., Katz, S.I. and Oppenheim, J.J., J. Immunol. 127, 1493, 1981.
9. Fontana, A., Kristensen, F., Dubs, R., Gemsa, D. and Weber, E., J. Immunol. 129, 2413, 1982.
10. Lovett, D.H., Ryan, J.L. and Sterzel, R.B., J. Immunol. 130, 1796, 1983.
11. Roska, A.K., Johnson, A.R. and Lipsky, P.E., J. Immunol. 132, 136, 1984.
12. Matsushima, K., Procopio, A., Abe, H., Scala, G., Ortaldo, J.R. and Oppenheim, J.J., J. Immunol. 135, 1132, 1985.

SYNGENEIC AND ALLOGENEIC T CELL REACTIVITY TO I-REGION DETERMINANTS ON RAT INTESTINAL EPITHELIAL CELLS

P.W. Bland

Department of Veterinary Medicine
University of Bristol
Langford House, Langford, Bristol BS18 7DU, U.K.

INTRODUCTION

Class II (Ia) molecules of the major histocompatibility complex (MHC) are integral membrane glycoproteins found, in normal circumstances, on cells of various lineages throughout the body. Their expression may be induced on other cell types however, by inflammatory mediators, for example, γ interferon (1). They function in the immune response to restrict the presentation of protein antigens to immunoregulatory T cells (2). They also act as auto- and allo-antigens in mixed lymphocyte responses (3).

In the normal adult small intestine, class II molecules are expressed on fully-differentiated epithelial cells (EC) in the mouse (4), the rat (5) and humans (6). In the rat, Ia antigens of both I-A and I-E specificities are expressed (5). They are not normally found on immature crypt cells (5) or on large bowel epithelia (personal observation). The density of EC Ia expression has been shown qualitatively to vary between inbred rat strains (5). Increased Ia density on columnar cells and aberrant Ia expression on crypt cells has been reported in experimentally-induced inflammation and graft-versus-host disease (7), and clinically, on large bowel epithelia in inflammatory bowel disease (8).

Ia antigens have been shown to be essential for the presentation of protein antigens by isolated rat EC to immune T cells *in vitro* (9). Experiments are described here to define the capacity for EC Ia antigens to mediate syngeneic and allogeneic 'mixed lymphocyte' type responses.

METHODS

Male WF ($RT1^u$), F344 $(RT1)^1$, BUF ($RT1^b$) and ACI ($RT1^a$) rats were used at seven to ten weeks of age.

All cultures were carried out in RPMI 1640 medium supplemented with 10% heat-inactivated FCS, 2 mM L-glutamine, 1 mM sodium pyruvate, 50 μg 2-ME, 100 u/ml penicillin, 100 μg/ml streptomycin, 40 μg/ml gentamycin and 20 mM HEPES.

EC were isolated from unimmunized rats by brief stirring of duodenal/ jejunal sacs in 0.5 mM EDTA, as previously described (9). T cells were derived from two successive nylon wool column treatments of pooled inguinal, mesenteric, popliteal and brachial lymph node cells from unimmunized rats.

T cells and irradiated (2,000 rads) EC were co-cultured in 35 mm wells for 18 h at 37°C at a T cell:EC ratio of 5:1. T cells were then separated from EC on Ficoll-Hypaque and cultured alone for 96 h and proliferative responses were determined by ^{3}H-TdR incorporation following a four hour pulse.

IL-2 was prepared by incubation of unfractionated WF spleen cells (5×10^6) in RPMI 1640 + 2 μg/ml concanavalin A for 24 h at 37°C. The supernatant was de-lectinized using Sephadex G-50 and dialyzed against RPMI 1640.

RESULTS

Syngeneic responsiveness

The response of T cells to autologous EC Ia antigens were evaluated for the four strains of rats. Figure 1 (left) shows that no significant autologous responses were detected. An attempt was then made to amplify possible weak autologous responses by the addition of exogenous IL-2. This treatment did not reveal significant responses (Fig. 1 right).

Allogeneic responsiveness

T cell responses to allogeneic EC Ia were then investigated by allogeneic T cell-EC co-culture. Figure 2 shows that significant T cell

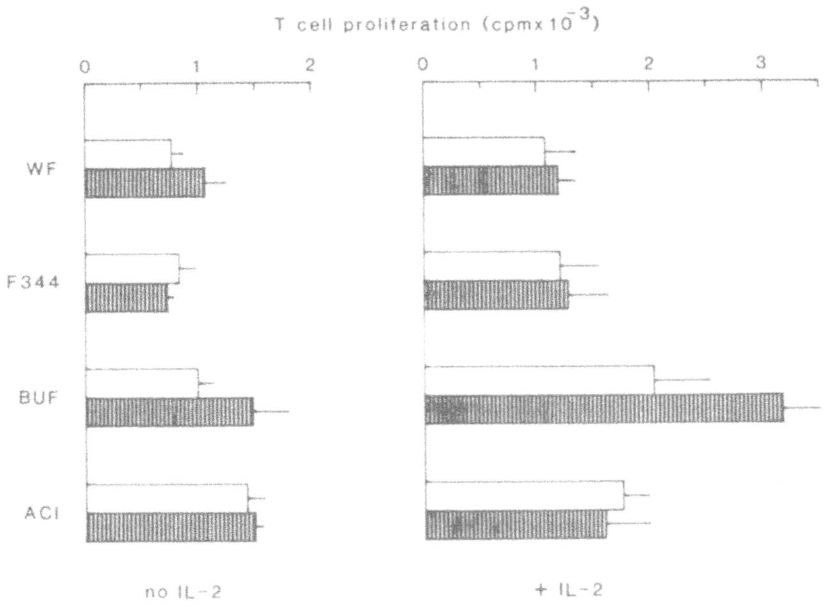

Figure 1. Responsiveness of rat lymph node T cells to syngeneic epithelial cells (EC). (□), T cells only; (▥), T cells + syngeneic EC.

proliferative responses were observed towards allogeneic epithelial cells in certain cases. Specifically, WF T cells were responsive to F344 and BUF, EC, BUF against F344 EC and ACI against BUF EC. The pattern of responsiveness did not reveal clear trends, although F344 and BUF were the only EC initiating significant proliferation in response to allo-antigens and F344 T cells were clearly unresponsive to all three allogeneic combinations.

Ia dependency of allo-responsiveness

The demonstration of allo-responsiveness demonstrated above is not, in itself, an unequivocal indication of T cell activity to EC Ia antigens. A range of foreign antigens on the allogeneic EC, or even factors secreted by EC could contribute to T cell activation. To define the role of EC Ia in the allogeneic responses, therefore, blocking experiments were carried out using the mouse monoclonal antiserum MRC OX 6 which recognizes polymorphic Ia determinants on all rat strains. The monoclonal mouse anti-human HLA-A,B,C antiserum which does not recognize rat determinants was used as a control. Figure 3 shows that partial, but significant, blocking of the BUF and ACI T cell responses to F344 and BUF EC, respectively, was achieved using this antiserum. However, the residual T cell responses

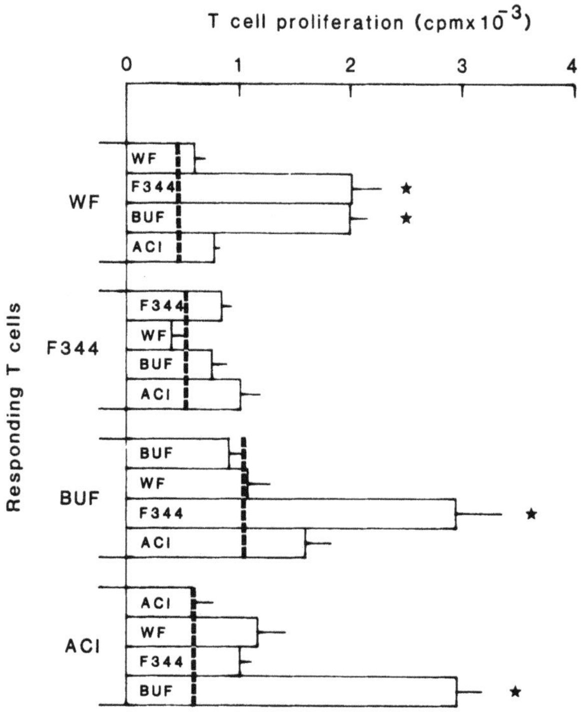

Figure 2. Responsiveness of rat lymph node T cells to allogeneic epithelial cells. Source of epithelial stimulator cells is shown in boxes. ★, $p < 0.05$; dotted line, responding T cells cultured alone.

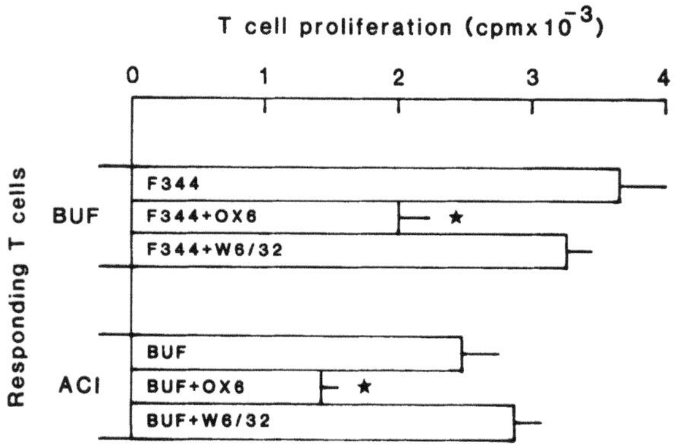

Figure 3. Blocking of epithelial cell-induced T cell allo-responsiveness using anti-Ia antiserum. Antisera were added at 1 in 2,000 throughout the 18 h induction culture. ★, $p < 0.05$.

were still significantly greater than those of BUF and ACI T cells cultured alone in the induction culture, suggesting that although a response was undoubtedly mounted against allogeneic Ia, other enterocyte-related factors were responsible for the residual response, or that MRC OX 6 binds to and blocks only a portion of the reactive epitope recognized by the allogeneic T cell receptor.

DISCUSSION

Although significant syngeneic responses were not initiated by EC, the allo-responsiveness confirms that EC Ia molecules can act as T cell antigens and can stimulate a 'mixed lymphocyte' type response. Quantitative data are not available to define the density of Ia molecules on EC. However, in unpublished studies using radioimmunoassay for cell-bound Ia, we have preliminary results indicating that the density of Ia antigens on EC isolated from normal rats is, in many cases, comparable, on a cell-to-cell basis with that on unfractionated spleen cells. It is unlikely, then, that the lack of auto-reactivity can be attributed to a simple low dose unresponsiveness. On the other hand, one could speculate that enhanced EC Ia expression seen in gut inflammation could promote reactivity to self EC Ia with possible damaging consequences.

CONCLUSIONS

No evidence was found for T cell reactivity towards self EC Ia antigens. However, significant T cell proliferation resulted from stimulation with allogeneic EC Ia in at least some cross-over combinations and this proliferative response was partially blocked using an anti-Ia monoclonal antiserum.

ACKNOWLEDGEMENTS

This work was supported by a grant from the National Foundation for Ileitis and Colitis.

REFERENCES

1. Beller, D.I. and Unanue, E.R., J. Immunol. 126, 263, 1981.
2. Shevach, E. and Rosenthal, A., J. Exp. Med. 138, 1213, 1973.
3. Schwartz, R.H., Fathman, C.G. and Sachs, D.H., J. Immunol. 116, 929, 1976.
4. Parr, E.L. and McKensie, I.F.C., Immunogenetics 8, 499, 1979.
5. Mayrhofer, G., Pugh, C.W. and Barclay, A.N., Eur. J. Immunol. 13, 112, 1983.

6. Scott, H., Solheim, B.G., Brandtzaeg, P. and Thorsby, E., Scand. J. Immunol. 12, 77, 1980.
7. Barclay, A.N. and Mason, D.W., J. Exp. Med. 156, 1665, 1982.
8. Selby, W.S., Janossy, G., Mason, D.Y. and Jewell, D.P., Clin. Exp. Immunol. 53, 614, 1983.
9. Bland, P.W. and Warren, L.G., Immunology 58, 1, 1986.

DIFFERENTIAL TISSUE DISTRIBUTION OF HLA-DR, -DP AND -DQ ANTIGENS

U. Forsum, K. Claesson, R. Jonsson, A. Karlsson-Parra, L. Klareskog, A. Scheynius and U. Tjernlund

Department of Clinical Bacteriology, Karolinska Institute, Stockholm, and Department of Oral Pathology, University of Göteborg, Institute of Clinical Bacteriology and Departments of Medical and Physiological Chemistry, Urology and Dermatology, University of Uppsala, Sweden

INTRODUCTION

At least three chromosomal loci code for class II transplantation antigens in humans; HLA-DR, -DP and -DQ. These antigens have been implicated to be critical restriction elements in various immune reactions. It is, however, far from clear how and where the class II antigens perform their functions. Available *in vivo* and *in vitro* data suggest that class II antigens are constitive cell membrane components on certain types of cells such as dendritic cells of the spleen and the Langerhans cell of the epidermis (1,2). Furthermore, class II antigens can be induced by gamma interferon and other stimuli on a variety of epithelial and endothelial cells that do not always express these antigens (3).

In the search for a role of class II antigens as restriction elements in various immune regulatory events, one possible approach is to define which cells in various organs of the body that express the different class II molecules normally and in various diseases. Such a mapping can take into consideration the time course of the reaction, the antigen involved, the cell types expressing class II or induced to express class II antigens and the lymphoid cells involved (4). It is logical to postulate that such investigations will give important information on how local immune reactions are regulated.

Earlier studies have revealed a differential distribution of HLA-DR and -DQ antigens in some tissues and conditions (5-7). The current study is aimed at comparing the distribution of HLA-DP molecules as detected by monoclonal antibodies in addition to HLA-DR and -DQ molecules in normal and pathological tissues. The results indicate that HLA-DP molecules have a different distribution as compared to the other class II molecules and that these differences could be of interest in further studies of local immune reactions.

MATERIALS AND METHODS

Biopsies were obtained from normal and diseased organs, immediately transported to the laboratory in Histocon®, frozen and stored at -70°C until further processed. Acetone fixed cryostat sections, 4 microns thick, were investigated by means of a PAP technique or by ABC-staining (8,9). Mouse monoclonal antibodies anti HLA-DR, anti Leu-10 and anti HLA-DP were obtained from Becton Dickinson, Sunnyvale, CA. The appropriate dilutions of the antibodies, 1.5 microg./ml, were determined on sections of normal skin and normal lymph nodes. Specificity tests included omission of the primary antibodies and replacement of the monoclonal antibodies by irrelevant antibodies. Staining was not observed in these tests. Single epidermal cell suspension of normal human skin obtained at plastic surgery or within 24 hr postmortem was prepared as described (10) with the modification of a 10 fold increase of deoxyribonuclease (Sigma) to 0.25%. The viability was about 85% as determined by trypan blue exclusion. The cells were processed for immunocytochemistry as previously described (11).

RESULTS

Skin cells

In normal epidermis HLA-DR, -DP and -DQ antigens were found on Langerhans cells. HLA-DP and -DQ seemed to be less pronounced on the dendrites. No expression of either antigen was observed on the keratinocytes. Cell suspensions from normal epidermis contained about 2% positive cells of either specificity. In the DP^+ and DQ^+ cell populations, a subpopulation, roughly 10%, stained stronger with anti -DP and -DQ, respectively, than the rest of the -DP and -DQ reactive cells. In biopsies from healthy volunteers with positive tuberculin reaction (d 6, n = 3), patients with mycosis fungoides (n = 1), lichen planus (n = 1) and in two biopsies from a patient with Borrelia spirochete manifestation acrodermatitis chronica atrophicans a differential expression of the various class II antigens was observed. In the tuberculin reaction, mycosis fungoides and lichen planus keratinocytes were $-DR^+$ and $-DQ^-$, $-DP^-$ whereas keratinocytes from the site of acrodermatitis lesions were $-DR^+$, $-DP^+$ and $-DQ^+$ as well (Fig. 1). In the dermis the number of $-DP^+$ and $-DQ^+$ cells was less than $-DR^+$ cells both in normal and lesional skin.

Liver

In needle biopsy liver sections from 5 patients with primary biliary cirrhosis, a large number of cells within typical portal mononuclear cell infiltrates expressed HLA-DR and -DQ. The DP- expression was generally weaker and the number of $-DP^+$ cells was less than $-DR^+$ and $-DQ^+$ cells. Some $-DR^+$, $-DP^-$ and $-DQ^+$ bile ducts were also identified.

Salivary glands

The expression of class II antigens in labial salivary gland biopsy specimens from 10 patients with Sjögren's syndrome showed a varied intensity of staining of the glandular epithelium. A clear hierarchy of expression followed the pattern -DR > -DP > -DQ and was related to the severity of inflammation measured by focal score determination (Fig. 1). Thus, more cases were $-DR^+$ than $-DP^+$ while -DQ on the whole was only expressed on dendritic cells in the glands. Class II antigen staining was particularly seen on the ductal epithelial cells and to a less extent on acinar cells.

Synovium

In biopsies from human knee joints (n = 6) obtained from patients with rheumatoid arthritis more lining cells were stained for -DR than for -DP or -DQ. A substantial number of lining cells as well as cells deeper in the synovium had, however, a strong expression of class II antigens coded from all three loci.

Kidney

Normal kidneys (n = 4) and kidneys from cases of transplantectomy due to rejection (n = 4) of the graft or infection (n = 2) were also studied. Strong -DR but no -DP or -DQ staining was seen in varying proportions of proximal tubules in all kidneys.

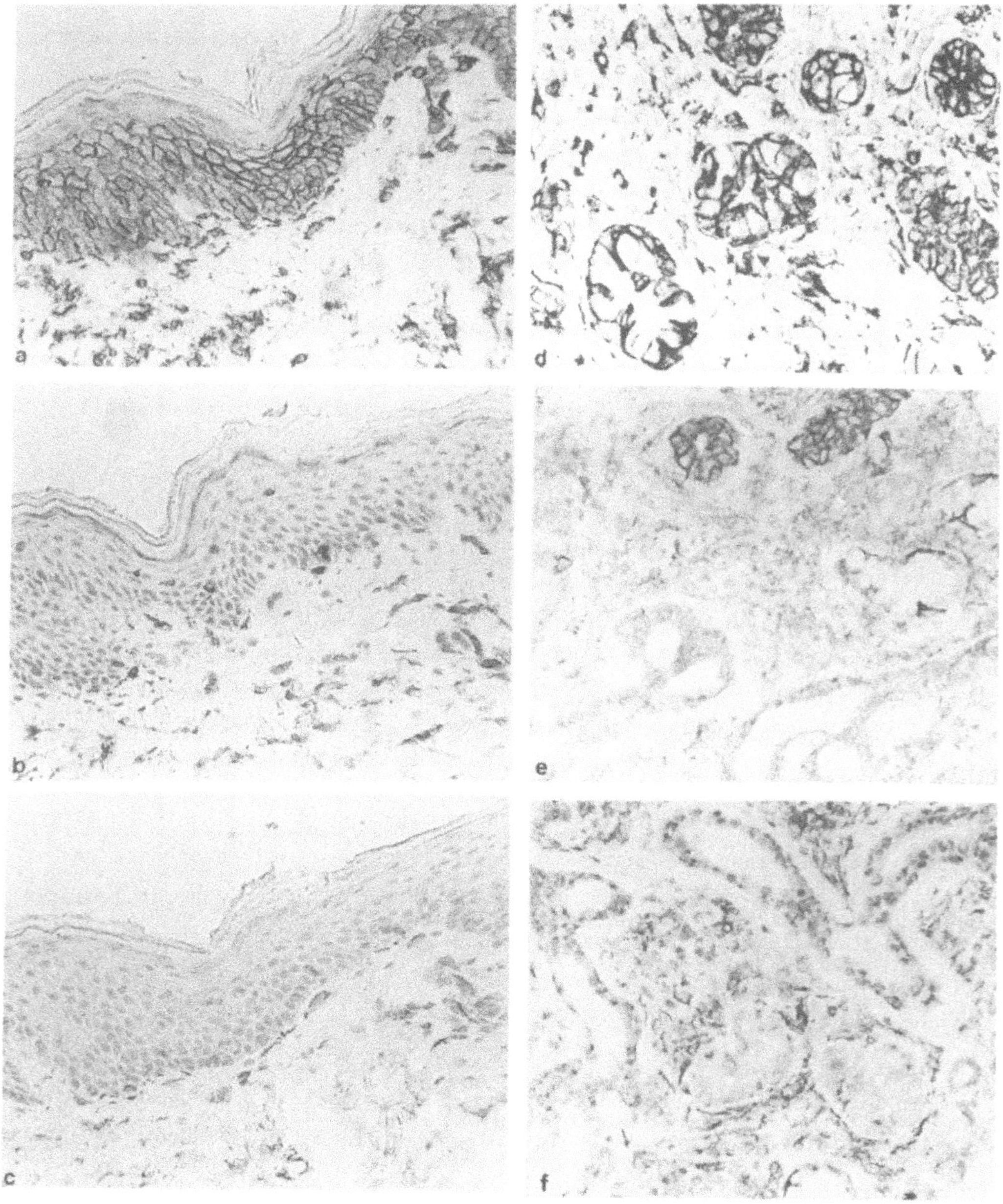

Figure 1. Immunohistochemical staining of positive tuberculin reaction (a-c) and labial salivary gland from a case of Sjögrenś syndrome (d-f). a and d stained with anti HLA-DR; b and e with anti HLA-DP; and c and f with anti HLA-DQ.

DISCUSSION

A major problem in defining the distribution of class II antigens in tissues is the variability of the antibodies used (12). Despite the fact that the genetic region coding for the human class II antigens is described in some detail, most monoclonal and polyclonal antibodies used to detect class II antigens have not been defined as to their reactivity with distinct molecules. In addition, monoclonal anti class II antibodies can react with two or more different chains coded by the class II genes (13). Available data, however, support the notion that the anti class II antibodies used in this study predominantly react with polymorphic determinants on the -DR, -DP and -DQ molecules, respectively (14,15). The present study indicates that the distribution of class II molecules in various organs varies between normal and diseased organs. These findings may indicate different functional roles for the different molecules encoded by the class II region.

First, the staining pattern observed in the skin biopsies indicates that the distribution of class II molecules on various cell types might vary with the condition inducing keratinocyte expression of class II molecules. A more detailed mapping of the differential expression of class II antigens on keratinocytes might thus shed some more light on what locus that is involved in restricting the immune response to environmental agents such as bacteria.

Second, the kidney biopsies indicate that differential expression of class II antigens on tubular epithelial cells occurs in both normal, infected and rejected kidneys. Since many studies have shown -DR to be most abundantly induced it could be that -DR molecules are of special importance in restricting immune responses in the kidney, while products of other loci dominates in immune responses of other organs (4,5).

Third, biopsies from the autoimmune diseases showed expression of all specificities studied to a varying degree in all cases. The salivary gland biopsies showed that class II antigen expression clearly correlates with the severity of inflammation in labial glands. Further, mapping of class II antigens on epithelial cells in autoimmune disease thus seems necessary.

CONCLUSIONS

Constitutive expression of HLA-DR molecules occurs in many cells of bone marrow origin but in epithelial cells the antigen expression is transient and inducible. In particular, an enhanced expression can be demonstrated in autoimmune diseases, delayed hypersensitivity reactions, after organ transplantation and infections and also experimentally after administration of gamma interferon or hormones (3). One main conclusion would thus be that the variable and inducible amount of class II antigens seen on many nonlymphoid cells is part of the immune regulation of the body and thus deserves particular attention in studies of the normal physiology of body membranes.

REFERENCES

1. Rowden, G., CRC Critical Rev. Immunol. 3, 95, 1981.
2. Steinman, R.M., Transplantation 31, 151, 1981.
3. Halloran, P.F., Wadgymar, A. and Autenried, P., Transplantation 41, 413, 1986.
4. Forsum, U., Claesson, K., Hjelm, E., Karlsson-Parra, A., Klareskog, L., Scheynius, A. and Tjernlund, U., Scand. J. Immunol. 21, 389, 1985.
5. Claesson, K., Forsum, U., Tufveson, G. and Wahlberg, J., Transplant. Proc. 18, 9, 1986.
6. Müller, C., Ziegler, A., Muller, C., Hadam, M., Waller, H.D., Wernet, P. and Müller, G., Immunobiol. 169, 228, 1985.
7. Tjernlund, U., Scheynius, A., Asbrink, E. and Hovmark, A., Scand. J. Immunol. 23, 383, 1986.
8. Klareskog, L., Forsum, U., Wigren, A. and Wigzell, H., Scand. J. Immunol. 15, 501, 1982.
9. Lindahl, G., Hedfors, E., Klareskog, L. and Forsum, U., Clin. Exp. Immunol. 61, 475, 1985.
10. Tjernlund, U., Scheynius, A., Kabelitz, D. and Klareskog, L., Acta. Dermatovenereol. 61, 291, 1981.
11. Claesson-Welsh, L., Scheynius, A., Tjernlund, U. and Peterson, P.P., J. Immunol. 136, 484, 1986.
12. Guy, K. and Steel, C.M., Clin. Exp. Immunol. 59, 251, 1985.
13. Bodmer, J. and Bodmer, W., Immunol. Today 5, 251, 1984.
14. Chen, Y.X., Evans, R.L., Pollack, M.S., Lanier, L.L., Phillips, J.H., Rousso, C., Warner, N.L. and Brodsky, F.M., Human Immunol. 10, 221, 1984.

15. Watson, A.J., DeMars, R., Trowbridge, I.S. and Bach, F.H., Nature 304, 358, 1983.

16. Russ, G.R., Pascoe, V., dÁpice, A.J.F. and Seymour, A.E., Transplant. Proc. 18, 293, 1986.

MUCOSAL T LYMPHOCYTES IN HUMAN COLONIC SCHISTOSOMIASIS: RELATIONSHIP TO MHC ANTIGENS

S. Badr-el-Din, L.K. Trejdosiewicz, D.J. Oakes, R.V. Heatley, A. Abou-Khadr*, G. Janossy** and M.S. Losowsky

Department of Medicine, University of Leeds,
St. James's University Hospital, Leeds, U.K.; and
*Alexandria University, Alexandria, Egypt; and **Academic
Department of Immunology, Royal Free Hospital, London, U.K.

INTRODUCTION

Immunity to schistosomal infections has attracted considerable attention due to its endemic prevalence in the Third World, although much of the data available derives from animal models. Human studies have concentrated on systemic immunity, where it has long been known that chronic helminthic infections result in major perturbations (1). Mechanism of immunity in schistosomiasis are not fully understood, although recently it has been reported that circulatory T lymphocyte CD4:CD8 ratios are perturbed (2), and parasite-derived immunosuppressive factor(s) have been described (3), which may occur at both local and systemic levels.

A feature of the local immune response to egg deposition is granuloma formation, a reaction which diminishes in intensity to subsequent egg deposition ("spontaneous modulation") during the course of chronic infection (4,5). Animal studies suggest that granuloma formation and modulation depends on a fine balance between T helper and suppressor activity (6). It has been suggested that granuloma formation depends on T helper cell activity (7), and modulation is mediated by T suppressor cells (8). Whereas there have been some reports of granuloma formation in the human liver (e.g., 7), to our knowledge there have been no studies in humans of local immune system responses in the colon, one of the main organs affected by egg deposition. The aims of our study were, therefore, to examine T lymphocyte distribution in the colonic mucosae of patients with simple schistosomal colitis, and the more severe form, multiple colonic polyposis, which affects up to 20% of Egyptian patients, and which may arise due to coalescence of granulomata (9). A further aim was to study expression of MHC antigens in colonic epithelium in view of recent interest in class II expression, and implications for antigen presentation.

MATERIALS AND METHODS

Tissue samples

Thirteen patients with chronic schistosomal colitis (6 with colonic schistosomal polyposis) and 5 controls with non-inflammatory conditions (irritable bowel syndrome or diverticular disease) from Egypt were included in this study. Colonoscopy biopsies were obtained (including two actual polyps), snap-frozen in thawing isopentane, transported in dry ice to the U.K. and cryostat sectioned at 5 μm.

Indirect immunofluorescence

The techniques detailed elsewhere in this volume (10) were used. Routinely, 4 serial sections were double-labeled with one IgG-class and one IgM-class monoclonal antibody in the following combinations: UCHT1 (CD3) and RFT8 (CD8) to establish subset distribution (assuming $CD3^{+}/CD8^{-}$ cells to be $CD4^{+}$ helper/inducer); RFT1 (CD5) and RFT8 to examine distribution of the CD5 pan-T marker by the $CD8^{+}$ (cytotoxic/suppressor) cell subset; RFT2 (CD7) and RFT8 to examine expression of the CD7 40 Kdalton marker of stimulated T cells on the various subsets; and UCHT1 and RF-DR-2 (anti-HLA-DR to examine: (a) T cells for activation and (b) Class II antigen expression by colonic epithelium. Antibody binding was detected by absorbed class-specific fluorochrome-conjugated second layers (Southern Biotechnology Associates).

For some experiments, a CD4 antibody (Leu 3a) was used; however, the weak reaction with class-specific second layers consistently underestimated the CD4:CD8 ratio as determined by CD3/CD8 double-labeling. Also used were antibodies RF-DR-1 (anti-HLA-DQ) with RF-DR-2, and W6/32 (anti-HLA-A,B,C) with RF-DR-2 to further study MHC antigen expression by colonic epithelium.

Specimens were examined in a Zeiss microscope equipped with epifluorescent illumination, wide-aperature immersion objectives and selective filters. Each observation was made by two independent observers, and ratios were derived from counts averaged over at least 5 high-power (x40) fields. Lamina propria and intraepithelial cells were identified separately.

RESULTS

Controls

The results obtained are summarized in Table 1. In the intraepithelial compartment, there was approximately a 2:1 predominance of CD8 (cytotoxic/suppressor) to CD4 (helper/inducer) cells. However, only a minority of these CD8 cells co-expressed the CD5 pan-T antigen strongly, whereas the huge majority of these cells expressed the CD7 marker of stimulated cells. In the lamina propria, the CD4:CD8 ratio was approximately 2:1 in favor of the CD4 subset, and a significantly higher percentage of the CD8 cells co-expressed CD5, although there was no major difference in distribution of the CD7 marker.

Simple schistosomal colitis

In the intraepithelial compartment, there was a marked shift in CD4:CD8 subset ratios ($p < 0.05$) with the CD4 cells becoming almost as numerous as CD8 lymphocytes. A second change observed ($p < 0.05$) was the increased expression of the CD5 antigen by intraepithelial CD8 cells. Whereas, there was no real difference in expression of the CD7 marker by CD8 cells, in the CD4 subset, the percentage of cells co-expressing CD7 was significantly increased ($p < 0.05$). However, there was little difference in T cell subsets in the lamina propria of controls and patients with simple schistosomal colitis.

Schistosomal colonic polyposis

The continued shift in subset distribution in the epithelial compartment was maintained, with the ratio of CD4:CD8 cells just exceeding unity ($p < 0.02$). As in the patients with simple colitis, a significantly higher percentage of the CD4 cells ($p < 0.05$) expressed the CD7 antigen, and the trend for increased expression of the CD5 marker by the CD8 subset was also noted ($p < 0.01$). However, unlike the situation in simple colitis, there was a significant alteration of T cell subset distribution in the lamina propria, with a drop in CD4:CD8 ratio from 2:1 to 7:5 ($p < 0.05$), although no significant changes in terms of expression of CD5 and CD7 markers were seen.

Table 1. T cell phenotype analysis

	CD8/CD5	Lymphocyte Subset CD7/CD8	CD8/CD7	CD3/CD8	Ratio * CD4:CD8
		INTRAEPITHELIAL LYMPHOCYTES			
Controls (n=5)					
Mean	29.0	74.8	84.6	65.2	0.55:1
S.D.	2.55	14.5	9.29	7.95	0.19
Simple Schistosomal Colitis (n=7)					
Mean	41.6	53.9	90.4	55.4	0.83:1
S.D.	13.2	11.4	5.50	6.73	0.24
Schistosomal Colonic Polyposis (n=6)					
Mean	43.7	56.0	92.5	49.5	1.05:1
S.D.	4.59	8.72	3.99	6.09	0.24
Schistosomal Colonic Polyps (n=2)					
1.	55	38	95	63	0.59:1
2.	60	38	100	55	0.82:1
		LAMINA PROPRIA LYMPHOCYTES			
Controls (n=5)					
Mean	48.8	57.6	88.4	33.6	2.08:1
S.D.	11.3	14.2	9.56	6.54	0.67
Simple Schistosomal Colitis (n=7)					
Mean	46.1	54.0	82.4	34.6	1.99:1
S.D.	9.06	10.3	9.29	6.53	0.60
Schistosomal Colonic Polyposis (n=6)					
Mean	43.0	59.5	85.0	41.7	1.40:1
S.D.	9.19	3.08	7.54	1.50	0.09
Schistosomal Colonic Polyps (n=2)					
1.	46	39	68	12	7.33:1
2.	42	34	72	13	6.69:1

Lymphocyte phenotypes established by double-label immunofluorescence. The figures represent the percentage cells positive for the first marker (eg. CD8) which co-express the second marker (eg. CD5, first column).

*derived from % CD3+CD8- cells.

Schistosomal polyps

Although only two actual polyps were available for study, thus precluding meaningful statistical analysis, both specimens were very similar (Table 1). In the intraepithelial compartment, the CD4:CD8 ratio was closer to that of normal mucosa than the non-polyp mucosa from schistomiasis patients, although there was a large increase in expression of the CD5 antigen by the CD8 subset, and a considerable increase in the percentage of CD4 cells which co-expressed the CD7 marker. In the lamina propria, there was a dramatic increase in the CD4 (helper/inducer) population, resulting in a CD4:CD8 ratio of about 7:1 (cf. 7:5 in non-polyp mucosa of polyposis patients). Of the relatively infrequent lamina propria CD8 cells, a slightly smaller percentage expressed CD7, whereas there was a high percentage of the CD4 subset positive for this marker.

Expression of MHC antigens by colonic epithelium

Expression of Class I antigens (HLA-A,B,C) was strong throughout the normal colonic mucosa, including the epithelium. By contrast, there was no unequivocally detectable of class II (HLA-D region) antigen expression by enterocytes in any of the control specimens examined.

In patients with schistosomiasis, there was no apparent dimunition of labeling for Class I antigens, and in all specimens examined, enterocytes were strongly positive for HLA-DR and HLA-DQ. The labeling was observed throughout the epithelium, being found in surface cells (including in the polyps), crypts and glands to approximately an equal extent.

DISCUSSION

T lymphocytes in normal human colon have not been extensively studied; our data from Egyptian controls show quite marked differences compared with published observations of U.K. controls (11,12) and the 21 U.K. controls we have studied (in preparation), thus emphasizing the need to use control patients from the same environmental background.

Our data shows that there are marked changes in T cell populations in the colon of patients with schistosomal colitis, some of these changes being related to the presence of multiple colonic polyps. Whereas colonic polyposis is an uncommon complication of schistosomal infection in most endemic areas, it is seen in up to 20% of Egyptian farmers with colonic schistosomiasis (13). The cause of polyp formation is unclear, although they may form as a consequence of granuloma coalescence (9), and might thus be regarded as the most severe manifestation of colonic schistosomiasis.

In respect of the intraepithelial compartment, the changes observed in T cells in schistosomiasis were most marked in the polyposis patients. There appeared to be an infiltration of the epithelium with CD4 (helper/inducer) cells, and increased proportion of which expressed the 40 Kdalton CD7 antigen particularly associated with stimulated T cells (see 14). This is consistent with our observation that the epithelium of all schistosomal patients was strongly HLA-DR$^+$, in view of the now-accepted hypothesis that class II expression in epithelia is induced by gamma-interferon, a lymphokine particularly associated with activated T helper cells. These data further suggest that the very high percentage of intraepithelial CD8$^+$

(cytotoxic/suppressor) cells which express CD7, both in control and schistosomal mucosae, are not involved in interferon production, as judged by the absence of class II expression by enterocytes of uninfected colon. Nevertheless, there was a significant increase in the percentage of CD8 cells co-expressing the CD5 (T1) antigen. Whereas the significance of CD5 expression by gut mucosal $CD8^+$ cells remains obscure, recent data linking expression of CD5 antigen with cell-cell interactions suggests that the $CD8^+CD5^+$ subset may be committed suppressor cells (see 10), maintaining a regulatory balance in aposition to a more numerous or active $CD4^+CD7^+$ population. It is worth noting that all these changes in intraepithelial colonic T cells resemble closely the changes associated with coeliac disease (14).

By contrast, the only perturbations in lamina propria T cells were observed in patients with polyposis, where two apparently paradoxical effects occurred: a drop in CD4:CD8 ratio in the general mucosa, and a massive increase in the actual polyps. Although this could be due to selective depletion of CD4 cells as a consequence of migration into the polyps, it assumes that no proliferation of T cells had occurred in response to antigenic stimulation. Alternatively, the decreased lamina propria CD4:CD8 ratio could reflect an increase in absolute numbers of CD8 (suppressor/inducer) cells. We suggest that this latter explanation better fits our observations and that the increase in percentage CD8 cells reflects a defensive response aimed at reducing granuloma hypersensitivity (8). However, we suggest that granuloma modulation fails to occur (or occurs too late) possibly either due to genetic or other factors, or because the CD8 response is inappropriate, consisting of cytotoxic cells rather than suppressor cells. Whereas, there is some evidence that CD8 cells mediate cytotoxicity to schistosomules (15), there is no evidence that they are effective against deposited eggs. If our hypothesis is correct, then left unregulated, the granulomas would continue to attract more and more CD4 cells, thereby exacerbating the problem (resulting in granuloma coalescence and polyp formation), whereas CD8 cells would continue to accumulate in the non-polypoid colonic mucosa. This hypothesis accords with other experimental observations (7).

CONCLUSIONS

1. Local cell-mediated immunity is considerably altered in schistosomal colitis.

2. The increase of intraepithelial stimulated ($CD7^+$) T helper/inducer cells probably represents an inappropriate response, designed to combat luminal pathogens.

3. Expression of class II antigens by colonic epithelium probably reflects the ongoing immune response, and may be a direct consequence of increased intraepithelial T helper/inducer cell activity.

4. In polyposis, we suggest that granuloma modulation (due to increased T suppressor/cytotoxic cells) fails to occur in the actual polyps, resulting in a massive influx of T helper/inducer cells.

ACKNOWLEDGEMENTS

This work was supported, in part, by the Egyptial Cultural Bureau.

REFERENCES

1. Colley, D.G., Cook, J.A., Freeman, G.L., Bartholemew, R.K. and Jordan, P., Int. Arch. Allergy Appl. Immunol. 53, 420, 1977.
2. Gastl, G.A., Feldmeier, H., Doehring, E., Kortmann, C., Daffalla, A.A., and Peter, H.H., Scand. J. Immunol. 19, 469, 1984.
3. Mazingue, C., Dessaint, J.P., Scmitt-Verhulst, A.M., Cerottini, J.C. and Capron, A., Int. Arch. Allergy Appl. Immunol. 72, 22, 1984.
4. Warren, K.S., in Parasites in the Immunized Host: Mechanisms of Survival, Ciba Foundation Symposium 25, 243, 1974.
5. Rocklin, R.E., Brown, A.P., Warren, K.S., Pelley, L.P., Houba, V., Siongok, T.K.A., Ouma, J., Sturrock, R.F. and Butterworth, A.E., J. Immunol. 125, 1916, 1980.
6. Phillips, S.M. and Fox, E.G., Cont. Top. Immunobiol. 12, 421, 1984.
7. Doughty, B.L., Ottensen, E.A., Nash, T.E. and Phillips, S.M., J. Immunol. 133, 993, 1984.
8. Damian, T.R., Cont. Top. Immunobiol. 12, 359, 184.
9. Edington, G.E. and Gilles, H.M., in Pathology in the Tropics, p. 138, Arnold Ltd (London), 1979.

10. Trejdosiewicz, L.K., Malizia, G., Badr-el-Din, S., Smart, C.J., Oakes, D.J., Southgate, J., Howdle, P.D., Janossy, G., Poulter, L.W. and Losowsky, M.S., (this volume).

11. Selby, W.S., Janossy, G., Goldstein, G. and Jewell, D.P., Clin. Exp. Immunol. 44, 453, 1981.

12. Selby, W.S., Janossy, G., Bofill, M. and Jewell, D.P., Gut 25, 32, 1984.

13. Cheever, A.W. and Andrade, Z.A., Trans. Royal Soc. Trop. Med. Hyg. 61, 626, 1967.

14. Malizia, G., Trejdosiewicz, L.K., Wood, G.M., Howdle, P.D., Janossy, G. and Losowsky, M.S., Clin. Exp. Immunol. 60, 437, 1985.

15. Ellner, J.J., Olds, G.R., Lee, C.W., Kleinheinz, M.L. and Edmonds, K.L., J. Clin. Invest. 70, 369, 1982.

CANINE PEYER'S PATCHES: MACROSCOPIC, LIGHT MICROSCOPIC, SCANNING ELECTRON MICROSCOPIC AND IMMUNOHISTOCHEMICAL INVESTIGATIONS

H. HogenEsch, J.M. Housman and P.J. Felsburg

Department of Veterinary Pathobiology
University of Illinois, Urbana, IL USA

INTRODUCTION

In 1928, Carlens reported on his detailed investigations of the morphology and ontogeny of lymphoid tissue in the intestinal tract of large domestic animals (1). He observed that the morphology and development of the ileal Peyer's patch (PP) was different from the PP in the rest of the small intestine. Recent studies in sheep (2), cattle (3) and swine (4) have confirmed and expanded Carlens' observations. The ileal PP has been shown to be functionally different from the jejunal PP and may represent the bursa-equivalent in sheep and cattle (3,5). In contrast, morphologic studies in mice (6), rats (7) and humans (8) do not indicate the existence of these regional differences of PP.

It is well established in laboratory rodents and rabbits that PP are the primary source of precursors of IgA secreting plasma cells (9). The recent finding of selective IgA deficiency in beagles (10) has stimulated our interest in the canine PP. Because of the scarcity of information on the morphology of the PP in the dog, we are currently studying their macroscopic, light microscopic, electron microscopic, and immunohistochemical features. Here we present preliminary data from our studies.

MATERIALS AND METHODS

Macroscopic examination

Intestine were removed from young adult dogs (1/2 to 1 year) and opened lengthwise along the mesenteric attachment. They were extensively rinsed in cold water to remove intestinal contents and mucus and fixed in 2% acetic acid for 24 h. The PP were counted and their surface area was measured.

Light microscopy

PP from the duodenum, jejunum and ileum of young adult dogs were fixed in 10% formalin. Paraffin embedded 6 μm sections were stained with H & E and PAS.

Scanning electron microscopy

PP from the duodenum of young adult dogs that had been fasted overnight were spread out and pinned down on a paraffin board and gently rinsed with phosphate buffered saline. They were fixed in modified Karnovsky's solution for 1 h at room temperature. The PP were then dissected in small blocks and kept overnight in fresh modified Karnovsky's solution. The tissues were secondarily fixed in osmium tetraoxide, dehydrated and critical point dried. The blocks were mounted, sputter coated with gold/palladium and examined with an ISI DS 130 microscope.

Immunohistochemistry

Sections of sublimate-formaldehyde fixed, paraffin embedded tissue were deparaffinized, rehydrated and stained for cytoplasmic IgM and IgA (cIgM and cIgA) with the PAP method. Peroxidase activity was visualized with 3,3-diaminobenzidine and the slides were counterstained with acid hematoxylin.

RESULTS

Macroscopic examination

The intestines contained 26 to 29 PP. The PP were randomly distributed with a large variation between the individual dogs, except for the first four or five PP in the proximal duodenum and the single PP in the ileum. The first PP was present at 8.5 to 10.6 cm from the pylorus and the next three or four PP followed at short (1-3 cm) intervals. The PP were cross oval or round proximally and became more elongate towards the ileum. They varied in size from 2 x 10 to 36 x 14 mm. The ileal PP was much larger. It was 256 - 299 mm long and its surface area accounted for 77 to 80.5% of the total surface area of the PP. The ileal PP began proximally as a band of 10 mm wide at the anti-mesenteric side of the ileum. After 100 to 140 mm the band gradually became broader and it involved the entire circumference of the ileum over the distal 65 to 105 mm. The PP ended at the ileocecal junction.

Light microscopy

Marked differences between the single ileal PP and the duodenal and jejunal PP were observed (Fig. 1). The duodenal PP contained large pear-shaped lymphoid follices, a large dome and a sizable densely cellular interfollicular area (IFA). The follicles were located in the submucosa, while the domes extended through the thick muscularis mucosae into the mucosa. The domes reached 1/2 to 3/4 of the length of the villi. The follicles had a germinal center composed of a light area that occupied the center of the follicle and a dark area at the base of the follicle. The light area contained follicular dendritic cells, large lymphoblasts and tingible body macrophages. In the dark area lymphoblasts and small lymphocytes were present. Mitotic figures were predominantly found in the dark area. A zone of densely packed small lymphocytes, the corona, separated the germinal center from the dome and the IFA. The dome contained a mixed population of cells, predominantly plasma cells, lymphocytes and macrophages. The dome epithelium (DE) was characterized by the presence of numerous intra-epithelial leukocytes and sparsity of goblet cells. Cross sections of intestinal crypts were present in the dome and corona, frequently extending

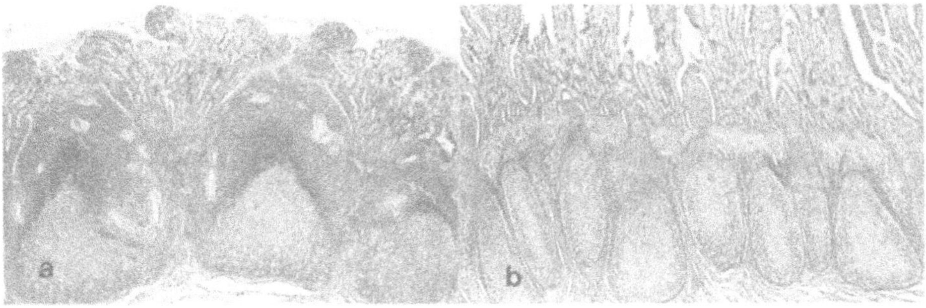

Figure 1. Duodenal (a) and ileal (b) Peyer's patch (H & E, x 22). The duodenal PP is characterized by lymphoid nodules with a large dome and corona, a densely cellular interfollicular area and the presence of intrafollicular intestinal crypts. The lymphoid nodules of the ileal PP have a small dome and corona and are separated by small interfollicular areas. They lack intrafollicular intestinal crypts.

into the submucosa. The epithelium of these crypts was similar to the DE. The IFA mainly contained small lymphocytes. High endothelial venules were found in these areas.

The architecture of the jejunal PP was similar to the duodenal PP. The lymphoid nodules were more elongate and the domes rarely exceeded 1/3 of the length of the villi. In contrast to the duodenal PP, intestinal crypts never extended into the submucosa and were only incidentally present in the domes of the lymphoid nodules.

The lymphoid nodules of the ileal PP were smaller than those of the duodenal and jejunal PP and sharply delineated with an exiguous IFA. The follicles had a large germinal center and a thin corona. The domes were small and serial sectioning revealed that the domes of only a few follicles extended into the mucosa. They never reached the base of the villi. The DE was similar to the DE of the duodenal and jejunal PP. The IFA was sparsely populated by small lymphocytes. High endothelial venules appeared rare.

Scanning electron microscopy

Examination of the DE of the follicle of a duodenal PP revealed a smooth surface largely composed of hexagonal epithelial cells with fine regular microvilli. Interspersed between these cells oval to hexagonal depressed areas, approximately one third of the size of the surface of an epithelial cell, were present (Fig. 2). Tufts of coarse microvilli were present on these depressed areas, which resemble the surface of M cells. These cells were present in low numbers and evenly distributed in the DE.

Immunohistochemistry

Many cIgA-positive cells and a few IgM-positive cells were present in the lamina propria around the lymphoid nodules of the PP. cIgA-positive cells were most numerous in the villi and sparsely present around the base of the crypts. The germinal centers rarely contained cIgA-positive cells, but a moderate to large number of cIgA-positive cells were found in the domes (Fig. 3). They were most numerous at the tip of the domes and decreased in number towards the muscularis mucosae. cIgM-positive cells were commonly present in the germinal center. In addition, marked extracellular staining of IgM was found in the germinal center.

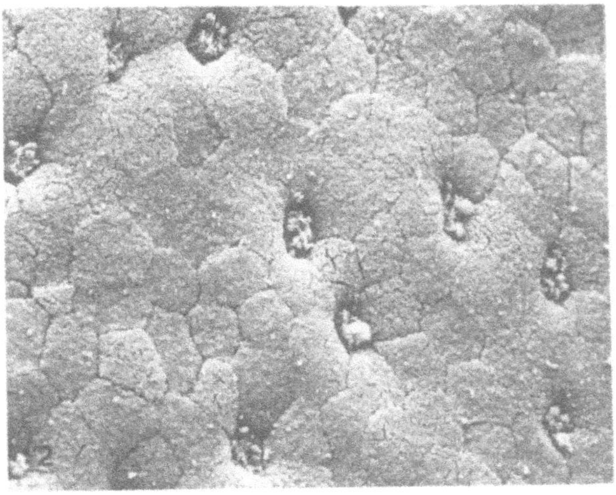

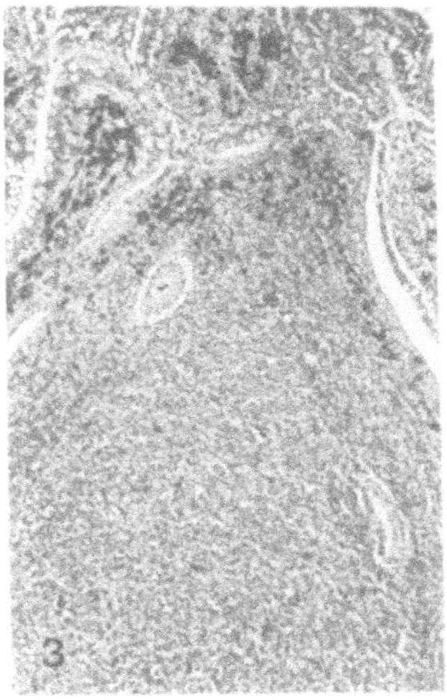

Figure 2 (left). Scanning electron microscopy of the dome epithelium of a duodenal PP. Cells, resembling M cells are characterized by depression of the surface and the presence of coarse microvilli (x 1720).

Figure 3 (right). IgA-containing cells in the dome of a lymphoid nodule of a duodenal PP.

DISCUSSION

The total number of PP varies widely between examined species and individual animals, from 1 - 10 in rabbits (11,12) to 245 - 320 in horses (1). We found 26 - 29 PP in the small intestine of the dog, which is in accordance with previous investigations (13). Similar to cattle, sheep and swine, the dog has a large typically shaped ileal PP, which contains the bulk of the total PP tissue.

The general histologic architecture of the PP appears similar in all examined animal species (14) and the dog is no exception. Based upon differences in the distribution of different cell types, a lymphoid nodule of the PP can be divided into a follicle, composed of a germinal center with a light and dark area and a corona and a dome. The follicles are separated by the IFA. Recent reports have demonstrated morphologic, developmental and functional differences between jejunal and ileal PP in ruminants and swine (2-5). Similarly, the canine ileal PP was characterized by a small dome and corona and a sparsely populated IFA, compared to duodenal and jejunal PP. No information is yet available on the ontogeny and function of canine PP from different parts of the small intestine.

In addition, in the dog the duodenal PP could be distinguished from the jejunal PP by the presence of intrafollicular intestinal crypts that extend through the muscularis mucosae into the submucosa. Solitary lymphoid nodules surrounding crypts that penetrate into the submucosa are numerous in the cecum and colon of man (8), dog (15,16) and other species of animals (1,16). These lymphoglandular complexes or "lymphatischen Darmkrypten" have also been described in the small intestine of swine, cattle, sheep and dogs (16). The author found these crypts in solitary nodules as well as PP without mentioning the distribution of the involved PP. The crypts probably improve the uptake of antigen from the gut by enlarging the surface area of the epithelium. Light microscopic examination suggests that the crypt epithelium is similar to the DE. The presence of a large dome and corona and the presence of crypts, in addition to their strategic location in the proximal part of the intestine, indicates an important role for the duodenal PP in the intestinal immune response.

Scanning electron microscopy of the DE of a duodenal PP revealed the presence of cells which were characterized by a depression of the surface and the presence of tufts of coarse microvilli. These cells strongly resemble the M cells that have been found in humans (17) and several animal species (18). Whether the cells are indeed M cells awaits confirmation by transmission electron microscopy. The occurrence of M cells in canine PP has been mentioned in earlier work (18).

Studies in rabbits and laboratory rodents (7,11,19) have demonstrated an absence of cIgA-positive cells in the lymphoid nodules of PP. It is thought that B cells, which have undergone an isotype switch towards IgA, leave the PP and undergo further maturation in the mesenteric lymph node and/or after returning to the lamina propria. How the IgA plasma cells reach their final location in the lamina propria is not well understood. The presence of many IgA plasma cells around high endothelial venules in PP of rats may indicate that the cells preferentially leave the circulation via the high endothelial venules and migrate to the lamina propria along the muscularis mucosa (7). On the other hand, Husband (20) has shown in rats that cIgA-positive cells enter the lamina propria diffusely throughout the villi. A recent study demonstrated cIgA-positive cells in the dome of human PP and it was proposed that B cells mature to IgA plasma cells in the PP and subsequently migrate to the lamina propria (21). In the present study, cIgA positive cells were also found in the dome of canine PP. This suggests that, different from rabbits and laboratory rodents, complete maturation of B cells into IgA plasma cells can occur in canine

PP. However, direct migration from the PP seems not likely to be a major source of IgA plasma cells in the lamina propria, because of the paucity of cIgA-positive cells along the muscularis mucosa and around the base of the crypts. Most of the IgA committed B cells probably migrate via the circulation to the lamina propria, similar to other animal species (7,22), while relatively few mature into plasma cells in the dome of the PP.

ACKNOWLEDGEMENTS

These studies were supported by a grant from the American Veterinary Medical Association Research Foundation and by grant AI 20860 from the National Institutes of Health.

REFERENCES

1. Carlens, O., Z. Anat. Entw. 86, 393, 1928.
2. Reynolds, J., Pabst, R. and Bordmann, G., Adv. Exp. Biol. Med. 186, 101, 1985.
3. Landsverk, T., Acta. Path. Microbiol. Immun. Scand. A. 92, 77, 1984.
4. Binns, R.M. and Licence, S.T., Adv. Exp. Biol. Med. 186, 661, 1985.
5. Reynolds, J.D. and Morris, B., Eur. J. Immunol. 13, 627, 1983.
6. Abe, K. and Ito, T., Arch. Histol. Jap. 40, 407, 1977.
7. Sminia, T. and Plesch, B.E.C., Virch. Arch. (Cell Path.) 40, 181, 1982.
8. Cornes, J.S., Gut 6, 225, 1965.
9. Craig, S.W. and Cebra, J.J., J. Exp. Med. 134, 188, 1971.
10. Felsburg, P.J., Glickman, L.T. and Jezyk, P.F., Clin. Immun. Immunopath. 36, 297, 1985.
11. Faulk, W.P., McCormick, J.N., Goodman, J.R., Yoffey, J.M. and Fudenberg, H.H., Cell. Immunol. 1, 500, 1971.
12. Sackmann, W., Acta. Anat. 97, 109, 1977.
13. Titkemeyer, C.W. and Calhoun, L., Am. J. Vet. Res. 16, 152, 1955.
14. Waksman, B.H., Ozer, H. and Blythman, H.E., Lab. Invest. 28, 614, 1973.
15. Atkins, A.M. and Schofield, G.C., J. Anat. 113, 169, 1972.
16. Hebel, R., Anat. Anz. 109, 7, 1960.
17. Owen, R.L. and Jones, A.L., Gastroenterology 66, 189, 1974.
18. Owen, R.L. and Nemanic, P., Scanning Electron Microscopy 11, 367, 1978.

19. Bienenstock, J. and Dolezel, J., J. Immunol. 106, 938, 1971.
20. Husband, A.J., J. Immunol. 128, 1355, 1982.
21. Spencer, J., Finn, T. and Isaacson, P.G., Gut 27, 405, 1986.
22. Husband, A.J., Beh, K.J. and Lascelles, A.K., Immunology 37, 597, 1979.

THE ROLE OF PEYER'S PATCHES IN INTESTINAL HUMORAL IMMUNE RESPONSES IS LIMITED TO MEMORY FORMATION

S.H.M. Jeurissen, G. Kraal and T. Sminia

Department of Histology, Medical Faculty
Free University, P.O. Box 7161, 1007 MC
Amsterdam, The Netherlands

INTRODUCTION

The interaction of antigens with the mucosal immune system in the gut has been studied extensively. It has become clear that depending on the type of antigen, the dose and the frequency of administration the immune response can vary between a state of tolerance (1,2) and extensive cellular or humoral reactivity (3-5). Peyer's patches (PP) are thought to play a crucial role in the regulation of these immune responses. This function has been attributed to PP, e.g., by the presence of M cells (specialized epithelial cells in the follicle associated epithelium), which sample antigens from the gut lumen (6).

The humoral immune response to intestinal antigens is characterized by the production of predominantly IgA immunoglobulins. Precursor cells of the IgA-producing plasma cells were shown to be derived from PP (7). In migration studies in which IgA lymphoblasts and plasma cells obtained from MLN and PP are intravenously injected, it was shown that these cells preferentially home into mucosa-associated lymphoid tissues (8). The induction of IgA committed B cells is thought to be regulated by IgA-specific T helper cells in PP (9). So far, little attention has been paid to the IgM response towards intestinal antigens as well as to the events leading to memory formation. In this paper we have further elucidated the role of PP in humoral immune responses to intestinal antigens and present evidence for a specific function in memory formation.

MATERIALS AND METHODS

Animals

Adult Wistar rats and Swiss mice (TNO, Zeist, The Netherlands) were used to study antigen uptake in the gut. To investigate the intestinal immune response $(C_3D_2)F_1$ mice (G.O. Bomholtgard Ltd., Glostrup, Denmark) were used.

Antigen uptake

Latex particles (Ø 1.09 μm, Dow-Latex, Heidelberg, FRG) and India ink (Pelikan Spezialtusche CII/1431a) were mixed into their drinking water. Horseradish peroxidase (HRP, Merck, Darmstadt, FRG) and HRP-coated latex were injected directly into the lumen of the small intestines (intra-intestinally, i.i.) of anesthetized animals (Hypnorm, Duphar, Weesp, The Netherlands). Carboxylated latex (COOH-latex, Ø 0.48 μm, Serva, Heidelberg, FRG) was coated with HRP according to the method of covalent binding of proteins to CH-Sepharose 4B (Pharmacia, Uppsala, Sweden). After 2, 6, 24 and 48 h PP, mesenteric lymph nodes (MLN) and gut segments were removed and snap-frozen in liquid nitrogen.

Detection of antigens

Cryostat sections, about 8 μm thick, were air-dried and fixed for 10 min in pure acetone. When HRP or HRP-coated latex were used, the slides were treated for 15 min with 3,3'-diaminobenzidine-HCl (DAB, Sigma, St. Louis, MO) in 0.5 mg/ml Tris-HCl buffer, pH 7.6, containing 0.01% H_2O_2. To demonstrate acid phosphatase the Burstone method (10) was used, with naphthol AS-BI-phosphate as substrate and hexazotized pararosaniline as diazonium salt.

Immunization procedure

To evoke a primary immune response 500 μg alum-precipitated keyhole limpet haemocyanin coupled to trinitrophenyl (KLH-TNP) was injected into the lumen of the proximal jejunum (i.i.) of anesthetized mice (Hypnorm in combination with ether). This dose of antigen had been found optimal in previous experiments. To study the secondary immune response, mice were given 500 μg KLH-TNP i.i. without adjuvant 14 d after priming.

In situ detection of anti-TNP antibody-containing cells

Five days after antigen administration, spleen, MLN and PP were removed and snap-frozen in liquid nitrogen. Specific anti-TNP antibody-containing cells were demonstrated as described by Claassen and van Rooijen (11,12). Briefly, 8 μm thick cryostat sections were dried and fixed for 10 min in pure acetone. The sections were horizontally incubated with TNP-conjugated to alkaline phosphatase (TNP-AP) or with TNP-conjugated to poly-L-lysine-HRP (TNP-POLY-HRP) overnight at 4°C. Slides were washed three times in PBS. When incubated with TNP-AP the slides were treated for alkaline phosphatase according to Burstone (10) with fast blue BB salt (no. F0250, Sigma) and naphthol-AS-MX-phosphate for 30 min at 37°C. After incubation with TNP-POLY-HRP slides were treated for 10 min with 3-amino-9-ethylcarbazole (AEC, Sigma) as substrate, containing 0.01% H_2O_2.

Quantification of anti-TNP antibody-producing cells by plaque-forming cell (PFC) assay

To determine total numbers of specific IgM-producing cells, the direct PFC assay was used. Cell suspensions of spleen, MLN and PP were mixed with TNP-coated sheep red blood cells and fresh guinea pig serum and after 4 h incubation at 37°C antigen-specific IgM plaques were counted. To obtain IgG-anti-TNP cells or IgA-anti-TNP cells indirect PFC assays were performed with IgG or IgA developing antisera (a kind gift of Prof. dr. R. Benner, Rotterdam). The mean value and standard deviation were calculated as described by Benner et al. (13).

RESULTS

Uptake of antigens

Native and HRP-coated latex particles were found shortly after administration directly beneath the PP follicle epithelium and in the germinal center. The majority of particles were taken up by macrophages, as demonstrated by combination with histochemistry for acid phosphatase. It appeared that coating the outer surface of latex particles with protein did not result in an altered uptake. India ink was selectively taken up in PP as well, where, in contrast to latex, it was also demonstrated in the interfollicular T cell area.

Two h after i.i. administration of HRP, numerous vacuoles in the villi enterocytes contained HRP and also in the lamina propria branched cells contained the antigen (Fig. 1). In contrast, little HRP was visible in the epithelial cells of PP. Using monoclonal antibodies against MHC class I antigens, anti-Ia, in combination with acid phosphatase staining, it was demonstrated that in the lamina propria of the villi, Ia-positive cells are present. These cells have the morphological characteristics of antigen-presenting cells *in situ*. In addition, many Ia-negative macrophages are also present.

Primary anti-TNP response

After a single i.i. injection, many anti-TNP antibodies containing cells had localized in the white pulp of the spleen (Fig. 2). In MLN some anti-TNP-containing cells were seen in the medulla. However, in all experiments performed we could never demonstrate specific antibody-containing cells in the lamina propria or PP. In contrast, anti-TNP antibodies were found in PP as immune complexes (Fig. 3). These complexes could also be demonstrated in the MLN, albeit to a much lesser extent, but were never found in the follicles of the spleen. The PFC assay for spleen, MLN and PP revealed that the antibodies produced were of the IgM class (Fig. 4).

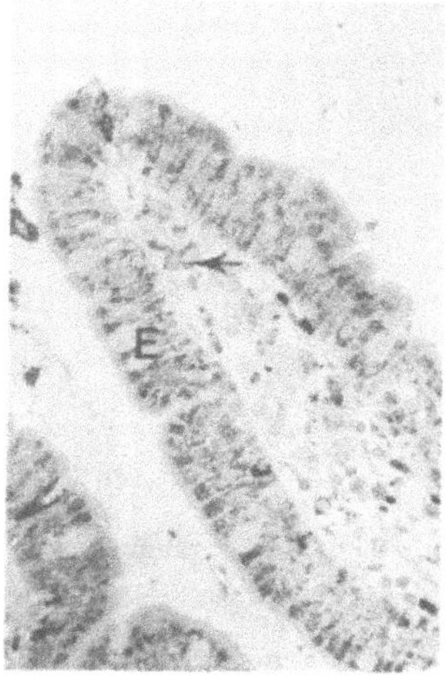

Figure 1. Two h after i.i. administration epithelial cells (E) of the villi contained HRP. In the lamina propria branched cells (arrow) with the antigen were present.

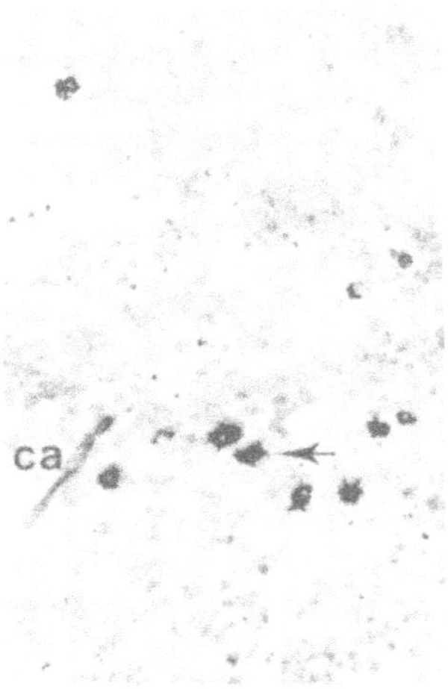

Figure 2. Anti-TNP antibody-containing cells (arrow) were demonstrated in the spleen at 5 d after i.i. priming by incubation of sections with TNP-AP followed by alkaline phosphatase reaction. c.a. = central artery.

Secondary anti-TNP response

The i.i. booster gave rise to an augmented number of specific antibody-containing cells in the spleen and MLN (Fig. 5). The splenic anti-TNP plasma cells produced antibodies of the IgM, IgG, and IgA classes. MLN appeared to differ from the spleen, because the PFC, which were present in rather low numbers produced only IgA antibodies. In PP, immune complex-like staining could be demonstrated with the in situ detection method whereas in PFC assays no anti-TNP producing cells were detected above background levels. The lamina propria of the villi contained low numbers of anti-TNP-containing cells.

DISCUSSION

To further elucidate the role of PP in humoral immune responses to intestinal antigens, we investigated the uptake of antigens from the gut lumen and the kinetics of the immune response. The experiments concerning the uptake of particulate and soluble antigens clearly showed that PP are not the only sites of entry. As described earlier by others (14,15), particulate antigens like India ink, latex and bacteria are absorbed by M cells of the follicle epithelium. These antigens are transported to the germinal center where they reside for long periods within the tingible

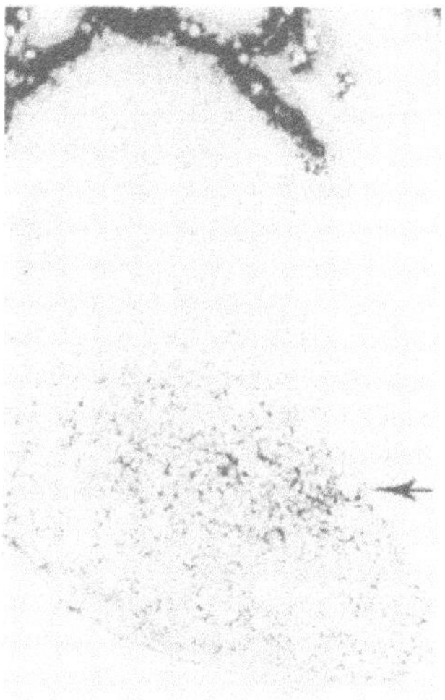

Figure 3. *In situ* detection of anti-TNP antibodies demonstrated an immune complex-like staining in follicle centers of PP (arrow). The PP epithelium is stained because of its endogenous alkaline phosphatase activity.

body macrophages (16). In contrast, soluble antigens are taken up in PP only in small numbers, whereas the bulk of these antigens are absorbed by the epithelium of the villi. Such differential uptake will probably influence the immune response against these antigens. Antigens present in PP will be transported to MLN via the lymphatics. In the villus epithelium antigens will pass to the underlying lamina propria, where Ia-positive, acid phosphatase-containing cells are present which represent antigen-presenting cells. Free antigen or antigen bound to antigen-presenting cells will then reach the systemic circulation via blood vessels, e.g. portal veins as has been shown by others (17,18).

The results of the present immunization experiments reflect the different antigen routes. After a single i.i. injection with KLH-TNP, anti-TNP cells of the IgM class were detected in the spleen. This can be explained by the fact that the first lymphoid organ that antigens in portal veins encounter will be the spleen. In this organ no immune complexes could be demonstrated in contrast to PP where they were abundantly present. Because no plasma cells of any Ig class can be found in PP, these complexes have to be formed from serum-borne antibody produced in the spleen and local antigen which is present in relatively high concentrations in PP follicles due to the antigen-transporting activity of M-cells.

When a secondary response was evoked, this again was predominantly located in the spleen. In contrast to single or repeated intravenous

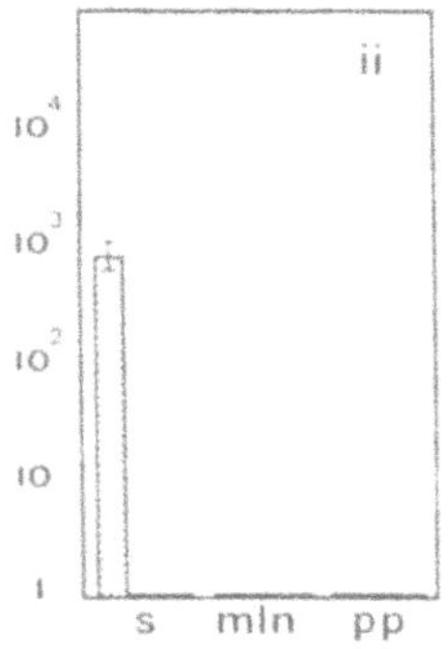

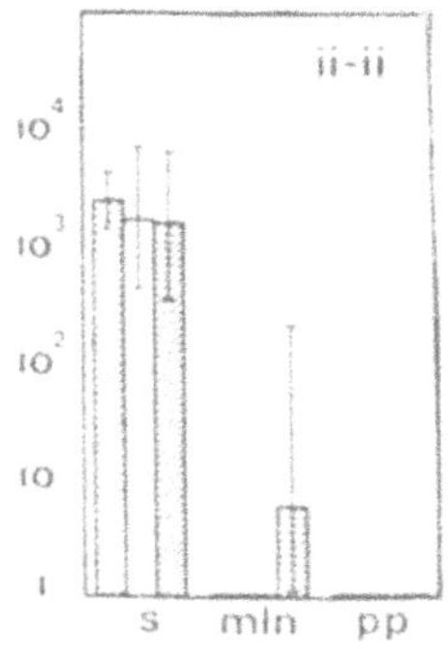

Figure 4 (left). Detection of the primary anti-TNP response with a plaque-forming cell assay 5 d after i.i. priming in spleen (S), MLN and PP. The dotted, white and striped bars, respectively, represent IgM, IgG and IgA plaque-forming cells.

Figure 5 (right). Detection of the secondary anti-TNP response with a plaque-forming cell assay, after i.i. priming and booster in S, MLN and PP. The dotted, white and striped bars, respectively, represent IgM, IgG and IgA plaque-forming cells.

injections, a large number of IgA-producing plasma cells could be demonstrated. In MLN, a moderate number of IgA anti-TNP cells were present, whereas no anti-TNP cells could be demonstrated in PP. Other experiments have shown that following i.i. priming antigen-specific IgA plasma cells can be evoked throughout the body wherever they encounter the same antigen again (19). These results imply that although the intestinal immune responses in terms of antibody-producing cells are predominantly located in the spleen, at the same time an IgA specific regulation mechanism is triggered, probably in PP.

In view of our results we believe that the occurrence of immune complexes in PP is a crucial phenomenon. These immune complexes, which are formed in PP, are trapped on follicular dendritic cells present in germinal centers. It has been demonstrated that follicular dendritic cells in PP are phenotypically different from those at other lymphoid tissues (20). Germinal centers have been shown to be the exclusive sites where memory formation (21,22) and heavy chain class switching (23) occur. Due to the IgA-specific T helper cells (9) present in PP, the differentiating memory B cells will be precommitted to produce IgA. These memory cells migrate throughout the body and will give rise to IgA-producing plasma cells upon renewed encounter with the appropriate antigen.

CONCLUSIONS

1. PP are not involved in local antibody formation following intestinal immunizations.

2. PP are the major site of IgA memory formation.

REFERENCES

1. Chase, M.W., Proc. Soc. Exp. Biol. Med. 61, 257, 1946.
2. Kagnoff, M.F., J. Immunol. 120, 1509, 1978.
3. Andrè, C., Bazin, H. and Heremans, J.F., Digestion 9, 166, 1973.
4. Asherson, G.L., Zembala, M., Perera, H.A.C.A. and Mayhew, B., Cell. Immunol. 33, 145, 1977.
5. Weisz-Carrington, P., Roux, M.E., McWilliams, M., Phillips-Quagliata, J.H. and Lamm, M.E., J. Immunol. 123, 1705, 1979.
6. Owen, R.L. and Jones, A.L., Gastroenterology 66, 189, 1974.
7. Craig, S.W. and Cebra, J.J., J. Exp. Med. 134, 188, 1971.
8. Roux, M.E., McWilliams, M., Phillips-Quagliata, J.M. and Lamm, M.E., Cell. Immunol. 61, 141, 1981.
9. Kawanishi, H., Saltzman, L.E. and Strober, W., J. Exp. Med. 157, 433, 1983.
10. Burstone, M.S., J. Nat. Cancer Inst. 20, 601, 1958.
11. Claassen, E. and van Rooijen, N., J. Immunol. Meth. 75, 181, 1984.
12. Claassen, E. and van Rooijen, N., J. Histochem. Cytochem. 33, 840, 1985.
13. Benner, R., Meima, F., van der Meulen, G.M. and van Muiswinkel, W.B., Immunology 26, 247, 1974.
14. Owen, R.L., Allen, C.L. and Stevens, D.P., Infect. Immun. 33, 591, 1981.
15. LeFevre, M.E., Warren, J.B. and Joel, D.D., Expl. Cell Biol. 53, 121, 1985.
16. Joel, D.D., Laissue, J.A. and LeFevre, M.E., J. Reticuloendothel. Soc. 24, 477, 1978.
17. Warshaw, A.L., Walker, W.A., Cornell, R.C. and Isselbacher, K.J., Lab. Invest. 25, 675, 1971.

18. Matsuno, K., Schaffner, T., Gerber, H.A., Ruchti, C., Hess, M.W. and Cottier, H., J. Reticuloendothel. Soc. 33, 263, 1983.
19. Jeurissen, S.H.M., Claassen, E., van Rooijen, N. and Kraal, G., Immunology 56, 417, 1985.
20. Jeurissen, S.H.M. and Dijkstra, C.D., Eur. J. Immunol. 16, 562, 1986.
21. Klaus, G.G.B., Humphrey, J.H., Kunkl, A. and Dongworth, D.W., Immunol. Rev. 53, 3, 1980.
22. Kraal, G., Weissman, I.L. and Butcher, E.C., Adv. Exp. Med. Biol. 186, 145, 1985.
23. Kraal, G., Weissman, I.L. and Butcher, E.C., Nature 298, 377, 1982.

MURINE PEYER'S PATCHES ARE CAPABLE OF GENERATING A CYTOTOXIC T CELL (CTL) RESPONSE TO NOMINAL ANTIGENS

S.D. London, D.H. Rubin and J.J. Cebra

Department of Biology, University of Pennsylvania, Philadelphia, PA; *Departments of Medicine and Microbiology, Veterans Administration Medical Center and University of Pennsylvania, Philadelphia, PA USA

INTRODUCTION

The experiments described in this report were designed to determine whether murine Peyer's patches are capable of generating a cytotoxic T cell (CTL) response to nominal (non-MHC encoded) antigens. To date, Kagnoff (1) is the only researcher who has been able to directly demonstrate CTL activity in Peyer's patches. He demonstrated that a cytotoxic T cell response could be detected in Peyer's patches from mice chronically fed tumor cells that were mismatched at the major histocompatibility locus. However, he was unable to demonstrate a similar response in Peyer's patches when mice were chronically fed tumor cells bearing minor histocompatibility differences. While his study demonstrated that a CTL response could occur in Peyer's patches, the generation of allospecific CTL's, whose precursors are present at high frequency among normal T cells (2), may not be representative of the potential of Peyer's patches to generate CTL activity directed to nominal antigens. We have utilized reovirus serotype 1 (reo 1) as a model nominal antigen to determine whether intraduodenally applied virus induces a detectable CTL response in murine Peyer's patches. Reo 1 was chosen for these studies for the following reasons: (a) reo 1 is a naturally occurring enteric virus that is stable within the gastrointestinal tract (3); (b) Finberg and co-workers (4) have demonstrated that a CTL response to reovirus can be elicited from splenocytes after intraperitoneal immunization. In this system, detection of a virus-specific CTL response is dependent upon <u>in vitro</u> restimulation of primed splenocytes; (c) reo 1 exclusively binds to and is transported from the intestinal lumen into Peyer's patches through M cells (5), thereby allowing interactions to occur within the Peyer's patch between virus, antigen-presenting cells, and lymphocytes; and (d) we have shown that intraduodenal application of reo 1 causes a detectable frequency of virus-specific B cells in the patch and in distal lymphoid tissues similar to the frequencies observed after parenteral inoculation. However, only the intraduodenal route of priming resulted in a high percentage of clones, obtained from either the spleen or Peyer's patches, which are precommitted to IgA production when their precursors are stimulated in vitro in the splenic focus assay (Cebra et al., this volume). Because of these findings, we have utilized the reo 1 system as a probe for the cytotoxic potential of Peyer's patches. Using this system, we report here that Peyer's patches from mice intraduodenally primed with reo 1 contain precursor CTL's (pCTL's) that generate Thy 1^+, Lyt 2^+, MHC-restricted effector CTL's upon in vitro restimulation with virus. This is first report that murine Peyer's patches can generate a CTL response to a nominal antigen. The implications of these findings are discussed in the final section of this communication.

MATERIALS AND METHODS

Viruses

Third passage, CsCl gradient-purified reovirus serotype 1/Lang or 3/ Dearing were used in all experiments.

Immunizations

Male C3Heb/FeJ ($H\text{-}2^k$) or DBA/2J ($H\text{-}2^d$) mice, obtained from The Jackson Laboratory (Bar Harbor, ME), were immunized with either 3×10^7 plaque forming units (PFU) of reo 1 or gelatin-containing saline by the indicated routes (intraduodenal or intraperitoneal injection).

Generation of cytotoxic effector cells

Peyer's patch or peripheral lymph node lymphocytes (PLN) were cultured for six days with syngeneic peritoneal exudate cells (PEC) (virus-pulsed where indicated) and 10% rat Concanavalin A (Con A)-conditioned medium containing alpha-methyl-mannoside. Splenocytes were pulsed with reo 1 and cultured without the addition of peritoneal exudate cells.

Cytotoxicity assays

A standard 5 hour ^{51}Cr release assay was used to calculate the lytic activity present in cultured effector populations. The following targets were used in these studies: L-929 fibroblast cells, the B10.D2 SV40 transformed kidney line KD2SV, C3H or BALB/c LPS blasts, the A/Sn derived Moloney virus-transformed T cell lymphoma YAC-1 or the DBA/2J mastocytoma P-815.

Frequency estimation of reovirus specific pCTL's

Individual microculture wells containing virus-pulsed syngeneic PEC's were seeded with limiting numbers of responding lymphocytes in the presence of 10% Con A supernatant and cultured for 8 days. Individual cultures were split and assayed for the ability to kill infected or uninfected L cells. Microcultures that lyse infected, but not uninfected, L cells three standard deviations greater than spontaneous release rates were considered positive. Frequency estimates and statistical significance was determined using the maximum likelihood method (6).

RESULTS

Generation of virus-specific cytotoxic and helper activity in murine Peyer's patches after intraduodenal application of reo 1

Peyer's patch lymphocytes obtained six days after a single intraduodenal application of 3×10^7 PFU of reo 1, generate a significant cytotoxic response against reo 1 infected L cell targets (Fig. 1). The generation of this virus-specific cytotoxic response is dependent upon *in vivo* viral priming. In addition, antigenic stimulation *in vitro* is necessary for the generation of this virus-specific cytotoxic response (not shown). Control (saline primed) Peyer's patches, cultured under identical conditions, do not generate virus-specific cytotoxic activity even after *in vitro* stimulation with reo 1 (Fig. 1).

The addition of an exogenous source of IL-2 (Con A-conditioned medium) increased the level of virus-specific lysis generated in these non-limiting cultures, although its presence was not an absolute requirement (Fig. 1A vs. 1B) However, in limiting dilution cultures, the generation of a virus-specific response was shown to be absolutely dependent upon factors present in Con A supernatants. Individual microcultures seeded with limiting input

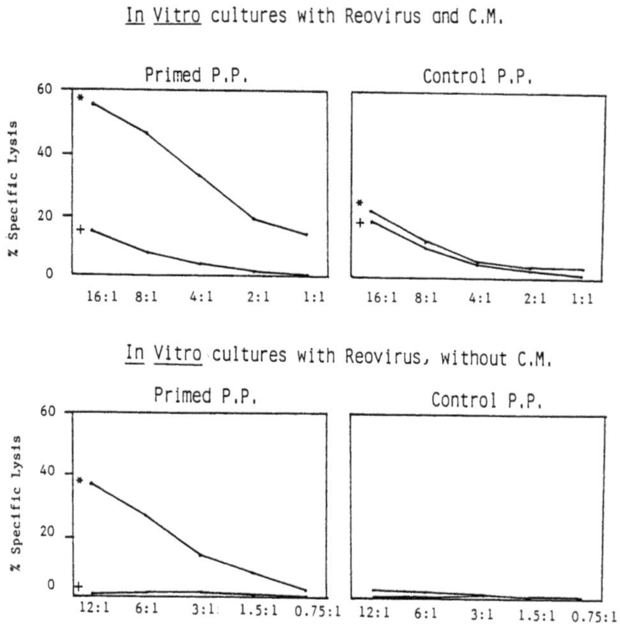

Figure 1. Peyer's patch lymphocytes obtained six days after the intraduodenal application of reovirus or saline, were cultured as indicated. Effectors were harvested and assayed for cytotoxic activity against reo 1 infected L cells (*) or uninfected L cells (+).

doses of primed Peyer's patch lymphocytes were assayed for the generation of virus-specific cytotoxic activity. Low input numbers of responding cells (60,000 cells/well) did not generate virus-specific cytotoxicity when cultured in the absence of Con A supernatant. However, 100% of such microcultures generated virus-specific cytotoxicity when cultured in the presence of 10% Con A supernatant (not shown). That non-limiting cultures of primed Peyer's patches can generate virus-specific cytotoxic activity without the addition of helper factors strongly suggests that virus-responsive helper cells, as well as pCTL's, are present in the patch six days after intraduodenal stimulation.

Characterization of the cytotoxic potential of Peyer's patch lymphocytes

Peyer's patch lymphocytes primed *in vivo* and *in vitro* with reo 1, were tested for cytotoxic activity against a panel of virus-infected or non-infected targets. Both reo 1 and 3 infected L cell targets were lysed, whereas uninfected L cells, syngeneic (C3H), or allogeneic (BALB/c) LPS blasts were not lysed. These *in vitro* cultured lymphocytes also generated cytotoxic activity to the classic natural killer (NK) target, YAC-1 and the spontaneous cytotoxic (SC) target, P-815 (Fig. 2). This pattern of target

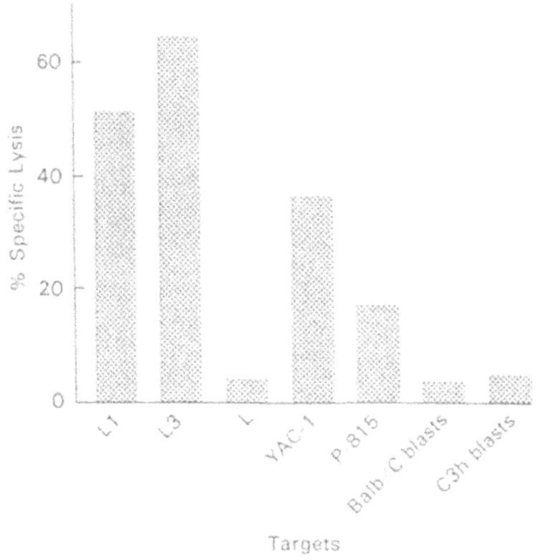

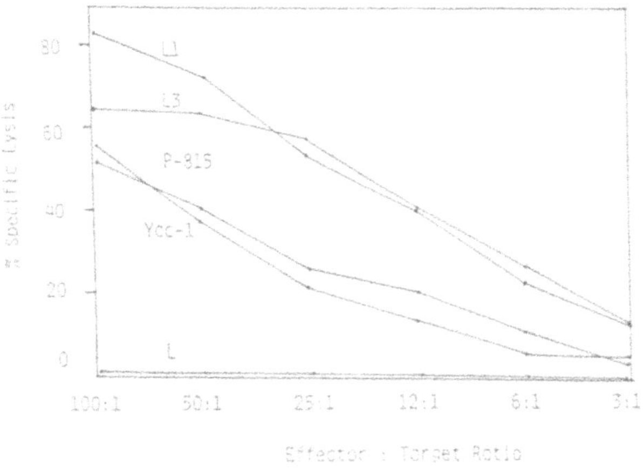

Figure 2 (top). Effectors obtained from *in vitro* cultures of six day intraduodenally primed Peyer's patches were assayed for cytotoxic activity against the indicated targets.

Figure 3 (bottom). Effectors obtained from *in vitro* cultures of six day intraperitoneally primed splenocytes were assayed for cytotoxic activity against the indicated targets.

lysis was not unique to virus-primed Peyer's patch lymphocytes. Splenocytes obtained from mice intraperitoneally primed with reo 1 also generate a similar pattern of lysis against either reo 1 or 3 infected L cells as well as NK/SC targets (Fig. 3). Furthermore, while the generation of virus-specific cytotoxic activity is dependent upon *in vivo* viral priming, the generation of NK/SC cytotoxic activity occurs in *in vitro* cultured Peyer's patch lymphocytes regardless of prior virus-priming (Fig. 4).

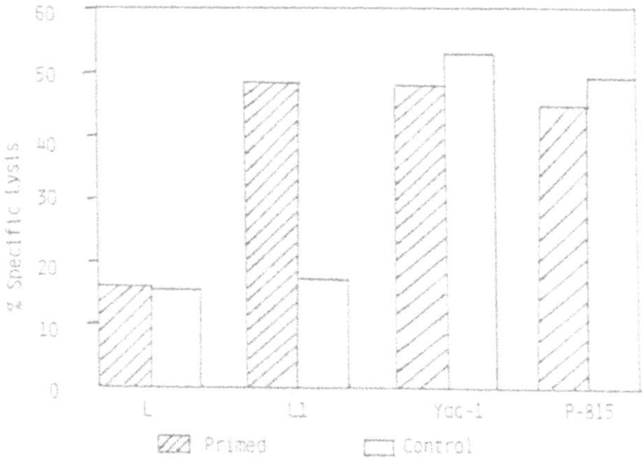

Figure 4. Six day intraduodenally primed or control Peyer's patches. Effectors obtained from primed or control mice were assayed against the indicated targets.

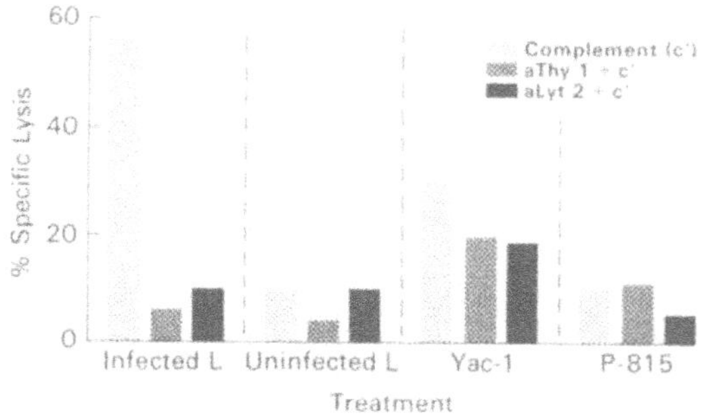

Figure 5. Intraduodenally primed Peyer's patches: phenotype of cultured effectors. The phenotype of effectors was determined by pretreatment with cytotoxic monoclonal antibodies plus complement.

The phenotype of the virus-specific effector cells was shown to be Thy 1^+, Lyt 2^+ by treatment of the in vitro generated effectors with cytotoxic monoclonal antibodies plus complement (Fig. 5). Finally, we determined that the virus-specific cytotoxic response is H-2 restricted. Reo 1 primed DBA/2 (H-2^d) Peyer's patch lymphocytes lyse H-2^d (KD2SV) but not H-2^k (L) infected targets, whereas the converse is true of C3H (H-2^k) effectors (Fig. 6).

Frequency analysis of 6 day or 6 month intraduodenally primed Peyer's patches and peripheral lymph nodes

We determined the frequency of virus-specific pCTL's present in either Peyer's patches or peripheral lymph nodes six days (Table 1) or six months

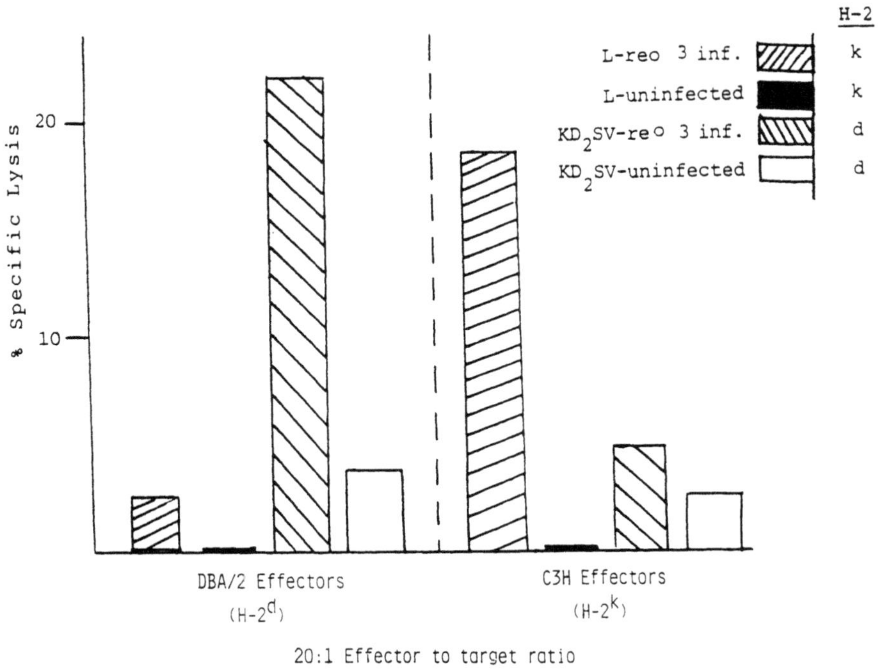

Figure 6. H-2 restriction of six day intraduodenally primed Peyer's patch lymphocytes was demonstrated using the strains of mice and targets indicated.

(Table 2) after a single intraduodenal application of reo 1. While we do not detect virus-specific pCTL's from control animals (Peyer's patches or peripheral lymph nodes), we can routinely detect and determine the frequency of virus-specific pCTL's present in various tissues after _in vivo_ priming. At either six days or six months following intraduodenal inoculation, a higher frequency of virus-specific pCTL's was present in Peyer's patches as compared to peripheral lymph nodes. When precursor frequencies are normalized relative to the proportion of Thy 1^+ or Lyt 2^+ cells that

Table 1. Six day intraduodenally primed tissues. Frequencies[a] normalized to cell type

Tissue	Lymphocytes	Thy 1^+	Lyt 2^+
PP	67	270	1675
PLN	5	6	17

[a]Frequency/10^6 cells.

Table 2. Six month intraduodenally primed tissues. Frequencies[a] normalized to cell type

Tissue	Lymphocytes	Thy 1^+	Lyt 2^+
PP	50	200	1235
PLN	23	28	85

[a]Frequency/10^6 cells.

are present in the tissues evaluated, the divergence in precursor frequencies becomes more pronounced. Because of the low proportion of Thy 1^+ and Lyt 2^+ cells present in Peyer's patches (25% and 5%, respectively) as compared to peripheral lymph nodes (80% and 25%, respectively), one observes a 4 fold to 20 fold increase in precursor frequency when Peyer's patch lymphocytes are normalized to Thy 1^+ or Lyt 2^+ cells, respectively. In contrast, there is only a 1.25 to 4 fold increase in frequency in peripheral lymph nodes.

DISCUSSION

We have demonstrated that murine Peyer's patches are capable of generating a CTL response to the nominal antigen reovirus serotype 1 after intraduodenal priming. We have defined a reo-specific CTL response to be one in which reo-infected, but not uninfected, L cells are lysed in a standard ^{51}Cr release assay. Lysis of reo infected targets occurs only in Peyer's patches obtained from mice intraduodenally primed with virus. The necessity for in vivo virus priming suggests that the cytotoxic activity that is generated in in vitro cultures is not a manifestation of naturally cytotoxic populations. That this is the case is supported by our observation that the generation of virus-specific cytotoxic activity does not occur in control patches, even when these populations generate substantial NK/SC activity upon in vitro culture. The virus-specific lysis is H-2 restricted and mediated by Thy 1^+, Lyt 2^+ effector cells. These observations define the virus-specific effector cells as being cytotoxic T lymphocytes. We have found that Peyer's patch-derived virus-specific CTL's are capable of lysing both reo 1 and 3 infected L cell targets. Since Finberg and coworkers (4,7) have published that reo-specific CTL's predominantly recognize serotypically unique determinants expressed on the viral hemagglutinin, we examined the lytic capability of intraperitoneally primed splenocytes following his published protocol. As with Peyer's patch-derived CTL's intraperitoneally primed splenocytes were also able to lyse both reo 1 and 3 infected L cells. Therefore, in our laboratory, the finding of reo specific CTL's that lyse reo 1 and 3 infected L cell targets are also found in the spleen and do not appear to be a unique feature of Peyer's patch lymphocytes.

Peyer's patches have been described as containing undetectable levels of NK activity (8) (SC levels have not been examined) when assayed without in vitro culturing. However, in this report, we have found that Peyer's patch lymphocytes are capable of generating NK or SC cytotoxic activity upon in vitro culture with Con A supernatant. NK or SC activity is generated from primed as well as control Peyer's patches. The finding of this type of activity from in vitro cultured Peyer's patches indicates that precursor populations for these non-specific cytotoxic cells occur in Peyer's patches. It is possible that these precursor populations, when activated in the patch, migrate and develop into functionally competent lytic cells in other tissues. If this is the case, it would be similar to the observation that Peyer's patches lack terminally differentiated B cells (plasma cells) even though they are capable of generating antibody-secreting cells in in vitro cultures (9).

The finding of CTL's responsive to nominal antigens in Peyer's patches has allowed us to hypothesize that gut-primed CTL's may comprise a unique subset of CTL's that differ in tissue lodging capability as compared to CTL's primed in the periphery. That the CTL's observed in Peyer's patches were locally generated is supported by the following data. Six days after intraduodenal immunization, significantly higher frequencies of pCTL's in Peyer's patches as compared to peripheral lymph nodes were observed. This suggests that enteric application of virus preferentially generates responsive pCTL's in the organized lymphoid tissues most proximal to the site of inoculation. We found 14-100 fold higher precursor frequencies (14 fold higher compared to total lymphocytes, 45 fold higher compared to Thy 1^+ and 100 fold higher compared to Lyt 2^+ lymphocytes) in Peyer's patches as compared to peripheral lymph nodes at this time point. We have also observed that this discrepancy in the distribution of precursors also occurs two days after intraduodenal priming (not shown). Conversely, two days after subcutaneous inoculation, we found that the predominant response is in the draining lymph nodes as compared to distal lymph nodes and Peyer's patches (not shown). Recently, a number of investigators have obtained evidence in the sheep (10) and mouse (11) that there may exist a preferential recirculation pattern to the gut-associated lymphoid tissues (GALT) from GALT-derived T lymphocytes. Our studies also support this hypothesis. Six months after the intraduodenal application of reovirus, a 2-15 fold higher frequency of precursors is maintained in the patch as compared to peripheral lymph nodes (2 fold higher compared to total lymphocytes, 7 fold higher compared to Thy 1^+ and 15 fold higher compared to Lyt 2^+ lymphocytes). The finding of a higher frequency of pCTL's in Peyer's patches as compared to peripheral lymph nodes six months after enteric inoculation offers further evidence that the route of inoculation may be an important determinant in preferentially repopulating mucosal vs. distal tissues with pCTL's. Whether reovirus specific CTL activity is generated in the gut mucosa (lamina propria or intraepithelial compartments) after intraduodenal application of virus, and whether the mucosal application of virus is more effective at generating a response in these locations is currently under investigation. The ability of gut- vs. systemically-derived lymphocytes to bind to lymph node vs. Peyer's patch high endothelial venules (HEV) after intraduodenal vs. parenteral priming will be investigated by examining the levels of MEL 14 antigen expressed on these populations. As the MEL 14 antigen is associated with the ability to bind to peripheral lymph node HEV (12), we would expect gut derived CTL's to bear low levels of this antigen.

The reovirus system offers a unique opportunity to investigate whether mucosally-derived CTL's are effective in conferring protection against a reovirus infection of the gastrointestinal tract. Two models of reovirus infection are available for studies of these types. The first model would determine whether mucosal vs. non-mucosal populations containing reovirus specific CTL activity, when adoptively transferred, can prevent the fatal encephalitis caused by the peroral inoculation of reo 3 to neonatal mice (13). A second model uses a reo 3 variant developed by Dr. Rubin which replicates to high titers in adult intestinal tissues. We will use this system to determine the ability of mucosally- vs. systemically-derived CTL populations to limit the intestinal replication of this newly isolated reo 3 variant in adult mice. Both these studies are feasible since reovirus-specific CTL's are not serotype specific and therefore cross react with reo 1 or 3 infected targets.

Finally, for viruses that initially impinge on the wet epithelium, the presence of virus-specific CTL's in this location could result in the local containment of the infectious agent prior to its dissemination. This would be advantageous to the host since sequella associated with infection at distal sites could thus be prevented from occurring. Therefore, the generation of a mucosally-associated CTL response may be advantageous in effective vaccine regimens for mucosal pathogens.

CONCLUSIONS

1. Reovirus-specific cytotoxic activity can be detected from intraduodenally primed Peyer's patch lymphocytes.

2. This cytotoxic activity is H-2 restricted and mediated by Thy 1^+, Lyt 2^+ T cells.

3. It appears that virus-specific helper cells are also generated in Peyer's patches after intraduodenal application of reovirus.

4. The route of virus inoculation may be an important determinant for the generation of a mucosal vs. systemic CTL response.

5. Peyer's patch lymphocytes, either virus-primed or control, can generate NK activity when cultured in vitro in the presence of Con A-conditioned medium.

ACKNOWLEDGEMENTS

We thank Al Chaney, Jennifer Kennedy and Alec McKay for their excellent technical assistance. This work was supported by grants DE 07085, AI 17997, CA 15822, AI 18554 and AI 11855. D.H. Rubin is supported by a Veterans Administration career development award.

REFERENCES

1. Kagnoff, M.F., J. Immunol. 120, 395, 1978.
2. Lindahl, K.F. and Wilson, D.B., J. Exp. Med. 145, 500, 1977.
3. Rubin, D.H. and Fields, B.N., J. Exp. Med. 152, 853, 1980.
4. Finberg, R., Weiner, H.L., Fields, B.N., Benacerraf, B. and Burakoff, S.J., Proc. Natl. Acad. Sci. USA 76, 442, 1979.
5. Wolf, J.L., Rubin, D.H., Finberg, R., Kauffman, R.S., Sharpe, A.H., Trier, J.S. and Fields, B.N., Science 212, 471, 1981.
6. Fazekas De St. Groth, S., J. Immunol. Meth. 49, R11, 1982.
7. Finberg, R., Spriggs, D.R. and Fields, B.N., J. Immunol. 129, 2235, 1982.
8. Tagliabue, A., Villa, L., Scapigliati, G. and Boraschi, D., Nat. Immun. Cell Growth Regul. 3, 95, 1983/1984.
9. Kiyono, H., McGhee, J.R., Wannemuehler, M.J., Frangakis, M.V., Spalding, D.M., Michalek, S.M. and Koopman, W.J., Proc. Natl. Acad. Sci. USA 79, 596, 1982.
10. Reynolds, J., Dudler, H.L. and Trnka, Z., Immunology 47, 415, 1982.
11. McDermott, M.R., Horsewood, P., Clark, D.A. and Bienenstock, J., Immunology 57, 213, 1986.
12. Gallatin, W.M., Weissman, I.L. and Butcher, E.C., Nature 304, 30, 1983.
13. Fields, B.N., Arch. Virol. 71, 95, 1982.

IMMUNOCYTOCHEMICAL STUDIES OF THE VASCULAR ENDOTHELIAL CELLS IN HUMAN PEYER'S PATCHES AND SOLITARY LYMPHOID FOLLICLES

H. Nagura and Y. Sumi

Laboratory of Germfree Life, Research Institute for
Disease Mechanism and Control, Nagoya University
School of Medicine, Nagoya 466 Japan

INTRODUCTION

The organized mucosal lymphoid tissues of the mammalian small intestine comprise Peyer's patches and lymphoid follicles. They are recognized as an essential component of mucosal organs in which mucosal immune responses are generated. Several recent reports have suggested that Peyer's patches routinely remove large numbers of lymphocytes from the blood circulation, perhaps because the postcapillary venules (PCV) in the thymus-dependent areas have a specialized high endothelium to which these lymphocytes adhere and then penetrate (1). In addition, since PCV are a unique vascular site for the selective passage of not only T- (2), but also of B-lymphocytes (3), the specific interaction between lymphocytes and PCV may be mediated through surface binding molecules (4). Lymphocytes-PCV interaction has primarily been defined by an *in vitro* assay, but the morphology, ultrastructure and immunohistochemistry of these lymphocytes and PCV have been studied less extensively.

Moreover, endothelial cells have previously been shown to have the capacity to express a number of functions of cells of the monocyte/macrophage lineage (5,6). The present investigation was undertaken to define immunohistochemically the ultrastructure and phenotypic characteristics of lymphoid cells and vascular endothelial cells in human Peyer's patches and solitary lymphoid follicles, and thereby aid in understanding the interactions between the endothelial cells and patch-derived lymphocytes.

MATERIALS AND METHODS

Portions of eight histologically normal specimens obtained from surgically removed ileum were used. The tissues were promptly fixed in periodate-lysine-paraformaldehyde (PLP) for 5-6 h at 4°C, embedded in Tissue-Tek OCT compound, frozen in dry-ice ethanol, and sectioned in a cryostat. In these sections, the indirect peroxidase-labeled antibody method was used for immunocytochemical staining with monoclonal antibodies (MoAb), and the direct peroxidase-labeled antibody method was employed for the conventional (polyclonal) antisera (6). Leu-1, Leu-2a, Leu-3a, Leu-4 and Leu-14 MoAb, and MoAb to HLA-DR and IL-2 receptor were obtained from Becton-Dickinson (Fujisawa Pharmaceutical Co., Tokyo, Japan); OK-M1 and OK-M5 MoAb were from Ortho Pharmaceutical Co. (Ortho Japan, Tokyo), and B2 MoAb was from Coulter Co. (Nikkaki Co., Tokyo, Japan). $F(ab')_2$ fragments of rabbit anti-mouse IgG labeled with horseradish peroxidase (HRP) (Tago, Inc., Cosmo Bio Co., Tokyo) were used as the second antibody. Antisera to immunoglobulins and Factor VIII related antigen were purchased from Dako (Kyowa Medics, Tokyo, Japan). The Fab' fragments of the γ-globulin fractions of these antisera were labeled with HRP.

RESULTS

The structure and cellular composition of solitary lymphoid follicles were similar to Peyer's patches.

Light microscopy

Venules with tall endothelial cells termed postcapillary venule (PCV) were found to dominate the vasculature of the interfollicular areas; in addition, there were numerous capillaries. Large concentrations of T-lymphocytes expressing the Leu-3a$^+$ helper/inducer phenotype were observed in the restricted territory surrounding PCV's. Several Leu-14$^+$ B-lymphocytes and a few IgA- and IgM-bearing cells also were present. In addition, both T- and B-lymphocytes (Leu-1$^+$ or Leu-14$^+$, but B2$^-$) and immunoglobulin-bearing cells were found, not only in the immediate vicinity of the PCV, but also in the walls and lumens. The IL-2 receptor was expressed on many lymphocytes around the PCV. The endothelial cells in PCV reacted with OK-M5 and with antibodies to HLA-DR, IgA, IgM, IgG and Factor VIII related antigen (von Willebrand factor, F8RAg), but not with OK-M1, whereas the capillaries in the follicular and interfollicular areas were HLA-DR$^+$ and OK-M5$^+$ but F8RAg$^-$ (Fig. 1).

The villi surrounding Peyer's patches termed patch-associated villi (PAV) were essentially similar to the villi of the absorptive mucosa. However, PCV in the interfollicular areas originated from venules in PAV. A dense capillary network was found immediately under the epithelium, and one or two small veins arose from the superficial capillary networks and

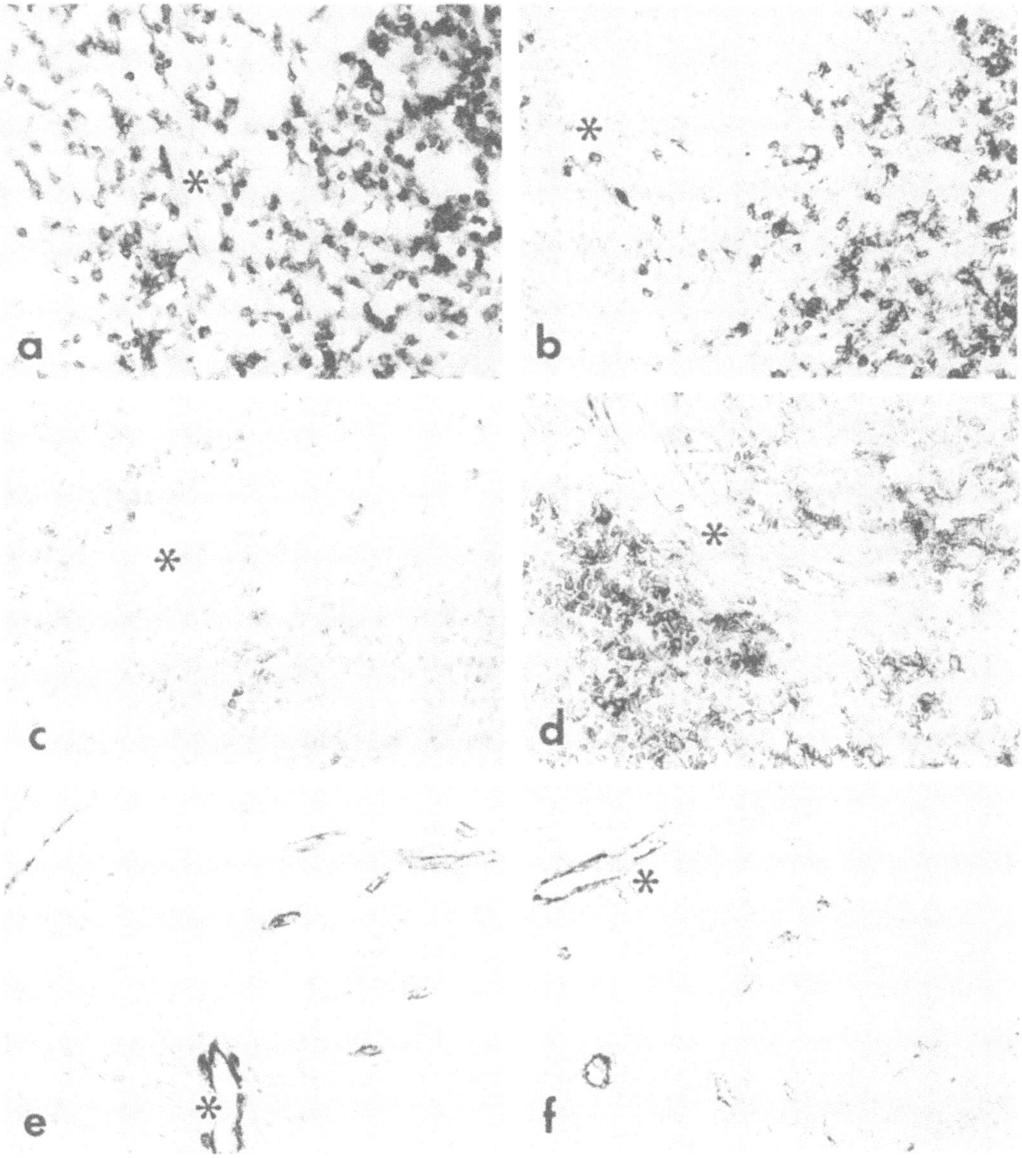

Figure 1. Light micrographs of human solitary lymphoid follicles reacted with Leu-4 (a), Leu-14 (b), IL-2 receptor (c), HLA-DR (d), OK-M5 (e) and Factor VIII related antigen (f). ✱ : PCV. (See text.)

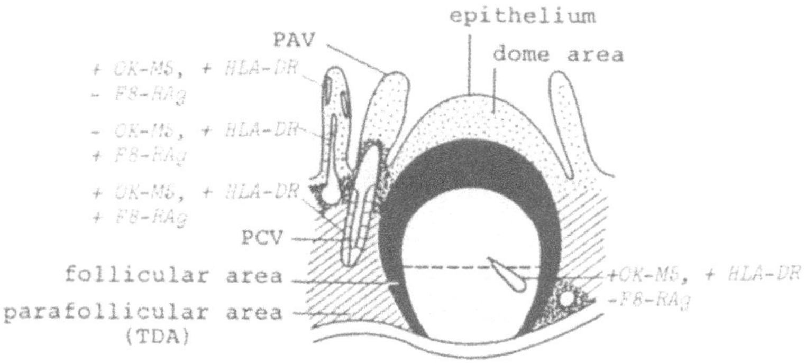

Figure 2. The surface phenotype of the endothelial cells in the Peyer's patch and solitary lymphoid follicle.

extended downward. The endothelium of the capillaries was HLA-DR$^+$ and OK-M5$^+$. It was negative or weekly positive for F8RAg, and gradually turned to F8RAg$^+$ as shown in PCV.

The results of the immunohistochemical characterization of endothelial cells in the Peyer's patch were schematically summarized in Figure 2.

Electron microscopy

The walls of the PCV were constituted by a monolayer of polygonal endothelial cells. However, the cell shape was often distorted due to the traversing lymphocytes. They frequently were attached to the luminal surface of the PCV endothelium, and attachment sites usually were far from the intercellular junction which was classified as desmosomes. Occasionally, the lymphocytes were captured by long cytoplasmic projections of endothelial cells or were entirely surrounded by their cytoplasm. There was a narrow, but definite, space between lymphocyte and endothelial cells. Occasionally, the cell coats of the two cell membranes were in close contact.

OK-M5 reacted with the luminal border of the endothelial cells, and occasionally with the inner surface of the cytoplasmic projections facing the traversing lymphocyte, and on the intercellular surfaces (Fig. 3). IgA, IgM or IgG were seen on the cell surface of the traversing lymphocyte, on the luminal border of endothelial cells and in the intercellular space

Figure 3. Electron micrograph of PCV endothelial cells reacted with OK-M5. The antigen detected by OK-M5 is present on the surface of endothelial cells (◀). A lymphocyte (Ly) is entirely surrounded by their cytoplasm.

between these two cells (Fig. 4). Leu-1 and Leu-14 were found only on the surface of the lymphocytes. Some of the lymphocytes in the vicinity of the PCV carried IL-2 receptors in the perinuclear spaces and poorly developed endoplasmic reticulum and on the cell surface. HLA-DR was expressed on the entire surface of endothelial cells and traversing lymphocytes, and some of HLA-DR^+ lymphocytes were in close contact with processes of HLA-DR^+ interdigitating cells.

Figure 4. Electron micrograph of PCV endothelial cells reacted with HRP-labeled anti-human IgM. IgM is present on the surface of a lymphocyte (Ly) and on the luminal border of endothelial cells (◀). A lymphocyte is captured by long cytoplasmic projections of the endothelial cell (→).

DISCUSSION

The present immunocytochemical observations of the PCV of human Peyer's patches and solitary lymphoid follicles have clearly demonstrated that the endothelial cells of the PCV express antigens found on a monocyte/macrophage lineage, and provided ultrastructural evidence that the selective passage of both T- and B-lymphocytes takes place through the cytoplasm of the endothelial cells.

The organ specificity of lymphocyte migration is known to be determined largely by selective interaction of circulating lymphocytes with endothelial cells of PCV, and the molecular basis of the lymphocyte-endothelium interaction has been well documented. Butcher et al. (7) have suggested that endothelial cells in mucosal and peripheral lymphoid tissues express distinctive determinants or factor for lymphocyte recognition, and recently Rosen et al. (4) have speculated that sialic acid on endothelial cells is a responsible factor for the organ-specific recognition of lymphocyte attachment. From a different point of view, Syrjanen (8) postulated that the endothelium-associated IgG could be involved in the regulation of T-lymphocyte passage through the PCV. Although such organ-specific lymphocyte migration mechanism is largely responsible for the unique feature of the mucosal immune responses, immunologic functions of the PCV endothelium are poorly understood.

It is generally accepted that human vascular endothelial cells carry the HLA-DR antigen (9), which are required for antigen presentation and lymphoproliferative response of the T-lymphocyte to soluble protein antigens. Moreover, the cells were shown in recent immunohistochemical studies using OK-M1 and OK-M5 MoAb to share antigens with the peripheral blood monocyte subset that possess the capacity to present self antigens in autologous mixed lymphocyte reactions (10,11). The present study proved that the PCV endothelium also carries the HLA-DR antigen and the antigen detected by OK-M5, suggesting that it is capable of substituting for macrophages in immune responses. In fact, large concentrations of T-lymphocytes are present in the restricted territory surrounding the PCV, and IL-2 receptor, which is detected on the surface of activated lymphocytes *in vitro* (12), is expressed on parts of these lymphocytes.

In the present study, some evidence of B lymphocyte passage through the PCV also has been present. The B lymphocytes traversing through the

PCV endothelium carry surface immunoglobulins and Leu-14 antigen, but not B2 antigen which is known to be expressed on immature follicular B lymphocytes. In other words, B lymphocytes generated in the germinal center of Peyer's patches and solitary lymphoid follicles reach the PCV via the blood circulation after considerable maturation, and traverse the wall of the PCV into the thymus-dependent areas. It might be speculated that the immunologic interaction between T and B lymphocytes occurs in the restricted territory surrounding the PCV.

These findings suggest that the surface antigens on the PCV epithelium could be the factors responsible for lymphocyte proliferation, as well as for the regulation of the lymphocyte passage through the venules.

Concerning the route used by the lymphocytes in traversing the PCV, it is still controversial whether this passage takes place through the cytoplasm of the endothelial cells (13) or through intercellular spaces (14). The present ultrastructural results suggest that passage occurs through the endothelial cells: (a) very intimate contact between the PCV endothelium and T and B lymphocytes was found; (b) attachment sites of lymphocytes usually were far from the intercellular junctions; (c) lymphocytes entirely surrounded by the cytoplasm of endothelial cells were occasionally seen; and (d) the surface of endothelial projections facing lymphocytes were positive for immunoglobulin just as was the luminal surface of the endothelial cells. The presence of lymphocytes situated between endothelial cells, however, might be interpreted as evidence that the lymphocytes had crossed the intercellular junctions. It seems unlikely, though, that they could have taken this route, since the desmosomes appeared intact, rather these cells might have passed through endothelial cells, then migrated to the intercellular spaces. However, one cannot definitely exclude the possibility that cells migrate by the intercellular route.

SUMMARY

The present immunohistochemical study of human Peyer's patches and solitary lymphoid follicles have revealed that the PCV in these thymus-dependent areas has a specialized endothelium to which T and B lymphocytes generated in these follicles selectively adhere and then penetrate. The PCV endothelium shares antigens with a peripheral monocyte or macrophage subset which is HLA-DR^+, OK-$M5^+$ and OK-$M1^-$. The presence of such antigens could be responsible for regulation of the lymphocyte passage through the venules, and for lymphocyte maturation, activation and proliferation during the migration. A possible route used by the lymphocytes traversing the PCV endothelium is discussed.

ACKNOWLEDGEMENTS

We thank Dr. William R. Brown for helpful discussion and critical evaluation of the manuscript.

REFERENCES

1. Gowans, J.L. and Knight, E.J., Proc. Roy. Soc. Biol. 159, 257, 1964.
2. Syrjanen, K.J., Exp. Mol. Pathol. 29, 291, 1978.
3. Kotani, M., Nawa, Y., Fujii, H., Fukumoto, T., Miyamoto, M. and Yamashita, A., Cell Tiss. Res. 152, 299, 1974.
4. Rosen, S.D., Singer, M.S. and Yednock, T.A., Science 228, 1005, 1985.
5. Knowles, D.M., Tolidjian, B., Marboe, C., D'Agati, V., Grimes, M. and Chess, L., J. Immunol. 132, 2170, 1984.
6. Nagura, H., Koshikawa, T., Fukuda, Y. and Asai, J., Virchows. Arch. (Pathol. Anat.), 409, 407, 1986.
7. Butcher, E.C., Stevens, S.K., Reichert, R.A., Scallay, R.G. and Weissmann, I.L., in Recent Advances in Mucosal Immunity (Edited by Strober, W., Hanson, L.Å. and Sell, K.W.), p. 3, Raven Press, New York, 1982.
8. Syrjanen, K.J., Exp. Path. 17, 40, 1979.
9. Hirshberg, H., Bergh, O.J. and Thorsby, E., J. Exp. Med. 152, 249s, 1980.
10. Breard, J., Reiherz, E.L., Kung, P.C., Goldstein, G. and Schlossman, S.R., J. Immunol. 124, 1943, 1984.
11. Shen, H.H., Talle, M.A., Goldstein, G. and Chess, L., J. Immunol. 130, 687, 1983.
12. Uchiyama, T., Nelson, D.L., Fleisher, T.A. and Waldmann, T.A., J. Immunol. 126, 1398, 1981.
13. Marchesi, V.T. and Gowans, J.L., Proc. Roy. Soc. Biol. 159, 283, 1964.
14. Ohmann, H.B., Cell Tiss. Res. 212, 465, 1980.

MIGRATION OF PEYER'S PATCH IgA PRECURSOR CELLS

J. Tseng

Department of Experimental Pathology, Division of Pathology, Walter Reed Army Institute of Research Washington, D.C. USA

INTRODUCTION

It is generally accepted that Peyer's patches (PP) are an enriched source of precursor cells for the IgA plasma cells in the gut lamina propria (GLP) (1,2). The IgA precursor cells migrate to the mesenteric lymph nodes (MLN), enter the blood circulation via the thoracic duct, and eventually arrive in the GLP where they become resident plasma cells (3-5). In an attempt to understand this migration journey more clearly, we studied the migration, lodging and differentiation properties of the IgA precursor cells by transferring lymphoid cells between syngeneic and Ig allotype congenic mice and examining the Ig isotype expression potential for the lymphoid cells of the gut-associated lymphoid tissue (GALT). The results led to a migration outline highlighted with asynchronized differentiations. The results are briefly reviewed in this paper.

RESULTS

Characteristics of PP IgA precursor cells

By passive transfer of lymphoid cells between Ig allotype congenic mice (CB-20 and BALB/c), we confirmed the finding of Craig and Cebra (1) that PP are indeed the most enriched source of IgA precursor cells (2). The CB-20 PP IgA precursor cells can repopulate the IgA plasma cells in the GLP of the irradiated BALB/c recipients, which begins at day 6 and reaches the maximum at days 12-14 after cell transfer. By separating cells according to their membrane Ig isotype using rosetting techniques (6), we found that IgM-IgD double-bearing cells are responsible for the repopulation. The IgA-bearing cells are also capable of repopulation; however, their efficiency is unexpectedly low. The IgM-IgD double bearing cells are small resting lymphocytes. They do not migrate directly to the GLP. Instead, they migrate to the spleen where they stay for at least 5 days for expansion and differentiation and then to the GLP where they differentiate into plasma cells and lodge there for the rest of their lives (2). The IgM-IgD double-bearing cells are the majority of the emigrating PP IgA precursor cells which also include IgA bearing cells and IgA blasts (3-5).

Asynchronized differentiation during migration

By passive transfer of lymphoid cells between Ig allotype congenic mice (2), lymphoid cells from the MLN, as those from PP, are also capable of repopulating the IgA plasma cells in the GLP. These IgA precursor cells show essentially the same characteristics as those of PP, i.e., they are small, resting IgM-IgD double-bearing cells and show the same time course of repopulation. On the other hand, IgA precursor cells from the GLP show a broad spectrum of differentiation (8). When transferred into Ig allotype congenic mice, they immediately appeared and continued to be present in the GLP from day 1 up to at least day 21 after transfer. Two population peaks were seen: the early one at approximately day 3 and a late one at days 12-15. The early repopulation peak is probably manifested by the lymphoblasts and well differentiated IgA precursors other than the IgM-IgD double-bearing cells which seem to be responsible for the late repopulation peak. This is based on the similarities those IgA precursors shared with PP IgA precursors, mainly, the same repopulation time course and a similar effect which occurs after splenectomy.

When B cells in the GALT are enumerated (Table 1), most B cells are IgM-IgD cells; IgA-bearing cells are always a minor population. When the lymphoid cells are cultured with pokeweed mitogen (PWM) which is the best among mitogens tested for generating IgA-containing cells (9), approximately 50, 80 and 0% of IgA-containing cells in the MLN, spleen and GLP cell cultures, respectively, are IgM-IgA double precursors (Table 2). These double producers are undoubtedly derived from IgM bearing cells. When the numbers

Table 1. B cells of the gut-associated lymphoid tissue

Cells	% Cells in tissues: PP	MLN	GLP	Spleen
Ig-bearing	55 (100)[a]	40 (100)	18 (100)	51 (100)
IgM only	7 (13)	7 (18)	8 (43)	4 (7)
IgM-IgD	40 (72)	30 (76)	7 (40)	46 (91)
IgA only	4 (7)	0.5 (1)	1 (7)	<0.01 (0)
IgA-IgD	0.2 (0.3)	0.8 (2)	<0.01 (0)	<0.01 (0)
IgG2 only	2 (4)	0.3 (0.8)	<0.01 (0)	0.6 (0.3)
Ig-containing	0.6 (100)	2 (100)	22 (100)	2 (100)
cIgA	0.2 (32)	1 (57)	21 (95)	0.1 (5)
cIgM	0.4 (65)	0.8 (40)	0.3 (1)	1 (50)
cIgG2	0.01 (2)	0.04 (2)	0.6 (3)	0.8 (38)

[a]Numbers in parentheses are % relative to total Ig-bearing or Ig-containing cells.

of the IgA-containing cells in the PWM stimulated cultures are compared with IgA-bearing cells in preparations fresh from the tissues, the former cells are significantly more than the later (Tables 1 and 2). These results, together with those of passive transfer studies, strongly suggest that the PP IgA precursor cells (IgM-IgD bearing) differentiate asynchronously during migration to the GLP, i.e., in the MLN and spleen, some IgM-IgD cells remain resting while others differentiate into precursor cells of the IgA single and IgM-IgA double producers. The precursors of these cells can further differentiate into IgA blasts which migrate directly to the GLP and other mucosal tissues. In the GLP, although some of the PP IgM-IgD cells may remain resting, most of them may differentiate into precursors of IgA single producers and blasts which lodge there permanently.

Lodging in the GLP

It has been found that IgA blasts from the GALT have the propensity to migrate to and lodge in the GLP and other mucosal tissues (3-5). When CB-20 PP cells were transferred into irradiated BALB/c recipients, most of the cells migrate to the spleen where they divide further and then

Table 2. Ig-containing cells generated by pokeweed mitogen in culture

Cell culture	PWM	Total cells with: IgM	IgA	IgG2	Double producers: IgM-IgA		IgM-IgG2	
PP	-	8	1.2	0.2	0.2	(15)[a]	0.03	(15)
	+	11	7	2	0.6	(10)	0.1	(5)
MLN	-	14	0.3	0.05	0.15	(50)	0.03	(50)
	+	13	3	0.2	1.5	(50)	0.1	(50)
Spleen	-	10	0.8	0.1	0.6	(80)	0.07	(70)
	+	24	2	3.5	0.6	(80)	2.5	(70)
GLP	-	0.02	4.3	0.01	< 0.01	(0)	< 0.01	(0)
	+	0.2	8.0	0.01	< 0.01	(0)	< 0.01	(0)

[a]Numbers in parentheses are % relative to total IgA- or IgG2-containing cells.

migrate quickly to the GLP (2). In the MLN and spleen of these recipients, dividing cells have the propensity to migrate directly to the GLP. Thus, at a certain phase of the cell division cycle, the IgA precursor cells and possibly other kinds of lymphoid cells migrate to and lodge in the GLP. To test this possibility, we generated B and T cell blasts in culture with concanavalin A (Con A) and bacterial lipopolysaccharide (LPS). When these lymphoblasts are tranferred into syngeneic mice, a large population migrates directly to and lodges in the GLP (Fig. 1). Lymphoblasts from all the peripheral lymphoid tissues share these characteristics. Since both Con A and LPS are potent differentiation inducers, differentiation stages of the lodging blasts also seem critical in determining the lodging.

Peanut agglutinin (PNA) and the MEL-14 monoclonal antibody have been used to study lymphocyte migration in the mouse (10,11). Lymphoid cells reactive to PNA and MEL-14 are sessile and circulating cells, respectively. In the GLP, there are no PNA reactive cells and MEL-14 reactive cells are in relatively small numbers (Table 3). Among the IgA-containing cells, MEL-14 reactive cells are mainly blasts. Thus, PNA reactivity may not be involved in the lodging while loss of MEL-14 reactive determinants seems to be important.

Table 3. MEL-14 reactive lymphoid cells in the gut-associated lymphoid tissue

	MEL-14 reactive cells among:	
Cells	Total cells (%)	Ig-containing cells (%)
PP	55	< 0.1
MLN	57	< 0.1
GLP	14	22

[a]Enumerated by fluorescence microscopy.

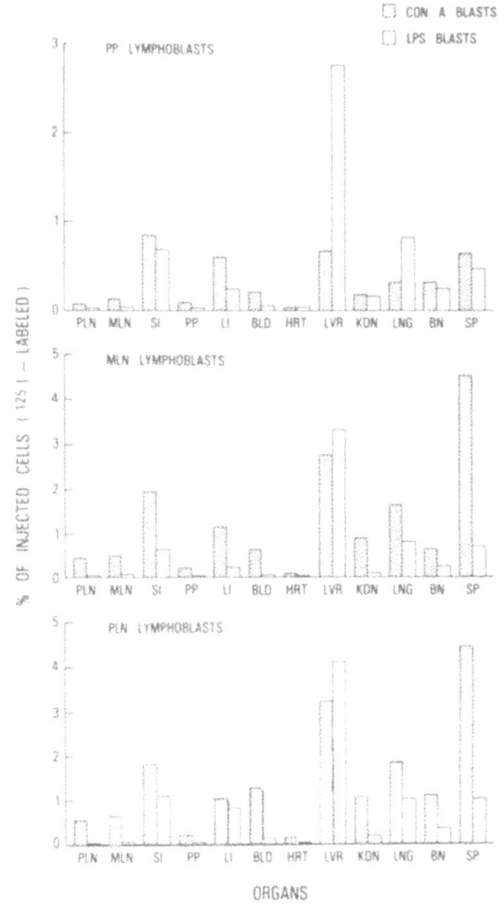

Figure 1. Preferential lodging of mitogen-induced lymphoblasts in the gut. CB-20 lymphoid cells were cultured with Con A (4 μg/ml) and LPS (25 μg/ml) for 3 days. Two hours before harvest, the lymphoblasts were labeled with ^{125}IUDR and injected into syngeneic CB-20 mice. Radioactivity was determined for the tissues 18-24 hours later. PLN, peripheral lymph nodes (inguinal, axillary and brachial nodes); MLN, mesenteric lymph nodes; SI, small intestine; PP, Peyer's patches; LI, large intestine; BLD, blood (1 ml); HRT, heart; LVR, liver; KDN, kidney; LNG, lung; BN, bone; SP, spleen.

Recirculation

Gowans and Knight (12) found that small resting lymphocytes in the thoracic duct are recirculating cells while lymphoblasts are sessile cells migrating dirctly to and lodging in the GLP. Similarly, IgA-containing blasts and small IgA-bearing cells in the thoracic duct were later found to be sessile and recirculating cells, respectively (13). In our passive transfer studies using Ig allotype congenic mice (2), dividing IgA-containing cells and IgA-bearing cells were found in the MLN of the recipients during days 6-10 (Fig. 2). The IgA blasts disappeared quickly, possibly

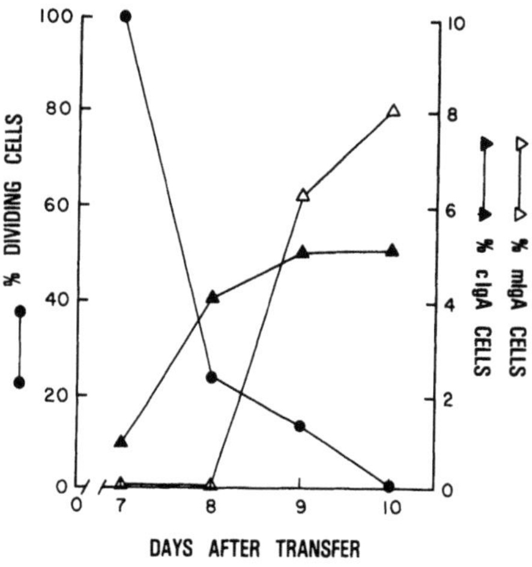

Figure 2. Dividing cells, IgA-bearing cells, and IgA-containing cells in the MLN of the BALB/c recipients 6-10 days after PP cell transfer. CB-20 PP cells were transferred into irradiated (400 R) BALB/c mice. At days 6-7, ^{3}H-thymidine (20 μC/mouse, 3 doses at 10 hours interval) was injected into the recipients. At days 7-10, MLN cells were examined by immunofluorescence microscopy and radioautography.

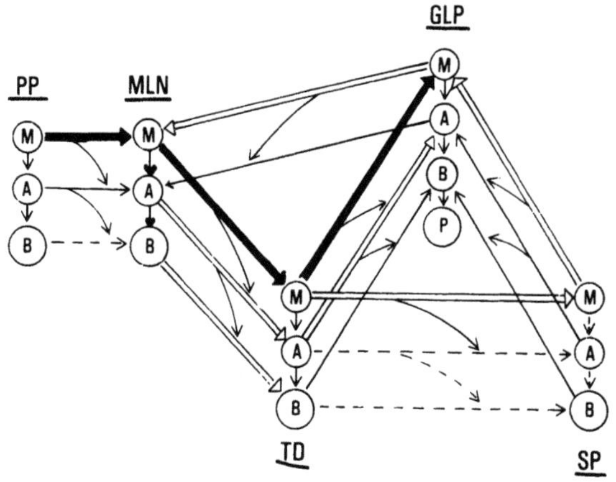

Figure 3. The migration journey of PP IgA precursor cells. Differentiation of IgM → IgA → IgA blasts occurs asynchronously en route to the gut lamina propria during the migration and recirculation.

to the GLP since an exponential increase of these cells were seen in the GLP (2). The IgA-containing cells and IgA-bearing cells increased exponentially during days 7-10 and 8-10, respectively. Because only a few IgA-bearing cells were seen in the PP of the recipients and essentially none were seen in the spleen, most of these IgA-bearing cells may be recirculating PP IgA precursors. Thus, the PP IgM-IgD double-bearing cells, the major IgA precursors, may recirculate in the gut lymphatics after passage through the GLP and switch to IgA-bearing cells and IgA blasts.

CONCLUSIONS

In the emigrating PP IgA precursor cells, IgM-IgD double-bearing cells are the majority, IgA-bearing cells and IgA blasts are the minor and minute population, respectively (Fig. 3). The IgA blasts migrate directly to the GLP and other mucosal tissues. While some of the PP IgM-IgD double-bearing cells remain resting, others may differentiate into IgA-bearing cells and then into IgA blasts as they migrate. The IgA blasts migrate directly to and lodge in the GLP and other mucosal tissues. The resting IgM-IgD double-bearing cells and the IgA-bearing cells are recirculating cells; they lodge in the GLP after differentiation into IgA blasts and then plasma cells. The lodging may occur at a certain stage of the cell division cycle and loss of MEL-14 reactive determinants may be involved.

ACKNOLWEDGEMENTS

The technical assistance of Mr. Michael Williams is heartily appreciated.

REFERENCES

1. Craig, S.W. and Cebra, J.J., J. Exp. Med. 134, 188, 1971.
2. Tseng, J., J. Immunol. 127, 2039, 1981.
3. Guy-Grand, D., Gricelli, C. and Vasalli, P., Eur. J. Immunol. 4, 435, 1975.
4. McWilliams, M., Phillips-Quagliata, J. and Lamm, M.E., J. Immunol. 115, 54, 1975.

5. Pierce, N.F. and Gowans, J.L., J. Exp. Med. 142, 1550, 1975.
6. Tseng, J., J. Immunol. 132, 2730, 1984.
7. Craig, S.W. and Cebra, J.J., J. Immunol. 114, 492, 1975.
8. Tseng, J., Eur. J. Immunol. 14, 420, 1984.
9. Tseng, J., J. Immunol. 128, 2719, 1982.
10. Gallatin, W.M., Weissman, I.L. and Butcher, E.C., Nature 304, 30, 1983.
11. Reichert, R.A., Gallatin, W.M., Weissman, I.L. and Butcher, E.C., J. Exp. Med. 157, 813, 1983.
12. Gowans, J.L. and Knight, E.J., Proc. R. Soc. Lond. (Biol.) 159, 257, 1964.
13. Husband, A.J. and Gowans, J.L., J. Exp. Med. 148, 1164, 1978.

MIGRATION OF INDIVIDUAL LYMPHOCYTES INTO PEYER'S PATCHES *IN VIVO*

C.A. Ottaway, H.P. Cheng and M.L. Bjerknes

Departments of Medicine and Anatomy
University of Toronto
Toronto, Canada M5S 1A8

INTRODUCTION

Peyer's patches are macroscopically recognizable aggregates of lymphoid tissue within the intestinal mucosa which function as major sites of antigen sampling, immune response generation and lymphocyte traffic. Morphologically, these patches contain nodules comprised primarily of B cells and inter-nodular corridors where T cells predominate. Peyer's patches collect T and B lymphocytes continuously and in large numbers from the blood stream. It is well recognized that the collection of blood-borne lymphocytes in Peyer's patches occurs, as it does in lymph nodes, at the level of the post-capillary venules. The anatomy of these vessels appears to be highly specialized to perform this function (1,2), and there is now strong evidence that the interaction of lymphocytes with the specialized high endothelium of these vessels is mediated by specific surface determinants of both the lymphocyte and the endothelial cells (3-9).

Our current concepts about lymphocyte traffic and the role of lymphocyte-endothelial interactions have emerged largely from two types of investigation. Migration *in vivo* is most frequently studied by assessing the distribution of transferred lymphocyte populations that bear some label. Their accumulation in organs or lymph reflects the number-averaged and time-averaged outcome of a complicated series of events, and provides indirect information about the processes involved. Such studies have been complemented over the last decade by another approach originated by Woodruff and colleagues (10) in which the potential interaction of lymphocytes with postcapillary venules of lymphoid tissues is assessed *in vitro* on fixed or frozen sections. This has led to new and important concepts, and has provided results that, to a large extent, accord with in vivo observations, but the extent to which the interactions that occur in vitro reflect those that occur under physiological conditions is not known.

The purpose of this paper is to describe studies in which the emigration behaviour of individual blood-borne lymphocytes from the postcapillary venules of Peyer's patches was directly visualized using in vivo microscopy. At the meeting, the results were presented in video format.

METHODS

Female BALB/c mice (6-8 wk old) (Canadian Breeding Laboratories, Montreal) were used throughout. Recipient animals were anesthetized with intraperitoneal pentobarbital (60 mg/Kg), the abdomen and peritoneum were opened and jejunal loops bearing Peyer's patches were gently exteriorized in saline. Single cell suspensions of lymphocytes from mesenteric lymph nodes were prepared from syngeneic donors and were labeled with tetramethylrhodamine isothyocyanate (RITC) (Research Organics, Cleveland, OH) using 4 ug RITC/5 x 10^7 cells/ml in RPMI-1640 with 5% fetal calf serum (FCS) for 15 min at 22°C (11). The labeled cells were centrifuged through FCS, washed and resuspended in RPMI 1640 without FCS and transferred to recipient animals via a lateral tail vein.

The tissues were examined using an epifluorescence equipped Zeiss ACM microscope and a silicon-intensified target television camera with simultaneous output to a TV monitor and video recorder. Video recordings were made at 60 frames/sec. Field excitation using blue light was used to examine autofluorescence. Green light was used to excite rhodamine fluorescence.

RESULTS AND DISCUSSION

The lymphoid nodules and vasculature of Peyer's patches are readily seen with epi-illumination because there is substantial autofluorescence within gut tissues (Figs. 1 and 2). The nodules are richly vascular and venous networks surround them (Fig. 1). Many of the venules draining the nodules and the internodular corridors are recognizable as high-endothelial venules (HV) through which lymphocytes extravasate (Figs. 1 and 2), because

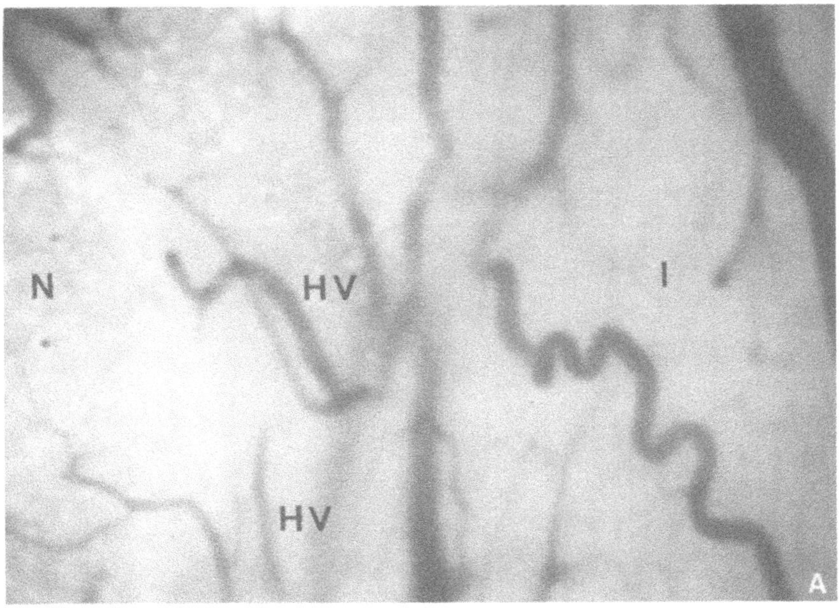

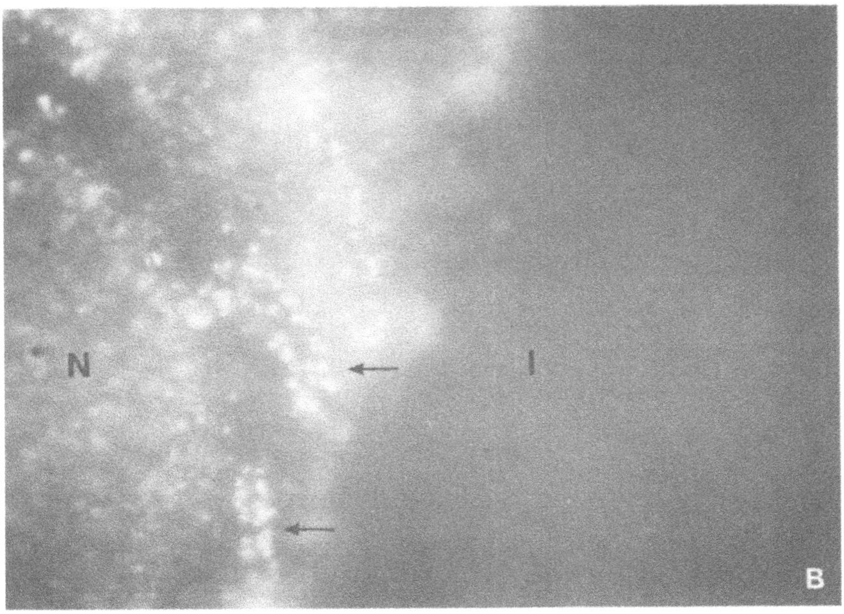

Figure 1. Boundary area of a Peyer's patch (24x objective). (A) Autofluorescence with blue light illumination showing nodule (N) and high endothelial venules (HV). Vessels of similar caliber can be seen in the neighboring region of absorptive epithelium (I). (B) Same as (A) but under green light showing rhodamine labeled lymphocytes in the HV (80 minutes after cell transfer). Note the absence of cells in the area of absorptive intestine.

large numbers of transferred rhodamine-labeled lymphocytes could be found in and around these vessels. In the living tissue, these venules can be recognized even with autofluorescence alone because they appear more

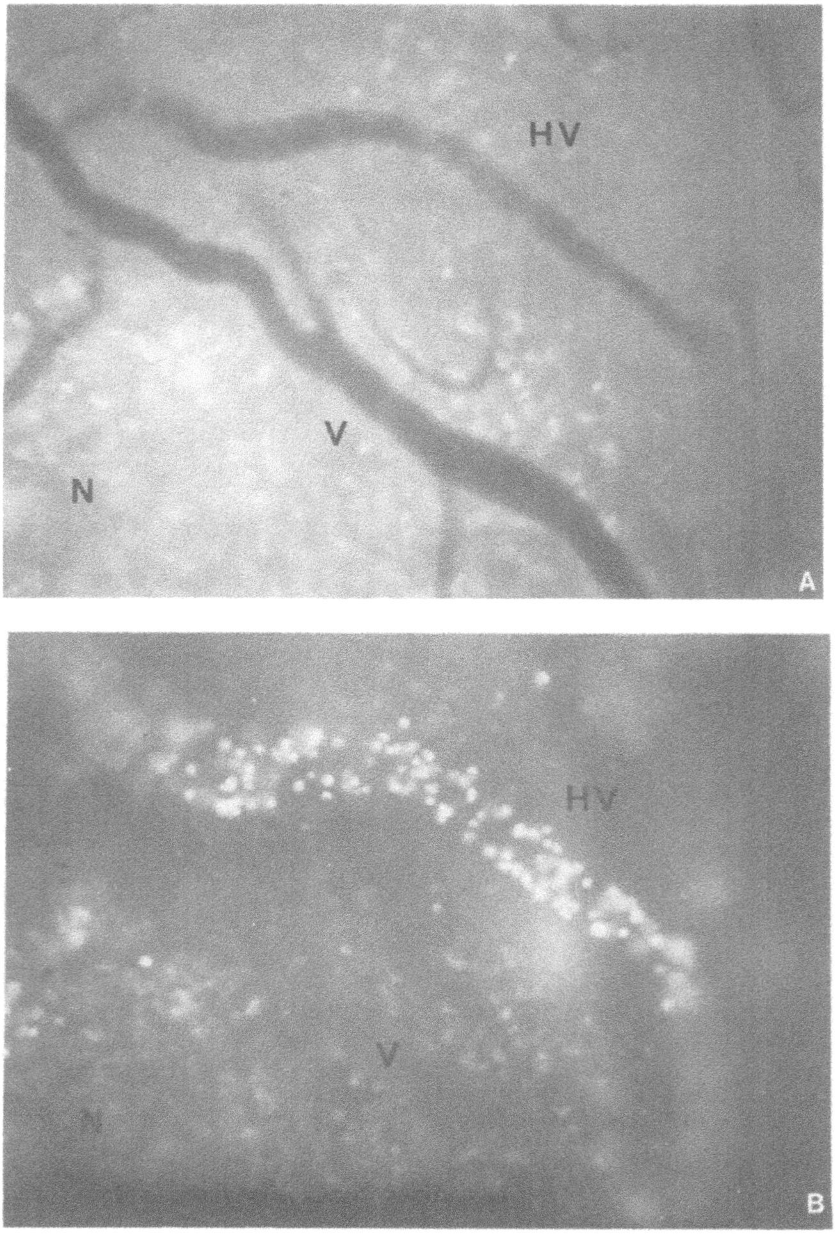

Figure 2. View of vessels (40x objective) surrounding a nodule (N) within Peyer's patch. (A) Autofluorescence showing opalescent high endothelial venule (HV) and nearby vein (V). (B) With green excitation of the same area showing rhodamine labeled lymphocytes in HV (75 min after cell transfer).

opalescent and have a more corrugated lumenal outline than other venules (Fig. 2). These specialized venules are only seen, however, in the vicinity of the lymphoid nodules and inter-nodular areas. At boundary areas between lymphoid and absorptive regions of intestine, vessels of comparable size in the non-lymphoid intestine did not collect lymphocytes to any appreciable extent (Fig. 1).

RITC-labeled lymphocytes can be seen within the vessels of the tissue within seconds of their transfer, they accumulate within the HV within minutes, and can be observed therafter. This permits the direct examination of at least two important processes involved in lymphocyte migration, specifically adherence and extravasation.

Adherence events

We have reported elsewhere (12) on aspects of the dynamics of lymphocytes within the HV. Those studies showed that 63% of all the labeled lymphocytes entering an HV adhered to the vessel wall, but the majority (79%) of those adherences were only temporary. Most of the cells (70%) detach within a second after adherence and about 10% detached between 1 and 10 seconds after adherence. An important finding was that after detaching and returning to the stream, the cells have a very high chance of adhering again, and overall about 60% of all the cells that enter the vessel adhere to the endothelium two or more times. One consequence of the recurrent nature of ths process is that the collection of lymphocytes within an HV was more efficient than if collection were dependent upon only a single trial of adhesion. For example, 13% of the entering lymphocytes were collected at their first adherence episode, but 26% of the entering lymphocytes were collected over the course of the venule.

Thus, the collision frequency and the collection frequency of lymphocytes within these venules is very high *in vivo* and appears to be specific for these specialized vessels. This supports our current concepts regarding the effectiveness of lymphocyte-endothelial interactions in these regions, and suggests that these interactions are even more pronounced *in vivo* than they are on *in vitro* sections. The contribution of collision frequency to the behavior of the cells, however, suggests that the hemodynamics of these vessels also makes an important contribution to the physiological effectiveness of the cell-cell surface interactions at the endothelium (13).

Extravasation events

To migrate through the Peyer's patch, a lymphocyte that is collected

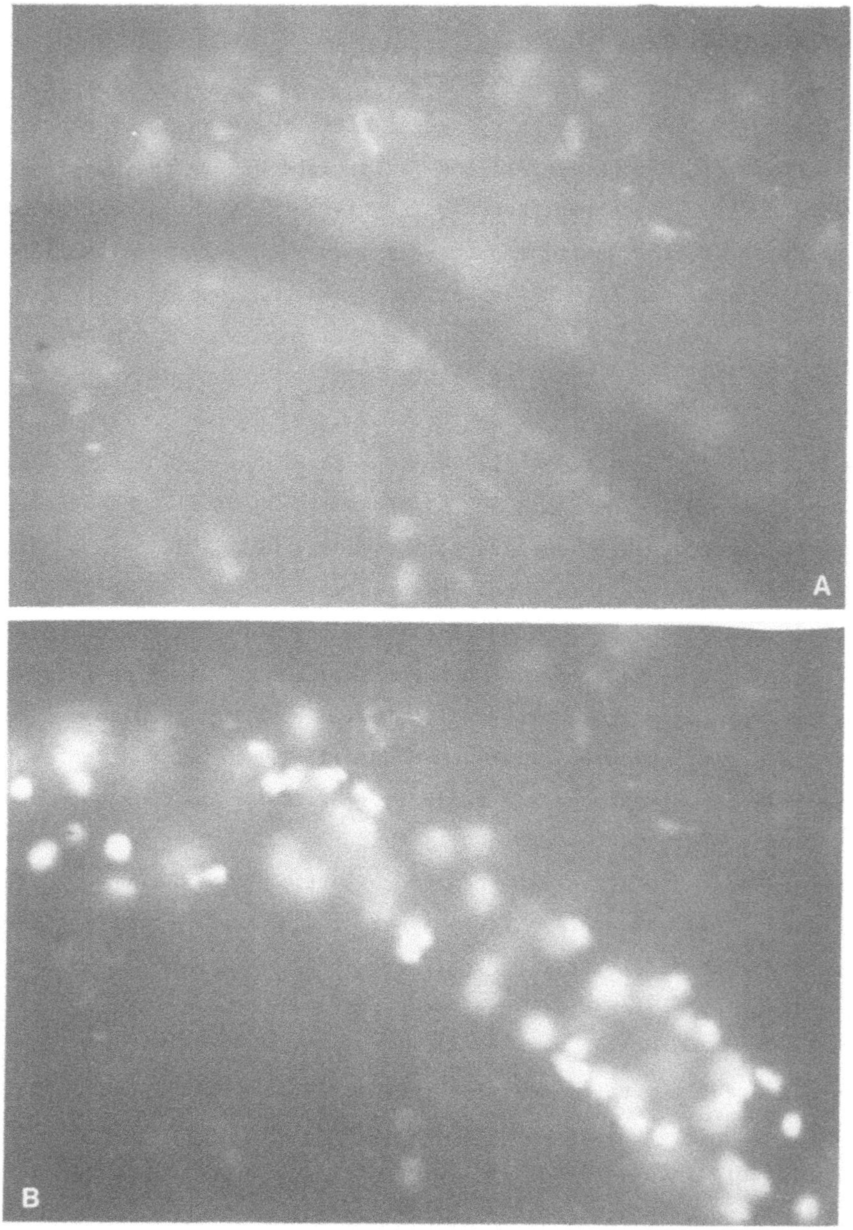

Figure 3. View of high endothelial venule (64x objective) in Peyer's patch. (A) Autofluorescence. (B) Same as (A) but with green excitation showing labeled lymphocytes. Many demonstrate locomotor morphology (75 minutes after cell transfer).

from the blood stream must make its way between endothelial cells and cross the basement membrane of the endothelium (1,2). The lymphocyte then must somehow detach itself so that it can make its way within the parenchyma of the tissue. The bulk of what is known about the locomotor capabilities

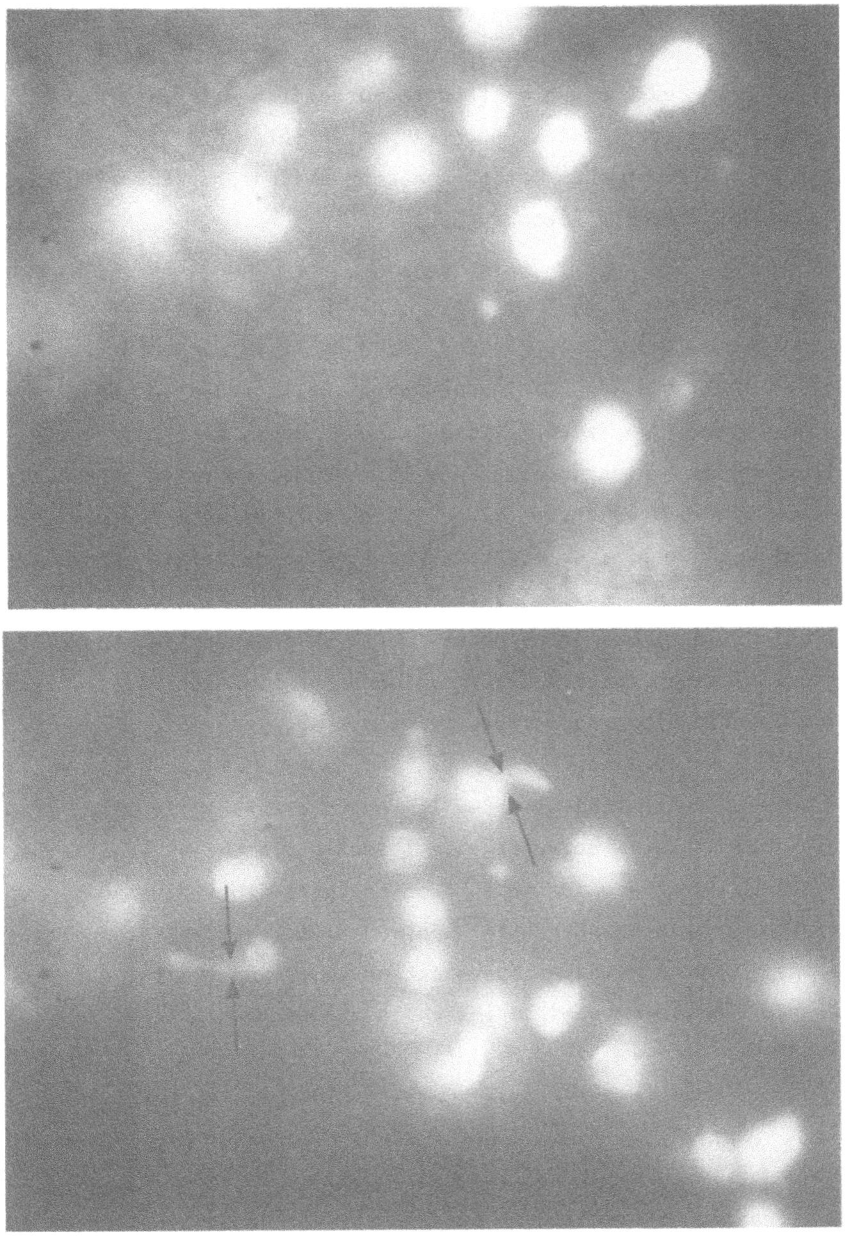

Figure 4. High magnification of rhodamine labeled lymphocytes extravasating into Peyer's patch (100x objective) (80 minutes after cell transfer). (A) A number of cells show bleb-like formations. (B) A number of cells show constriction rings (arrows) and uropod formation.

of lymphocytes has arisen from *in vitro* rather than *in vivo* studies (14). A characteristic polarized locomotor morphology has been recognized for lymphocytes *in vitro* for more than 50 years (15). The features of this locomotor morphology include the so-called hand-mirror shape, the constriction ring (a contracted band of cytoplasm through which the lymphocyte appears to move), and the uropod or tail of the moving lymphocyte (14-16). These features have attracted attention for many years, and occasionally lymphocytes have been caught in this morphology during ultrastructural studies of their passage across the postcapillary venules of lymph nodes and Peyer's patches (1,2).

It was, therefore, of interest to examine the morphology of extravasating lymphocytes in vivo as they made their way from the postcapillary venules (Figs. 3 and 4). Large numbers of cells could be seen in various states of asymmetry. Recent cinematographic studies of lymphocyte locomotion in three-dimensional collagen gels have demonstrated that during locomotion lymphocytes extend bleb-like structures into the collagen matrix, the cells then developed a constriction ring which remains fixed with respect to the external environment and the cell moves forward through the constriction (16). The lymphocytes in Figure 4 demonstrate morphological features including apparent constriction rings that are remarkably similar to those described by those investigators.

It is well recognized that few lymphocytes freshly isolated from blood or tissue demonstrate locomotor activities in vitro (14), but it seems likely that a large proportion of those exiting from the blood in vivo are undergoing active locomotion. This activity may be very pertinent to the way in which lymphocytes select or sample particular microenvironment within Peyer's patches during their migration.

CONCLUSIONS

1. The adherence of individual lymphocytes to the endothelium of postcapillary venules and the subsequent extravasation of these lymphocytes can be directly examined in intact Peyer's patches using in vivo microscopy.

2. The process by which lymphocytes are collected from the blood in the postcapillary venules is rapid, repetitive and efficient.

3. During extravasation, a large proportion of the migrating lymphocytes appear to be actively locomoting.

ACKNOWLEDGEMENTS

This work was supported by the Medical Research Council of Canada and the Canadian Foundation for Ileitis and Colitis.

REFERENCES

1. Schoefl, G.I., J. Exp. Med. 136, 568, 1972.
2. Anderson, A.O. and Anderson, N.D., Immunology 31, 731, 1970.
3. Stevens, S.K., Weissman, I.L. and Butcher, E.C., J. Immunol. 128, 844, 1982.
4. Chin, Y.-H., Carey, G.D. and Woodruff, J.J., J. Immunol. 129, 1911, 1983.
5. Gallatin, W.M., Weissman, I.L. and Butcher, E.C., Nature 304, 30, 1983.
6. Stoolman, L.M., Tenaforde, T.S. and Rosen, S.D., J. Cell. Biol. 99, 1535, 1984.
7. Chin, Y.-H., Rasmussen, R., Gokhan Cakiroglu, A. and Woodruff, J.J., J. Immunol. 133, 2961, 1984.
8. Rosen, S.D., Singer, M.S., Yednock, T.A. and Stoolman, L.M., Science 228, 1005, 1985.
9. Rasmussen, R., Chin, Y.-H. and Woodruff, J.J., J. Immunol. 135, 19, 1985.
10. Stamper, H.B. and Woodruff, J.J., J. Exp. Med. 144, 828, 1976.
11. Butcher, E.C. and Weissman, I.L., J. Immunol. Methods 37, 97, 1980.
12. Bjerknes, M., Cheng, H. and Ottaway, C.A., Science 231, 402, 1986.
13. Ottaway, C.A., in Migration and Homing of Lymphoid Cells, (Edited by Husband, A.J.), CRC Press, Boca Raton, FL, 1987 (in press).
14. Parrott, D.M.V. and Wilkinson, P.C., Prog. Allergy 28, 193, 1981.
15. Lewis, W.H., Bull. Johns Hopkins Hosp. 49, 29, 1931.
16. Haston, W.S. and Shields, J.M., J. Cell. Science 68, 227, 1984.

CHEMOTAXIS AS A MECHANISM FOR RECRUITMENT OF MUCOSAL PLASMA CELL PRECURSORS

S.J. Czinn, J. Robinson and M.E. Lamm

Institute of Pathology and Department of Pediatrics
Case Western Reserve University
Cleveland, Ohio USA

INTRODUCTION

Precursor cells in mucosal-associated lymphoid tissue travel via the lymphatic system to the regional lymph nodes, proceed to the blood and then preferentially home to a number of sites, including the gut, respiratory tract, and during lactation, the mammary glands where they complete their differentiation into IgA plasma cells (1-6). The basis of the selective homing of these cells to secondary sites is not understood. The objective of the current work is to begin to examine chemotaxis as a possible mechanism.

Investigators have previously evaluated the role of antigens, secretory component and blood flow as possible mechanisms to account for the homing of IgA lymphocytes (2,3,7-10). However, the literature does not support any of these as fundamental. Another mechanism that could be responsible for lymphocyte migration is chemotaxis. In terms of mucosal immunity, a putative chemotactic agent could well be a secretory product of the differentiated epithelium of the mucous membrane. Because there is good evidence for a common mucosal immune system, it seems reasonable to assume initially that the same basic homing mechanism operates at all mucosal sites. Mouse milk was selected for examination as a source of such a chemotactic factor because it is an exocrine secretion whose production correlates with the time of migration of circulating IgA lymphocytes to the mammary gland, it is available, and the mouse is a good animal in which to study cellular homing. Such a factor would be predicted to be secreted from the mammary epithelial cells into the underlying stroma, and since the lactating mammary gland is an apocrine gland, intact as well as fragments of secretory epithelial cells are released into milk during lactation (11). Therefore, if a chemotactic factor for IgA lymphocytes is produced by mammary epithelial cells and is present in breast tissue during lactation, the factor could be present in milk as well. In this study, mesenteric lymph node (MN) surface IgA-positive lymphocytes, purified by cell "panning", were used in a micropore filter Boyden chamber assay to evaluate milk as a potential source of the putative chemotactic factor.

METHODS

Animals

Male (C57Bl/6 x DBA/2) F1 mice (6-12 weeks old) were obtained from The Jackson Laboratory (Bar Harbor, ME).

Preparation of cells

MN or peripheral nodes (PN) (inguinal, axillary) were teased into single-cell suspensions in Hanks' balanced salt solution (HBSS) with Hepes buffer and antibiotics (Grand Island Biological Co., Grand Island, New York). The cell suspensions were treated with 0.83% ammonium chloride to lyse red cells, and were washed three times with prewarmed HBSS, incubated for 5 min at 37°C and rapidly filtered twice through nylon wool to remove dead cells and debris.

Separation of lymphocyte subsets

Lymphocytes were separated on the basis of surface markers by panning (12). 100 x 15 mm polystyrene Petri dishes (Falcon Lab, Oxnard, CA) were coated with rabbit or goat anti-mouse IgA, IgM or IgG (Gateway Immunosera, St. Louis, MO; and Litton Bionetics, Charleston, SC). 3×10^7 lymphocytes in 3 ml PBS/5% fetal calf serum were added to each dish, incubated for 40 min at 5°C, swirled for 30 seconds, reincubated for 30 min, and the dish was gently washed five times with PBS. The bound cells, either surface IgA-, IgM- or IgG-positive, were recovered by gently flushing the surface of the plate with 3 ml PBS/1% fetal calf serum,using a Pasteur pipette. Purified populatons of T cells were obtained by negative selection after coating plates with a combination of anti-mouse IgA, IgG and IgM.

The purity of the lymphocyte populations was determined by immunofluorescence with fluorescein-conjugated goat anti-mouse IgA and IgG (Cappel Labs, Malvern, PA) and rabbit anti-mouse IgM for B cells and anti-mouse brain (Litton Bionetics) for T cells.

Lymphocyte migration assay

Lymphocyte migration assays were performed in modified Boyden chambers (13-15) with the leading front technique (16). The assay uses two compartments separated by an 8 μ pore nitrocellulose membrane (Sartorius, Gottingen, West Germany). Chambers containing 2.5 x 10^5 lymphocytes in HBSS in the upper compartment were incubated for 3 h at 37°C, after which the membranes were fixed in formaldehyde, stained and cleared with xylene (13). Migration into the membrane was measured with the microscope micrometer by determining the distance to the leading front, defined as the farthest microscope field containing three cells, in five vertical zones of the membrane chosen at random. Migration was expressed as an index (MI), the ratio of distance migrated with the factor present to the distance migrated in the presence of medium alone.

Chemotaxis is directional locomotion under the influence of a concentration gradient. When movement is toward a higher concentration of chemotactic factor, chemotaxis is said to be positive. With cells in the upper compartment, positive chemotaxis is maximal when the chemotactic factor is present only in the lower compartment, compared to having the factor in the upper or both compartments. Chemokinesis is a random increase of locomotion without a directional component, that is determined by the absolute local concentration of a factor. Placing a chemokinetic factor in the upper compartment alone with the lymphocytes gives maximal migration. In order to differentiate chemotaxis from chemokinesis, a variation of the checkerboard assay was performed (16). The varying effect on lymphocyte migration of placing the test factor in the upper, lower or both compartments of the chamber was ascertained.

RESULTS AND DISCUSSION

In the first experiment, skim milk was fractionated into acid-soluble whey and acid-insoluble casein and tested in the Boyden chamber The response of MN IgA lymphocytes to the whey fraction was chemotactic, i.e., maximal migration occurred when the whey fraction was only in the lower compartment, compared to migration when the whey was in the upper or both compartments ($p < 0.05$). In contrast, the response of MN IgA lymphocytes to casein was chemokinetic since migration was greater when the factor was in the upper compartment than in the lower compartment ($p < 0.05$). In multiple experiments, of which Table 1 is representative, the chemotactic effect of the whey fraction and the chemokinetic effect of casein were clearly and consistently demonstrated.

In the second experiment, homogeneous populations of murine mesenteric node IgA-, IgG-, IgM-bearing and T lymphocytes were obtained by panning and tested in the Boyden chamber. Table 2 illustrates the response of the various MN lymphocyte populations to the whey fraction. The response of both the surface IgA- and surface IgG-positive MN lymphocytes was chemotactic. In contrast, surface IgM-positive lymphocytes gave indeterminate results, with no suggestion of chemotaxis. The response of the T lymphocytes was chemokinetic.

The third experiment was designed to determine whether this chemotactic effect applied selectively to cells from mucosal-associated lymphoid tissue. Surface IgG-positive lymphocytes from MN and PN were purified by panning and then tested in the chemotactic assay. Table 3 shows data from one experiment. The MN IgG lymphocytes again responded in a chemotactic fashion; in marked contrast, however, the PN IgG lymphocytes exhibited no directional movement. These results suggest that the chemotactic activity in the whey fraction is specific for subsets of lymphocytes derived from mucosal

Table 1. Migration index of IgA lymphocytes from mesenteric nodes exposed to whey and casein fractions

Milk fraction	Compartment containing the milk fraction		
	Upper	Both	Lower
Whey	1.2 ± 0.2	1.5 ± 0.2	2.2 ± 0.2[a]
Casein	1.6 ± 0.2[b]	1.7 ± 0.2	1.1 ± 0.2

[a]Different ($p<0.05$) from migration index with whey fraction in upper or both compartments.

[b]Different ($p<0.05$) from migration index with casein in lower compartment.

Table 2. Migration of index of subsets of mesenteric node lymphocytes to whey

Surface Marker	Compartment containing the whey fraction		
	Upper	Both	Lower
IgA	1.2 ± 0.03	1.5 ± 0.03	2.1 ± 0.03[a]
IgG	1.1 ± 0.03	1.3 ± 0.03	2.6 ± 0.03[a]
IgM	1.8 ± 0.03	1.6 ± 0.03	1.7 ± 0.03
Thy-1	1.4 ± 0.03[b]	1.4 ± 0.03	0.9 ± 0.03

[a]Different ($p<0.05$) from migration index with whey fraction in upper or both compartments.

[b]Different ($p<0.05$) from migration index with whey fraction in lower compartment.

associated lymphoid tissue. In PN, the number of IgA lymphocytes is too few to allow purification and comparison to MN IgA cells in a similar fashion.

An additional set of experiments was done to inquire whether the chemotactic factor in milk is locally produced by examining whether mouse serum is also chemotactic (Table 4). The effect is indeterminate. Because no chemotactic effect on IgA lymphocytes is seen with serum, the experiments suggest the existence of a locally produced chemotactic factor for IgA (and IgG) lymphocytes in milk.

In the above work, we pursued the idea that homing IgA lymphocytes may be attracted or retained by a secretory product of differentiated epithelium which acts chemotactically and locally. In support of the hypothesis, we were able to demonstrate that mouse milk contains a chemotactic activity for MN derived, surface IgA positive lymphocytes that is not present in serum. This chemotactic effect was also seen for IgG lymphocytes from MN, although IgG cells from PN did not respond. This is consistent with cell traffic studies which suggest that precursor cells from MN can also give rise to a minor population of intestinal IgG plasma cells (4).

Additional work (not shown) has demonstrated that the factor is nondialyzable and precipitates in 50% saturated ammonium sulfate. It has

Table 3. Migration index of mesenteric and peripheral node IgG-bearing lymphocytes exposed to whey

IgG Lymphocytes	Compartment containing the whey fraction		
	Upper	Both	Lower
Mesenteric node	1.5 ± 0.3	1.9 ± 0.3	3.0 ± 0.3[a]
Peripheral node	1.7 ± 0.3	1.7 ± 0.3	1.7 ± 0.3

[a]Different ($p<0.05$) from migration index with whey fraction in upper or both compartments.

Table 4. Migration of mesenteric node IgA and IgG lymphocytes to the globulin fraction from lactating as well as normal mouse serum

Surface marker	Compartment containing lactating mouse serum		
	Upper	Both	Lower
IgA	1.0 ± 0.1	ND[a]	1.1 ± 0.1
IgG	1.0 ± 0.1	ND	1.0 ± 0.1
	Compartment containing normal mouse serum		
IgA	1.1 ± 0.1	ND	1.0 ± 0.1
IgG	1.0 ± 0.1	ND	1.0 ± 0.1

[a]ND = not done.

an apparent molecular weight between 20-60 KDa as determined by gel filtration, and is inactivated by trypsin and heat (75°C for 30 min or 100°C for 2 min).

CONCLUSIONS

These studies suggest that a chemotactic factor for IgA-positive lymphocytes in mucosal associated lymphoid tissue is present in the whey fraction of milk. This factor could be responsible for the selective homing of IgA lymphocytes to the lactating mammary gland and other secretory sites.

ACKNOWLEDGEMENTS

This work was supported by National Institutes of Health grant CA 32582.

REFERENCES

1. Lamm, M.E., Adv. Immunol. 22, 223, 1976.
2. Guy-Grand, D., Griscelli, C., Vassalli, P., Eur. J. Immunol. 4, 435, 1974.
3. McWilliams, M., Phillips-Quagliata, J.M., Lamm, M.E., J. Immunol. 115, 54, 1975.
4. McDermott, M.R., Bienenstock, J., J. Immunol. 122, 1892, 1979.
5. Montgomery, P.C., Ayyildiz, A., Lemaitre-Coelho, I.M. and Vaerman, J.-P., Ann. N.Y. Acad. Sci. 409, 428, 1983.
6. Roux, M.E., McWilliams, M., Phillips-Quagliata, J.M., Weisz-Carrington, P. and Lamm, M.E., J. Exp. Med. 146, 1311, 1977.
7. Parrott, D.M.V., Ferguson, A., Immunology 26, 571, 1974.
8. Hall, J.G., Hopkins, J., Orlans, E., Eur. J. Immunol. 7, 30, 1977.
9. Stevens, S.K., Weissman, I.L. and Butcher, E.C., J. Immunol. 128, 844, 1982.
10. Ottaway, C.A., Bruce, R.G. and Parrott, D.M.V., Immunology 49, 641, 1983.
11. Larson, B.L., J. Dairy Res. 46, 161, 1979.
12. Wysocki, L.J. and Sato, V.L., Proc. Natl. Acad. Sci. USA 75, 2844, 1978.
13. El-Naggar, A.K., Van Epps,D.E. and Williams, R.C., Cell. Immunol. 60, 43, 1981.
14. Ward, P.A., Unanue, E.R., Goralnick, S.J. and Shreiner, G.F., J. Immunol. 119, 416, 1977.
15. Wilkinson, P.C., Parrott, D.M., Russell, R.J. and Sless, F., J. Exp. Med. 145, 1158, 1977.
16. Zigmond, S.H. and Hirsch, J.G., J. Exp. Med. 137, 387, 1973.

PROPERTIES OF HUMAN B CELLS TERMINATING IN NORMAL GUT-ASSOCIATED LYMPHOID TISSUE, INCLUDING PEYER'S PATCHES

K. Bjerke and P. Brandtzaeg

Laboratory of Immunohistochemistry and Immunopathology, Institute of Pathology, University of Oslo, The National Hospital, Rikshospitalet, Oslo, Norway

INTRODUCTION

The intestinal secretory IgA system is quantitatively the most important humoral immune system of the body - about 10^{10} Ig-producing cells being present per metre of gut (1). The precursors of these immunocytes are apparently generated largely in the Peyer's patches owing to specialized mechanisms of antigen uptake and immune regulation (2,3). Lymphoid follicles of the appendix and solitary follicles scattered throughout the small and large bowel mucosa, show comparable features and may function as a part of the gut-associated lymphoid tissue (GALT). A comparative study of the immunoglobulin (Ig) isotype expression of B cells associated with lymphoid follicles of the appendix, colon and ileum mucosa and in Peyer's patches was therefore carried out. Cytoplasmic J chain was included as a marker of clonal immaturity (4) to study the extent of terminal B cell maturation *in situ*.

METHODS

Tissue specimens of normal human intestinal mucosa were extracted in cold isotonic phosphate-buffered saline to remove extracellular diffusible Ig components before processing by fixation in ethanol and paraffin embedding (5). Serial sections (6 μm) were evaluated by paired immunofluorescence staining with isotype-specific rabbit IgG conjugates. Before costaining of cytoplasmic Ig isotype and J chain the sections were pretreated with acid (pH 3.2) 6 M urea. The density of Ig-producing cells was determined by morphometry, and three tissue compartments related to lymphoid follicles were subjected to evaluation: germinal centre, subepithelial dome, and lamina propria adjacent to the follicle. With regard to J chain expression, also the lamina propria distant to lymphoid follicles were examined in the appendix and ileum mucosa.

RESULTS

The density of Ig-producing cells in the dome area and alongside the lymphoid follicles was higher than in the distant lamina propria. This was ascribed to a significantly raised number of IgG immunocytes (Table 1, Fig. 1); the percentages of IgA and IgG immunocytes were quite similar adjacent to the follicles (Fig. 2). Ig-producing cells were sparse in the germinal centres (Fig. 3), particularly in those of solitary follicles of the colon and ileum (Fig. 2). IgM, and to a lesser extent IgG, immunocytes predominated in the follicles of the appendix and Peyer's patches - both isotypes being significantly more represented than IgA ($p = 0.03$). IgD- and IgE-producing cells were absent in all tissue compartments.

The most frequent cytoplasmic J chain expression was seen in the distant lamina propria where on an average 97% of the IgA, 73% of the IgG and 100% of the IgM immunocytes were positive (Fig. 4). The proportion

Table 1. Density (cells/mm^2) of IgA- and IgG-producing immunocytes in dome area and lamina propria adjacent to lymphoid follicles of appendix mucosa compared with overall lamina propria (median and range)

Tissue compartments	IgA Cells	IgG Cells
Overall lamina propria	1259 (753-2163)	95 (9-356)
Follicle-associated lamina propria:		
adjacent zone	838 (377-1712)	869 (338-2304)
dome area	977 (160-1857)	508 (327-2429)

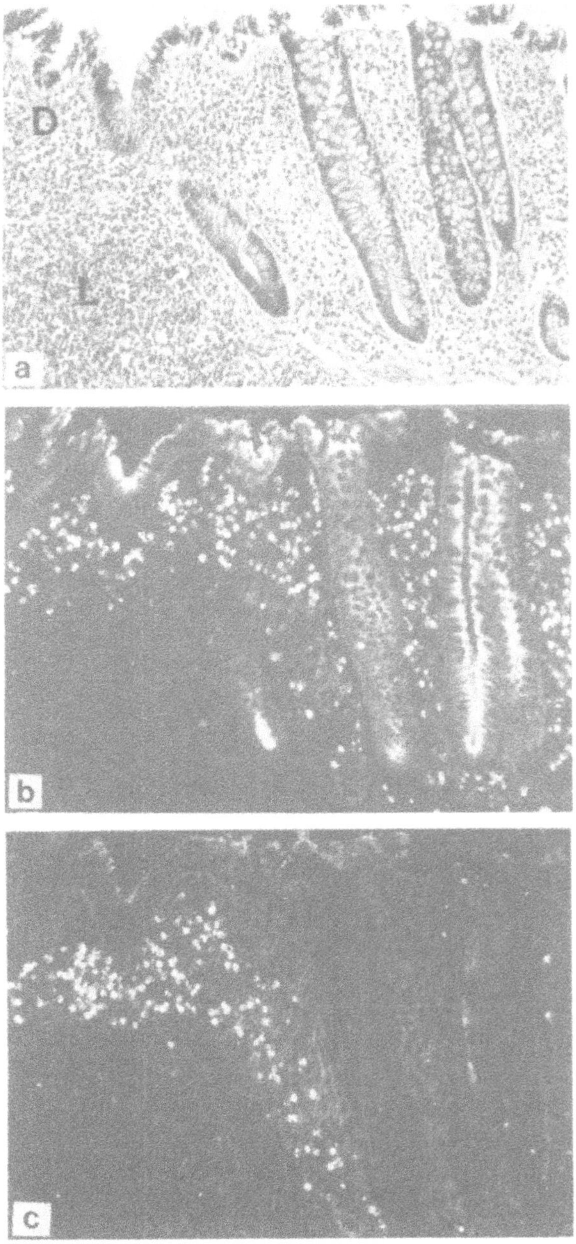

Figure 1. Two adjacent sections of pre-washed and ethanol-fixed normal appendix mucosa. (a) H & E-stained section for orientation. L = lymphoid follicle. D = dome. (ab) Comparable field from section subjected to paired staining for IgA (b, red fluorescence) and IgG (c, green fluorescence). Note preferential accumulation of IgG-producing cells in the dome and alongside the follicle, whereas IgA-producing cells are abundant also between the crypts on the right. Both crypt and surface epithelium show selective uptake of IgA in columnar cells, signifying external transport of this isotype.

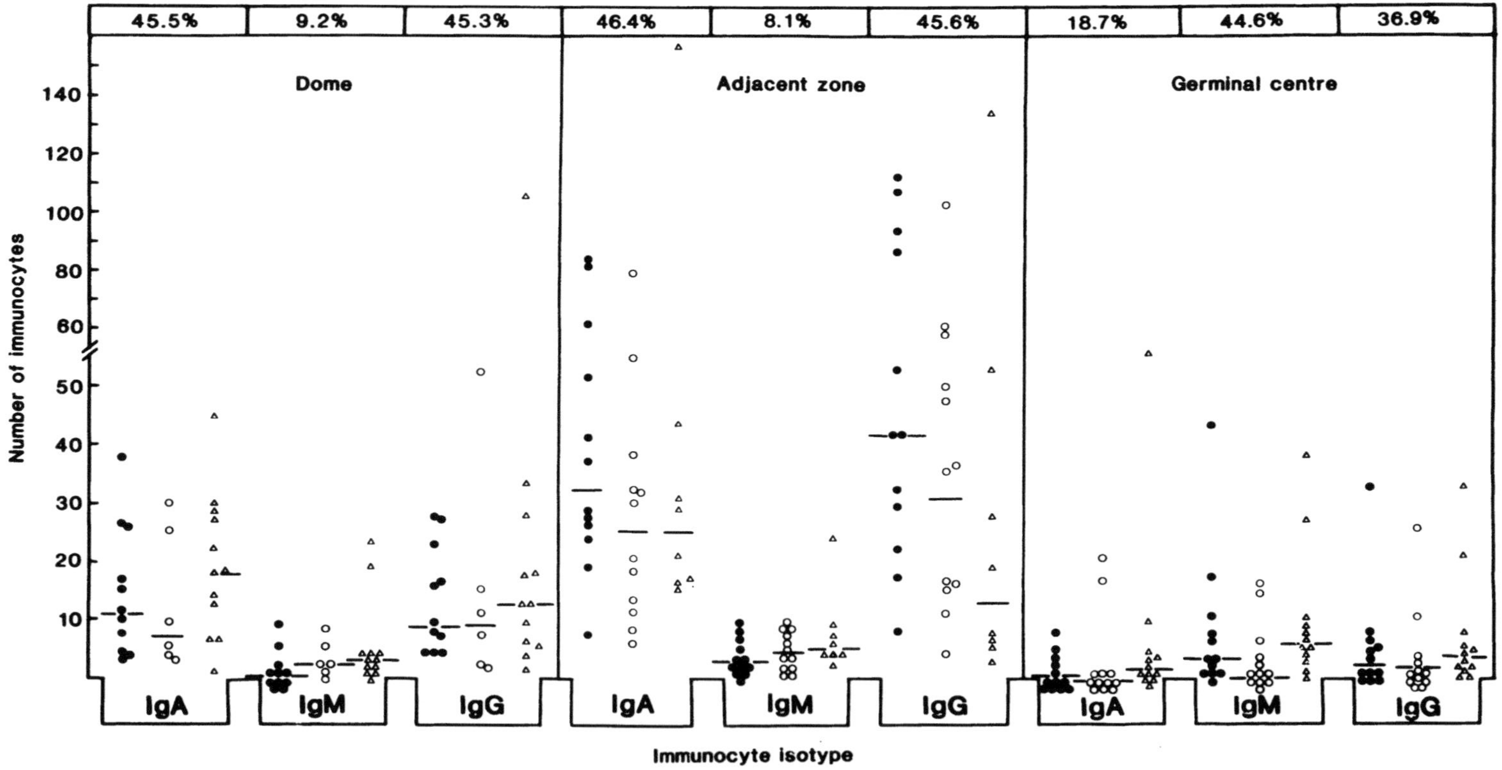

Figure 2. Distribution of IgA-, IgM- and IgG-producing immunocytes in three follicle-associated tissue compartments from appendix (●), colon and ileum (○) and Peyer's patches (△).

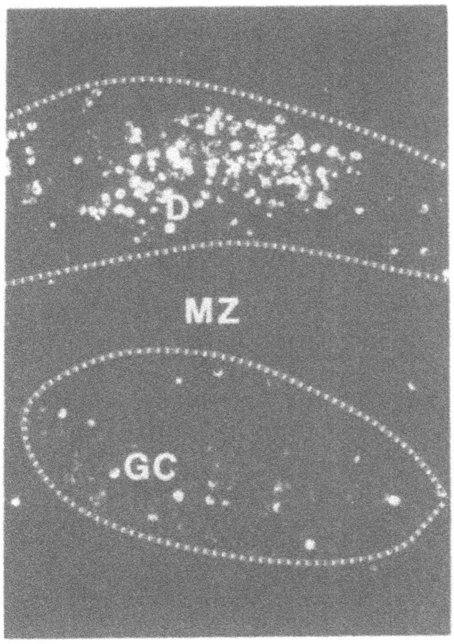

Figure 3. Section of prewashed and ethanol-fixed Peyer's patch subjected to direct immunofluorescence staining for cytoplasmic IgG. Broken lines delineate different tissue compartments (D = dome; MZ = mantle zone; and GC = germinal centre). Note relatively few immunocytes in GC and accumulation in D. Gut lumen at the top.

of J chain-positive IgG immunocytes was significantly reduced in the dome ($p < 0.05$) as well as alongside the lymphoid follicles ($p < 0.03$) (Fig. 5). The J chain positivity in the germinal centres was on an average 50%, 60% and 25% for IgA, IgM and IgG cells, respectively. This percentage for the two former isotypes was significantly lower than in the dome area ($p < 0.02$).

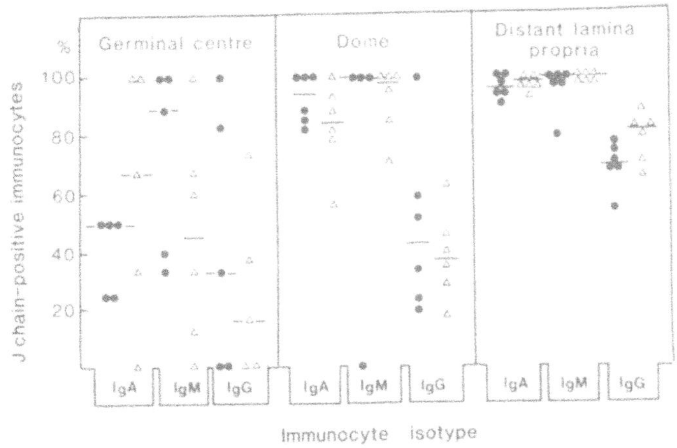

Figure 4. Distribution of J chain-positive immunocytes according to cytoplasmic isotype in three tissue compartments of appendix (●) and Peyer's patches (△).

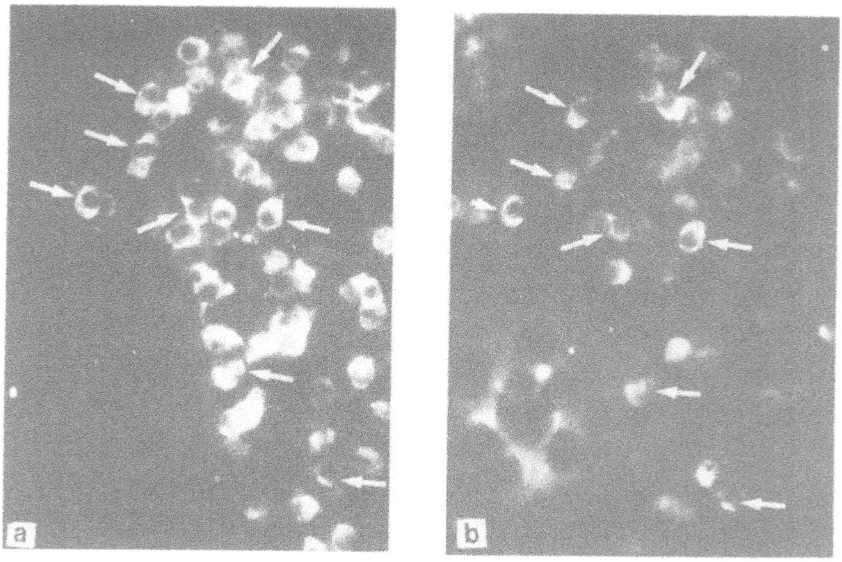

Figure 5. Acid urea-treated section of prewashed and ethanol-fixed appendix mucosa subjected to paired immunofluorescence staining for IgG (a, green fluorescence) and J chain (b, red fluorescence) in the zone between crypt (C) on the left and lymphoid follicle on the right (not shown). Note that relatively few IgG-producing cells are J chain-positive (examples indicated by arrows). The other J chain-positive cells represent IgA (or IgM) immunocytes; the crypt epithelium is stained for J chain because it contains secretory IgA (and secretory IgM).

DISCUSSION AND CONCLUSIONS

Human Peyer's patches could not be distinguished from solitary lymphoid follicles in the ileum, colon, and appendix mucosa on the basis of the functional B cell characteristics identified in this immunohistochemical study.

Since most B cells after terminal maturation at secretory sites express J chain, regardless of concomitant cytoplasmic isotype, they may collectively belong to a population of relatively early memory clones (4,6). Conversely, the population of follicle-associated immunocytes which showed prominent IgG expression and down-regulated J chain synthesis most likely consists mainly of mature memory clones. This observation indicated that the migration route preferred by B cells of mature clones is directly from the follicle into the nearby lamina propria.

Accumulation of members of such mature memory clones with down-regulated J chain expression is, however, much more pronounced in peripheral lymph nodes and tonsils (7); this difference may explain that GALT is quantitatively the most important origin of B cells seeding distant secretory sites; such cells escape terminal maturation in situ and end up mainly as immunocytes producing J chain-containing dimeric IgA adjacent to glandular structures. The immunoregulatory basis for this is fundamental to secretory immunity as J chain is a key factor for external Ig transport (4).

REFERENCES

1. Brandtzaeg, P., Valnes, K., Scott, H., Rognum, T.O., Bjerke, K. and Baklien, K., Scand. J. Gastroenterol. 20 (Suppl. 114), 17, 1985.
2. Elson, C.O., Scand. J. Gastroenterol. 20 (Suppl. 114), 1, 1985.
3. Brandtzaeg, P., Scand. J. Gastroenterol. 20 (Suppl. 114), 137, 1985.
4. Brandtzaeg, P., Scand. J. Immunol. 22, 111, 1985.
5. Brandtzaeg, P., Immunology 26, 1101, 1974.
6. Brandtzaeg, P. and Korsrud, F.R., Clin. Exp. Immunol. 58, 709, 1984.
7. Korsrud, F.R. and Brandtzaeg, P., Scand. J. Immunol. 13, 271, 1981.

SUBCLASS DISTRIBUTION OF IgG- AND IgA-PRODUCING CELLS IN SECRETORY TISSUES AND ALTERATIONS RELATED TO GUT DISEASES

P. Brandtzaeg, K. Kett and T.O. Rognum

Laboratory for Immunohistochemistry and Immunopathology
Institute of Pathology, and Institute of Forensic Medicine
The National Hospital
Rikshospitalet, 0027 Oslo 1, Norway

INTRODUCTION

Both serum IgA and secretory IgA (sIgA) consist of two subclasses, IgA1 and IgA2, which differ in primary structure, carbohydrate composition, and antigenic properties (1). While IgA1 predominates (about 90%) in normal serum, exocrine secretions have been reported to contain a relatively large proportion (30-50%) of IgA2 (2,3). It is not known how IgA subclass production is regulated; apparently contradictory information about the influence of antigenic stimuli has been published (4-7).

B lymphocytes co-expressing either IgA1 or IgA2 along with IgM were found in about equal numbers in peripheral blood of newborns, whereas a preferential shift towards IgA1-positive B cells without IgM (about 80%) occurred with increasing age (8). Nevertheless, about equal proportions of IgA1- and IgA2-producing cells developed after stimulation of circulating B lymphocytes from adults; this finding was in part ascribed to an enrichment of IgA2 precursors in the IgM-positive B lymphocyte population, whereas there was no evidence for switching from IgA1 to IgA2 expression (9).

All human secretory tissues normally contain a significant, but varying number of IgM-, IgG- and IgD-producing cells in addition to the predominating IgA immunocytes (10-12). The fraction of IgG cells is small (3-5%) in normal intestinal mucosa but considerably larger in respiratory mucosa. In inflammatory disease, the number of IgG immunocytes increases significantly (10,12). The distribution of the four IgG subclasses among the mucosal immunocytes is unknown, however, both in health and disease. Knowledge about this is important because previous studies have indicated a marked IgG subclass restriction of specific antibodies, depending on the nature of the antigen (7,13). T cells may regulate IgG subclass responses by enhancing the differentiation of precommitted B cells (14), but there is no information as to whether this regulation differs in various secretory tissues and mucosal diseases.

This paper reviews recent immunohistochemical studies performed in our laboratory (15-20) to map the subclass distribution of IgG and IgA immunocytes in various secretory tissues including normal and diseased gut mucosa.

MATERIALS AND METHODS

Tissue specimens

The selected tissue blocks were deemed to be normal by conventional histological examination, with the exception of gastric and nasal specimens, some of which showed mild chronic inflammation. In addition, specimens of cervical and inguinal lymph nodes showed minor non-specific reactive lymphadenopathy.

Specimens of the following categories of intestinal disorders (adult patients) were included: ulcerative colitis and Crohn's disease (colonic specimens); untreated coeliac disease, treated coeliac disease (gluten-free diet), and established food allergy (jejunal specimens showing a substantial number of IgG-producing cells when preliminarily examined.

Immunohistochemistry

Fresh tissue specimens were prepared as thin slices which were extracted in cold phosphate-buffered isotonic saline for 48 h prior to ethanol fixation and paraffin embedding (21). Serial sections were cut at 6 μm, dewaxed and subjected to paired immunofluorescence staining.

The sections were first incubated with one of the subclass-specific murine monoclonal antibodies and, thereafter, with a mixture of fluorescein-labeled rabbit anti-mouse IgG and rhodamine-labeled rabbit anti-human IgG or IgA. Both incubations took place at room temperature for 20 h.

The four IgG subclass-specific antibodies (Clones 2C7, GOM2, CB1-AH7 and RJ4) were selected on the basis of the recently published results of an international collaborative study of such reagents (22). The two IgA subclass-specific antibodies (Clones 69-11.4 and 16-512-H5) were provided by Drs. J. Radl and J.J. Haaijman (23). The anti-mouse reagent was either obtained from Dakopatts, Copenhagen (F224, lot 0980; absorbed with polymerized human serum) or prepared in our laboratory. The latter was also true for the reagents specific for human IgG or IgA. Details about working concentrations and conjugate characteristics have been published elsewhere (15).

Microscopy and cell counting

Cells were observed in mounted sections (15) under a Leitz Orthoplan fluorescence microscope equipped with a Ploem-type vertical illuminator for selective observation of green (fluorescein) or red (rhodamine) staining. Several hundred red cells were usually examined in every tissue specimen for concomitant green cytoplasmic fluorescence. The proportion of cells containing one of the subclasses was calculated in relation to the total number of IgG- or IgA-producing immunocytes detected in the evaluated area of the same section. For each tissue category the counts of green cells were only slightly overestimated (101-105%) in relation to the 100% red internal reference. Differences between medians of results were calculated by Wilcoxon's two-tailed test for unpaired samples.

RESULTS

IgG subclasses

Performance testing of the paired immunofluorescence method on sections of tonsillar tissue afforded clear-cut identification of immunocytes producing each of the four IgG subclasses, the IgG1 isotype being strikingly predominant (Fig. 1). Also, all secretory tissues examined (nasal, jejunal and colonic mucosa) contained mainly IgG1-producing cells. In nasal mucosa the median IgG3 subclass proportion was significantly higher than that of IgG2 ($p < 0.04$), but there were large individual variations (Fig. 2). In a group of 10 patients with selective IgA deficiency, relatively more nasal IgG2 cells were seen than in the control material (19% vs 10%); this difference was significant ($p < 0.02$) for five patients who showed marked compensatory IgM rather than IgD response in their nasal mucosa (16).

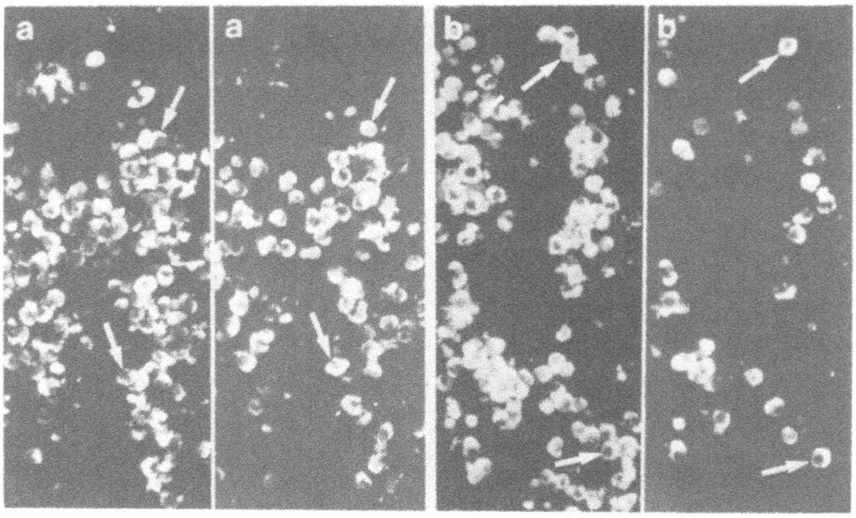

Figure 1. Paired immunofluorescence staining for IgG (left panel, rhodamine) and IgG subclass (right panel, fluorescein) in comparable fields from two serial sections of palatine tonsil. (a) IgG/IgG1; (b) IgG/IgG2. Note predominance of IgG1-producing cells beneath epithelium (indicated by dark areas). Examples of identical cells labeled with arrows in paired pictures (x200).

Because of the small number of IgG-producing cells present in control gut mucosa we have not as yet obtained confident data for the normal intestinal IgG subclass distribution. However, in the mucosal biopsy material we have studied, including jejunal specimens from patients with treated coeliac disease (see below), a preponderance of IgG2 over IgG3 immunocytes was seen. The same held true in the dome areas of normal Peyer's patches (Bjerke α Brandtzaeg, unpublished).

IgA subclasses

The IgA subclass profile of the various immunocyte populations evaluated appears in Figure 3. All non-secretory lymphoid tissues showed, as expected, a marked predominance of IgA1-producing cells. However, striking differences were noted among the secretory tissue sites. Nasal mucosa was fairly similar to the non-secretory tissues in that the proportion of IgA1 immunocytes was 91-100% (Fig. 3). We have recently evaluated another material of eight nasal specimens and found a slightly lower median (90%) of IgA1-producing cells (range, 74-97%). It was noteworthy that the IgA1 isotype predominated even when the immunocytes were confined to the glandular stroma (Fig. 4a). An inflammatory reaction in nasal mucosa is evidenced by cellular infiltration of the stroma beneath the surface epithelium.

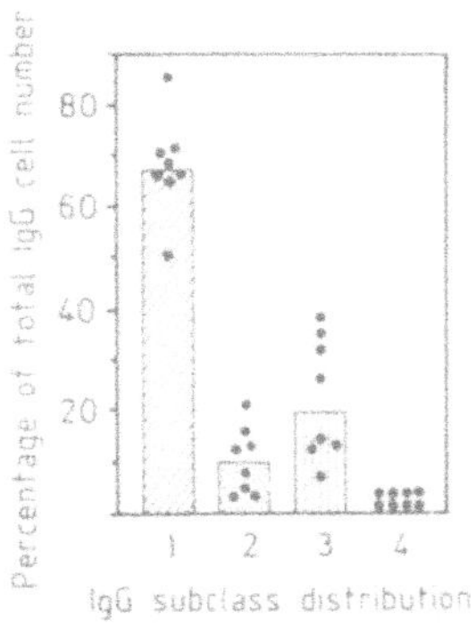

Figure 2. Proportions of IgG subclass-producing cells in eight specimens of nasal mucosa from patients with intact immune system.

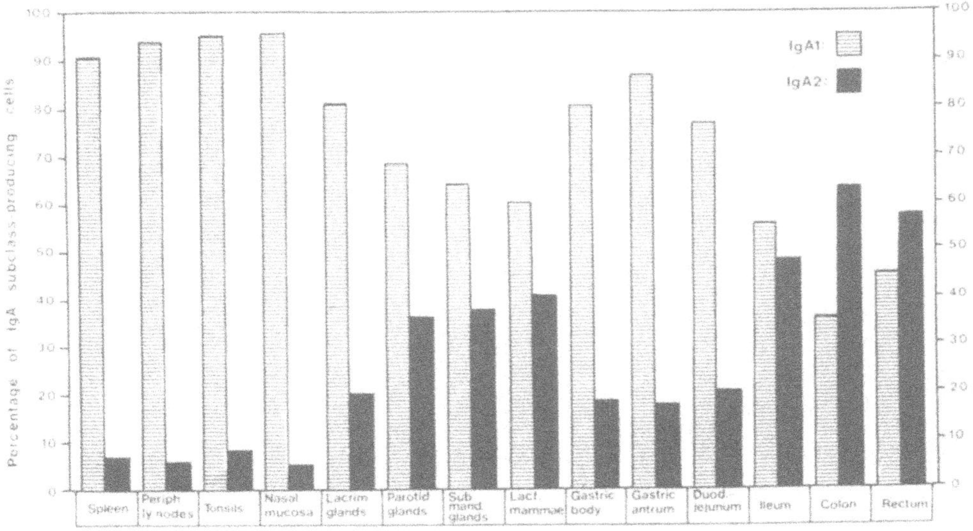

Figure 3. Subclass profile of IgA immunocytes in various human tissues as indicated.

Another immunohistochemical feature of interest in nasal mucosa was the virtual absence of staining for IgA2 in secretory epithelium, indicating minimal secretion of this isotype in most specimens. Distinct epithelial staining for IgA2 was seen only in specimens containing about 20% or more IgA2-producing immunocytes.

IgA1 immunocytes likewise predominated (63-86%) in lacrimal glands (Figs. 3 and 4b) and gastric mucosa (63-99%), and also in the proximal small intestinal mucosa (65-85%). The proportion of IgA1 cells was usually smaller in salivary and mammary glands (42-80%). In the distal small intestine, most specimens contained almost an equal number of IgA1 and IgA2 immunocytes, the median IgA1 ratio in ileum being 55% (42-70%). In the large bowel, almost all specimens contained more IgA2 than IgA1 cells (Fig. 4c), the median IgA1 proportion being 40% (25-66%). It was noteworthy that in the latter type of tissue epithelial staining signified external transport of both subclasses.

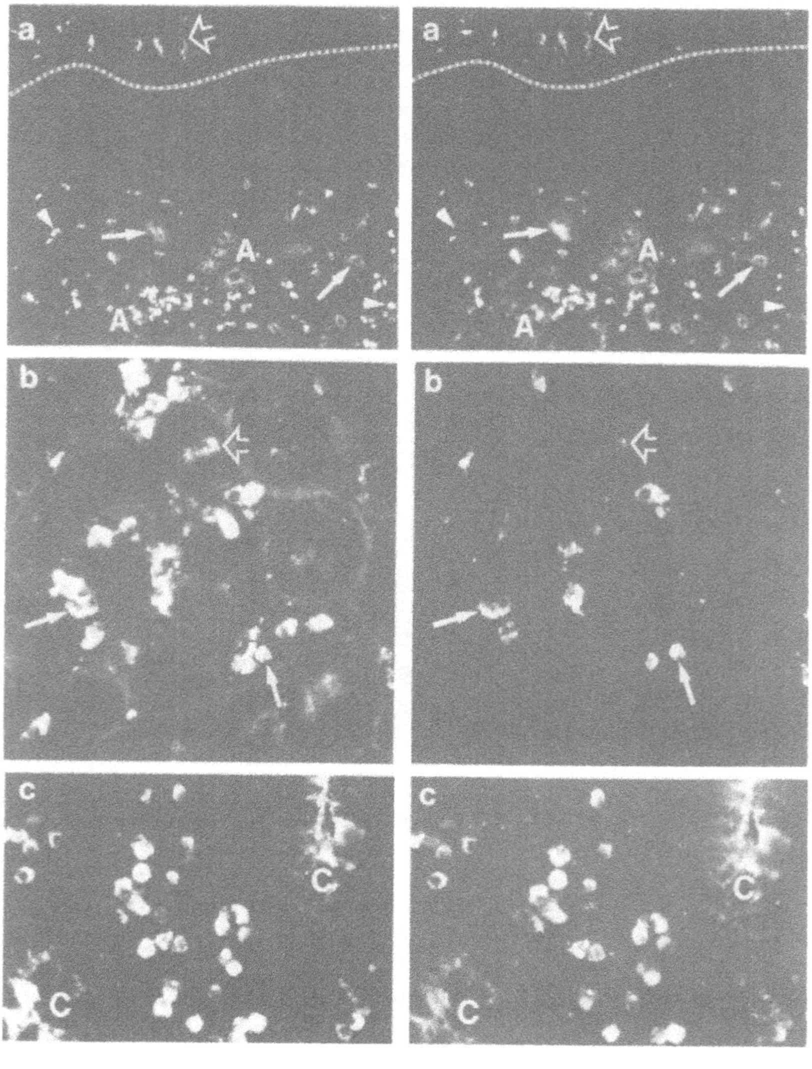

Figure 4. Paired immunofluorescence staining for IgA (left panel, rhodamine) and IgA subclass (right panel, fluorescein) in various secretory tissues. (a) Normal nasal mucosa: IgA/IgA1; immunocytes are present only in the glandular area between acini (A) which show abundant IgA1 uptake (closed arrows), whereas surface epithelium (above dashed line) contains relatively little IgA1 (open arrow); only a few cells (arrowheads) do not belong to the IgA1 subclass. (b) Normal lacrimal gland: IgA/IgA2; in this field IgA2-producing cells (arrows) amount to 33%, but there is little uptake of this isotype in acini (open arrow). (c) Normal colonic mucosa: IgA/IgA2; in this field IgA2-producing cells amount to 88% and there is abundant uptake of this isotype in crypt epithelium (C) (a, x80; b,c, x200).

Gut diseases

Our findings for IgG subclass-producing cells are summarized in Table 1. The median proportion of IgG1 immunocytes was significantly higher in ulcerative colitis than in Crohn colitis, whereas the reverse was true for the IgG2 subclass ($p < 0.02$). With regard to mucosal IgA-producing cells, the IgA1 subclass was significantly increased ($p < 0.008$) in both diseases, more so in ulcerative colitis (median, 71%; range, 62-83%) than in Crohn colitis (median, 57%; range, 40-68%).

The only significant ($p < 0.05$) alteration of the IgG subclass distribution in coeliac disease was observed for IgG2 cells; the proportion of such immunocytes was higher in untreated than in treated patients and also higher than in those with food allergy (Table 1).

Table 1. Subclass distribution (%) of IgG-producing cells in intestinal mucosa

Mucosal site	Disease	Median distribution (range)			
		IgG1	IgG2	IgG3	IgG4
Colon	Crohn's disease	66.5 (55-79)	24.9 (16-47)	3.8 (3.4-11)	2.1 (0-6)
Colon	Ulcerative colitis	81.3 (57-91)	9.4 (4.8-37)	4.1 (1.4-26)	0.8 (0-22)
Jejunum	Food allergy	71.2 (55-100)	8.2 (0-38)	6.2 (0-30)	6.0 (1.5-14)
Jejunum	Treated coeliac disease	78.5 (45-83)	12.3 (3.4-32)	6.0 (2-17)	1.7 (0-24)
Jejunum	Untreated coeliac disease	56.6 (31-75)	36.7 (34-65)	6.0 (1-11)	2.0 (0-19)

DISCUSSION

IgG subclasses

Since the normal subclass response of intestinal IgG immunocytes was not determined, it is difficult to know whether ulcerative colitis was associated with a marked local IgG1 response and a relatively reduced IgG2 response, or whether the reverse was true in Crohn colitis. A recent preliminary report based on study of cultured intestinal lymphocytes demonstrated a strikingly increased and preferential spontaneous secretion of IgG1 for cells from ulcerative colitis, whereas the increased IgG production in Crohn's disease showed subclass proportions comparable to controls, that is, IgG1 > IgG2 > IgG3 (24). A preponderance of IgG2 over IgG3 cells in jejunal mucosa with minimal lesions (treated coeliac disease or food allergy) likewise indicated that this is a general intestinal IgG response pattern.

Conversely, the IgG response in nasal mucosa tended to show a preference of IgG3 over IgG2 cells. This disparity between the two mucosal sites might reflect differences in antigen exposure. Previous studies of serum antibodies have shown that bacterial carbohydrates stimulate preferentially IgG2, whereas viral proteins induce IgG1/IgG3 (7,13,25-27)- IgG3 often appearing relatively early (28). The reason for a shift towards IgG2 producing cells in nasal mucosa of some IgA-deficient patients might be explained by infections with Streptococcus pneumoniae and/or Haemophilus influenzae which are known to stimulate preferentially IgG2 (25,29). However, this could not be the full explanation as most of the patients who compensated with a prominent nasal IgM response were without recurrent respiratory infections (16).

The disparity between ulcerative colitis and Crohn's disease of the colon in terms of the mucosal IgG-subclass response has pathogenetic implications; it may reflect dissimilar microbial exposure in the gut, different genetic "make-up" of the patients, or a combination of both. It is noteworthy in this context that certain mitogenic stimuli produce a coordinate IgG1 and IgG3 response or a selective IgG2 response, depending on the nature of the B cell population (30). It is, moreover, of interest that certain IgG1 and IgG3 heavy-chain markers are associated with Crohn's disease, namely those constituting the phenotype Gm(a,x,f;b,g) and the haplotype $Gm^{a,x;g}$ (31).

The raised frequency of mucosal IgG2-producing cells noted in untreated coeliac disease may likewise signify an interplay between genetic and immunological factors. Thus, those patients who lack HLA-B8 and HLA-DR3 always seem to have the phenotype Gm(f;n;b) (32); the IgG2 allotype marker G2m(n), moreover, is apparently associated with a persistent IgG response to gluten in treated patients (33).

IgA subclasses

A predominance of IgA2-producing cells in normal large bowel mucosa accords with previously reported findings in three specimens examined with the same monoclonal antibodies (34). Conversely, an earlier study based on polyclonal antibodies reported a fairly even distribution of IgA1 and IgA2 immunocytes throughout the gastrointestinal tract (35). Our demonstration of a preponderance of IgA1 cells in salivary glands and particularly so in lacrimal glands, contrasts significantly with previous data obtained with the same monoclonal antibodies (34,36). Technical problems may partly explain these discrepancies. We used an indirect method and an internal 100% reference (polyclonal anti-IgA) to ascertain comparable detection sensitivity for both subclasses. Moreover, our tissue specimens were prewashed to avoid interstitial staining caused by serum-derived and locally produced IgA1.

The substantial predominance of IgA1 immunocytes in lacrimal glands was in harmony with the observation that nasal mucosa contained mainly IgA1-producing cells. Moreover, when nasal secretions were analyzed for specific antibodies after topical application of live influenza virus in volunteers, the secondary immune response was found to be expressed preferentially by IgA1 (5). We have previously reported a remarkable similarity between lacrimal and nasal glandular tissue as to the composition of the local immunocyte population: both sites contain more IgD-producing cells than other secretory tissues, especially in IgA-deficiency (10,11).

Immunoregulatory implications

Switching mechanisms for the expression of isotypes are most likely involved in the differentiation of B cells within the secretory immune system. As reviewed elsewhere (37), there is much evidence that murine Peyer's patch cells can undergo T cell-regulated switching directly from IgM to IgA expression; observations on human B cells have indicated that

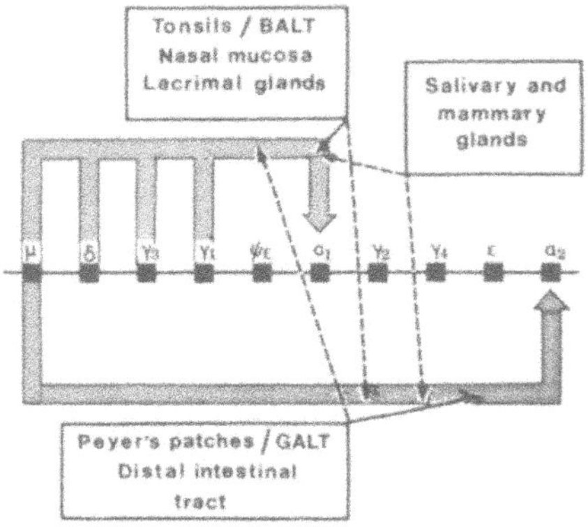

Figure 5. Putative C_H switching pathways leading to preferential production of IgA1 or IgA2 in the secretory immune system. It is proposed that sequential switching is preferred in tonsils and BALT, whereas direct switching from μ to α2 is preferred in GALT. The importance of these two pathways for the development of immunocyte populations in various secretory tissues is indicated by solid (preferential) and broken (subsidiary) arrows. Salivary and mammary glands apparently are in an intermediate position, probably because they are seeded by similar numbers of precursor cells from BALT and GALT (ref. 15).

this pathway leads preferentially to IgA2 production (9). Secretory sites seeded mainly by precursors from Peyer's patches and other gut-associated lymphoid tissues (GALT) may, hence, show preferential accumulation of IgA2 immunocytes, as observed by us for the distal intestinal tract (Fig. 5). However, sequential switching of the heavy chain constant (C_H) gene expression is probably also important (38). According to the arrangement of the human C_H region (39), IgA1 immunocytes may thus differentiate mainly from IgG1-expressing precursors; this has recently been suggested by studies of human myeloma cells (40). As IgG immunocytes are relatively frequent in nasal and gastric mucosa and mainly belong to the IgG1 subclass, frequent vectorial switching from IgG1 to IgA1 expression at these sites may explain the observed high proportion of IgA1 immunocytes. Perhaps switching from IgD to IgA expression may additionally contribute to a preferential local development of this isotype. Mayer et al. (41) recently described a malignant human T cell clone that afforded switching from IgM and IgD to both IgG and IgA expression.

The sequential pathway may be preferred by precursors from tonsils and bronchus-associated lymphoid tissues (BALT) and, thereby, also explain the predominance of IgA1 immunocytes in lacrimal glands (Fig. 5). This scheme would fit with our previously proposed dichotomy of the secretory immune system (11,37). Salivary and mammary glands probably receive precursor cells in similar numbers from GALT and BALT and are hence in an intermediate position, both with regard to the frequency of IgD immunocytes (42) and the development of IgA1- and IgA2-producing cells (17).

The regional differences in the secretory immune system were emphasized by the observation that only in severely inflamed colonic mucosa did the proportion of IgA1 immunocytes approach that found in normal nasal mucosa. The increased IgA1- to IgA2-producing cell ratio in inflammatory bowel disease probably reflected influx of cells representing systemic immunity; this was in keeping with decreased J chain expression as reported previously (43).

ACKNOWLEDGEMENTS

This work was supported by grants from the Norwegian Cancer Society, the Norwegian Research Council for Science and the Humanities, and Anders Jahre's Fund.

REFERENCES

1. Mestecky, J. and Russell, M.W., Monogr. Allergy 19, 277, 1986.
2. Grey, H.M., Abel, C.A., Yount, W.J. and Kunkel, H.G., J. Exp. Med. 128, 1223, 1968.
3. Delacroix, D.L., Dive, C., Rambaud, J.C. and Vaerman, J.-P., Immunology 47, 383, 1982.
4. Brown, T.A. and Mestecky, J., Infect. Immun. 49, 459, 1985.
5. Brown, T.A., Murphy, B.R., Radl, J., Haaijman, J.J. and Mestecky, J., J. Clin. Microbiol. 22, 259, 1985.
6. Conley, M.E. and Briles, D.E., Immunology 53, 419, 1984.
7. Hammarstrom, L., Persson, M.A.A. and Smith, C.I.E., Immunology 54, 821, 1985.
8. Conley, M.E., Kearney, J.F., Lawton, A.R. and Cooper, M.D., J. Immunol. 125, 2311, 1980.
9. Conley, M.E. and Bartelt, M.S., J. Immunol. 133, 2312, 1984.
10. Brandtzaeg, P., Prot. Biol. Fluids 32, 363, 1985.
11. Brandzaeg, P., Gjeruldsen, S.T., Korsrud, F., Baklien, K., Berdal, P. and Ek, J., J. Immunol. 122, 503, 1979.

12. Brandtzaeg, P., Valnes, K., Scott, H., Rognum, T.O., Bjerke, K. and Baklien, K., Scand. J. Gastroent. 20 (Suppl. 114), 17, 1985.
13. Shakib, F. and Stanworth, D.R., Ricerca Clin. Lab. 10, 561, 1980.
14. Maymui, M., Kuritani, T., Kubagawa, H. and Cooper, M.D., J. Immunol. 130, 671, 1983.
15. Brandtzaeg, P., Kett, K., Rognum, T.O., Söderstrom, R., Bjorkander, J., Söderstrom, T., Petruson, B. and Hanson, L.Å., Monogr. Allergy 20, 179, 1986.
16. Brandtzaeg, P., Karlsson, G., Hansson, G., Petruson, B., Bjorkander, J. and Hanson, L.Å., Clin. Exp. Immunol., 1987 (in press).
17. Kett, K., Brandtzaeg, P., Radl, J. and Haaijdman, J.J., J. Immunol. 136, 3631, 1986.
18. Kett, K., Rognum, T.O. and Brandtzaeg, P., Gastroenterology, 1987 (in press).
19. Kett, K. and Brandtzaeg, P., Gut, 1987 (in press).
20. Rognum, T.O., Kett, K., Bengtsson, U., Scott, H. and Brandtzaeg, P., Gut, 1987 (in press).
21. Brandtzaeg, P., Immunology 26, 1101, 1974.
22. Jefferis, R., Reimer, C.B., Skvaril, F., de Lange, G., Ling, N.R., Lowe, J., Walker, M.R., Phillips, D.J., Aloisio, C.H., Wells, T.W., Vaerman, J.-P., Magnusson, C.G., Kubagawa, H., Cooper, M., Vartdal, F., Vandvik, B., Haaijman, J.J., Makela, O., Sarnesto, A., Lando, Z., Gergely, J., Rajnavolgyi, E., Laszlo, G., Radl, J. and Molinaro, G.A., Immun. Letters 10, 223, 1985.
23. Valentijn, R.M., Radl, J., Haaijman, J.J., Vermeer, B.J., Weening, J.J., Kauffman, R.H., Daha, M.R. and van Es, L.A., Kidney Internat. 26, 760, 1984.
24. Scott, M.G., Macke, K., Nash, G., McDermott, R. and Nahm, M., Fed. Proc. 44, Abstr. No. 7631, 1985.
25. Freijd, A., Hammarstrom, L., Persson, M.A.A. and Smith, C.I.E., Clin. Exp. Immunol. 56, 233, 1984.
26. Linde, G.A., Hammarstrom, L., Persson, M.A.A., Smith, C.I.E., Sundqvist, V.A. and Wahren, B., Infect. Immun. 42, 237, 1983.
27. Skvaril, F. and Schilt, U., Clin. Exp. Immunol. 55, 671, 1984.
28. Hornsleth, A., Bech-Thomsen, N. and Friis, B., J. Med. Virol. 16, 321, 1985.
29. Siber, G.R., Schur, P.H., Aisenberg, A.C., Weitzman, S.A. and Schiffman, G., N. Engl. J. Med. 303, 178, 1980.
30. Scott, M.G. and Nahm, M.H., J. Immunol. 135, 2454, 1984.
31. Kagnoff, M.F., Brown, R.J. and Schanfield, M.S., Gastroenterology 85, 1044, 1983.

32. Kagnoff, M.F., Weiss, J.B., Brown, R.J., Lee, T. and Schanfield, M.S., Lancet 1, 952, 1983.
33. Weiss, J.B., Austin, R.K., Schanfield, M.S. and Kagnoff, M.F., J. Clin. Invest. 72, 96, 1983.
34. Crago, S.D., Kutteh, W.H., Moro, I., Allansmith, M.R., Radl, J., Haaijman, J.J. and Mestecky, J., J. Immunol. 132, 16, 1984.
35. Andre, C., Andre, F. and Fargier, M.C., Clin. Exp. Immunol. 33, 327, 1978.
36. Allansmith, M.R., Radl, J., Haaijman, J.J. and Mestecky, J., J. Allergy Clin. Immun. 76, 569, 1986.
37. Brandtzaeg, P., Scand. J. Gastroent. 20 (Suppl. 114), 137, 1985.
38. Cebra, J.J., Fuhrman, J.A., Horsfall, D.J. and Shahin, R.D., in Seminars in Infectious Disease, (Edited by Weinstein, L. and Fields, B.), Bacterial Vaccines, Vol. 4, (Edited by Robbins, J.B., Hill, J.C. and Sadoff, J.C.), p. 6, Thieme-Stratton, New York, 1982.
39. Flanagan, J.G. and Rabbits, T.H., Nature 300, 709, 1982.
40. Hammarstrom, L., Mellstedt, H., Persson, M.A.A., Smith, C.I.E. and Ahre, A., Acta. Path. Microbiol. Immunol. Scand. Sect. C 92, 207, 1984.
41. Mayer, L., Posnett, D.N. and Kunkel, H.G., J. Exp. Med. 161, 134, 1985.
42. Brandtzaeg, P., Ann. N.Y. Acad. Sci. 409, 353, 1983.
43. Brandtzaeg, P. and Korsrud, F.R., Clin. Exp. Immunol. 58, 709, 1984.

ALTERED PATTERNS OF SECRETION OF IgA AND IgG SUBCLASSES BY ULCERATIVE COLITIS AND CROHN'S DISEASE INTESTINAL MONONUCLEAR CELLS

R.P. MacDermott, G.S. Nash, M.G. Scott, M.H. Nahm, M.J. Bertovich and I.J. Kodner

Divisions of Gastroenterology and Laboratory Medicine
Departments of Medicine, Pathology and Surgery, Barnes and Jewish Hospitals, Washington University Medical Center
St. Louis, MO USA

INTRODUCTION

Ulcerative colitis (UC) and Crohn's disease (CD) are inflammatory bowel diseases (IBD) due to unknown etiologic and potentiating factors resulting in immune responses of a chronic inflammatory nature (1). There is an increase in cytoplasmic, surface, and secreted antibodies from IBD intestinal lymphocytes, due mainly to enhanced expression and production of IgG (2-4). In previous studies (5,6) we have found that immunoglobulin secretion patterns by peripheral blood and intestinal mononuclear cells (MNC) from inflammatory bowel disease patients is altered. IBD peripheral blood MNC reveal a markedly increased spontaneous secretion of IgA which is partially suppressed by PWM (5,6). Intestinal MNC from control specimens also spontaneously secrete large amounts of IgA, which is suppressed by PWM (5,6). In IBD patients, intestinal MNC exhibit decreased spontaneous IgA secretion, but have increased IgG secretion compared with control intestinal MNC (5-7). The changes in antibody secretion observed in IBD could be due to: (a) preferential proliferation of subpopulations of cells due to immunoregulatory alteration; (b) switching of the isotype and/or subclass of antibody secreted by the lymphocytes themselves; or (c) changes in the homing and trafficking patterns of the lymphocytes due to the inflammatory process. To investigate these possibilities, we have examined the nature of the subclasses of IgA and IgG secreted by intestinal MNC from IBD patients.

MATERIALS AND METHODS

Intestinal tissue (large or small bowel) was obtained at the time of surgery from patients with a variety of diagnoses, including adenocarcinoma, diverticulitis and inflammatory bowel disease. Tissues obtained from adenocarcinoma or diverticulitis specimens, were at least 10 cm from the area of pathology, and considered controls for investigational purposes. Tissues obtained from IBD specimens were primarily from involved sites. All patients with IBD had surgical resections because of intractability or complications of the bowel disease, and the majority were on steroid therapy at the time of surgery. MNC from human intestinal mucosa were isolated as previously described by Bull and Bookman (8) with modifications as we have described (5,9,10). Ribs were obtained at the time of surgery from patients undergoing thoracotomy and processed as previously described (11,12) in order to obtain pure human bone marrow MNC.

Intestinal, rib bone marrow, or peripheral blood MNC were cultured _in vitro_ in assay medium alone or in the presence of PWM, as previously described (5,6,13,14). Supernatants of cultured MNC were examined for the percent of dimeric and monomeric IgA (9) using High Performance Liquid Chromatography (HPLC; Beckman Instruments, Palo Alto, CA). For the HPLC separation, the samples were dialyzed into tris-phosphate buffer (0.1 M, pH 7.0) with 5% glycerol and 0.05 or 0.1 ml volumes were injected into a 7.5 x 300 mm TSK Gel 3000 SW column and eluted at 0.5 ml/min (9). Fractions of 0.25 ml were collected and assayed for IgA. IgA1 was measured by a liquid-phase double-antibody RIA (9) using modifications of previously described procedures (15). The assay required on day one: 0.01 ml of sample or standard, 0.2 ml of ^{125}I labeled IgA1 (25000 cpm) and 0.1 ml of the rabbit anti-IgA or anti-IgA1, (the generous gift of Dr. Dominique L. Delacroix and Dr. Jean-Pierre Vaerman; International Institute of Cellular and Molecular Pathology, Brussels, Belgium) all diluted in veronal-buffered saline with 10% PBS. On day two, 0.1 ml of normal rabbit serum (1:500) and 0.1 ml of goat anti-rabbit globulin (1:25) was added. On day three, 2 ml of veronal-buffered saline with 10% FBS was added and the tubes were harvested. Both IgA1 and total IgA were assayed simultaneously using the same reagents (except for the first antibody) as well as the same standards to minimize assay variation (9). The influence of the size of the IgA (15) was negligible in the IgA1 assay and, therefore, errors in determining the percentage of IgA1 due to technical differences could be avoided. IgA2 determinations were not performed because attempts to use monoclonal anti-IgA2 sublcass antibodies revealed major effects due to differences in the size of monomeric vs dimeric IgA molecules. Dimeric IgA2 was overestimated relative to monomeric IgA2 in assays using monoclonal antibodies by a factor of 50-150%. The solid phase RIA for total IgA and the liquid-phase double-antibody RIA for total IgA yielded similar results and employed the same IgA standards. The solid phase RIA (13) was used to analyze the Sephacryl S-300 and HPLC separated samples because of the large number of fractions for assay. The liquid phase double-antibody RIA (15) was used for the IgA1 subclass determinations because it employed much smaller amounts of anti-IgA1 antibody, which was in short supply.

IgG subclass specific antibodies were either monoclonal (IgG1, IgG3) or polyclonal (IgG2) and their production, purification and confirmation of specificity and sensitivity have been previously described (16). Concentrations of IgG4 were less than the sensitivity of the assay (100-200 ng/ml) in the intestinal MNC supernatants which is consistent with data from *in vitro* cultures of other human tissues (16). The purification and standardization of the human myeloma proteins used as standards in these assays were previously described, as was quantitation of the IgG subclasses, by a solid-phase inhibition-type radioimmunoassay (16). Briefly, 96-well flexible polyvinyl microtiter plates were coated with subclass specific antibodies, followed by a 1% solution of bovine serum albumin (10). Samples were then added at various dilutions. 10^5 cpm of proband myeloma protein (with a specific activity of approximately 10^7 cpm/ng) labeled with ^{125}I by the chloramine-T method was then added to each well. Following overnight incubation, wells were washed, separated and individually counted. The quantity of each subclass was calculated by comparing the inhibition produced by the experimental samples to standards (10,16). The sensitivity of an assay was the amount of standard protein that resulted in 50% inhibition of maximum binding. The assays had sensitivities of 50-200 ng/ml and demonstrated at least 100 fold specificity compared to control assays (16). For the 27 samples on which all three IgG subclass assays, as well as the total IgG assay were performed (10), the sum of the subclass assays yielded equivalent results to the independently-performed total IgG assay with a correlation coefficient of r=0.88, y=0.98x - 2.15.

RESULTS

Initially, we studied IgA secretion (Table 1) and found that, in comparison with control peripheral blood MNC (0.4 μg/ml), isolated control

Table 1. Spontaneous IgA Secretion

	Total IgA (μg/ml)	% Monomeric IgA	% IgA1
Control PB MNC (N)	0.4 $\overset{\times}{\div}$ 1.1 (154)	54.0 ± 7% (4)	88 ± 2% (21)
Control Int MNC (N)	25.1 $\overset{\times}{\div}$ 1.3 (53)	31.0 ± 3% (10)	61 ± 2% (22)
UC Int MNC (N)	9.0 $\overset{\times}{\div}$ 1.6 (20)	53.0 ± 8% (8)	74 ± 4% (13)
CD Int MNC (N)	7.4 $\overset{\times}{\div}$ 1.6 (35)	43.0 ± 6% (10)	71 ± 3% (19)
Rib Bone Marrow (N)	11.8 $\overset{\times}{\div}$ 1.2 (34)	81.0 ± 7% (4)	85 ± 2% (19)

intestinal lamina propria MNC exhibited very high spontaneous secretion of IgA (25.1 μg/ml). Compared to control intestinal MNC, secretion of IgA (Table 1) by ulcerative colitis intestinal MNC (9.0 μg/ml) and Crohn's disease intestinal MNC (7.4 μg/ml) was decreased (9). Human bone marrow MNC also exhibited a markedly increased spontaneous secretion of IgA (11.8 μg/ml).

The IgA spontaneously secreted by human bone marrow MNC was predominantly monomeric (81%) while control peripheral blood MNC secreted 54% of their IgA in the monomeric form (Table 1). Control intestinal MNC secreted predominantly dimeric IgA, while 31% of their IgA was monomeric IgA (Table 1). Intestinal MNC from IBD specimens (9) exhibited an increase in the proportion of IgA secreted as monomeric IgA, with 43% of IgA from Crohn's disease intestinal MNC and 53% of IgA from ulcerative colitis intestinal MNC, being monomeric (Table 1). IgA1 is the predominant form of IgA secreted by human bone marrow (85%) and control peripheral blood MNC (88%), while control intestinal MNC secrete 61% of their IgA as IgA1 (Table 1). In examination of 19 Crohn's disease specimens, the intestinal lamina propria MNC were found to secrete 71% of their IgA as IgA1, and intestinal MNC from 13 ulcerative colitis specimens were found to secrete 74% of their IgA as IgA1 (9).

Control intestinal MNC spontaneously secrete more IgG (3.0 μg/ml) than did control peripheral blood MNC (0.4 μg/ml). When compared with control intestinal MNC (10), a further increase in spontaneous secretion of IgG was observed with IBD MNC (Table 2). The most marked alteration in IgG synthesis was seen with ulcerative colitis intestinal MNC which exhibited a significant ($p < 0.01$) increase in spontaneous IgG secretion (15.7 μg/ml) in comparison with control intestinal MNC (10). Crohn's disease intestinal MNC revealed moderately increased spontaneous secretion of IgG (7.6 μg/ml).

Examination of IgG subclass secretion (Table 2), revealed that control intestinal MNC synthesized and secreted appreciable amounts of IgG1 (1.8 μg/ml) and IgG2 (1.3 μg/ml), and modest amounts of IgG3 (0.2 μg/ml). The most marked change in IgG2 subclass secretion (Table 2) was observed in ulcerative colitis intestinal MNC (10) which spontaneously secreted large amounts of IgG1 (13.4 μg/ml: 7.5 times that of control intestinal MNC, $p < 0.001$ and 3.7 times that of Crohn's disease intestinal MNC $p < 0.05$). IgG2 secretion by ulcerative colitis intestinal MNC (1.9 μg/ml) was not significantly different from control intestinal MNC, while IgG3 secretion (0.8 μg/ml) demonstrated a fourfold increase over controls ($p < 0.01$). The Crohn's disease intestinal MNC samples (10) exhibited a different pattern (Table 2), with increased IgG secretion predominantly seen in the IgG2 subclass but also involving all three subclasses measured. CD intestinal MNC IgG1 secretion (3.6 μg/ml) was increased twofold over controls; IgG2 secretion (2.9 μg/ml) was increased 2.2 times that of the control value and 1.5 times that of UC IgG2 secretion; and IgG3 secretion (0.5 μg/ml) was increased 2.5 times that of controls. Calculation of the mean of individual percentages of total IgG for each subclass revealed a marked increased in the proportion of IgG1 (77.8%) secreted by UC intestinal MNC in comparison with controls (51.4%) and CD (47.9%) intestinal MNC. Because Crohn's disease intestinal MNC demonstrated elevations in all three subclasses, the pattern of IgG subclass secretion, when expressed as percentages, was virtually identical to control intestinal MNC.

DISCUSSION

Our previous studies have demonstrated that intestinal MNC have unique capabilities and differ in their functional characteristics when compared to peripheral blood MNC (5,6,9,10,17). Intestinal MNC have an increased spontaneous secretion of immunoglobulins compared to peripheral blood MNC. We have focused our studies on spontaneous antibody secretion, in particular, because PWM nonspecifically causes suppression of activated intestinal B cells, as well as activated peripheral blood B cells from CD and UC patients

Table 2. Spontaneous IgG Secretion (μg/ml)

	IgG (total)	IgG1	IgG2	IgG3
Control PB MNC (N)	$0.4 \overset{\times}{\div} 1.1$ (155)	$0.3 \overset{\times}{\div} 1.5$ (5)	$0.2 \overset{\times}{\div} 1.4$ (5)	$0.1 \overset{\times}{\div} 1.6$ (5)
Control Int MNC (N)	$3.0 \overset{\times}{\div} 1.4$ (11)	$1.8 \overset{\times}{\div} 1.4$ (11)	$1.3 \overset{\times}{\div} 1.3$ (11)	$0.2 \overset{\times}{\div} 1.3$ (11)
UC Int MNC (N)	$15.7 \overset{\times}{\div} 1.4$ (12)	$13.4 \overset{\times}{\div} 1.4$ (12)	$1.9 \overset{\times}{\div} 1.4$ (12)	$0.8 \overset{\times}{\div} 1.4$ (12)
CD Int MNC (N)	$7.6 \overset{\times}{\div} 1.5$ (9)	$3.6 \overset{\times}{\div} 1.5$ (9)	$2.9 \overset{\times}{\div} 1.6$ (9)	$0.5 \overset{\times}{\div} 1.8$ (9)
Rib Bone Marrow MNC (N)	$6.2 \overset{\times}{\div} 1.5$ (7)	$3.9 \overset{\times}{\div} 1.5$ (7)	$1.5 \overset{\times}{\div} 1.6$ (7)	$0.5 \overset{\times}{\div} 1.4$ (7)

(5,6,9). Spontaneous antibody secretion *in vitro* may more closely reflect *in vivo* events than does overt, nonspecific PWM-induced suppression.

The increased spontaneous IgA secretion by control intestinal MNC is consistent with the intestinal lamina propria being a major source of IgA plasma cells which secrete dimeric IgA with J chain. Our results (9) also support the findings of Kutteh and coworkers (18,19), who demonstrated that human intestinal MNC secrete primarily dimeric IgA, that human bone marrow MNC secrete predominantly monomeric IgA, and that human peripheral blood MNC secrete large amounts of IgA1. IgA has two subclasses: IgA1 and IgA2. IgA1 is the major subclass in the serum (79% to 82%), while IgA2 is significantly increased in secretions (26% to 41% IgA2 in secretions compared to 18% to 21% in serum) (20). The data in the present study are, therefore, consistent with these observations in that peripheral blood MNC secreted 88% of its IgA as IgA1, while isolated intestinal MNC secreted 61% of its IgA as IgA1.

Previous studies by Brandtzaeg et al. (2) and by Baklien and Brandtzaeg (3,4) demonstrated a fourfold increase in the total number of intestinal lymphocytes in IBD. IgG-containing cells were increased 30 fold, IgA-containing cells twofold and IgM containing cells fivefold greater than normal (2-4). That IBD MNC should exhibit increased IgG and IgG subclass secretion *in vitro* (10) is not surprising in the light of these previous observations of increased number and altered ratios of intestinal lymphocytes and plasma cells in IBD. The increased secretion of IgG and IgG subclasses from IBD intestinal MNC (10), therefore, is most likely related to the increased percentage of IgG containing cells present in vivo in inflamed mucosa. The fourfold increase in total intestinal lymphocytes in IBD with only a twofold increase in IgA-containing cells could produce a dilutional effect leading to the apparent decrease in total IgA secretion that we have observed. However, Danis and coworkers (21) investigated intestinal mucosal immunoglobulin secretion by culturing colonoscopic biopsies and observed significant reductions in IgA secretion from both ulcerative colitis and Crohn's disease patients. These results, therefore, are consistent with our findings (5,6,9) in that we have also found decreased secretion of IgA from both CD and UC intestinal MNC, in comparison to control intestinal MNC.

The clinical importance of IgG subclasses and their regulation is demonstrated by reports of selectively altered subclass levels in immunodeficiencies and autoimmune diseases (22-25). Different antigens and mitogens induce antibody responses restricted to particular IgG subclasses in both murine and human studies (26-28). Recent studies by Scott and Nahm (16) have shown human IgG1 and IgG3 to be preferentially and coordinately stimulated in in vitro responses to mitogens, which may in part, account for the elevation of IgG3 secretion in conjunction with the increase in IgG1 secretion by UC intestinal MNC. Taken together, these studies strongly suggest that IgG subclasses are not randomly expressed. Subclass expression is complex and may depend on the nature of the antigenic signal, as well as on regulatory factors and possibly B cell subpopulations. Because IgG1 serum levels are elevated in several autoimmune diseases, it could be speculated that UC IgG1 antibodies participate in an autoimmune process by complement fixation and chemotaxis of accessory cells to the pathologic site. Delineation of the stimuli and antigens which induce the increased secretion of IgG subclasses in IBD may provide insight into possible etiologic and immunopathogenic aspects.

Our previous studies (5,6,9-14,17) and the present work have demonstrated that: (a) major alterations occur with regard to spontaneous antibody secretion in IBD; (b) PWM-induced suppressor cell generation is a nonspecific phenomenon; (c) the peripheral blood compartment often reflects secondary phenomena in IBD; (d) intestinal MNC comprise a unique immunologic compartment with separate immunobiologic capabilities; and (e) it is within the intestine involved with disease that major alterations in antibody secretion are occurring, particularly with regard to the IgA and IgG subclasses.

Therefore, alterations in spontaneous secretion of immunoglobulins in general and of IgA and IgG and their subclasses in particular, by isolated IBD intestinal MNC deserve increased attention.

On the basis of our results to date (9,10), we postulate the following sequence of events. In both ulcerative colitis and Crohn's disease, decreased IgA secretion may lead to a mucosal defense deficiency due to an inadequate dimeric IgA and IgA2 response. As part of a compensatory protective mechanism to make up for the loss of normal "gatekeeper" mucosal IgA function, increased monomeric IgA and IgA1 secretion may occur due to homing of B cells from the peripheral blood and/or the situation of local mucosal B cells. In ulcerative colitis an IgG1-mediated immune response and in Crohn's disease an IgG2-mediated immune response may result in either a normal immune protective response to specific agents or destructive immune effector events directed against intestinal cells. Because different antigens preferentially induce different subclasses, further examination of IgA and IgG subclasses in CD and UC may provide a clue concerning the nature of infectious agents or inducing signals involved.

CONCLUSIONS

Intestinal mononuclear cells from inflammatory bowel disease patients were found to demonstrate alterations in their patterns of spontaneous secretion. Control intestinal MNC had markedly heightened spontaneous secretion of IgA, while secretion of IgA by IBD intestinal MNC was decreased in comparison. Control intestinal MNC secreted predominantly dimeric IgA (only 31% monomeric IgA), while IBD intestinal MNC secreted increased amounts (43% to 53%) of monomeric IgA. Control intestinal MNC secreted 61% IgA subclass 1 (IgA1), while IBD intestinal MNC secreted increased amounts (71% to 74%) of IgA1. Therefore, intestinal MNC from involved IBD intestinal specimens spontaneously secrete increased percentages of monomeric IgA and IgA1 in comparison to control intestinal MNC. Intestinal MNC from IBD specimens spontaneously secreted more total IgG than did control intestinal MNC. This increased spontaneous IgG secretion by UC intestinal MNC was primarily due to markedly increased production of IgG1. Slightly increased secretion of IgG3, but not IgG2, by UC intestinal MNC was present when compared with control and CD intestinal MNC. In contrast, CD intestinal MNC exhibited modestly increased spontaneous secretion of IgG2 with slight increases in the other IgG subclasses. These observations may represent the normal mucosal IgA and IgG immune response to infectious agents or inducing factors of either a primary or secondary nature.

ACKNOWLEDGEMENTS

This work was supported in part by U.S.P.H.S. grants AM 21474, AI 15322 and AI 19676 and by a grant from the National Foundation for Ileitis and Colitis.

REFERENCES

1. Kirsner, J.B. and Shorter, R.G., N. Engl. J. Med. 306, 775, 1982.
2. Brandtzaeg, P., Baklien, K., Fausa, O. and Hoel, P.S., Gastroenterology 66, 1123, 1974.
3. Baklien, K. and Brandtzaeg, P., Clin. Exp. Immunol. 22, 197, 1975.
4. Baklien, K. and Brandtzaeg, P., Scand. J. Gastroent. 11, 447, 1976.
5. MacDermott, R.P., Nash, G.S., Bertovich, M.J., Seiden, M.V., Bragdon, M.J. and Beale, M.G., Gastroenterology 81, 844, 1981.
6. MacDermott, R.P., Beale, M.G., Alley, C.D., Nash, G.S., Bertovich, M.J. and Bragdon, M.J., Ann. N.Y. Acad. Sci. 409, 498, 1983.
7. Bookman, M.A. and Bull, D.M., Gastroenterology 77, 503, 1979.
8. Bull, D.M. and Bookman, M.A., J. Clin. Invest. 59, 966, 1977.
9. MacDermott, R.P., Nash, G.S., Bertovich, M.J., Mohrman, R.F., Kidner, I.J., Delacroix, D.L. and Vaerman, J.-P., Gastroenterology 91, 379, 1986.
10. Scott, M.G., Nahm, M.H., Macke, K., Nash, G.S., Bertovich, M.J. and MacDermott, R.P., Clin. Exp. Immunol. 66, 209, 1986.
11. Alley, C.D. and MacDermott, R.P., Blood 55, 669, 1980.
12. Alley, C.D., Nash, G.S. and MacDermott, R.P., J. Immunol. 128, 2804, 1982.
13. Nash, G.S., Seiden, M.V., Beale, M.G. and MacDermott, R.P., J. Immunol. Meth. 49, 261, 1982.
14. Beale, M.G., Nash, G.S., Bertovich, M.J. and MacDermott, R.P., J. Immunol. 128, 486, 1982.
15. Delacroix, D.L., Elkon, K.B., Geubel, A.P., Hodgson, H.F., Dive, C. and Vaerman, J.-P., J. Clin. Invest. 71, 358, 1983.

16. Scott, M.G. and Nahm, M.H., J. Immunol. 133, 2454, 1984.
17. MacDermott, R.P., in Recent Advances in Crohn's Disease, (Edited by Pena, A.S., Weterman, I.T., Booth, C.C. and Strober, W.), p. 439, Martinus Nijhoff Publishers, The Hague, 1981.
18. Kutteh, W.H., Prince, S.J. and Mestecky, J., J. Immunol. 128, 990, 1982.
19. Kutteh, W.H., Koopman, W.J., Conley, M.E., Egan, M.L. and Mestecky, J., J. Exp. Med. 152, 1424, 1980.
20. Delacroix, D.L., Dive, C., Rambaud, J.C. and Vaerman, J.-P., Immunology 47, 383, 1982.
21. Danis, V.A., Harries, A.D., and Heatley, R.V., Clin. Exp. Immunol. 56, 159, 1984.
22. Oxelius, V.A., Laurell, A.B., Lindquist, B., Golebiowaska, H., Axelsson, U., Bjorkander, J. and Hanson, L.Å., N. Engl. J. Med. 304, 1476, 1981.
23. Oxelius, V.A., Am. J. Med. 76, 7, 1984.
24. Waldmann, T.A., Broder, S., Goldman, C.K., Frost, K., Korsmeyer, S.J. and Medici, M.A., J. Clin. Invest. 71, 282, 1983.
25. Yount, W.J., N. Engl. J. Med. 306, 541, 1982.
26. Shakib, F. and Stanworth, D.R., La Ricerca Clin. Lab. 10, 561, 1980.
27. Slack, J., Der-Balian, G.P., Nahm, M.H. and Davie, J.M., J. Exp. Med. 151, 853, 1980.
28. Yount, W.J., Dorner, M.M., Kunkel, H.G. and Kabat, E.A., J. Exp. Med. 127, 633, 1968.

IMMUNOHISTOCHEMICAL ANALYSIS OF HUMAN INFLAMMATORY APPENDIX

G. Faure, G. Halbgewachs and M.C. Bene

Laboratoire d'Immunologie
UFR Sciences Medicales
Universite de Nancy I, BP 184
54500 Vandoeuvre les Nancy, France

INTRODUCTION

The digestive mucosal system of laboratory animals has been well studied, particularly in mice and rats where Peyer's patches are found in clusters clearly visible along the ileum. Most of our knowledge on digestive mucosal immunity has thus been derived from functional immunological studies or from immunohistochemistry in these species (1-3). To apply this information to human physiology is tempting, but remains disputable. Peyer's patches are macroscopically undetectable in human ileum and this area of the gut can only be obtained post-mortem or during hemicolectomy for a tumor of the right colon, usually in elderly patients (4-6). Although most of its physiological roles remain unknown, the appendix might be an organ useful in assessing the structure and function of the gut-associated lymphoid tissue in young humans. We report here an immunohistological study of the vermiform appendix from 20 patients, obtained at surgery for appendicitis.

METHODS

Fresh human appendices were obtained from 20 young male and female patients (age range 10 to 25 years old) undergoing surgery for acute appendicitis. The tissues were immediately snap frozen in liquid nitrogen and kept at -85°C in an ultra-low temperature freezer (Sanyo, Japan) until study. Serial 4 micrometer thick cryostat sections of samples conveniently and transversely oriented were obtained with a thermostated microtome at -30°C (Slee, London). The sections were air-dried, placed in humid chambers at room temperature and processed without further fixation. An orientative morphological study was carried out using toluidine blue rapid staining on the first slide. A comprehensive panel of polyclonal and monoclonal antibodies was used to stain the following sections. Briefly, direct immunofluorescence techniques were used with FITC polyclonal antibodies directed against Ig heavy (IgG, IgA, IgM, IgD) and light (κ,λ) chains, C3c, Fibrinogen (Behring, Marburg, FDA), human Fibronectin (Cappell, Cochranville, PA, USA). An indirect immunofluorescence technique was chosen with mouse monoclonal antibodies (Orthoclone, Raritan, NJ; Coulterclone, Hialeah, FL; Becton-Dickinson, Mountain View, CA, USA) directed against molecules specific for T and B cell surface antigens defining clusters CD1, 2, 3, 4, 8, 9, 11, 14, 19, 20 and 21, class II antigens (DR, DQ), NK cells, and CEA antigen (Hybritech, Liège, Belgique). FITC antimouse Ig serum (Institut Pasteur Production, Paris, France) was used as second layer. Incubation time was 30 min, and they were performed in humid chambers at room temperature. Staining periods were followed by 3 washings in PBS after which sections were covered with a PBS/glycerol mixture (7/3) intended to prevent dehydration and stored in human chambers at 4°C.

Stained sections were examined under UV light within 24 hours of processing, using a Leitz Orthoplan microscope equipped with a Ploem system of epi-illumination and phase contrast.

RESULTS

Different areas are usually described from morphological observation, in animal appendiceal mucosa (Fig. 1A):

- germinal centers,
- a surrounding mantle zone made of small lymphocytes,
- a zone beneath the epithelial dome, more heterogeneous, thought to be a predominantly B cell area,
- lateral and interfollicular zones, thought to be T cell areas,
- the lamina propria, in periluminar villi and among the glandular structures.

From a morphological point of view, the human appendiceal mucosa is less well individualized than Peyer's patches or appendix structures in rabbit or rat (Fig. 1B). In one case, an intraluminal parasite was visible.

Follicle centers were made of larger B cells similar to lymph nodes or tonsillar centrocytes: these cells bear the antigens defined by monoclonal antibodies of clusters CD 19 (+), 20 (+), 21 (B2 ++, BL13 +++). They expressed brightly class II antigens. They were stained in decreasing frequency with anti-IgM (76%), -IgA (42%), or -IgG (36%). Occasionally (in 2 cases), scattered Leu-7^+ cells and CD 2^+ cells were observed in the same region.

Mantle zone smaller cells were $sIgM^+$ - $sIgD^+$ B lymphocytes bearing antigens defined by monoclonal antibodies from clusters CD 19 and CD 20. They were also class II positive.

In the lateral and interfollicular zones, the lymphoid tissue mainly consisted of T cells (CD3+++), predominantly CD4 positive, with less numerous (1/10) CD8 positive cells. In 60% of cases, they brightly expressed class II antigens. Numerous eosinophils were clearly visible in most cases (60% of samples, up to 50 cells/field at X400 magnification). High endothelial venules were distinguishable in this area with anti-fibronectin antiserum.

The subepithelial dome area contained B cells ($CD19^+$), some IgA plasma cells, and numerous class II^+ interdigitating cells.

In the lamina propria, numerous plasma cells could be observed, containing usually IgA and less frequently IgM and IgG, with a 15/1 ratio. They were associated with T cells of a phenotype similar to that observed in another segment of the gut. Eosinophils were also seen in significant numbers in some patients.

We did not detect intraepithelial T cells with any of the previously described anti-T cell antibodies either in the dome epithelium or in the villi. All epithelial cells positively stained with CD 9 and anti-CEA monoclonal antibodies, and did not express class II molecules. The glandular epithelium usually contained IgA, while epithelium of the villi or the dome were negative.

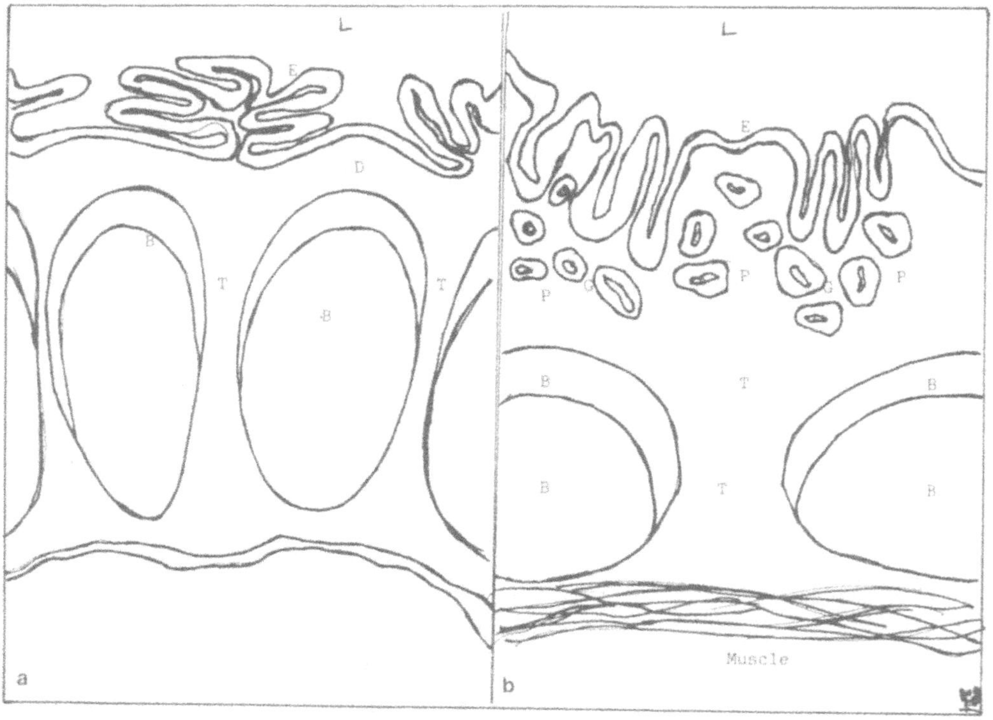

1a: RABBIT 1b: HUMAN

Figure 1. (a) Schematic representation of rabbit appendix. (b) Comparative schematic representation of human appendix. G, glands; B, B cell areas; T, T cell areas; P, plasma cell areas; E, epithelium; D, dome area; L, lumen.

CONCLUSIONS

This work describes the microarchitecture of inflammatory appendix using various antibodies directed against intracellular and cell-membrane molecules as well as some extracellular tissue material. Although most information obtained is quite similar, slight differences are noted, when compared with the very recently published results of studies on this "normal" organ (4-6,8,9). They might be explained by local inflammation phenomena.

These data are also essentially similar to those reported previously with animal tissues, in spite of the quite obvious morphological differences. Similarities can also be found with the immunohistological organization of Peyer's patches (5,10).

These data allow us to draw a clearer picture of the appendiceal organization in humans, with different functional areas more intricate than in rodent tissue. The appendix is clearly a mixture of a mucosal lymphoid tissue and secondary lymphoid organ, i.e., lymph nodes. The predominant presence of IgA-producing cells in lamina propria gut-like areas resembles the organization of jejunal areas. Few IgG plasma cells were observed in our study, and this has also been reported by others (6). The possible role of the appendix as a B cell reservoir or maturation organ is supported by the presence of all types of B cells and plasma cells. The origin and migration routes of these B cells remain, however, to be determined (11-15).

The occurrence of immune reactions is suggested by the abundance of antigenic debris, or even parasites in the lumen. This is also suggested because of the presence of class II-positive T cells in the vicinity of large secondary germinal centers. Macrophages seem to be less evidently localized in human appendix, while they appear prominent in rabbit tissue. The heterogeneity of their phenotypes could preclude the variety of their functions (4,5). The use of anti-class II reagents, however, allowed the observation of interdigitating cells in the lamina propria in significant numbers, although smaller than in jejunal samples (16). Another striking difference in class II expression in appendix compared to jejunal tissue, is the lack of both DR and DQ molecules on epithelial cells from glandular, villous, or dome regions (9,16-18). Finally, intra-epithelial lymphocytes were not observed in any of our 20 samples when determined by ultrastructural or immunological staining (3,8,10,18,19) and the precise lineage of these cells in normal appendicular tissue needs more documentation.

The human appendix thus appears as a relatively large lymphoid organ with every potential to develop immune responses, depending on age as other immunologically active tissues (20,21). Its physiological microarchitecture requires comparison in pathological conditions. This study did not show striking inflammatory phenomena, apart from the presence of eosinophils in rather large numbers as well as epithelial differences, although pathological changes were likely to be present in such a clinical acute situation (22,23). The rationale of appendicectomy cannot be discussed from the findings reported here. Our observations would rather sustain the comparison with tonsillectomy, where large amounts of immunocompetent tissue is removed.

ACKNOWLEDGEMENTS

This study was supported, in part, by CRE Inserm 84 3002 and by the Comité Lorraine de la Fondation pour la Recherche Médicale.

REFERENCES

1. Faulk, W.P., McCormick, J.N., Goodman, J.R., Yoffey, J.M. and Fudenberg, H.H., Cell. Immunol. 1, 500, 1971.
2. Sminia, T. and Plesch, B.E.C., Virchows Arch. (Cell. Pathol.) 40, 181, 1982.
3. Bockman, D.E., Arch. Histol. Jap. 46, 271, 1983.
4. Spencer, J., Finn, T. and Isaacson, P.G., Gut 26, 672, 1985.
5. Spencer, J., Finn, T. and Isaacson, P.G., Gut 27, 405, 1986.
6. Bjerke, K., Brandtzaeg, P. and Rognum, T.O., Gut 27, 667, 1986.
7. Anderson, K.C., Bates, M.P., Slaughenhoupt, B.L., Pinkus, G.L., Schlossman, S.F. and Nadler, L.M., Blood 63, 1424, 1984.
8. Selby, W.S., Janossy, G. and Jewell, D.P., Gut 22, 169, 1981.
9. Scott, H., Solheim, B.G., Brandtzaeg, P. and Thorsby, E., Scand. J. Immunol. 12, 77, 1980.
10. Bjerke, K. and Brandtzaeg, P., Scand. J. Immunol. 18, 71, 1983.
11. Sminia, T., Hendriks, H.R., Janse, M. and Van De Ende, M., Virchows Arch. (Cell. Pathol.) 47, 123, 1984.
12. Van der Jeijden, D., Nieweg, O., Rijkmans, B., Stikker, R., Opstelten, D. and Nieuwenhuis, P., Virchows Arch. (Cell. Pathol.) 34, 43, 1980.
13. Toma, V.A. and Retief, R.P., J. Immunol. Methods 20, 333, 1978.
14. Butcher, E.C., Rouse, R.V., Coffman, R.L., Nottenburg, C.N., Hardy, R.R. and Weissman, I.L., J. Immunol. 129, 2698, 1982.
15. Phillips-Quagliata, J.M., Roux, M.E., Arny, M., Kelly-Hatfield, P., McWilliams, M. and Lamm, M.E., Ann. N.Y. Acad. Sci. 409, 194, 1983.
16. Selby, W.S., Poulter, L.W., Hobbs, S., Jewell, D.P. and Janossy, G., J. Clin. Pathol. 36, 379, 1983.
17. Spencer, J., Finn, T. and Isaacson, P.G., Gut 27, 153, 1986.
18. Bene, M.C., Moneret-Vautrin, D.A. and Faure, G.C., 6th Int. Congress of Immunology, Toronto, 1.41.33 1986.
19. Cerf-Bensussan, N., Schneeberger, E.E. and Bhan, A.K., J. Immunol. 130, 2615, 1983.

20. Stein, H., Bonk, A., Tolksdorf, G., Lennert, K., Rodt, H. and Gerdes, J., J. Histochem. Cytochem. 28, 746, 1980.
21. Berry, J.A. and Lack, L.A.H., J. Anat. Physiol. 40. 247, 1905.
22. Butler, C., Human Pathol. 12, 870, 1981.
23. O'Brien, A. and O'Briain, D.S., Arch. Pathol. Lab. Med. 109, 680, 1985.

CHARACTERIZATION AND MITOGENIC RESPONSIVENESS OF MURINE MAMMARY GLAND MONONUCLEAR CELLS

E.T. Lally, R.C. Fiorini, C.A. Skandera*, I.M. Zitron* and P.C. Montgomery*

Department of Pathology, School of Dental Medicine, Center for Oral Health Research, University of Pennsylvania Philadelphia, PA USA; and *Department of Immunology and Microbiology, Wayne State University School of Medicine Detroit, MI USA

INTRODUCTION

Lymphocyte traffic from subcompartments of intestinal mucosal associated lymphoid tissue (MALT) to mammary (1), salivary (2) and lacrimal (3) glands is a characteristic feature of the mucosal network. With respect to glandular structures it is not clear whether these compartments function simply by providing an environment into which precommitted B cells migrate and terminally differentiate or whether they also contain the functional cell populations necessary to interact in the generation of local antibody responses. Numerous studies have demonstrated the presence of viable lymphocyte populations in the colostrum, milk and mammary secretions for a variety of animal species (4-17). These cell populations have been isolated and studied with respect to cell surface markers (10,15-17) and responsiveness to mitogens (4,6-9,11-14). However, it is not known whether the cells which were characterized in these studies are expressed only in secretions or represent the total mononuclear cell component of the gland. Since little is known about isolated glandular cell populations and because the mouse is a well-defined model for studying B cell ontogeny, T and B cell interactions and cell traffic, the present report examines the morphological characteristics, membrane marker distribution and mitogen responsiveness of mouse mammary gland cell populations.

MATERIALS AND METHODS

Animals

C57BL/6 mice of both sexes (Jackson Laboratory), 6-8 weeks of age, were bred in house. Nursing mothers, 4 to 8 days postpartum, were utilized as tissue donors.

Cell preparation

Peripheral blood cells were collected by bleeding from the retroorbital plexus into heparinized blood collection tubes. Spleen and thymus were removed, placed in cold Hanks' balanced salt solution (HBSS), minced and passed through 6 layers of surgical gauze to remove large fragments and capsular material. Before removing mammary gland tissue from the abdominal wall and thoracic areas, axillary and inguinal lymph nodes were excised to avoid contamination with non-mucosal lymphoid cells. The glandular tissue was placed in cold HBSS + 5% fetal calf serum (FCS), minced with scissors and fine forceps and pressed through a 40 mesh screen. The cells were washed twice in HBSS and large particles were allowed to settle out. All cell preparations were suspended at a concentration of 2×10^7 nucleated cells/ml, layered onto Lympholyte M (Accurate Chemical) and centrifuged at 500 x g for 20 min at room temperature. The cell layer at the interface was removed, washed twice in HBSS and once with RPMI 1640. For morphologic examination cell suspensions were subjected to cytocentrifugation and stained with Giemsa stain. Viability was determined by trypan blue exclusion. Cell preparations were routinely >95% viable with yields ranging from 10^5-10^6 cells per mouse.

In order to ensure that the Lympholyte M separation did not select for lymphocyte subpopulations, spleen cell suspensions were examined for surface marker distribution (as outlined below) before and after the Lympholyte M procedure. Since no significant differences were noted and this step was obligatory for mammary gland cells, all cell populations were prepared in this manner.

Thy-1, Lyt-1 and Lyt-2 bearing cells

Initially, mononuclear cells bearing Thy-1 isoantigen were enumerated by immunofluorescence and complement-mediated cytolysis, employing rabbit anti-mouse brain (RAMB) antiserum. RAMB was prepared by a modification (18) of the method of Golub (19). A 1:400 dilution of RAMB antiserum used in the immunofluorescence system stained 97% of thymus cells, 36% of spleen cells, 62% of mesenteric lymph node cells and 7% of bone marrow cells. When antibody-mediated complement-dependent killing was employed as a method for determining the Thy-1 marker, similar values were obtained (18). In subsequent studies, Thy-1, Lyt-1 and Lyt-2 bearing cells were enumerated by complement-mediated cytolysis employing commercial monoclonal reagents (Accurate Chemical). Final concentrations of anti-Thy-1.2 (culture supernatant; 1:20), anti-Lyt-1.2 (ascites 1:10) and anti-Lyt-2.2 (culture supernatant, 1:20) were determined by titration with C57BL/6 thymocytes.

Immunoglobulin bearing cells

Immunofluorescence and complement-mediated cytolysis were employed to enumerate mononuclear cells which displayed mIg. $F(ab')_2$ preparations of rabbit anti-mouse light chain reagents were used in all immunofluorescence studies to preclude Fc receptor binding (20).

Complement receptor bearing cells

Cells with complement receptors (C3) were enumerated employing the EAC-rosette technique using sheep erythrocytes sensitized with an IgM fraction of rabbit anti-Forssman antibody as described by Bianco et al. (21).

Fc receptor bearing cells

Cells bearing Fc receptors were detected utilizing the EA-rosette technique outlined by Parish and Hayward (22). The sheep erythrocytes were sensitized with IgG antibodies.

Macrophages

Macrophages were identified morphologically and by using nonspecific esterase staining detailed by Koski et al. (23).

Blastogenesis

Cell suspensions were made up in RPMI 1640 (containing 2 mM L-glutamine, 100 units penicillin - 100 μg streptomycin/ml, 10 μg/ml gentamicin, 0.01 M HEPES buffer, 0.23% sodium bicarbonate, 5% FCS and 5×10^{-5} M 2ME). Aliquots of 0.10 ml (containing 4×10^5 cells) were dispensed into 96 well, flat-bottom tissue cultures plates and 0.05 ml of various mitogens were added with final volume made up to 0.25 ml with RPMI. Initially, experiments were carried out using spleen cells over a range of cell and mitogen concentrations. For spleen cell concentrations of 4×10^5 cells/well, the optimal mitogen concentrations/ml of culture were 1.0 μg for Con A, 4.0 μg for PWM and 25 μg for LPS (*E. coli* 0111:B4). After incubating the cultures for 48 h at 37°C (5% CO_2), 0.63 μCi ^{3}H-thymidine was added to each well. Sixteen hours later the cells were harvested using an Otto Hiller Cell Harvester and the glass filter discs counted in 4.0 ml Aqueous Counting Scintillant (Amersham) using an LKB 1218 Rack Beta Scintillation Counter.

RESULTS

Mammary gland cell types

The results of the morphological examination of mammary gland cell preparations are presented in Table 1. The data are expressed as the percentage of each cell type in the total cell population. Although variability in the distribution of individual cell types was observed, cells exhibiting classical lymphocyte morphology predominated (78.2%). With respect to macrophages (15.3%), two different cell types were noted in these preparations. Cells containing a small, dense, centrally-located nucleus and a large vacuolated cytoplasm as well as cells exhibiting a more characteristic macrophage morphology were observed. Both cell types were positive when examined using the non-specific esterase stain (see Table 2). In addition, cell preparations contained epithelial cells (7.1%), polymorphonuclear leukocytes (2.8%) and in some cases fat-containing cells (<1%).

Percentage distribution of mononuclear cells in spleen, thymus, peripheral blood and mammary gland

Table 2 presents a detailed analysis of the percentage distribution of mononuclear cells in mammary gland, with values obtained for spleen,

Table 1. Mammary gland cell types after buoyant density centrifugation

Cell type[a]	Percent total population[b]
Lymphocytes	78.2 ± 13.3[c]
Macrophages	15.3 ± 4.7
Epithelial cells	7.1 ± 3.8
Polymorphonuclear leukocytes	2.8 ± 1.5

[a]Based on morphology.
[b]% of cells from 5 different mice; at least 250 cells/mouse were counted.
[c]Mean ± standard deviation.

Table 2. Percentage distribution of mononuclear cells in spleen, thymus, peripheral blood and mammary gland

	Spleen	Thymus	Peripheral Blood[a]	Mammary Gland
Thy-1 (cytolysis)	33.5 ± 6.0[b]	97.3 ± 2.2	66.4 ± 5.5	32.2 ± 6.8
Thy-1 (fluorescence)	36.3 ± 1.2	96.5 ± 2.2	N.D.	38.6 ± 4.0
Membrane Ig(cytolysis)	50.4 ± 5.7	5.9 ± 2.9	17.3 ± 4.7	38.3 ± 6.0
Membrane Ig(fluorescence)	42.9 ± 7.9	< 1	19.5 ± 5.0	27.8 ± 7.4
Fc Receptor	33.1 ± 6.7	2.1 ± 1.1	20.2 ± 4.2	43.1 ± 7.0
C3 Receptor	44.2 ± 3.0	< 1	18.8 ± 3.0	30.3 ± 4.5
Macrophages (esterase)	8.2 ± 5.1	N.D.	N.D.	12.0 ± 3.5

[a]Heparinized blood.
[b]Mean ± standard deviation, based on 5 or more determinations.

thymus and peripheral blood given for comparison. Complement-dependent lysis and fluorescence for the most part gave comparable results and the data indicated that the distribution of lymphocytes and macrophages in mammary gland cell isolates was similar to spleen cells. However, the percentages of cells bearing mIg and C3 receptors were higher in spleen than mammary gland.

T cell subset distribution in mammary gland and spleen

Monoclonal reagents were employed to assess the percentage of T cell subsets in spleen and mammary gland cell populations. These data are shown in Table 3. The percentage of Thy-1.2 bearing lymphocytes in this analysis was identical to the data obtained with the polyclonal reagent (see Table 2). In the splenic population, most of the Thy-1^+ cells exhibited either an Lyt-1^+,2^- or Lyt-1^-,2^+ phenotype. In contrast, in the mammary gland population, the sum of the Lyt-1^+ and Lyt-2^+ cells was greater than the percentage of Thy-1^+ cells, indicating a very different composition from spleen.

Mitogen responses of splenic and mammary gland lymphocytes

A comparative functional assessment of the splenic and mammary gland lymphocyte populations was carried out by assessing the blastogenic responses to Con A, PWM and LPS. Data obtained from two separate experiments

Table 3. Percentages of T cell subsets in spleen and mammary gland

	Spleen	Mammary gland
Thy-1.2	33.3 ± 8.3[a,b]	38.9 ± 1.2
Lyt-1.2	18.5 ± 3.6	34.2 ± 6.7
Lyt-2.2	16.4 ± 5.8	28.1 ± 6.4

[a]Mean ± standard deviation determined by antibody-mediated complement-dependent cytolysis, based on 5 or more determinations.

[b]Thy-1.2, spleen vs. mammary gland, not significant; Lyt-1.2, spleen vs. mammary gland, $0.02 < p < 0.025$; Lyt-2.2, spleen vs. mammary gland, $0.05 < p < 0.10$; p-values determined using two-tailed students t-test.

Table 4. Mitogenic responses of isolated spleen and mammary gland cells

	Control (no mitogen)	Con A (1.0 μg)	PWM (4.0 μg)	LPS (25.0 μg)
Experiment 1				
Spleen	1207 ± 209[b]	162887 ± 10752	41661 ± 4900	85433 ± 6832
		135[c]	35	71
Mammary gland	623 ± 103	74689 ± 7617	32729 ± 1991	57454 ± 1039
		120	53	92
Experiment 2				
Spleen	1785 ± 178	180723 ± 11587	34754 ± 3166	72919 ± 6480
		101	19	41
Mammary gland	2144 ± 1163	135067 ± 7824	32677 ± 1551	46450 ± 10447
		63	15	22

[a]Mitogen concentrations are expressed/ml of culture. Total culture volume was 0.25 ml.

[b]Mean ± standard deviation cpm determined on a minimum of 4 cultures containing 4×10^5 lymphocytes.

[c]Stimulation indices expressed as the ratio of mean cpm of experimental cultures to mean cpm of control cultures.

are presented in Table 4. The thymidine incorporation data showed that mammary gland populations were able to respond to the three test mitogens. The incorporation data indicated that the mammary gland lymphocyte mitogen responsiveness was generally comparable to spleen cells for Con A, PWM and LPS. A comparison of the stimulation indices further confirms this observation.

DISCUSSION

In general, it appears that colostrum contains approximately 10% lymphocytes (4-7,16) with the majority of other cell types being macrophages and polymorphonuclear leukocytes (16). Epithelial cells were rarely encountered (16). While it is difficult to make direct comparisons between cells appearing in mammary secretions and those isolated from glandular tissue, it is surprising that the majority of cell types obtained from 4-8 day postpartum mammary gland tissue were lymphocytes (78.2%). Macrophages with vacuolated cytoplasm observed in our glandular isolates were also noted previously in human colostral cell populations (4-7,16). While our overall percentages of macrophages are lower than previously noted for cell populations obtained from human colostrum (16), it is relevant to note that in a recent study, using both mechanical and enzymatic procedures (with no subsequent gradient enrichment), 3-10% of mouse salivary gland cell isolates were macrophages (24). Further investigation is necessary to determine if the differences in the distribution of cell types we observed can be attributed to species variation or the selectivity of the isolation procedures.

The data on cell surface distribution from mammary gland cells show distinct differences when compared with surface marker data of either thymus or peripheral blood cell populations. While some studies have suggested similarities (12), most have indicated that differences (8,11,15) exist between the percentage of T cells isolated from mammary gland secretions and peripheral blood. Our data obtained with either the polyclonal (Thy-1) or monoclonal (Thy-1.2) T cell reagents show that the percentages of total T cells in mammmary gland is similar to spleen. Variation exists between the T cell subsets present in mammary gland and spleen, the mammary gland apparently possessing a greater percentage of Lyt-1^+,2^+ cells than spleen. Finding Lyt-1^+ cells in mouse mammary gland cells is consistent with previous studies in rats showing the presence of W3/25^+ (helper/inducer) cells in both mammary (25) and lacrimal (26) gland populations. While our observation showing greater percentges of Lyt-1^+,2^+ cells in mammary gland cells may suggest a population of T cells less mature than, or functionally distinct from, those found in spleen, two-color fluorescent analysis is necessary to confirm co-expression. However, it is important to note in lacrimal gland isolates (26) that cells bearing OX-7 (Thy-1) predominated over those bearing W3/13 (pan-T cell marker). In rats (unlike mice) Thy-1 is not present on the majority of peripheral T cells and is considered to be a marker of immature T cells (27,28). The percentage of cells bearing immunoglobulin (B cells) in mammary gland was greater than that seen in peripheral blood or thymus, but lower than noted for spleen. The finding that fewer mammary gland cells possessed the C3 receptor (predominantly a B cell marker) is consistent with this observation.

The mitogen responses of lymphocytes obtained from mammary glands indicate that both functional T and B cells are present in the glandular tissue. The significance of the slightly diminished response of the mammary gland cells to Con A is open to speculation though it may simply reflect a variation in the cellular differentiation stage. Our data stand in sharp contrast to previous observations in which milk or colostral cells were shown to be hyporesponsive when compared to peripheral blood lymphocytes in humans (6-8,11,14), dog (9) or cow (9,12,13). While no such comparative response data is available for the mouse, it is clear that in our experimental system mammary gland lymphocyte populations contain mitogen responsive T and B cell populations.

While additional studies will be required to examine fully the capacity of glandular cell populations to respond to antigenic stimulation, it appears that the mouse mammary gland not only functions by providing a differentiative environment for precommitted B cells, but also contains a cellular apparatus with the potential to generate local antibody responses.

CONCLUSIONS

1. Cell populations prepared from murine mammary gland tissue by mechanical disruption and buoyant density centrifugation contained 78.2% lymphocytes, 15.3% macrophages, 7.1% epithelial cells and 2.8% polymorphonuclear leukocytes.

2. The distribution of mononuclear cells in mammary gland resembled spleen rather than thymus or peripheral blood populations with respect to Thy-1, membrane immunoglobulin, Fc and C3 receptor bearing cells and macrophage content.

3. With respect to T cell subsets, mammary gland appears to possess a greater percentage of Lyt-1^{+},2^{+} cells than spleen.

4. The Con A, PWM and LPS responses of mammary gland lymphocytes were comparable to those obtained with splenic lymphocyte populations.

ACKNOWLEDGEMENTS

This study was supported by U.S.P.H.S. grants EY 05133 and DE 02623. We thank Ms. A. Sabady for typing the manuscript.

REFERENCES

1. Roux, M.E., McWilliams, M., Phillips-Quagliata, J.M., Weiz-Carrington, P. and Lamm, M.E., J. Exp. Med. 146, 1311, 1977.
2. Jackson, D.E., Lally, E.T., Nakamura, M.C. and Montgomery, P.C., Cell. Immunol. 63, 203, 1981.
3. Montgomery, P.C., Ayyildiz, A., Lemaitre-Coelho, I.M., Vaerman, J.P. and Rockey, J.H., Ann. N.Y. Acad. Sci. 409, 428, 1983.
4. Smith, C.W. and Goldman, A.S., Pediatr. Res. 2, 103, 1968.
5. Mohr, J.A., Leu, R. and Mabry, W., J. Surg. Oncol. 2, 163, 1968.
6. Diaz-Jouanen, E. and Williams, R.C., Clin. Immunol. Immunopath. 3, 248, 1974.
7. Parmely, M.J., Beer, A.E. and Billingham, R.E., J. Exp. Med. 144, 358, 1976.
8. Parmely, M.J., Reath, D.B., Beer, A.E. and Billingham, R.E., Transpl. Proc. 9, 1477, 1977.
9. Smith, J.W. and Schultz, R.D., Cell. Immunol 29, 165, 1977.
10. Concha, C., Holmberg, O. and Morein, B., J. Dairy Res. 45, 287, 1978.
11. Ogra, S.S. and Ogra, P.L., J. Pediatr. 92, 550, 1978.
12. Concha, C., Holmberg, O. and Morein, B., J. Dairy Res. 47, 305, 1980.

13. Schore, C.E., Osburn, B.I., Jasper, D.E. and Tyler, D.E., J. Immunol. Immunopathol. 2, 561, 1971.
14. Oksenberg, J.R., Persitz, E. and Brautbar, C., Am. J. Reproduct. Immunol. 8, 125, 1985.
15. Maconi, P.E., Fadda, F.F., Cadoni, A., Cornaglia, P., Zaccheo, D. and Grifoni, V., Int. Archs. Allergy App. Immunol. 56, 385, 1978.
16. Crago, S.S., Prince, S.J., Pretlow, T.G., McGhee, J.R. and Mestecky, J., Clin. Exp. Immunol. 38, 585, 1979.
17. Bush, J.R. and Beer, A.E., Am. J. Obstet. Gynecol. 133, 708, 1979.
18. Lally, E.T., Zitron, I.M., Fiorini, R.C. and Montgomery, P.C., Adv. Exp. Med. Biol. 107, 143, 1978.
19. Golub, E.S., J. Exp. Med. 136, 369, 1972.
20. Winchester, R.J., Fu, S.M., Hoffman, T. and Kunkel, H.G., J. Immunol. 114, 1210, 1975.
21. Bianco, C., Patrick, R. and Nussenzweig, V., J. Exp. Med. 132, 702, 1970.
22. Parish, C.R. and Hayward, J.A., Proc. R. Soc. Lond. G. 187, 47, 1974.
23. Koski, I.R., Poplack, D.G. and Blaese, R.M., in In vitro Methods in Cell-Mediated and Tumor Immunity, (Edited by Bloom, B.R. and David, J.R.), p. 359, Academic Press, New York, 1976.
24. Oudghiri, M., Seguin, J. and Deslauriers, N., Eur. J. Immunol. 16, 281, 1986.
25. Parmely, M.J. and Manning, L.S., Ann. N.Y. Acad. Sci. 409, 517, 1983.
26. Montgomery, P.C., Peppard, J.V. and Skandera, C.A., Proc. Int. Symp. Immunol. Immunopathol. of the Eye, 1987 (in press).
27. Hunt, S.V., Eur. J. Immunol. 9, 853, 1979.
28. Gilman, S.C., Rosenberg, J.S. and Feldman, J.D., J. Immunol. 128, 644, 1982.

CLEARANCE, LOCALIZATION AND CATABOLISM OF INTRAVENOUSLY ADMINISTERED PROTEIN ANTIGENS IN LACTATING MICE

P.R. Harmatz, D.G. Hanson, M.K. Walsh, R.E. Kleinman,
K.J. Bloch and W.A. Walker

Departments of Pediatrics and Medicine, Harvard Medical School and the Combined Program in Pediatric Gastroenterology and Nutrition (Massachusetts General Hospital and Children's Hospital) and the Clinical Immunology and Allergy Units, Massachusetts General Hospital, Boston, MA USA

INTRODUCTION

Dietary protein antigens including wheat, cows milk proteins, and ovalbumin have been identified in breast milk of lactating women (1-3). The quantity of antigen reported has varied depending on the individual study. Wheat (3) and cows milk proteins (1) were detected by immunoprecipitation at concentrations of about 1 μg/ml, while ovalbumin (OVA) and beta-lactoglobulin (a specific cow's milk protein not present in human serum or milk) were detected in the range of 100 pg/ml to 6 ng/ml (2). Methodologic variations have been suggested to account for these differences in dietary antigen levels in breast milk (2). An alternate hypothesis is that inherent differences in the protein molecules themselves, in their processing in the lactating female or in their mechanism(s) of transport into breast milk, may account for the differences in reported concentrations. In the present experiments, we examined the pattern of clearance of four radiolabeled protein antigens from maternal circulation in the mouse, and their localization and catabolism within selected tissues.

METHODS

Animals

CD-1 timed-pregnant mice were placed on a diet free of bovine proteins and OVA (Purina Cat Chow), on day 15 of pregnancy. All experiments were performed on day 7-9 after delivery. Animals were given 0.01% potassium iodide in the drinking water beginning 48 hours before the experiment.

Preparation of radiolabeled antigen

Bovine serum albumin (BSA), OVA, bovine gammaglobulin (BGG) and beta-lactoglobulin (BLG) were labeled with ^{125}I by the chloramine-T method (9). All labeled proteins were 80-90% precipitable with specific rabbit antisera. The monomeric form of each protein was prepared by gel filtration chromatography. The approximate concentration of each protein was determined spectrophotometrically (5,6).

Clearance of radiolabeled antigens after intravenous injection

Lactating mice were injected intravenously (i.v.) with one of the four monomeric radiolabeled antigens. Each animal received 8.4×10^6 cpm (140 ug of protein) in normal saline. Blood was obtained prior to sacrifice at 1 min, 10 min, 1 h and 4 h. Liver, mammary tissue, kidney, spleen, stomach and small intestine were recovered at each time point. Radioactivity per gram of clotted blood was determined and serum recovered. Immunoreactive protein was identified by co-precipitation with specific rabbit antibody-antigen complexes.

Organ distribution of radioactivity

Total organ radioactivity was corrected for the amount of radioactivity associated with blood in the intravascular space (7). Organs were then homogenized and radioactivity in clarified supernatants was examined by co-precipitation with specific rabbit antibody-antigen complexes in the presence of protease inhibitors.

RESULTS

Clearance of radioactivity from the circulation of lactating mice

The amount of co-precipitable radioactivity remaining in the circulation after injection of the four proteins is shown in Figure 1. After injection of ^{125}I-BSA and ^{125}I-BGG coprecipitable radioactivity in the blood decreased less than 40% and 25%, respectively, over 4 hours. In contrast, the co-precipitable radioactivity in blood decreased rapidly after injection of ^{125}I-BLG and ^{125}I-OVA.

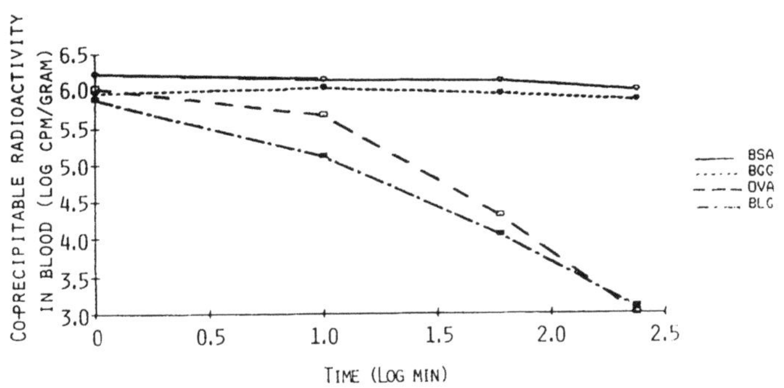

Figure 1. Clearance of immunoprecipitable radioactivity from the circulation of lactating mice injected with ^{125}I-labeled BSA, BGG, OVA or BLG. Each data point represents the mean of three animals.

Distribution of radioactivity in organs of lactating mice

Mammary tissue (Table 1) showed a progressive increase in radioactivity over the 4 h period after injection of ^{125}I-BSA and ^{125}I-BGG. After injection of ^{125}I-OVA and ^{125}I-BLG, radioactivity also increased in mammary tissue but reached its highest level at 1 h. In the liver, kidney and stomach, significant amounts of radioactivity were present only after injection of ^{125}I-OVA and ^{125}I-BLG, with peak levels occurring early in liver and kidney, and later in the stomach. In the small intestine, radioactivity accumulated over the 4 h after injection of ^{125}I-BSA and ^{125}I-BGG. In contrast, after injection of ^{125}I-OVA and ^{125}I-BLG, the radioactivity was elevated early (1 and 10 min) and declined thereafter.

After injection of ^{125}I-BSA and ^{125}I-BGG, the radioactivity remained immunoprecipitable in all organs except the stomach. In contrast, after injection of ^{125}I-OVA and ^{125}I-BLG, the radioactivity was poorly immunoprecipitable in all organs by 1 h.

Control experiments demonstrated that with the exception of BLG, the other 3 proteins remained specifically precipitable during tissue homogenization and analysis. In the presence of stomach and small-intestinal homogenates, BLG lost antigenic determinants under the conditions tested.

Table 1. Distribution and characterization of radioactivity in organs of lactating mice injected with ^{125}I-labeled BSA, OVA, BGG or BLG

	BSA				BGG				OVA				BLG			
	1min	10min	1hr	4hr	1min	10min	1hr	4hr	1min	10min	1hr	4hr	1min	10min	1hr	4hr
Mammary Gland																
	0.9[a]	3.09	6.52	9.35	1.70	1.61	3.89	6.96	1.14	4.63	7.61	3.26	2.31	4.50	17.8	14.1
	(97)[b]	(95)	(92)	(74)	(95)	(93)	(87)	(88)	(89)	(73)	(7)	(8)	(80)	(34)	(2)	(1)
Liver																
	0.0	0.0	0.0	0.0	0.62	0.11	0.51	0.0	1.59	5.64	1.07	0.20	0.84	3.50	0.62	0.35
	(95)	(93)	(93)	(88)	(90)	(89)	(89)	(88)	(83)	(72)	(48)	(10)	(72)	(56)	(18)	(13)
Stomach																
	0.27	0.30	0.57	0.16	0.28	0.28	0.64	0.61	0.18	0.08	2.56	1.83	0.97	2.15	4.76	3.51
	(80)	(76)	(42)	(42)	(93)	(89)	(48)	(35)	(78)	(22)	(2)	(1)	ND[c]	ND	ND	ND
Spleen																
	0.0	0.09	0.07	0.12	0.06	0.18	0.14	0.14	0.17	0.21	0.04	0.03	0.33	0.14	0.09	0.03
	(95)	(97)	(95)	(91)	(92)	(91)	(88)	(91)	(88)	(62)	(31)	(1)	(76)	(52)	(9)	(9)
Kidney																
	0.0	0.69	0.66	0.50	0.65	0.69	0.96	0.40	1.73	5.0	1.56	0.1	6.83	23.4	1.02	0.26
	(94)	(94)	(88)	(84)	(93)	(92)	(92)	(86)	(88)	(73)	(47)	(11)	(70)	(43)	(17)	(8)
Small Intestine																
	0.94	2.78	2.85	2.88	1.95	2.65	3.85	2.68	1.08	2.39	0.88	0.61	5.17	4.33	2.04	0.99
	(93)	(92)	(89)	(89)	(87)	(88)	(85)	(84)	(78)	(70)	(21)	(10)	ND	ND	ND	ND

a Mean organ radioactivity in counts per minute (10^{-5}) minus radioactivity due to estimated blood content of the organ; n=3 mice per data point.

b Percentage of total organ radioactivity co-precipitated by specific rabbit antibody-antigen complexes; total organ radioactivity includes tissue- and blood-associated counts.

c ND = not done.

DISCUSSION

Persistence of immunoprecipitable antigen in the maternal circulation (Fig. 1) was positively associated with accumulation of the antigen in mammary gland (Table 1). At present, it is unclear whether accumulation is primarily dependent on absolute concentration of antigen in maternal blood, the length of time that mammary tissue is exposed to circulating antigen, or on both factors. Selected organs, in addition to the mammary gland, were examined to define patterns of clearance and processing of the proteins that might influence transfer into the mammary gland (Table 1). After injection of ^{125}I-OVA and ^{125}I-BLG, total and immunoprecipitable radioactivity accumulated rapidly in liver, kidney, and small intestine, and then decreased during the next 4 h. A delayed peak of total radioactivity was observed at 1 h in the stomach extract; little of this material was imunoprecipitable (Table 1). These data suggest that intact protein (or large fragments thereof) first localized in liver, kidney and small intestine, and then underwent degradation, with release of ^{125}I from the organ. Small iodinated fragments or free ^{125}I then apparently accumulated in the stomach (8,9). Hepatic uptake of OVA, a glycoprotein with mannose or N-acetylglucosamine in the terminal position, may occur via a specific receptor for these carbohydrates on sinusoidal cells in the liver (10,11). This would not, however, explain the apparent hepatic accumulation of BLG. The role of the kidney in the metabolism of "small" proteins ($<$ 50 kD) has been well documented (12).

After injection of ^{125}I-BSA and ^{125}I-BGG, radioactivity accumulated in the small intestine. Total small-intestinal radioactivity stabilized after 10 min and remained immunoprecipitable through 4 h. We have no explanation for the accumulation of these labeled proteins in the intestine.

Four dietary protein antigens were shown to differ in their rates of clearance from the maternal circulation, and localization and catabolism within selected tissues. Persistence of immunoprecipitable antigen in the maternal circulation appeared to correlate with transfer of antigen into mammary tissue. Such differences in the amount and character of antigen localizing to mammary tissue are likely to influence the transfer and detectability of antigens in the milk.

CONCLUSIONS

1. BSA, BGG, BLG and OVA differ in their rates of clearance from the maternal circulation.

2. Accumulation of immunoreactive proteins in mammary tissue varied inversely with their rate of clearance from the maternal circulation.

3. The liver and kidney contribute to the rapid clearance of OVA and BLG from the maternal circulation.

ACKNOWLEDGEMENTS

This work was supported by grants from the National Institute of Health AM 33506, HD 12437, AM 01141 and AI 20865 and a grant from the Hood Foundation.

REFERENCES

1. Jakobsson, I. and Lindberg, T., Lancet ii, 437, 1978.
2. Kilshaw, P.J. and Cant, A.J., Int. Archs. Allergy Appl. Immun. 75, 8, 1984.
3 Kulangara, A.C., Med. Sci. Libr. Compend. 8, 19, 1980.
4. Hanson, D.G., Vaz, N.M., Maia, L.C.S., Hornbrook, M.M., Lynch, J. and Roy, C.A., Int. Archs. Allergy Appl. Immunol. 55, 526, 1977.
5. Fasman, G.D., Handbook of Biochemistry and Molecular Biology: Proteins, Vol. II, p. 383, CRC Press, Cleveland, OH, 1976.
6. Waddell, W.J., J. Lab. Clin. Med. 48, 311, 1956.
7. Kim, Y.W. and Halsey, J.F., J. Immunol. 129, 619, 1982.
8. Honour, A.J., Myant, N.B. and Rowlands, E.N., Clin. Sci. (London) 11, 447, 1952.
9. Jones, R.E., Proc. R. Soc. Lond. 199, 279, 1977.
10. Day, J.F., Thornburg, R.W., Thorpe, S.R. and Baynes, J.W., J. Biol. Chem. 255, 2360, 1980.
11. Stahl, P.D., Rodman, J.S., Miller, M.J. and Schlesinger, P.H., Proc. Natl. Acad. Sci. USA 75, 1399, 1978.
12. Cohen, J.J. and Kamm, E.E., in The Kidney, (Edited by Brenner, B.M. and Rector, F.C.), p. 144, W.B. Saunders, Philadelphia, PA, 1981.

SPECIFIC ANTIBACTERIAL ANTIBODY-PRODUCING CELLS IN HUMAN NASAL MUCOSA

M.-C. Béné, G. Faure, and M. Wayoff.

Laboratoire d'Immunologie and Clinique O.R.L.
UFR Sciences Médicales, Université Nancy I
54500 Vandoeuvre les Nancy
France

INTRODUCTION

Recurrent infections of the rhinopharyngeal area, common in young children, are elusive to most classical therapies. The use of local vaccines to enhance local immunity has been proposed since the sixties. Although these immunomodulators have been widely used, their mechanisms of action remain disputed. A likely hypothesis is that inactivated microbes could induce a specific local immune response against bacteria commonly found in the relevant area. This is supported by the demonstration of antigen-specific antibodies in the secretions. The precise site of synthesis of specific immunoglobulins is, however, not well documented in humans. Suitable technology allowing the detection of antibody-producing cells *in vivo* has been only recently developed and applied to animal models (1).

We report a study documenting the presence of specific immunoglobulin-producing cells in the nasal mucosa. The antigens tested are included in a local vaccine commercialized in France.

PATIENTS AND METHODS

Patients

The study included 7 males, 2 females (age range 23-60, mean 38) who reported to the ear-nose-throat clinic for chronic maxillar sinusitis. They had suffered recurrent episodes of infectious rhinorrhea for at least

2 years, but had no other local pathology (polyposis, dysplasia) or general disorder (atopy, systemic disease). Any local or general therapy such as antibiotics or antiinflammatory drugs was discontinued for at least one month before the onset of the study.

All patients received an IRS19° therapy which consisted of local intracavitar sprays or instillations, at least twice a day for 1 month. This local vaccine is a suspension containing 1.5×10^{10} bacteria per ml. Major strains are Streptococcus pneumoniae, Micrococcus pyogenes, Gaffkya tetragena, Klebsiella pneumoniae and Haemophilus influenzae as well as several members of the Streptococcus and Moraxella families.

Methods

Nasal mucosa samples were obtained with informed consent of the patients, before and one month after beginning the treatment. Biopsy specimens were immersed immediately in liquid nitrogen, forwarded to the laboratory and stored in a deep freezer (-80°C REVCO) until study. Four micron thick cryostat sections were collected on glass slides, air dried and processed without further fixation. One section was stained with toludene blue for histological observation and mast-cells detection. Serial sections were used for immunohistological examination. They were first incubated with the following antigenic suspensions either pure or diluted 1:10 in phosphate-buffered saline (PBS):

Streptococcus pneumoniae type 2 (138-20026)
Streptococcus pneumoniae type 3 (96-20102)
Streptococcus D19 (107-20776)
Klebsiella pneumoniae (20360)
Haemophilus influenzae type b (839-19159)

After three min washes in PBS, the sections were further incubated with fluorescein-conjugated antisera specific for each bacterial strain, at dilutions varying from 1/5 to 1/20 in PBS. Working dilutions had been initially tested on pure strain smears. Two dilutions were tested for each tissue sample. Incubations duration was 30 min, and they were performed in humid chambers at room temperature. Both strains and antisera were produced by Berri-Balzac Laboratories (France). The staining period was followed by 3 washings in PBS after which sections were covered with a PBS/glycerol mixture (7/3) intented to prevent dehydration, and stored in humid chambers at 4°C. Stained sections were examined within 24 h of processing, in a Leitz Orthoplan microscope equipped with a Ploem system of epiillumination for immunofluorescence and phase contrast. The small size of the samples impaired additional identification of plasma-cell isotypes.

Controls

Control sections were performed for each sample, omitting the initial incubation with antigenic material. These demonstrated the absence of non-specific finding of fluoresceinated antisera. A second series of controls demonstrated the absence of cross reactivities : sections incubated with a given strain were further stained with fluorochrome-labeled antiserum to another strain.

RESULTS

Histological examination of the sections showed epithelial and chorionic areas with usually moderate cellular infiltration. Cell density varied from one sample to another, but never displayed the characteristics of acute inflammation. Cell types observed were macrophages, plasma cells, mast cells and eosinophils. The presence of the latter cell type raised acute problems for UV light examination, because of their propensity to bind fluorescein-labeled reagents. Eosinophils were the only fluorescent cells on control slides. On test sections, their presence was confirmed by alternative observation under UV light and in phase contrast microscopy. Plasma cells thus were defined as UV-positive/phase contrast-negative cells. Plasma cells producing specific antibodies for the tested strains were observed before and after treatment in 6 patients. Their number was usually small: 2 to 3 specific Ig-producing cells per sample, but significant as compared to the total number of plasma cells in these small biopsies. Specific antibody-producing cells were mostly directed to Streptococcus D antigens, while plasma cells to Haemophilus influenzae were only observed in 3 patients. After local immunization, two patients had plasma cells to all 5 strains tested. In one patient, the number of positive cells was definitely higher in the post-therapy biopsy.

CONCLUSIONS

This work demonstrates the presence, in human nasal mucosa, of plasma cells synthetizing antibodies specific for antigens of 5 different bacterial strains contained in a nasal soluble vaccine. These were detected before and after one month of treatment, i.e., heavy immunogen exposure. At least for one patient, their number and spectrum increased significantly, although it might be difficult to interpret small samples from different locations. Quantitative immunohistomorphometry could not be performed due to the small size of most samples, representing .1 to .2 mm^2. The presence of numerous eosinophils and mast cells was a challenge, but the observation of serial sections and the use of phase-contrast microscopy allowed differentiation between these cell types and correct identification of the plasma cells (2).

This study provides a fundamental confirmation of the opportune choice of the bacterial strains contained in the local vaccine IRS19. It also demonstrates that nasal mucosa is a proper target for such therapy. The presence of potentially responsive B cells in this area supports an expected beneficial effect of local immunization. Clinical trials had previously established the efficiency of this rather widely used product, as well as a limited number of immunological studies, essentially performed on peripheral blood cells (3). The direct approach used in this work provides more direct evidence of local efficiency. Such studies have seldom been reported in humans (4). Providing that great care is taken in the interpretation of the fluorescent images, the availability of purified strains or antigens and relevant antisera opens an interesting field in the exploration of accessible mucosal territories.

ACKNOWLEDGEMENTS

The authors are grateful to Dr. N. Wierzbicki and Laboratoires Sarbach for initiating the study and providing reagents through the Société Berri Balzac. This work was supported in part by CRE Inserm 84 3002 and by the Comité Lorraine de la Fondation pour la Recherche Médicale.

REFERENCES

1. Van Rooijen, N., Kors, N., Van Nieuwmegen, R. and Eikelenboom, P., Anat. Rec. 206, 189, 1983.

2. Brandtzaeg, P. and Baklien, K., Lancet i, 1297, 1976.
3. Charon, J., Seidel, S. and Wray, D., Gaz. Med. 91, 1, 1984.
4. Van Rooijen, N. and Kors, N., J. Histochem. Cytochem. 33, 175, 1985.

INCIDENCE AND DISTRIBUTION OF IMMUNOCYTES IN THE MURINE ORAL MUCOSA

M. Lacasse, A. Collet*, W. Mourad and N. Deslauriers

Departement de Biochimie and Groupe de Recherche en Ecologie Buccale, and *Departement d'Anatomie, Faculté de Médecine Université Laval, Québec, Canada

INTRODUCTION

Specific mucosal defense mechanisms involve the mobilization of the secretory immune system. Even in a healthy individual, secretory immunity is involved in host-bacterial interactions at colonized mucosal surfaces. For example, in the oral cavity of SPF-inbred mice, the colonization and the growth of indigenous bacteria are under the continuous influence of salivary IgA antibodies (1,2). Conversely, it appears that, under normal conditions, the indigenous flora can effectively sensitize the secretory immune system. It is possible that the availability of oral microbial antigens, via retrograde passage through the secretory ducts of minor salivary glands (MSGs) (3), could potentiate IgA antibody production by inducing further proliferation and differentiation of GALT-derived precursor cells (4).

Initially, our knowledge about the immunological characteristics of the oral mucosal immune system in the BALB/c mouse was derived from a phenotypic characterization of oral mucosa cells in single-cell suspensions (5). It was established that the murine oral mucosa contains an efferent lymphoid compartment consisting of Ig-containing and Ig-secreting cells, and an afferent lymphoid compartment consisting of T and B lymphocytes. As the mucosa also contains a significant percentage of macrophages, we hypothesized that oral lymphoid tissue may function as an antigen-reactive system able to carry out the last stages of a local secretory immune response. We, therefore, investigated the spatial arrangement of these immunocytes in tissue sections of the buccal and palatine oral mucosae. This approach allows a comparison between the arrangement of the oral immune system in the healthy mouse and the architecture of this system in humans and primates.

MATERIALS AND METHODS

Animals

BALB/c male mice were obtained from Charles River Breeding Farms (St. Constant, Quebec) and used between 17 and 20 wk of age. We used 9 animals in this study (6 for paraffin sections and 3 for frozen sections).

Dissection of the oral mucosa

Mice were killed by exsanguination. The oral mucosa, including the cheeks and the soft palate, was excised in one piece from the underlying muscle tissue.

Staining of paraffin sections

The excised tissue was rinsed in Iscove medium (Flow Lab., Mississauga, Ontario) and then immediately placed in either 10% buffered formalin or Bouin fixative. Afterwards, the tissue was dehydrated in alcohol and embedded in paraffin. Sections (5 μm thick) were cut, mounted and stained in series with HαE, PAS and Giemsa stain. Cytochemical demonstration of nonspecific esterases was performed according to Stuart et al. (6) with minor modifications.

Immunofluorescent staining of frozen sections

After washing in Earle's balanced salt solution (EBSS), specimens were embedded in tragacanthe gum (Fisher Scientific) and snap-frozen in liquid N_2-cooled isopentate. Four to 6 μm cryostat sections were cut, fixed in acetone at -20°C for 5 min, then rinsed in 0.01 M phosphate buffered saline (PBS), pH 7.0. Sections were stained by a direct immunofluorescent procedure with dichlorotriazenyl-amino-fluorescein (DTAF)-labeled affinity-purified goat antibodies to mouse IgG (γ), IgM (μ) and IgA (α) (Kirkegaard and Perry Lab., Gaithesburg, MD) or fluorescein isothiocyanate (FITC)-labeled mouse monoclonal antibodies to Thy-1.2 antigen (Miles, Rexdale, Ontario) as already described (5).

RESULTS

Distribution of immunocytes in the murine oral mucosa

Superficially, the soft palate (oral side) and the cheeks were covered by a keratinized, stratified, squamous epithelium. The oral submucosa contained variable amounts of minor salivary glands (MSGs), these being more numerous in the soft palate. Immunocytes were found scattered throughout the lamina propria and the interglandular connective tissue. Usually, their number was relatively low (Fig. 1). However, some sites showed an increased cell concentration in the vicinity of MSGs, particularly in the connective tissue surrounding secretory ducts and between the glandular acini (Fig. 2 and 3). Lymphoid cells were often seen in these sites. Some small aggregations were also seen near the mucous glands (Fig. 4). Among the six animals used, only one larger aggregation was observed, but still in close association with the glands of the soft palate (Fig. 5).

Morphological and histochemical analysis of immunocytes in the oral mucosa

Lymphoid cells of different sizes, including typical small lymphocytes with round and hyperchromatic nuclei, were disseminated either in the periglandular area or between the acini of the MSGs.

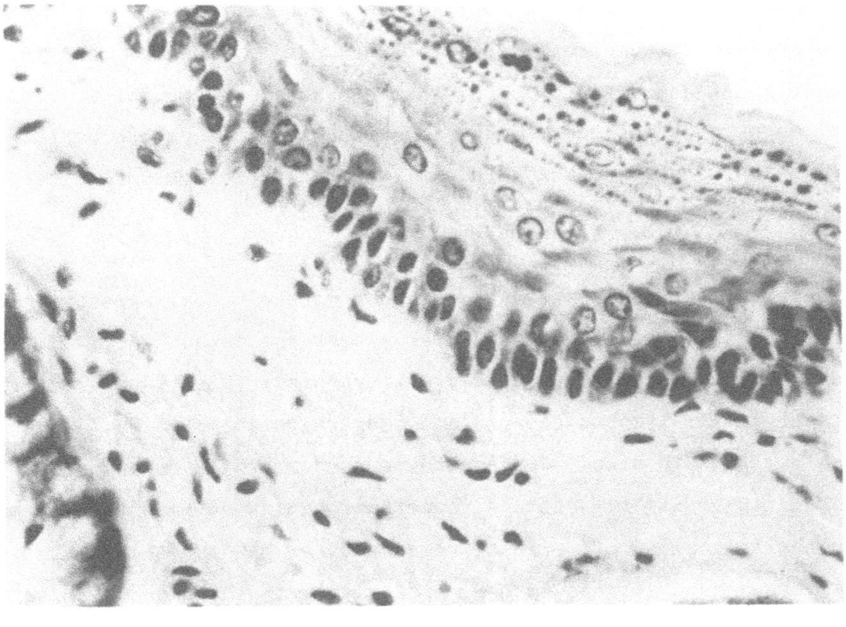

Figure 1. Low cell concentration in the lamina propria near MSGs in the soft palate. Cells with a clear halo are distinguishable along the basal layer of the keratinized epithelium Paraffin section, H&E (x900).

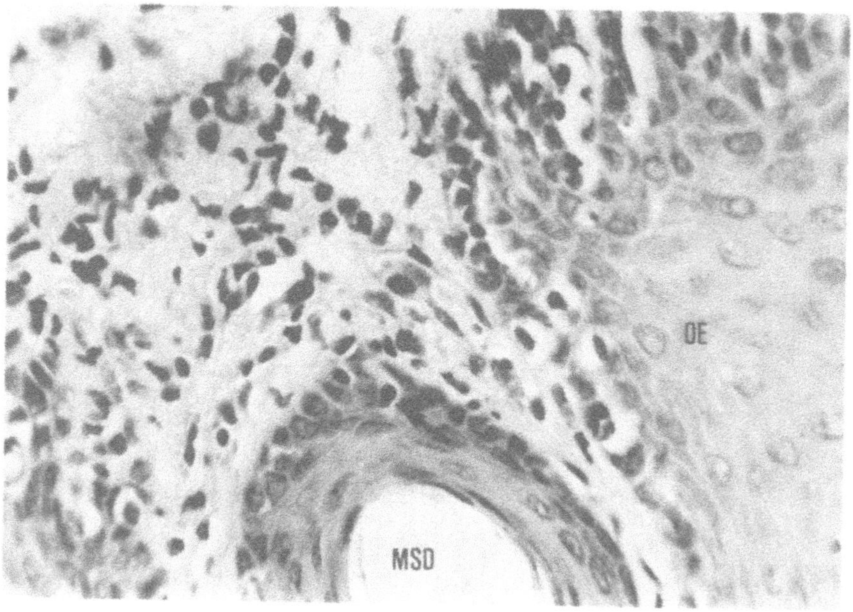

Figure 2. Increased cell concentration in the connective tissue surrounding a main secretory duct (MSD) underneath the oral epithelium (OE) of the soft palate. Some cells show a lymphoid appearance. Note cell with a dark round nucleus penetrating ductal epithelium (arrow). Paraffin section, H&E (x850).

The only large aggregation found closely associated with the MSGs (Fig. 5) was comprised of numerous, darkly stained nuclei. Unlike other sites of high cell concentration, many of them had an elongated shape. This atypical appearance left some doubt about the lymphoid nature of the cells. Lymphoid cells with round shaped nuclei were only present in limited numbers in this aggregation.

Intraepithelial cells showing different morphological aspects were observed within the oral epithelium, mostly near the basal layer. These cells shared one common feature: a clear cytoplasm (Fig. 6) characteristic of intraepithelial lymphocytes (7) and Langerhans cells (7,8). This typical clear halo varied in size. Corresponding round to oval nuclei were either hyperchromatic or lightly stained, sometimes having an indented appearance. Intraepithelial cells were regular components of the mucosal epithelium, being more numerous at some sites, particularly in the gland-rich soft palate. Identical cells were also observed in the epithelial layer of some MSG ducts; they are especially prominent when the epithelium remains stratified.

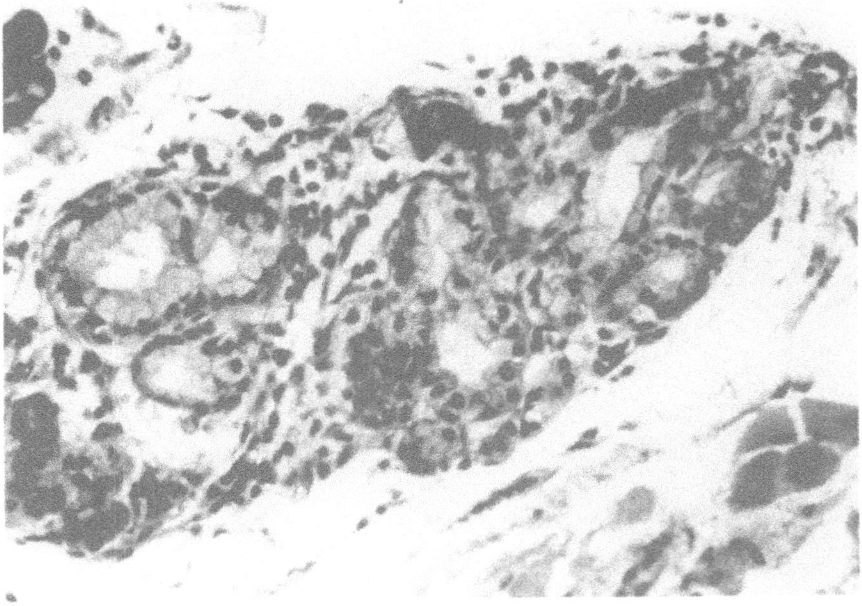

Figure 3. Lymphoid cells in the interacinar connective tissue of oral cheek mucosa. Paraffin section, H&E (x550).

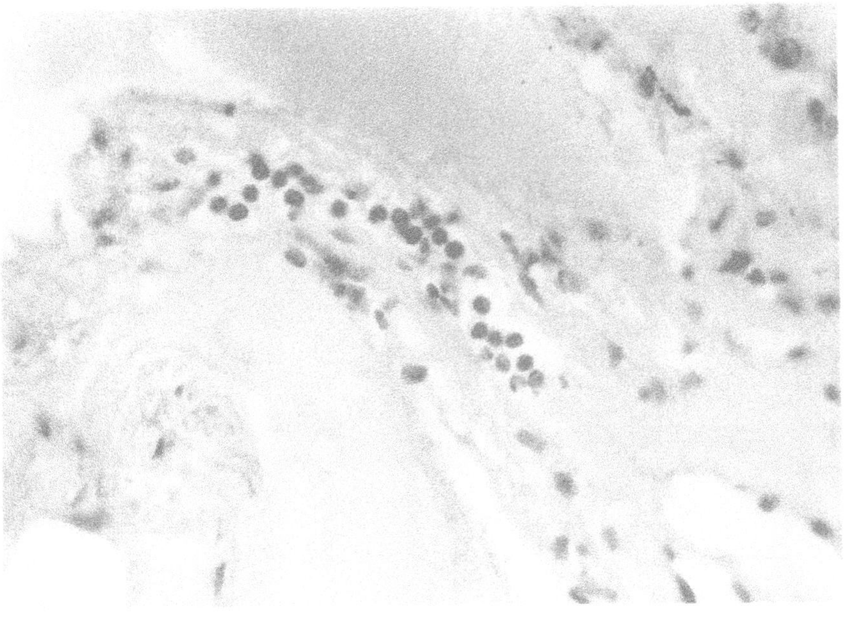

Figure 4. Small aggregation of lymphoid cells near the mucous glands in the cheek mucosa. Paraffin section, H&E (x850).

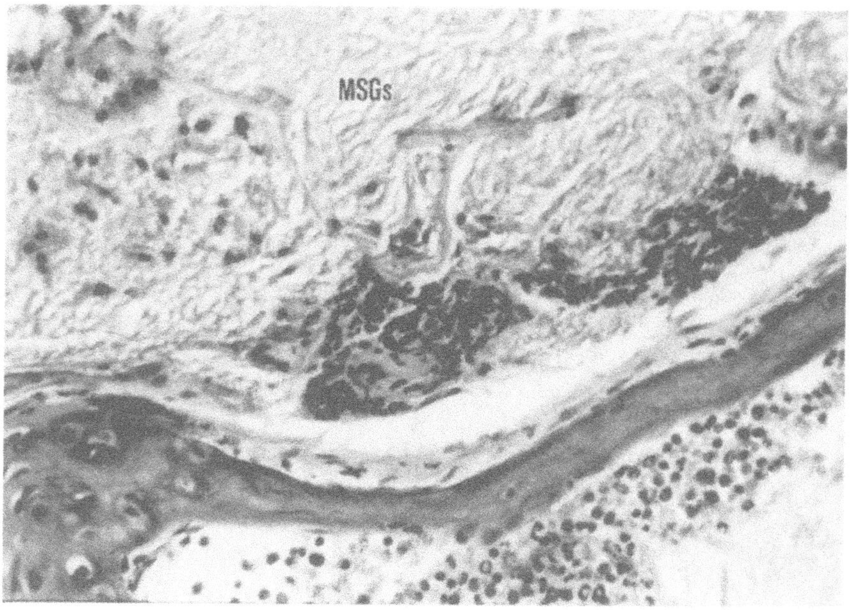

Figure 5. Large aggregation of cells closely associated with the MSGs in the soft palate. Cells show a more elongated nucleus than in small aggregations. The glandular epithelium is greatly attenuated in this area. Paraffin section, H&E (x600).

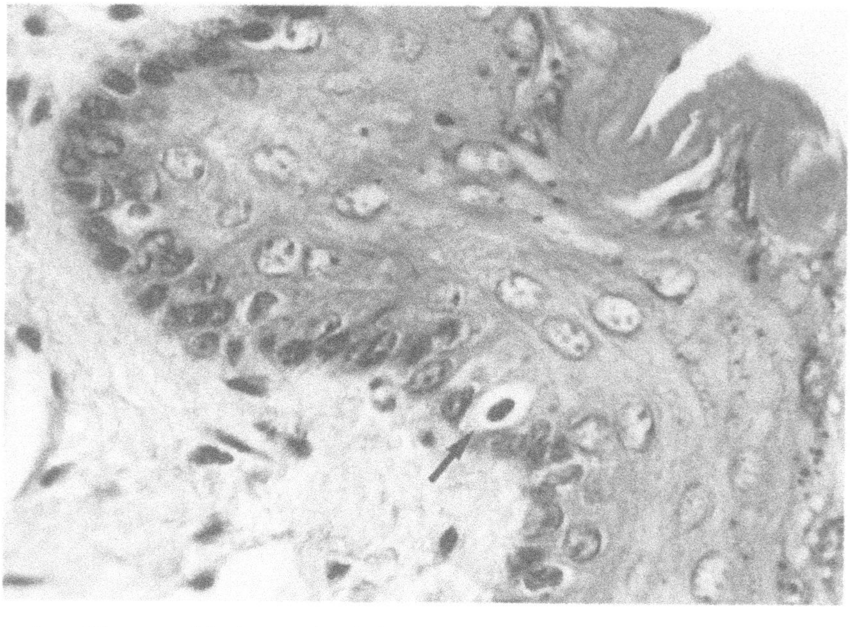

Figure 6. Clear cell (arrow) with a particularly prominent halo in the oral epithelium of the soft palate. Paraffin section, H&E (x1100).

A similar disposition was found in some ductal epithelia for esterase-positive cells (Fig. 7), these also occurring at a low frequency in the lamina propria.

A smaller population of mast cells, identified by a PAS reaction and/or HαE staining (Fig. 8) was irregularly found in individual animals, generally near blood vessels in the periphery of the glands, and occasionally in the interacinar connective tissue. Degranulation was sometimes observed.

Immunofluorescent staining of frozen tissue sections

Ig-synthesizing cells of the M, G and A isotypes were demonstrated by direct immunofluorescent staining of frozen tissue sections (Fig. 9). These were found almost exclusively either between the acini or in the periphery of the glands. In most sections, we noted a predominance of IgA-synthesizing cells over IgM- and IgG-containing cells. An interacinar and periacinar distribution of Thy-1-bearing cells was also observed but these were generally found beneath the epithelium (Fig. 10).

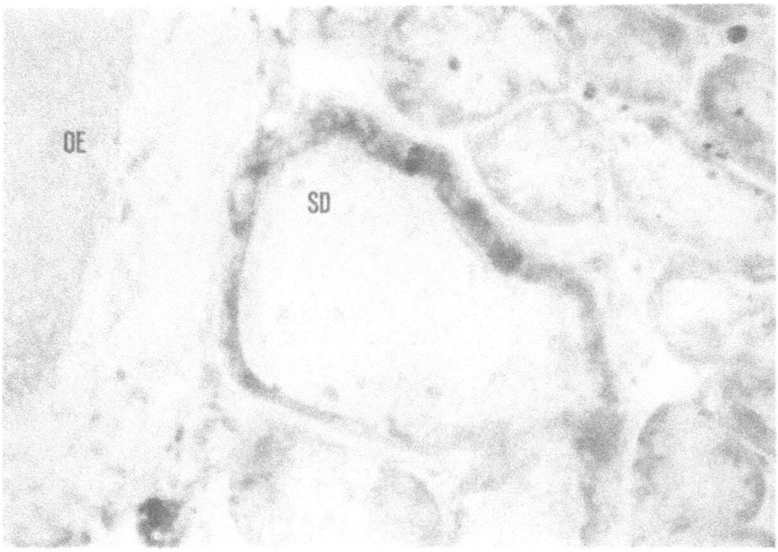

Figure 7. Esterase-positive cells in the epithelium of a secretory duct (SD) (OE = oral epithelium of the soft palate). Paraffin section, cytochemical demonstration of nonspecific esterases (x550).

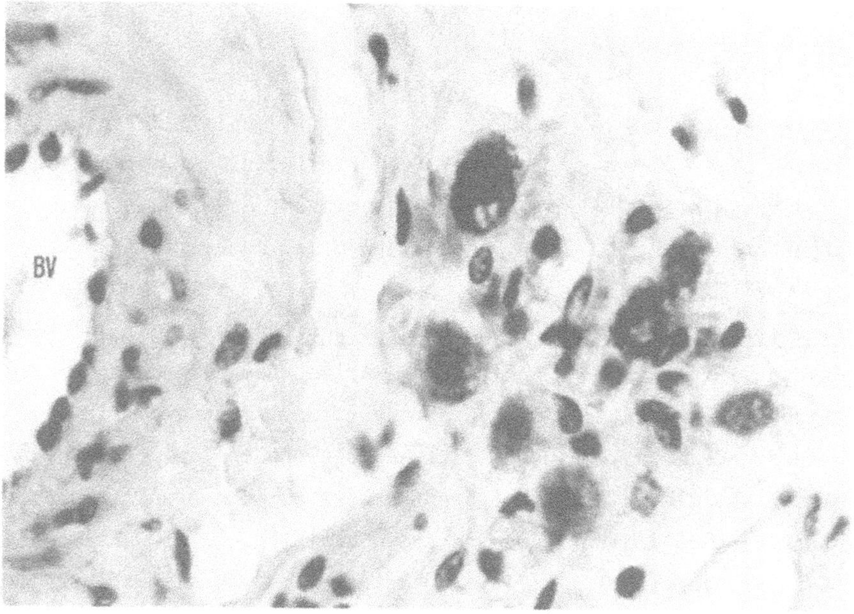

Figure 8. Mast cells near a blood vessel (BV) in the oral cheek mucosa. Paraffin section, H&E (x1250).

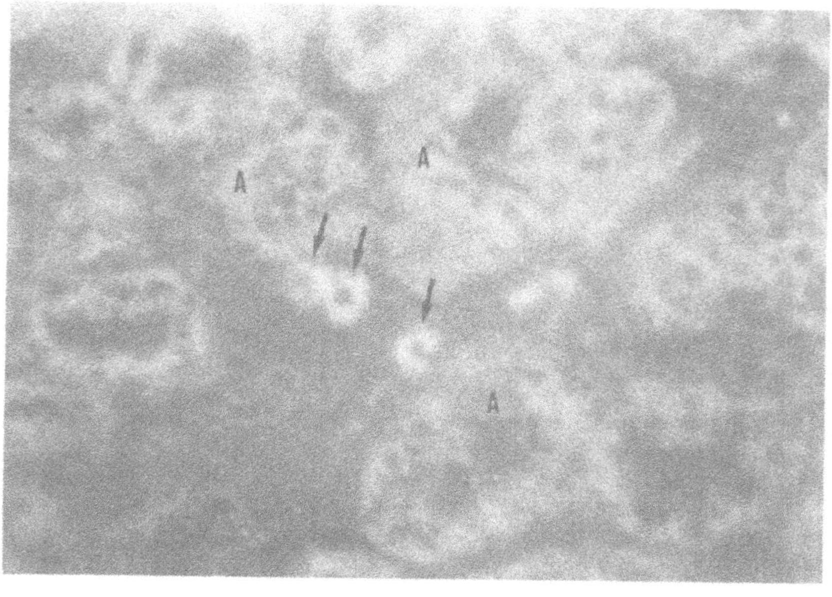

Figure 9. IgA-synthesizing cells (arrows) between the glandular acini (A) of the soft palate. Frozen tissue section, anti-IgA (DTAF) staining (x800).

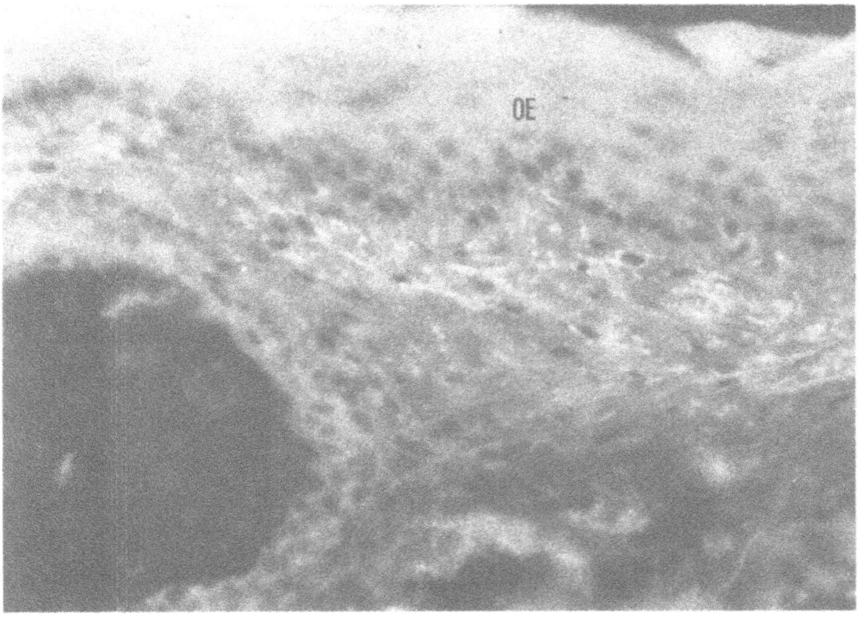

Figure 10. Thy-1-bearing cells beneath the oral epithelium (OE) of the soft palate. Frozen tissue section, anti-Thy-1.2 (FITC) staining (x550).

DISCUSSION

This study provides a general picture of the structure and composition of the oral mucosa in the healthy mouse. We summarize here the observations made in 9 animals under standardized experimental conditions of age, sex, diet and genetic background. Present data suggest that the murine oral immune system is mainly associated with the MSGs, and to some extent with the basal epithelium.

MSGs are important factors in salivary immunity. Physiological data showed that MSG secretions in the human contain high concentrations of secretory IgA (9). As most MSGs have short ducts and are located superficially throughout the lamina propria of the oral mucosa it has been suggested that they are continuously exposed to oral antigens. Nair and Schroeder have provided evidence of a natural retrograde flow of oral antigens to the MSG duct-associated lymphoid tissue (3,10). The oral lymphoid tissue has been reported to occur in dense aggregations at various sites in the oral mucosa in primates, but more often associated with the secretory ducts of MSGs (DALT) in monkeys (reviewed in 11). Such structures were not observed in our study of the murine oral mucosa. It is possible that these structures are not present in specific pathogen-free animals, since they are thought to undergo involution in clinically healthy humans (11). The absence of ductal follicles in the mouse does not appears to be age-related (11) since our preliminary observations on younger (6-8 wk old) animals did not show this characteristic arrangement of the lymphoid tissue.

As there are neither tonsils (12) nor DALT in the mouse, it appears that under normal physiological conditions the immune surveillance of the oral mucosa is effected by a specialized diffuse immune system. The incidence and distribution of immunocytes, observed in SPF animals, most probably represents the basal activity of the oral immune system. This basal activity is, in part, reflected by the distribution of differentiating B cells in single-cell suspensions of the mucosa (5): 40% of resident B lymphocytes were found to be in their resting state.

The fact that most of the oral mucosa is keratinized in rodents may be of functional relevance for the stimulation and the development of the local immune system. This specialized diffuse immune system may well share some similarities with the one present in the skin (13). This does not exclude the eventuality of a repeated local antigenic challenge brought about by a (replicating) mucosal pathogen (Deslauriers, Lacasse, Trudel, Collet and Auger: Oral candidosis in the mouse. XIV International Congress of Microbiology, Manchester, England, September, 1986).

CONCLUSIONS

1. In the mouse, the oral immune system is mainly associated with the MSGs. Sites of high lymphoid cell concentration were always close to glandular acini or MSG secretory ducts. Few lymphoid aggregations were present in the vicinity of MSGs. The cell concentration of the lamina propria remains low in the non-glandular regions, especially in the cheeks. This particular disposition may well reflect the availability of immunocytes against oral antigens entering secretory ducts.

2. The oral epithelium also contributes significantly to the oral immune system. Clear cells, isolated or in small clusters, were, for the most part, located near the epithelial basal layer. These cells most likely correspond to lymphocytes and Langerhans cells. However, a clear distinction between them is not possible under the light microscope.

3. As there are neither tonsils nor DALT in the mouse, it appears that under normal physiological conditions the immune surveillance of the oral mucosa is effected by a specialized diffuse immune system. The incidence and distribution of immunocytes observed in SPF animals most probably represent the basal activity of the oral immune system.

ACKNOWLEDGEMENTS

The authors wish to thank R. Delamare and A. Pusterla for excellent technical assistance, G. Bourgeau for correcting the English and C. Lacroix for typing the manuscript. This work was supported by Medical Research Council of Canada (grant MA 8934).

REFERENCES

1. Deslauriers, N., Oudghiri, M., Séguin, J. and Trudel, L., Immunol. Invest. 15, 4, 1986.
2. Deslauriers, N., Séguin, J. and Trudel, L., Microbiol. Immunol., 1987 (in press).
3. Schroeder, H.E., Moreillon, M.-C. and Nair, P.N.R., Arch. Oral Biol. 28, 133, 1983.
4. Genco, R.J., Linzer, R. and Evans, R.T., Ann. N.Y. Acad. Sci. 409, 650, 1983.
5. Deslauriers, N., Néron, S. and Mourad, W., Immunology 55, 391, 1985.
6. Stuart, A.E., Habeshaw, J.A. and Davidson, A.E., II, in Handbook of Experimental Immunology (Edited by Weir, D.M.), p. 31.22, Blackwell Scientific Publications, Oxford, 1978.
7. Bos, I.R. and Burkhardt, A., J. Oral Path. 9, 65, 1980.
8. Shelley, W.B. and Juhlin, L., Acta. Dermatovener. (Suppl)79, 7, 1978.
9. Crawford, J.M., Taubman, M.A. and Smith, D.J., Science 109, 1206, 1975.
10. Nair, P.N.R. and Schroeder, H.E., Arch. Oral Biol. 28, 145, 1983.
11. Nair, P.N.R. and Schroeder, H.E., Immunology 57, 171, 1986.
12. In Biology of the Laboratory Mouse (Edited by Green, E.L.), p. 251, McGraw-Hill, New York, p. 251, 1966.
13. Edelson, R.L. and Fink, J.M., Scientific American 252, 46, 1985.

CHARACTERIZATION OF LYMPHOID CELLS FROM THE HUMAN FALLOPIAN TUBE MUCOSA

M.D. Cooper, C. Dever, K. Tempel, E.J. Moticka, T. Hindman and D.S. Stephens

Departments of Medical Microbiology, Immunology and Pathology, Southern Illinois University School of Medicine, Springfield, IL; and Department of Medicine Emory University, Atlanta, GA USA

INTRODUCTION

Much information about the immune response available at mucosal surfaces has been derived through studies on the gut mucosa of man and animals (1,2). By contrast, relatively little is known about the immunocompetent cells and their activity from other mucosal surfaces. Several studies (3-6) have demonstrated differences between mucosal immune responses in different organs. One organ for which relatively little data is available is the human fallopian tube. Early studies by Tourville et. al. (7) on the localization of immunoglobulin producing cells in the human fallopian tube demonstrated the presence of IgG and IgA, but not IgM secreting cells in the lamina propria (LP) and along the basement membrane (BM). Biological consequences of the immunoglobulins produced by these cells is still speculative. In addition, immunocompenent cells other than B cells in the fallopian tube have not been identified or characterized. In order to increase our understanding of the types of immune responses which might take place at this important host-parasite interface, we initiated studies to determine the cell types present in Neisseria infected and uninfected organ culture models of human fallopian tubes.

MATERIALS AND METHODS

Human fallopian tube organ cultures (FTOC) and infections

Organ cultures were prepared from human fallopian tubes as previously described (13) and infected with *Neisseria gonorrhoeae* 192A, *Neisseria subflava* 19243 or *Neisseria meningitidis* RNP. Stocks of these cultures were maintained in defibrinated blood at -70°C. Inocula were prepared from organisms grown overnight at 37°C on GC agar (Difco Laboratories, Detroit, MI) containing 1% IsoVitalex (BBL Microbiology Systems, Cockeysville, MD) in 5% CO_2. The final concentration of the inoculum was 2×10^5 CFU/ml.

Immunocytochemical procedures

Tissues examined by immunofluorescence were fixed in 90% ETOH and processed according to the method of Sainte-Marie (8). In some studies, frozen sections were prepared. For frozen sections, the tissue was oriented, embedded in O.C.T. Compound (Miles Scientific, Naperville, IL) and frozen in 90% ETOH over liquid nitrogen. Three to five micron sections were prepared, fixed and used in an indirect fluorescent antibody test. Staining was accomplished by using a fluorochrome-conjugated polyclonal antibody (Cooper Biomedical, Inc., Cappel Lab, Malvern, PA) directed against either IgG, IgA or IgM or total Igs or monoclonal antibodies (Becton Dickinson, Oxnard, CA) directed against Leu-4, Leu-1, Leu-2a, Leu-3a and Leu-11b. Intraepithelial lymphocytes (IEL) were counted in 10 or more high power fields. A minimum of 200 or more lamina propria lymphocytes were counted in each section using the method of cumulative means described by Chalkley (9). Sections were examined under a Zeiss fluorescent microscope using a 40 x phase oil objective and an epifluorescence condensor with selective FITC filter.

Immunoperoxidase staining of tissue was accomplished using a modification of the procedure described by Sternberger (10) and Curran and Jones (11). In brief, tissues were deparaffinized in xylene and dehydrated in ETOH. Endogenous peroxidase was destroyed by incubation in H_2O_2 in MEOH. Tissues were then hydrated and nonspecific binding sites were blocked by incubation with normal swine serum. Following an overnight incubation in the primary antisera the tissue was washed and swine anti-rabbit sera applied. This was followed by incubation with rabbit peroxidase anti-peroxidase and reaction with 3-3' diaminobenzidine tetrahydrochloride.

The tissue was counterstained with hematoxylin dehydrated through ETOH and xylene, mounted using a synthetic mounting media, and observed using light microscopy.

Cell suspensions

Single cell suspensions of the fallopian tube mucosa were obtained using a modification of the method described by Tagliabue et al. (4). Briefly, the tubes were cleaned and incubated in 1 mM dithiothreitol (DTT) in Hanks' balanced salt solution for 15 min. Following incubation, the tissue was cut in 2 mm square pieces and incubated for 2 h in collagenase/ dispase [(5:5 mg/ml) (5 ml/g tissue)]. The treated tissue was then filtered through a 100 μ wire screen, and incubated for 15 min in the presence of RNase and DNase. Following this, the cells were incubated overnight in RPMI 1640 + 20% FCS and then fractionated over discontinuous Percoll density gradients with cells collected at the interface of the 20 to 60% layer. These cells were assessed for surface phenotype using surface markers defined by FITC-conjugated monoclonal antibodies to Igs, Leu-4 and Leu-11b (Becton-Dickinson, Mountain View, CA). Numbers of macrophages were estimated by nonspecific esterase staining.

RESULTS

Immunocytochemical studies of infected and noninfected mucosal tissues

Infected and noninfected fallopian tube organ cultures were examined by peroxidase anti-peroxidase and immunofluorescence techniques for the presence of immunoglobulins. Tissues examined immediately after removal from patients stained so intensely in the lamina propria (LP) by either technique that individual lymphocytes could not be discriminated from free Ig in the tissue. Further, it was observed that there was a noticeable lack of staining in the epithelium (data not shown). In organ cultures infected for 24 h with *Neisseria* there were noticeable changes when compared with uninfected tissue. Numerous lymphocytes (plasma cells) were positive for individual immunoglobulins and were in evidence near the epithelial layer (Fig. 1b and 1c). There was also further staining along the basement membrane particularly for IgA (Fig. 1a and 1b arrows).

Epithelial cells of infected fallopian tube mucosa were compared with uninfected tubes for numbers of Ig surface positive cells. Results are

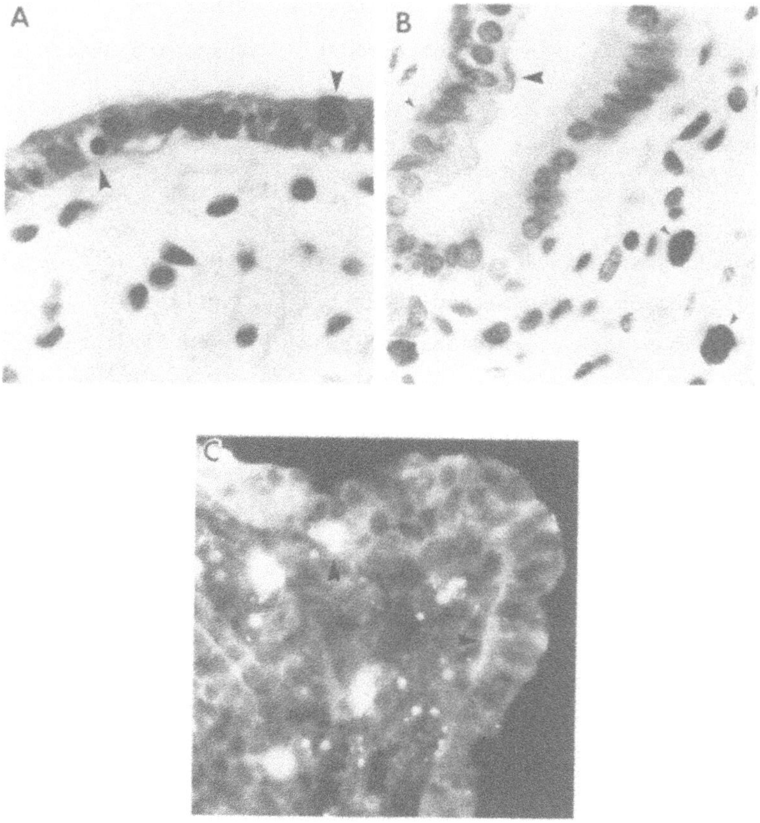

Figure 1. (A) PAP staining of Neisseria infected FTOC at 24 h. Top arrow indicates presence of cell with sIgA staining. Bottom arrow shows presence of unstained IEL. (B) PAP staining of FTOC at 48 h post infection. Note the presence of IgA-positive plasma cells in the LP (small arrows) and the presence of sIgA on the luminal surface of the epithelial cells (large arrows). (C) Immunofluorescence of 48 h post infected FTOC. Arrows indicate the IgA positive basement membrane and plasma cells.

depicted in Table 1. Epithelial cells containing secretory component (SC) of sIgA were significantly increased in infected tissues when compared to uninfected controls by 12 h ($p < 0.05$). The number of SC and sIgA positive cells increased at both 24 and 48 h compared to uninfected controls and was significant for both SC ($p < 0.001$) and sIgA ($p < 0.01$). However, the numbers of surface IgA-positive cells did not increase and were not significantly different when infected and noninfected tissues were compared.

Table 1. Distribution of immunoglobulin surface positive cells in human fallopian tube mucosal epithelial cells of Neisseria infected and noninfected FTOC

	Secretory component % + cells		sIgA % + cells		IgG % + cells	
Time (h)	I	NI	I	NI	I	NI
0	-	< 0.2	-	0.6	-	0.8
12	1.11	1.6	9.4	3.3	1.2	2.3
24	15.1	< 0.2	25.3	6.2	0.8	6.9
48	34.5	13.9	40.3	11.3	0.6	0.6

I = Infected.
NI = Noninfected.

Cell separation of lymphoid cells from human fallopian tubes

Single cell suspensions were prepared following enzymatic digestion of the fallopian tube mucosa. Cells were analyzed for presence of surface markers and the results are shown in Table 2. It is apparent that the cells which were recovered from the 60% Percoll interface contained a mixture of lymphoid cells normally found in the fallopian tube. There is a higher percentage of T cells (~26%) than B cells (~6%). This is consistent with results reported for other mucosal tissues. It is also of interest to note that there is a significant population of lymphoid cells which express the NK marker Leu-11b (8.25%). The population of esterase-positive cells is low as was expected since these cells have undergone plastic adherence prior to the Percoll gradient centrifugation. We are also aware that our total percentages are less than 100% of the total cell population. It should be noted that these populations were not purified previously other than an overnight incubation on plastic surfaces and there are probably cells other than those of lymphoid linage which migrated at the same density as the lymphocytes. The transition between 20 and 60% Percoll is rather abrupt and not selective. We are presently in the process of further refining the limits of our gradient banding for better purification.

Table 2. Distribution of lymphoid cells from human fallopian mucosa fractionated over 60% Percoll gradients.

Surface Ig^+	Leu-4^+	Leu-$11b^+$	Esterase
Percent Positive Cells $\pm$ SEM[a]			
5.7 $\pm$ 2.1	26.15 $\pm$ 4.6	8.25 $\pm$ 0.7	2.8 $\pm$ 1.6

[a]SEM - Standard error of the mean.

DISCUSSION

Much of our knowledge of lymphoid cells of the mucosal immune system has been derived from experiments on gut mucosa. The majority of lymphocyte preparations from the gut in both human and experimental animals has produced lymphoid cell mixtures containing both IEL and LPL (12). Several reports have indicated that these cells perform a variety of functions (i.e., cytotoxic T cells, ADCC, NK activity and antibody formation). It is apparent from morphological examination of the mucosa of the human fallopian tube that anatomically it is similar to the mucosa of the gut. It is widely known that the gut has the ancillary immunological structures known as Peyer's patches. However, the human fallopian tube does not have any structures which are analogous to these. In other respects, the two mucosae appear similar. There is a wide distribution of lymphoid cells in the mucosa of human fallopian tissue (Table 2). There are also IELs present in the mucosal epithelium (Fig. 1A). However, when one begins to isolate and characterize the lymphocytes from the mucosa of the human fallopian tube the differences between the gut and fallopian tube mucosa become apparent.

We have initiated studies on the immunocompetent cell populations of the fallopian tube mucosa. Our results indicate that the distribution of immunoglobulin-bearing cells is similar to that of the gut mucosa as described by Tourville et al. (6). Further, this distribution was similar to that of normal human female reproductive tracts reported by Tourville et al. (7). When tissue from Neisseria infected organ cultures was examined for immunoglobulin-producing cells it was observed that there was a significant increase in the numbers of IgA-bearing plasma cells in the LP when compared to the uninfected controls. We have also reported previously that the human fallopian tube organ cultures are capable of the de novo synthesis of measurable amounts of IgA with increased levels in Neisseria infected organ cultures (13). This increase is most likely a nonspecific response to the bacteria products present. Neisseria, being gram-negative bacteria, are known producers of lipopolysaccharide (LPS) and this substance is a polyclonal B cell activator. Further, from our other studies (14), LPS has been shown to attach to and penetrate epithelial cells and, therefore, probably acts as a nonspecific mitogen.

In attempts to characterize the total lymphoid cell population of the human fallopian tube mucosa, we have used discontinuous Percoll gradients to separate the lymphoid cells. These cells express B, T and NK surface markers and the ratio of B cells to T cells is approximately 1:4. These numbers are similar to those reported for other mucosal sites. It is of interest to note a significant number of cells express NK surface markers. This is most likely the result of cell preparations containing IELs which have a high percentage of cells expressing the NK phenotype and which are responsible for local NK activity. The fact that the fallopian tube mucosa has a significant NK population leads to some interesting speculation as to their potential function in local defense mechanisms.

CONCLUSIONS

1. Human fallopian tube mucosa possesses Ig-bearing plasma cells which are distributed in a manner similar to that seen in gut mucosa.

2. Infection with Neisseria increases the numbers of SC and IgA positive cells over noninfected control tissue.

3. Percoll gradient separation of fallopian tube-associated lymphoid cells revealed the presence of B and T cells and a surprisingly large number of NK cells.

ACKNOWLEDGEMENT

This investigation was supported by U.S.P.H.S. research grant AI 20603.

REFERENCES

1. Tomasi, T.B. and Plaut, A.G., in Advances in Host Defense Mechanisms, (Editors, Gallin, J.I. and Fauci, A.S.), p. 31, Raven Press, New York, 1985.
2. Bull, D.M. and Bookman, M.A., J. Clin. Invest. 59, 966, 1977.
3. Arnaud-Battandier, F., Bundy, B.M., O'Neill, M., Bienenstock, J. and Nelson, D.L., J. Immunol. 121, 1059, 1978.
4. Tagliabue, A., Befus, A.D., Clark, D.A. and Bienenstock, J., J. Exp. Med. 155, 1785, 1982.
5. Watt, P.J. and Ward, K.A., Trans. Opthalmol. Soc. U.K. 104, 367, 1985.
6. Tourville, D.R., Adler, R.H., Bienenstock, J. and Tomasi, T.B., J. Exp. Med. 129, 411, 1969.
7. Tourville, D.R., Ogra, S.S., Lippes, J. and Tomasi, T.B., Amer. J. Obstet. Gynec. 108, 1102, 1970.
8. Sainte-Marie, G., J. Histochem. Cytochem. 10, 250, 1962.
9. Chalkley, H.W., J. Natl. Cancer Inst. 4, 47, 1943.
10. Sternberger, L.A., in Immunocytochemistry, p. 104, J. Wiley, New York, 1979.
11. Curran, R.C. and Jones, E.L., Clin. Exp. Immunol. 28, 103, 1977.
12. Parrot, D.M.V., Tait, C., MacKenzie, S., Mowat, A.McI., Davies, M.D.J. and Micklem, H.S., Ann. N.Y. Acad. Sci. 409, 307, 1983.
13. Cooper, M.D., McGee, Z.A., Mulks, M.H., Koomey, J.M. and Hindman, T.L., J. Infect. Dis. 150, 737, 1984.
14. Cooper, M.D., McGraw, P.A. and Melly, M.A., Infect. Immun. 51, 425, 1986.

ULTRASTRUCTURAL LOCALIZATION OF IgA AND IgG IN UTERINE EPITHELIAL CELLS FOLLOWING ESTRADIOL ADMINISTRATION

K.H. Templeman and C.R. Wira

Department of Physiology, Dartmouth Medical School
Hanover, New Hampshire USA

INTRODUCTION

The secretory immune system in the reproductive tract of the female mammal is acutely sensitive to stimulation by estradiol (1). Within three hours of each of three daily doses of estradiol to the ovariectomized rat, IgG enters the uterine lumen (2) concomitant with the fluid imbibition phase of estrogen stimulation of the uterus. The levels of IgA in the uterine lumen, on the other hand, do not rise significantly until 32-48 hours of estradiol stimulation (2,3). In order to characterize the morphologic nature of the process of immunoglobulin transport in this polarized epithelial system, we analyzed the distribution patterns of post-embedment immunogold labeling assays of IgA and IgG in uterine epithelial cells at various times of estradiol stimulation.

MATERIALS AND METHODS

Adult female Sprague Dawley rats (Charles River Breeding Laboratories, Wilmington, MA) were ovariectomized 9 days prior to use. Animals received either estradiol (1 μg/day for three days) or saline carrier injections prepared in the same manner as the hormone (2). A maximum of three injections was given at 24 h intervals, with tissues examined at 3, 52 and 72 hours from the time of the first injection. Saline-injected controls were examined at the 52 h stage.

Tissues at each time interval were prepared by perfusion of the uterine vessels via the abdominal aorta with Dulbecco's phosphate-buffered saline (pH 7.4) followed by fixative consisting of 2% glutaraldehyde, 2% paraformaldehyde, 2% sucrose in 0.1 M cacodylate buffer with 1 mM $CaCl_2$. Uterine horns were excised, further cut into 1 mm^3 blocks, and either postfixed in 1% OsO_4 for embedment in Epon, or without postfixation for embedment in Lowicryl K4M® (Chemische Werke Lowi) according to the manufacturers instructions. To facilitate polymerization of a large series of blocks, a simple specimen carrier was designed (4).

The assay of IgA was performed on fresh Lowicryl thin sections mounted on uncoated nickel grids. To reduce nonspecific binding, the grids were blocked with 0.1% bovine serum albumin (BSA) and 5% normal goat serum in Tris-buffered saline (TBS) at pH 7.4, incubated for one hour with 50 μg/ml of an IgA-specific mouse monoclonal antibody (5), rinsed in buffer with 0.1% BSA, and finally incubated with a 1:25 dilution of goat anti-mouse IgG immunogold conjugate (particle size 10 nm; Janssen Life Sciences, Inc.). Control assays were companion-run with the substitution of isotype-matched mouse IgG1 monoclonal antibody for the IgA-specific primary antibody. For Epon-embedded samples, thin sections were etched with saturated aqueous sodium metaperiodate (6) or 3% hydrogen peroxide for 30 min prior to the immunogold assay.

In the IgG immunogold assay, normal rabbit serum was absorbed against freshly perfused rat brain immediately prior to use in order to decrease nonspecific binding by serum components. To serve as a control for the ammonium sulfate cut of goat antiserum specific for rat heavy chain of IgG (Miles Laboratories, Elkhart, ID), normal goat serum was precipitated with ammonium sulfate and dialyzed against PBS. Another control consisted of absorption of the anti-heavy chain reagent with ChromPure rat IgG agarose (Jackson ImmunoResearch Laboratories). The sections were blocked with 5% absorbed rabbit serum with 0.1% BSA in TBS, pH 7.4, briefly rinsed in goat serum block before incubation for 2 h with a 1:100 dilution of antiserum, then postlabeled with a 1:25 dilution of rabbit anti-goat immunogold conjugate (particle size 5 nm; Janssen Life Sciences, Inc.). Grids were stained with uranyl acetate and briefly (15 sec) with leads citrate prior to examination.

Grain concentrations were quantified by counting the number and organelle association of gold particles in areas representing 15 μm^2 in continuous montage electron micrographs. In assigning organelle association, any questionable patterns were judged to be noncytoplasmic and assigned to the nearest organelle.

RESULTS

IgA localization

Immunoglobulin A is found within uterine luminal epithelial cells both prior to and following estradiol stimulation. As seen in Figure 1, when tissue specimens from rats treated with estradiol for 52 h were embedded in Lowicryl and examined with a nonspecific first antibody, very few, if any, gold grains were present. When a first antibody specific for IgA was used (Fig. 2), considerable amounts of IgA were found distributed throughout the uterine cells. In other studies (not shown), we have found that IgA is present within uterine cells both prior to (saline-treated) and at 3 h and 72 h after the time of first treatment with estradiol.

Analysis of the distribution of IgA within uterine epithelial cells following Lowicryl processing as well as Epon embedment with etching treatment indicated that the majority of IgA was cytoplasmic and not membrane-associated. Both prior to and following estradiol stimulation, the percentage of grains associated with vesicular cell components (including coated vesicles, smooth vesicles, multivesicular bodies and endoplasmic reticulum) ranged from 0-1% of the total grains counted. In contrast, the level of IgA labeling that was clearly cytoplasmic ranged from 50-92%.

To further clarify the cytoplasmic distribution of IgA in uterine epithelial cells, tissues were analyzed by stereo microscopy. When labeled specimens were examined, IgA grains were localized in small homogeneous foci in the ground substance, almost always connected to from one to several intermediate filaments that were 10 nm in diameter, and not in association with coated vesicles. We also observed that IgA staining did not penetrate tissue sections and was confined to the surface of each section.

IgG localization

IgG was found in low concentration in the uterine epithelial cells of saline control tissue, and became stronger in response to hormone treatment. Within the epithelium the labeling pattern suggested that IgG might

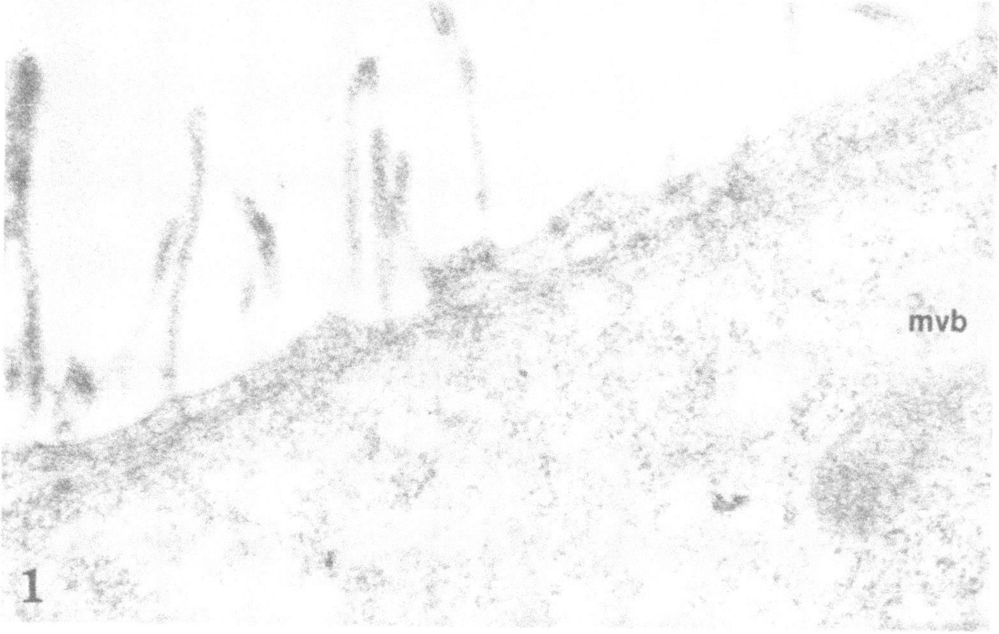

Figure 1. Luminal surface of a rat uterine epithelial cell at 52 h of estradiol stimulation. In this immunogold control treatment of a Lowicryl-embedded, unosmicated sample, the specific antibody against rat IgA was replaced with a nonspecific isotype of monoclonal antibody. No gold grains are found in the micrograph. mvb, multivesicular body. (Magnification x60,000)

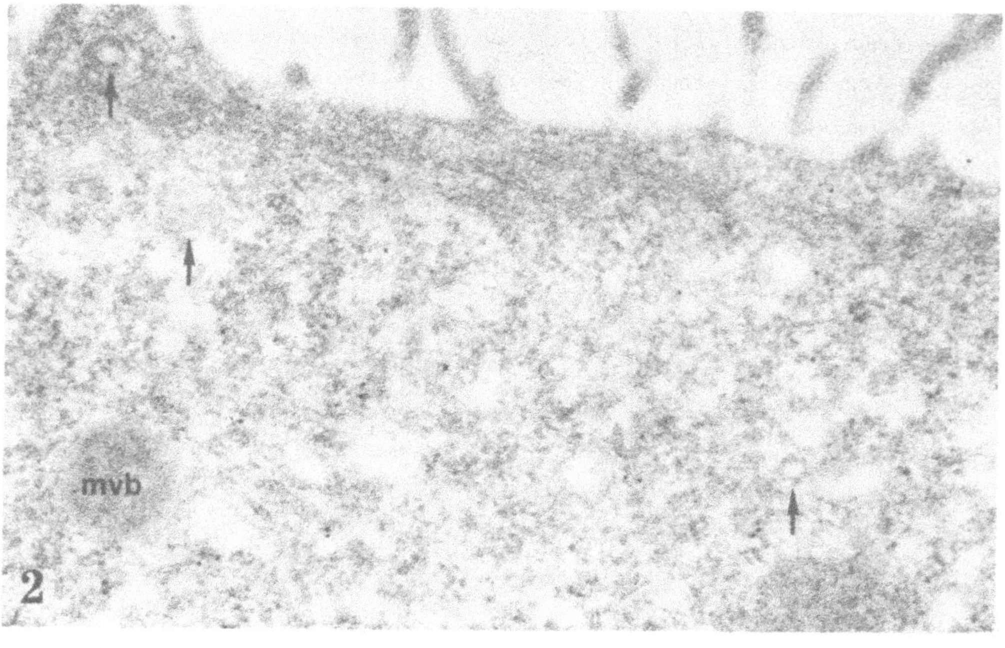

Figure 2. Immunogold labeling of the luminal surface of a rat uterine epithelial cell at 52 h of estradiol stimulation, prepared as in Fig. 1, except for the use of a specific anti-IgA monoclonal antibody in the assay. Small dense dots of the gold probe are found distributed throughout the cytosol, and not in association with the vesicles (arrows), typical of the apical cytoplasm. (x60,000)

be infrequently associated with discrete uncoated vesicles and reticular elements. In contrast to the IgA experiments, IgG attachment to intermediate filaments was not observed. Stereopsis suggested some labeling of the supranuclear Golgi components. As was the case with IgA, label was found extending along the microvilli, and was not associated with surface pits or coated vesicles. At no time was label for either IgG or IgA found in the intercellular spaces. Unlike IgA, strong labeling of IgG was observed throughout the stroma and in vascular lumina of the endometrium. Eosinophils, which migrate into the uterus and invade the epithelium by 72 h, were also strongly labeled for both IgA and IgG.

DISCUSSION

The results of the present study indicate that IgA and IgG are present in uterine epithelial cells both prior to and following estradiol stimulation, and that the movement of both immunoglobulins is directly through epithelial cells rather than between them. Moreover, from an analysis of the organelle association of intracellular IgA, our findings suggest that IgA movement is consistently associated with intermediate filaments and not with coated vesicles. In contrast, IgG movement is distinct from IgA in that it is not microfilament-associated, but rather is diffusely distributed or occasionally found associated with small vesicular and reticular elements.

Our approach in these studies was to use postembedment immunolabeling which has been used previously as an effective technique to characterize macromolecular transport phenomena *in situ* (7). It avoids the risk of a target molecule being routed along an alternative pathway of receptor-mediated endocytosis, which could occur with ligand damage or alteration by iodination reagents or reductive methylation, and in the metabolic pathways usually followed by certain viruses (8), horseradish peroxidase (9) and colloidal gold (10). Another major advantage of the procedure is the ability to companion-run multiple samples for later analysis.

Our finding that the foci of IgA-positive labeling are usually associated with intermediate filaments may explain why others have found that IgA sediments with larger membrane components during cellular fractionation (11,12). That IgA transport is not disrupted by cytochalasin B (13) can be explained by the property of this agent to depolymerize actin-like filaments, while intermediate filaments are often unaffected.

These studies at the ultrastructural level provide support for the previous biochemical evidence from this laboratory that IgA moves into the uterine lumen against a concentration gradient, while IgG moves down a gradient (14). The differences in transport of the two immunoglobulins are underscored in this study by their distinctive structural associations within the epithelial cytoplasm.

CONCLUSIONS

1. Immunoglobulins A and G are found in the uterine epithelium at all stages of estradiol stimulation as well as in the saline-injected ovariectomized controls.

2. Movement of the immunoglobulins does not occur intercellularly, but take place directly through the epithelial cytoplasm.

3. The ultrastructure of labeled cytoplasmic elements suggests differences in the IgG and IgA transport mechanisms, with IgA being associated with intermediate filaments.

ACKNOWLEDGEMENTS

This research was supported by grant AI 13541 from the National Institutes of Health.

REFERENCES

1. Wira, C.R. and Sandoe, C.P., Endocrinology 106, 1020, 1980.
2. Sullivan, D.A. and Wira, C.R., Endocrinology 112, 260, 1982.
3. Sullivan, D. and Wira, C.R., Endocrinology 114, 650, 1984.
4. Templeman, K.H. and Wira, C.R., J. Electron Microscopy Technique 4, 73, 1986.

5. Sullivan, D., Colby, E.B., Hann, L.E., Allansmith, M.R. and Wira, C.R., J. Immunol. Methods 15, 311, 1986.
6. Bendayan, M. and Zollinger, M., J. Histochem. Cytochem. 31, 101, 1983.
7. Roth, J., Histochem. J. 14, 791, 1982.
8. Simons, K. and Warren, G., Advances in Protein Chem. 36, 79, 1984.
9. Steinman, R.M., in In Vitro Methods in Cell-Mediated and Tumor Immunity (Edited by Bloom, B.R. and David, J.R.), p. 379, Academic Press, New York, 1976.
10. Gosselin, R.E., Fed. Proc. 26, 987, 1967.
11. Tolleshaug, H., Brandtzaeg, P. and Holte, K., Scand. J. Immunol. 13, 47, 1981.
12. Mullock, B.M., Hinton, R.H., Dobrota, M., Peppard, J. and Orlans, E., Biochim. Biophys. Acta. 587, 381, 1979.
13. Nagura, H., Nakane, P.K. and Brown, W.R., J. Immunol. 123, 2359, 1979.
14. Wira, C.R., Sullivan, D.A. and Sandoe, C.P., J. Steroid Biochem. 19, 469, 1983.

ORIGIN OF IgA AND IgG ANTIBODIES IN THE FEMALE REPRODUCTIVE TRACT: REGULATION OF THE GENITAL RESPONSE BY ESTRADIOL

C.R. Wira and C.P. Sandoe

Department of Physiology, Dartmouth Medical School
Hanover, New Hampshire USA

INTRODUCTION

Despite extensive studies, venereal disease remains a major world wide health problem which has devastating effects on both adults and newborns (1-3). The rise of gonococcus, herpes, group B streptococcus and pelvic inflammatory diseases during the past decade emphasizes the need for a renewed effort to develop an effective and lasting approach to immunological protection.

Others have previously shown that the female reproductive tract is a part of the mucosal immune system (4,5) and that antibodies to a variety of microbial antigens are present in secretions of the genital tract (6). Host defenses against these microbes may arise either from immune responsiveness to local infection or by lymphoblast migration from other mucosal sites to the genital tract (7).

We have previously described the effects of estradiol and progesterone on the presence of immunoglobulins and secretory component in the female reproductive tract of the rat (8-10) and human (11). Acting through distinct mechanisms which include lymphocyte migration (12) serum transudation (13, 14) and immunoglobulin transport (10,15), estradiol stimulates both IgA and IgG movement into the uterine secretions. Hormone regulation of these immunoglobulins has the opposite effect in cervico-vaginal secretions in that both estradiol and progesterone lower IgA, IgG and SC levels (16).

In the present study, we have utilized our rat model to determine the origin of specific antibodies in the reproductive tract and to analyze the role of estradiol in regulating the accumulation of these specific antibodies in the uterus and vagina. Specifically, our goals were (a) to determine whether immunization via the gastrointestinal tract of rats results in the appearance of specifically directed IgA and IgG antibodies in uterine and vaginal secretions and (b) to examine the regulatory role of estradiol in the stimulation and/or suppression of these antibodies in genital tract secretions.

METHODS

Adult female Sprague Dawley rats (Charles River Breeding Laboratories, Wilmington, MA) were maintained in constant temperature rooms under 12 hr intervals of light and dark. Ovariectomies were performed 7-10 days before each experiment. Estradiol, purchased from Calbiochem (La Jolla, CA), was dissolved in ethanol and resuspended in saline (0.9%). Control animals received only saline. At the time of immunization, animals were ether anesthetized and following a midline incision, intestinal segments were exteriorized to permit injection (27 gauge needle) of saline washed (2x) sheep erythrocytes (SRBC; Gibco Laboratories, Grand Island, New York; 100 µl of packed cells, 1 x 10^{10} cells/ml) into Peyer's patches (PP; 5-10 µl SRBC/PP; 15-20 PP/animal). For reproductive tract immunizations, uterine horns were exposed by a suprapubic incision. Following intraluminal instillation of 20-25 µl of packed SRBC into uterine horns with a 27 gauge needle, the utero-cervical junction was doubly ligated to prevent leakage. Vaginae of all rats were flushed with saline prior to hormone treatment as described previously (16). At the time of sacrifice, vaginal secretions were collected prior to anesthesia by flushing with saline (0.2 ml). Animals were anesthetized with sodium pentobarbital (60 mg/kg body weight, Abbott Laboratories, Chicago, IL) and injected with pilocarpine (1.0 mg/rat; Sigma Chemical Co., St. Louis, MO) to stimulte saliva flow. Saliva was collected from the oral cavity. Blood was collected by direct cardiac puncture, allowed to clot (1 h at room temperature followed by 24 h at 3°C) and then centrifuged (20,000 xg for 4 min) to collect serum. Following vascular perfusion with saline, uterine secretions were obtained by luminal flushing as described previously (9).

Radioimmunoassays to measure IgA and IgG antibodies specifically directed against SRBC were developed using purified mouse monoclonal anti-rat IgA (17) and heavy-chain specific goat anti-rat IgG (Miles Laboratories, Elkhart, IN) which was further purified by Protein A chromatography. Specificity of antibodies was demonstrated by immunoelectrophoresis and radioimmunoassay criteria. Both antibodies were iodinated by the Iodo-GEN method (13). To measure IgA and IgG antibodies, secretions or sera were diluted in Dulbecco's buffer (PBS/BPA; 0.15 M NaCl, 2.7 mM KCl, 1.5 mM $KH_2 PO_4$, 6.5 mM $Na_2 HPO_4$, pH 7.1) containing bovine plasma albumin (1 mg/ml). Samples (50 µl) were incubated for 1 h at room temperature with SRBC (100 µl, 1×10^9 cells/tube) in Eppendorf tubes on a vibrator mixer. Following incubation, tubes were centrifuged (3,000 x g for 6 sec), supernatants were removed, and cells were washed by vortex resuspension with 1 ml PBS/BPA. After recentrifugation and removal of wash supernatants, 100 µl of either ^{125}I labeled mouse anti-rat IgA or goat anti-rat IgG were added to the pellets. Sheep RBCs were resuspended and incubated for an additional 2 h as described above. At the completion of incubation, assay tubes were centrifuged and cells washed with either PBS/BPA (1.0 ml/tube; IgA assay) or 0.9% saline containing Tween 20 (0.05%, Sigma; IgG assay). Following a final centrifugation (12,000 x g for 2 min), cell pellets were counted in a Packard Multiprias autogamma counter (Packard Company, Downers Grove, IL). Analysis of both assays indicated that longer incubations (up to 8 h) or additional SRBC washes at each stage of the assays, did not enhance antibody binding or lower nonspecific background levels.

For each assay, unlabeled antibody (anti-IgA or -IgG) was added to radiolabeled antibody to cause a 20% displacement of iodinated material from SRBC pretreated with IgA or IgG antibodies. Prior to analysis of each experimental unknown (uterine fluid, serum, etc.), a pooled sample was serially diluted in PBS/BPA and analyzed to ensure that antibody levels fell on the linear portion of the assay curve. Statistical analysis was performed by utilizing the Student's _t_ test.

RESULTS

Estradiol regulation of immunoglobulin levels in the female genital tract

Figure 1 shows the effect of estradiol on immunoglobulin A and G levels in uterine and vaginal secretions of adult-ovariectomized rats. As we

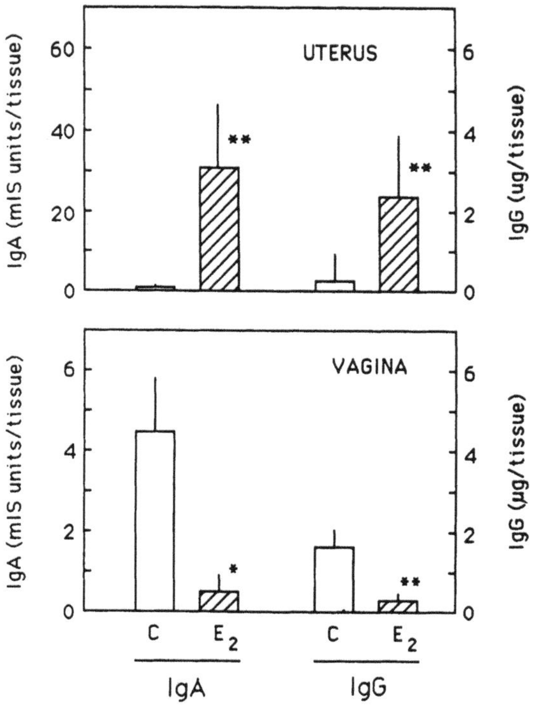

Figure 1. The influence of estradiol on Immunoglobulin A and G levels in uterine and vaginal secretions. Ovariectomized rats were injected with estradiol (1 µg/day) or saline for 3 days prior to sacrifice 24 h after the third injection. Each bar represents the mean value of 5-7 animals per group. The vertical line on each bar represents the standard error (SE). *Significantly different ($p < 0.05$) from control (saline). **Significantly different ($p < 0.01$) from control.

have reported previously (8,9), in the absence of estradiol (controls), very little if any, IgA and IgG can be measured in uterine secretions. With hormone treatment, uterine levels are markedly elevated (10-20 fold) when estradiol is administered at doses comparable to those measured during the estrous cycle. Of special interest was our finding that estradiol had an opposite effect on immunoglobulin levels in vaginal secretions. As seen in Figure 1, estradiol reduced the levels of both IgA and IgG in vaginal secretions relative to saline-injected controls. In other studies, we have found that this effect is separate and distinct from that observed in the uterus (16).

The role of estradiol in the presence of specific antibodies in genital tract secretions following Peyer's patch and uterine immunization

Studies from several laboratories have shown that oral immunization can give rise to the presence of antibodies at several mucosal surfaces (18)

including the female reproductive tract (7). Our approach in the present experiments was to determine whether gastrointestinal immunization would result in the presence of IgA- and IgG-specific antibodies in the rat and to establish the role of estradiol in regulating their presence in genital tract secretions. We utilized the experimental approach of Andrew and Hall (18) and injected sheep erythrocytes (SRBC) into Peyer's patches. This approach elicits antibody responses in bile and sera that are comparable to feeding SRBC but results in less variation within groups. As seen in Figure 2, Peyer's patch primary immunization and boost (PP/PP) followed by estradiol treatment for 3 days prior to sacrifice resulted in a marked accumulation of both SRBC-specific IgA an IgG antibodies in uterine secretions. In the absence of estradiol, specific antibody levels were either low or absent. In time course studies (not shown), we have found that the magnitude of this estradiol effect varies with the time after secondary immunization. The presence of antibodies was also determined following primary immunization to Peyer's patches followed by a boost to the uterus

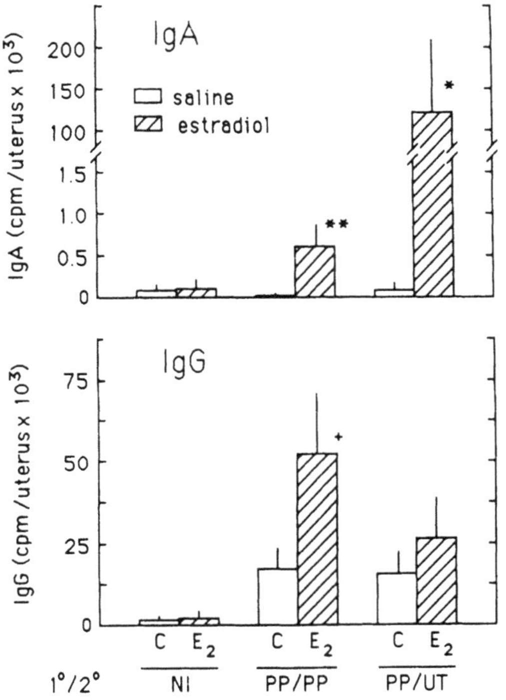

Figure 2. Effect of estradiol on uterine levels of IgA and IgG antibodies to SRBC following primary Peyer's patch and secondary Peyer's patch or uterine immunization. Ovariectomized animals received secondary immunization 13 days after initial exposure. Each animal received 3 daily treatments of estradiol (1 μg/day) or saline and was killed 24 h after the last injection. The time of sacrifice was 13 days after the secondary immunization. Each bar represents the mean $\pm$ SE (4 animals/group). *Significantly greater ($p < 0.05$) than control. ($\pm$) Significantly greater ($p < 0.06$) than control. **Significantly greater ($p < 0.02$) than control.

(PP/UT). Under these conditions, we found that uterine IgA antibody levels following estradiol treatment were significantly higher than control animals. No differences, however, were observed in uterine IgG antibody levels following estradiol treatment of PP/UT immunized animals. In other studies (not shown), however, we have found that IgG antibody levels are sometimes higher than controls. Of particular interest was our finding that IgG, but not IgA, antibodies were present in the uterine lumina of both PP/PP and PP/UT immunized animals in the absence of estradiol. One explanation for this may be that our assay measured only those uterine IgG antibodies that are not destroyed or cleared as a part of the genital tract response to intraluminal instillation of SRBC. Since SRBC in the uterine lumen following PP/UT immunization are lysed, our measurements of IgG antibody levels most likely represent an underestimation of IgG present.

To determine whether specific antibodies appear in the vagina following Peyer's patch immunization, vaginal secretions were also analyzed. As illustrated in Figure 3, IgA and IgG antibodies againt SRBC were measured in the vaginae of rats following both PP/PP and PP/UT immunization. In contrast

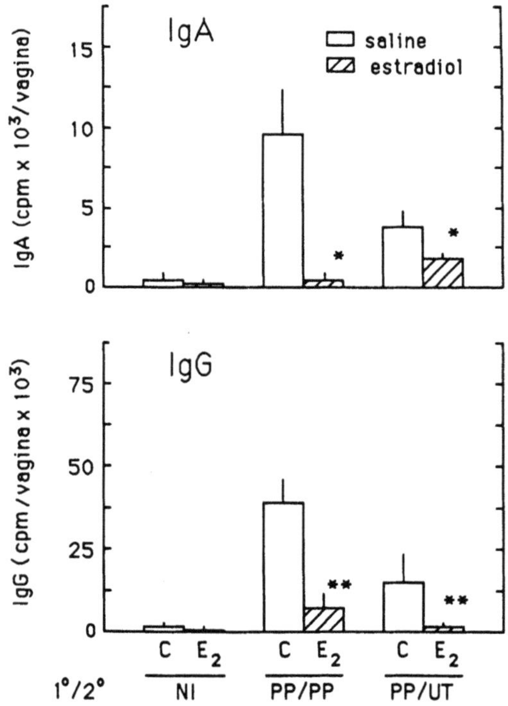

Figure 3. Vaginal IgA and IgG antibody levels in ovariectomized rats immunized with SRBC as described in Fig. 1. Vaginal flushings were collected 24 h after the third injection of estradiol (1 μg/day for 3 days) just prior to sacrifice. Bars represent mean $\pm$ SE. *Significantly lower ($p < 0.05$) than saline-treated groups. **Significantly lower ($p < 0.03$) than saline-treated animals.

to the uterus, levels of vaginal IgA- and IgG-anti SRBC antibodies were either markedly reduced or not detectable following estradiol administration. In other studies (not shown), we have observed that estradiol has a suppressive effect on vaginal IgA and IgG antibodies following primary as well as secondary immunization.

DISCUSSION

Previous studies from our laboratory have shown that IgA and IgG in the female reproductive tract are under hormonal control and that, depending on the tissue examined, estradiol may have either stimulatory (uterus) or inhibitory (vagina) effects (19). The present study extends these observations in two ways. First, by utilizing the approach of Peyer's patch immunization, it demonstrates that at least some of the immunoglobulins present in uterine and vaginal secretions are of gastrointestinal origin. Second, it indicates that estradiol, in addition to regulating total immunoglobulin levels in the genital tract, markedly influences the presence of specific gut-derived IgA and IgG antibodies in uterine and vaginal secretions.

The mechanisms that lead to antibodies in uterine and vaginal secretions are probably unique for each class of immunoglobulin. Our earlier observations as well as those of others have shown that IgA-lymphocytes concentrate in the uterus in response to estradiol (12) and migrate from mesenteric lymph nodes to the reproductive tract during the estrous cycle (20). More recently, we have experimentally induced elevated serum polymeric IgA levels by portocaval anastomosis and failed to see an estradiol-stimulated increase in uterine IgA levels beyond that present in sham-operated animals (21). If uterine polymeric IgA was of serum origin, then we would have expected to see a rise in uterine IgA levels comparable to those seen in serum. These studies suggest that uterine IgA is not derived from serum but most likely due to local synthesis, derived at least in part, from the gastrointestinal tract. In contrast, we have previously shown that in response to estradiol, IgG is transferred from blood to tissue to lumen at a time that coincides with estradiol stimulation of fluid inbibition (13,14). Our inability to detect IgG lymphocytes further suggests that IgG antibodies are not synthesized locally, but rather are of serum origin (12). Studies are presently underway to clarify the mechanism(s) involved in IgA and IgG antibody accumulation in the genital tract.

Immune responsiveness in the female genital tract can be elicited by both oral immunization and direct instillation of antigen into the genital tract. In response to intrauterine, intravaginal and oral immunization of human volunteers with inactivated poliovaccine, Ogra et al. (7) obtained evidence for both gastrointestinal tract induced and local immunity in the genital tract. More recent studies have confirmed these observations and demonstrated that both oral immunization and vaginal application of antigen can either confer protection against venereal pathogens (6,22-24) or result in problems of infertility (25). Our study demonstrates that immune responsiveness in the female reproductive tract is unique in its sensitivity to female reproductive hormonal changes. Further, it indicates that estradiol acts through different mechanisms in different parts of the genital tract to selectively stimulate as well as suppress antibody levels following gastrointestinal immunization.

These findings have practical implications with regard to the possible treatment and/or prevention of venereal disease. A large body of information clearly has shown that venereal diseases have increased 10-15 fold over the past two decades (1,2). Despite extensive studies to prepare vaccines, much still remains to be done to elicit an effective response and confer lasting protection. Our studies indicate that experimental protocols need to include factors such as site of immunization and endocrine balance at the time of secretion sampling. Recognizing that hormones play an important role in regulating the genital tract immune system, an awareness of endocrine influences on immune responsiveness during the menstrual cycle or during endocrine therapy, is essential to the effective use of potential vaccines.

CONCLUSIONS

1. Immunization via the gastrointestinal tract of rats results in the appearance of SRBC specific antibodies in secretions of the uterus and vagina.

2. The presence of these antibodies is dependent on estradiol. In the absence of this hormone, vaginal IgA and IgG antibodies are present, while antibodies in uterine secretions are very low or cannot be detected. With estradiol treatment, uterine antibody levels increase markedly, while vaginal levels are inhibited.

3. These findings indicate that immunization route, hormone balance and site of antibody recovery are critical factors when eliciting an antibody response in the female reproductive tract.

ACKNOWLEDGEMENTS

This investigation was supported by U.S.P.H.S. research grant AI 13541.

REFERENCES

1. Weisner, P.L., in Sexually Transmitted Diseases, NIH Publication #81, 2213, 21, 1980.
2. Becker, T.M., Stone, K.M. and Cates, W., Jr., Reprod. Med. 31, 359, 1986.
3. Franciosi, R.A., Knostman, J.D. and Fummerman, R.A., J. Pediat. 82, 707, 1973.
4. Tomasi, T. and Bienenstock, J., Adv. Immunol. 9, 1, 1968.
5. Tourville, D., Ogra, S., Lippes, J. and Tomasi, T., Am. J. Obstet. Gynecol. 108, 1102, 1970.
6. Chipperfield, E.J. and Evans, B.A., Infect. Immunity 11, 215, 1975.
7. Ogra, P. and Ogra, S.S., J. Immunol. 110, 1307, 1973.
8. Wira, C.R. and Sandoe, C.P., Nature 268, 534, 1977.
9. Wira, C.R. and Sandoe, C.P., Endocrinol. 106, 1020, 1980.
10. Sullivan, D.A., Underdown, B.J. and Wira, C.R., Immunol. 49, 379, 1983.
11. Sullivan, D.A., Richardson, G.S., MacLaughlin, D.T. and Wira, C.R., J. Steroid Biochem. 20, 509, 1984.
12. Wira, C.R., Hyde, E., Sandoe, C.P., Sullivan, D. and Spencer, S., J. Steroid Biochem. 12, 451, 1980.
13. Sullivan, D.A. and Wira, C.R., Endocrinol. 112, 260, 1983.
14. Sullivan, D.A. and Wira, C.R., Endocrinol. 114, 650, 1984.
15. Wira, C.R., Sullivan, D.A. and Sandoe, C.P., J. Steroid Biochem. 19, 469, 1983.
16. Wira, C.R. and Sullivan, D.A., Biol. Reprod. 32, 90, 1985.
17. Sullivan, D.A., Colby, E., Hann, L., Allansmith, M.R. and Wira, C.R., Immunol. Invest. 15, 311, 1986.
18. Andrew, E. and Hall, J.G., Immunol. 45, 169, 1982.
19. Wira, C.R., Sullivan, D.A. and Sandoe, C.P., Ann. N.Y. Acad. Sci. 409, 534, 1983.

20. McDermott, M.R., Clark, D.A. and Bienenstock, J., J. Immunol. 124, 2536, 1980.

21. Wira, C.R. and Stern, J., J. Steroid Biochem. 24, 33, 1986.

22. Sturn, B. and Schneweis, K.-E., Med. Microbiol. Immunol. 165, 119, 1978.

23. Yang, S.-L. and Schumacher, G., Fert. Steril. 32, 588, 1979.

24. McDermott, M.R., Smiley, J.R., Brais, L.J., Rudzroga, H.E. and Bienenstock, J., J. Virology 51, 747, 1984.

25. Allardyce, R.A., J. Exp. Med. 159, 1548, 1984.

CHOLECYSTOKININ-INDUCED RELEASE OF IgA ANTIBODIES IN RAT INTESTINE

S. Freier, M. Eran and A. Abrahamov

Department of Pediatrics and Institute of
Gastroenterology, Shaare Zedek Hospital
Jerusalem

INTRODUCTION

It has been shown previously that the intravenous (i.v.) injection of cholecystokinin (CCK) into healthy adult volunteers will result in a rise of antibodies belonging to the A, M, E and D classes of immunoglobulins (1,2). It appeared likely that these antibodies were derived largely, if not wholly, from the gall bladder and the pancreas, as CCK is known to cause gall bladder contraction and to promote secretion of pancreatic enzymes. It could, however, not be excluded that CCK had a direct effect on the intestinal release of immunoglobulins. This report, therefore, deals with the effect of CCK on the release of IgA in an isolated perfused loop of rat intestine.

METHODS

Rats of the Hooded-Lister strain weighing 160-180 g were used. The rats were immunized by intraperitoneal injection (i.p.) of 250 μg of ovalbumin (OA) in 0.1 ml saline mixed with an equal volume of Freund's complete adjuvant. Fourteen days later, a booster injection of 10 μg OA in 0.1 ml in 0.9% NaCl mixed with an equal volume of Freund's complete adjuvant was given by the same route. On the 21st day, the rats were anesthetized with thiopentone and a loop of small intestine 10 cm distal to the pylorus and 10 cm long was severed at both end and isolated _in situ_. This loop did not, therefore, receive any biliary or pancreatic secretions but the blood supply remained intact. The loop was perfused with saline at a rate of 0.2 ml/min. After flushing the loop for 30 min, collection of specimens was begun. Two and one-half min aliquots were collected, four for base line determinations and the others after the intravenous administration of cholecystokinin octapeptide (CCK-OP) ("SINCALIDE" Squibb, Princeton, NJ). Control animals received 0.2 ml saline i.v.

Dose response curves showed that CCK-OP produces a rise of IgA antibodies at doses of 10, 20, 40 and 80 ng. The time of onset of the response and its potency were similar for all doses used, but the duration of the response was less with a dose of 10 ng. In the definitive experiments, therefore, a dose of 20 ng in 0.2 ml of normal saline was given.

The possibility of proteolytic effect was excluded by estimating total tryptic activity (3) as well as total proteolytic activity in the perfused fluid.

Enzyme linked immunosorbent assay (ELISA)

Specific anti OA-IgA antibodies (AB) were measured by the ELISA technique: Ovalbumin (Sigman Chemical Co., St. Louis, MO) was dissolved in sodium bicarbonate buffer (pH 9.6 flat bottom NUNC Immuno II, Roskilde, Denmark) were filled with 200 μl of phosphate buffered saline (PBS). The plates were left overnight at room temperature, washed 3 times with PBS-Tween "20" and dried. Then, 200 μl of the perfusion fluid was added to the wells, left at 37°C for 60 min and at room temperature overnight. The wells were again washed 3 times with PBS Tween "20" and dried. Goat anti-rat secretory IgA (Sigma Chemical Co.) in a concentration of 1:500 was added and incubated for 40 min at 37°C. The wells were washed 3 times with a solution of 0.25% BSA in PBS and dried. Alkaline phosphate anti-goat IgG (Sigma) diluted to 1:1000 in PBS with 0.5% BSA was added and left for one hour at 37°C. After 3 more washes with PBS Tween "20", diethanolamine with paranitro-phenolphosphate 1 mg/ml was added and incubated for 30 min at 37°C. The reaction was stopped by adding 50 μl of 4N NaOH and was read in a Dynatech photometer (Dynatech, Alexandria, VA) at 405 nm. All tests were run in duplicate.

As basal antibody levels varied between rats, all results were expressed as percentages. The mean of four 2.5 min aliquots, during the baseline period was designated 100%. Subsequent readings in O.D. were compared with this baseline and expressed as a percentage of it. For each group, therefore, pre- and post-injection (or instillation) periods were compared, and, in addition, control and test groups were compared. The Mann-Whitney test and Student's _t_ test were used for statistical analysis.

RESULTS

The injection of CCK-OP resulted in a significant ($p < 0.001$) rise of IgA antibodies by 2.5 min and a maximum level by 5 min (Fig. 1). By 10 min, IgA antibodies were still significantly higher than in the controls ($p < 0.005$). In the control group IgA antibodies remained at baseline level in the first 2.5 min and then steadily declined.

DISCUSSION

The purpose of this experiment was to establish whether CCK accelerates the release of IgA from the gastrointestinal mucosa. From our data, it appears that this does in fact take place. The duration of the response appeared to be related to the dose. How this effect is brought about is not known. There is evidence from the literature that the injection of atropine (a cholinergic antagonist) reduces the baseline secretion of IgA by 50% (4), while the cholinergic agonists pilocarpine and bethanechol augment IgA release. It appears, therefore, that both the cholinergic

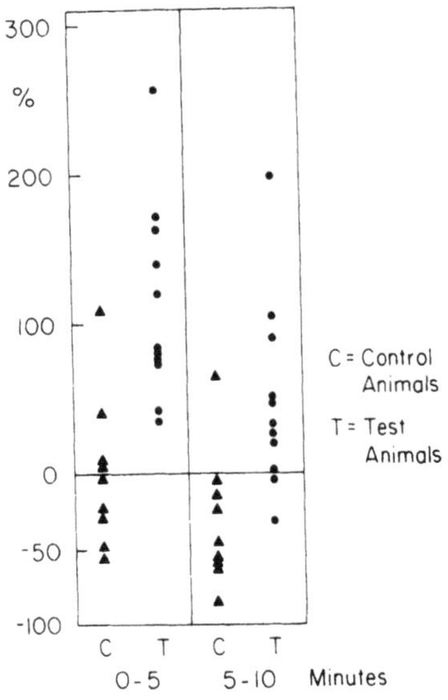

Figure 1. This figure shows the change (in percent) in IgA concentration at 5 and 10 min following injection of CCK-OP.

nervous sytem, as well as the neuromodulator CCK are involved in the rate of immunoglobulin secretion.

The mechansims of CCK-induced IgA release are not known. Several possibilities can be suggested. First, a purely mechanical effect may be at play. The antibodies detected may already have been released into the crypts and may be expressed from them by increased motility of the intestine brought about by CCK.

Second, it is possible that CCK-induced vasodilation results in immunoglublin release. It is known that CCK acts as a vasodilator in the pancreas (5).

The speed with which IgA appears in the intestine following the injection of CCK makes it unlikely that the effect observed is due to de novo synthesis in the lamina propria plasma cells. However, the possibility that CCK effects the receptor mediated transport within the enterocyte must be entertained.

Finally, a specific secretory mechanism cannot be excluded. In pancreatic acinar cells, CCK causes an outflux of intracellular calcium and stimulation of cyclic GMP (6), which is followed by pancreatic enzyme release. A similar mechanism may therefore be postulated for immunoglobulin release.

Whatever the mechanism which brings about this release of IgA, it may have physiological significance in the process of food digestion. The presence of food-specific antibodies may play a role in the immune exclusion of food at the mucosal surface. Furthermore, it may improve the efficiency of digestion of anchoring IgA food complexes to the mucosa (7).

REFERENCES

1. Shah, P.C., Freier, S., Park, B.H., Lee, P.C. and Lebenthal, E., Gastroenterology 83, 916, 1982.
2. Freier, S., Lebenthal, E., Freier, M., Shah, P.C., Park, B.H. and Lee, P.C., Immunology 49, 69, 1983.
3. Townes, P.L., J. Pediatr. 75, 221, 1969.

4. Dodd-Wilson, I., Saltis, R.D., Olson, R.E. and Erlandson, S.L., Gastroenterology 83, 881, 1982.
5. Chou, C.C., Hsieh, C.P. and Dabney, J.M., Am. J. Physiol. 232, H103, 1977.
6. Gardner, J.D. and Jensen, R.T., Am. J. Physiol. 238, 963, 1980.
7. Walker, W.A. and Isselbacher, K.J., New Engl. J. Med. 297, 767, 1977.

A MODEL FOR PANETH CELL STUDY: TISSUE CULTURE OF THE HYPERPLASTIC PANETH CELL POPULATION OF RABBIT THIRY-VELLA ILEAL LOOPS

S.E. Kern, D.F. Keren, T.F. Beals* and J. Varani

Department of Pathology, The University of Michigan Medical School; and *The Veterans Administration Medical Center, Ann Arbor, Michigan USA

INTRODUCTION

Paneth cells are characteristically located at the bases of the crypts of Lieberkühn in the small intestine and contain prominent eosinophilic granules. Early studies associated them with a digestive purpose (1,2) and Paneth cells are curiously absent from the mucosa of some carnivores (3). More recent studies have suggested an antibacterial role. The secretory granules of the Paneth cells contain lysozyme (4,5), an enzyme with antibacterial properties (6,7). With ultrastructural studies, Erlandsen identified microorganisms in stages of digestion within phagolysosomes of rat Paneth cells (8,9).

The mucosa of chronic isolated (Thiry-Vella) ileal loops in rabbits is characterized by marked villus atrophy, increased crypt depth, and prominent Paneth cell hyperplasia (10). We took advantage of the increased numbers of Paneth cells in this preparation to enrich for Paneth cells in tissue cultures prepared from the mucosa of these loops. These cultures were studied by light and electron microscopy.

MATERIALS AND METHODS

Tissue culture technique

Thiry-Vella loops were created in female New Zealand white rabbits as previously described (10). After at least two weeks (necessary for development of Paneth cell hyperplasia), rabbits were sacrificed, and the loops removed. One loop was adequate for a tissue culture preparation. Each loop was inverted by forceps to expose the mucosa. Visible mucus was removed by blotting. The inverted loop was cut in 3 cm lengths, and trypsinized in two 50 ml changes of trypsinizing solution containing 0.25% trypsin (1:250, Difco, Detroit), 15 mM HEPES buffer (Research Organics, Inc., Cleveland), 500 units/ml penicillin G (Pfizer, New York), and 20 μg/ml gentamycin (Schering Pharmaceuticals, Kenilworth, NJ) in balanced salt solution. The trypsin digests were filtered through cotton gauze and then through 110 μm nylon mesh, to remove aggregates of tissue and mucus. The filtrate was centrifuged at 400 x g for 10 min, and the pellet resuspended in 32 ml of culture medium composed of RPMI 1640 (Gibco, Grand Island, NY) with 10% fetal calf serum, 20 μg/ml gentamycin, and 1% antibiotic-antimycotic (Gibco). Three ml of this plating solution were added to each 35 mm tissue culture dish (Corning, Corning, NY). Placement of sterile glass coverslips in the culture dishes did not affect numbers of cells attaching, and allowed easy removal and handling for light microscopy. Hemocytometer and Coulter counts were done on the plating solution. The tissue cultures were incubated at 37°C in a 5% CO_2/95% air atmosphere. Culture medium was changed every two days.

Light microscopic and ultrastructural studies

Human and rabbit normal ileum, formalin-fixed and paraffin-embedded, were stained with various histologic techniques, as were coverslips from tissue cultures.

Intact normal ileum, Thiry-Vella loops, trypsin digests and tissue cultures were fixed in formaldehyde-glutaraldehyde (Tousimis, Rockville, MD), for examination by transmission electron microscopy (TEM). Postfixation in 1% osmium tetroxide (with potassium ferrocyanide) was followed with *en bloc* uranyl acetate staining. Dehydration in increasing concentrations of ethanol was followed by propylene oxide as a transition to a mixture of Araldite and Poly/Bed 812 monomers (Polysciences, Warrington, PA). Polymerization of the plastic was at 65°C. Thin sections were stained with both lead citrate and uranyl acetate. Tissue cultures were studied at days 1, 4, and 9.

RESULTS

Tissue culture technique

Histologic study of the trypsinized rabbit loop ileum revealed three hour trypsinization to effect digestion of most of the lamina propria, without significant digestion of muscularis mucosa, serosa, or intervening layers. Hemocytometer counts on plating solution generally revealed a total yield of 80-160 million nucleated cells. Coulter counts after hemolysin treatment were considerably higher, attributable to tissue and mucus debris. Cell viability was consistently 90% or greater by trypan blue exclusion. (EDTA as an alternative to trypsinization produced lower viability). Plating efficiency as measured by counts of attached cells in d 1 culture varied widely, but was less than 1%. Cultures were proliferating on d 4, and confluent epithelioid (as opposed to fibroblast-like) cultures, when present, developed by d 9.

Light microscopic studies

H & E stained d 1 cultures on glass coverslips contained a mixed cell population (Fig. 1). While polymorphonuclear cells were the major population, mononuclear cells with prominent eosinophilic granules were numerous, some closely resembling Paneth cells (Fig. 1, inset). The heterophils and eosinophils of the rabbit also contain eosinophilic granules, and although nuclear characteristics were often helpful, we could not always distinguish between these two cell types. Large spreading cells, probably macrophages, often contained phagocytized debris which caused their phagolysosomes to be eosinophilic, as evidenced by the common finding of phagocytosis of entire heterophils. The thickness of many cells and the frequent occurrence of cytoplasmic blebs further impaired distinctions between heterophils, macrophages and Paneth cells.

Other staining techniques were studied in an attempt to specifically identify Paneth cells. Masson's trichrome, phosphotungstic acid-hematoxylin, and periodic acid Schiff-Alcian blue were not specific for Paneth granules. Beibrich scarlet at pH = 8.7, and phloxine-tartrazine each specifically stained Paneth granules in human tissue, but not in rabbit tissue. Anti-human lysozyme did not stain rabbit Paneth cells; while we did not have an anti-rabbit lysozyme available, lysozyme would not be expected to be specific since macrophages also contain the enzyme. Staining with unconjugated rhodamine at 3 μg/ml combined with fluorescence microscopy was the most useful method in identifying Paneth cells in both formalin-fixed

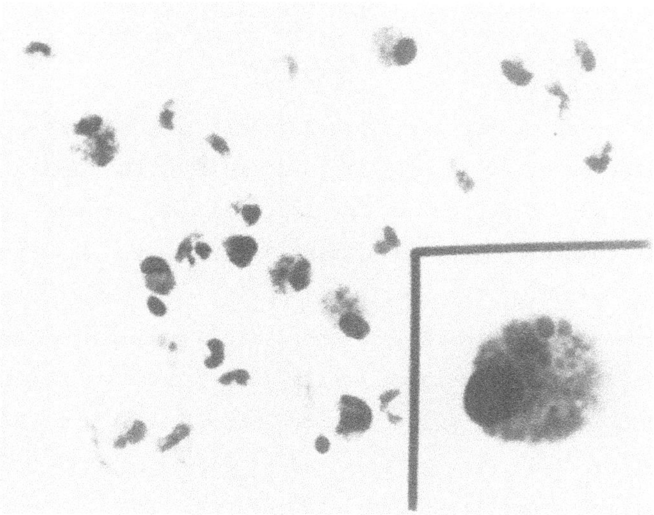

Figure 1. Day one tissue cultures contain a mixed cell population. (H & E, x330) Inset: The large cells of early cultures often resemble Paneth cells, with prominent eosinophilic granules and a single eccentric round nucleus. (H & E, x1320)

paraffin-embedded sections and in cytologic preparations; rhodamine stained rabbit Paneth granules more reliably than eosin, but the staining was not entirely specific.

Ultrastructural studies

Paneth cells had ultrastructural characteristics which allowed their identification (Fig. 2). Paneth cells contain prominent secretory granules which could be distinguished from lipid granules. Rough endoplasmic reticulum was abundant and Golgi complexes were numerous. Electron-dense inclusions were present within phagolysosomes, but this feature was not specific, as we found similar inclusions within lamina propria macrophages. Desmosomes joined Paneth cells.

We identified Paneth cells in the trypsin digest, and in d 1 and d 4 cultures (Figs. 3 and 4). In culture, Paneth cells exhibited microvilli, or a ruffled or smooth surface. Although confluent d 9 cultures contained cells with few small eosinophilic granules, the cells in these older cultures showed no differentiating ultrastructural features. Many polymorphonuclear cells were found to contain crystalline (or rod-like) inclusions within their granules, and were common in d 1 cultures. Some macrophages of d 1 or d 4 cultures contained ingested cells within phagolysosomes. Mucus-secreting cells, erythrocytes, fibroblasts, as well as many degenerating cells, were present within d 1 cultures.

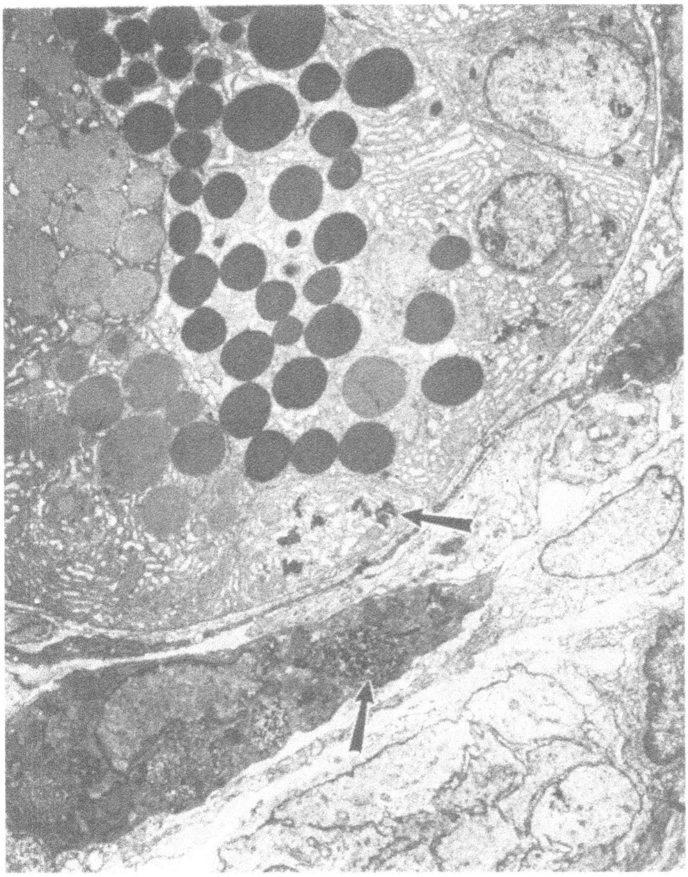

Figure 2. Ultrastructure of the base of a crypt. Paneth cells with prominent apical secretory granules and a single basal nucleus occupy most of the field. Electron dense inclusions (arrows) are present within both Paneth cells and lamina propria macrophages (TEM, x4200).

DISCUSSION

Paneth cells are known to secrete lysozyme (4,5) and to phagocytize microorganisms (8,9), and a significant role for them in regulating the microbial flora of the intestinal crypts has been postulated (8). Other possible functions have also been proposed, such as roles in zinc or amino acid metabolism (11). Generally, Paneth cell research has been hampered by both the difficulty of studying intact bowel, and the inability to demonstrate them in tissue culture or isolate them for other *in vitro* studies.

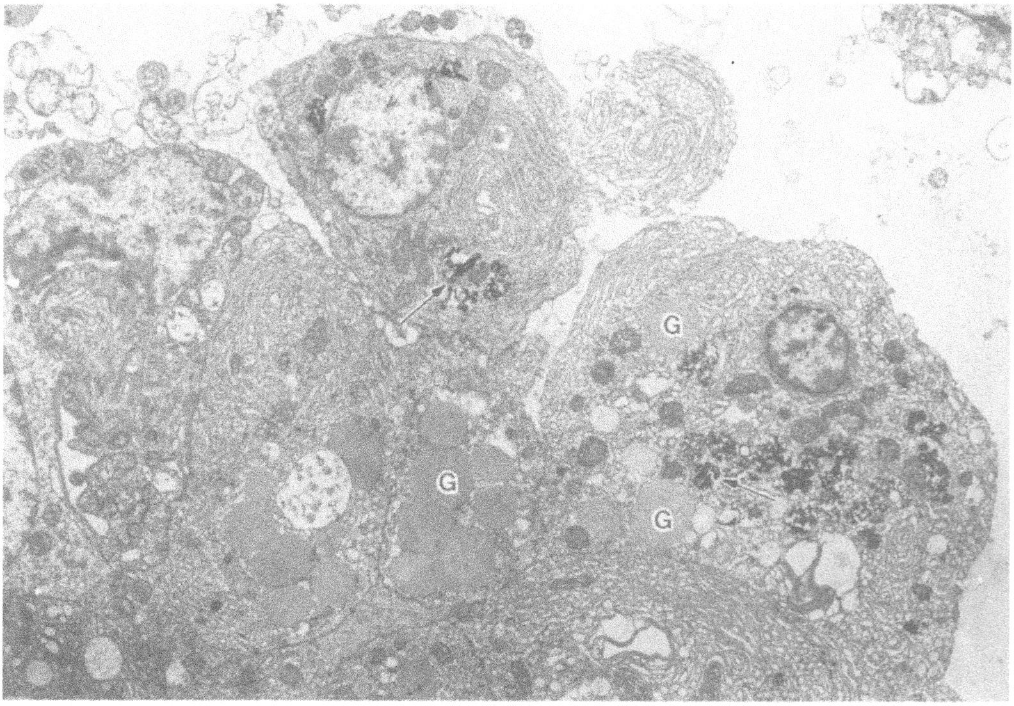

Figure 3. Trypsin digest contains Paneth cells both in aggregates (shown here) and as single cells. Granules (G) and electron dense inclusions (arrows). (TEM, x6880)

Using the hyperplastic Paneth cell population of the rabbit Thiry-Vella loop model, we have been able to identify Paneth cells ultrastructurally in trypsin digests of the ileal mucosa, as well as in d 1 and d 4 tissue culture. Due to the undifferentiated appearance of older cultures, it is anticipated that future <u>in vitro</u> studies of Paneth cells will make greatest use of their presence in the trypsin digests and acute cultures. Day 1 cultures may have an advantage over fresh digest in that residual mucus can be washed from the attached cells, allowing improved conditions for cell separation techniques.

Paneth cells are readily distinguished from other cell types in routine histologic preparations, but in tissue culture the light microscopic appearance does not allow satisfactory distinction between cell types. Rabbit Paneth cells, heterophils, eosinophils, and macrophages can overlap in appearance, and both artifacts of fixation and dead cells are associated with eosinophilic granularity. Although other investigations have described a variety of histochemical stains for Paneth cells in humans and rats, we have not found any of these to be specific for identification of rabbit

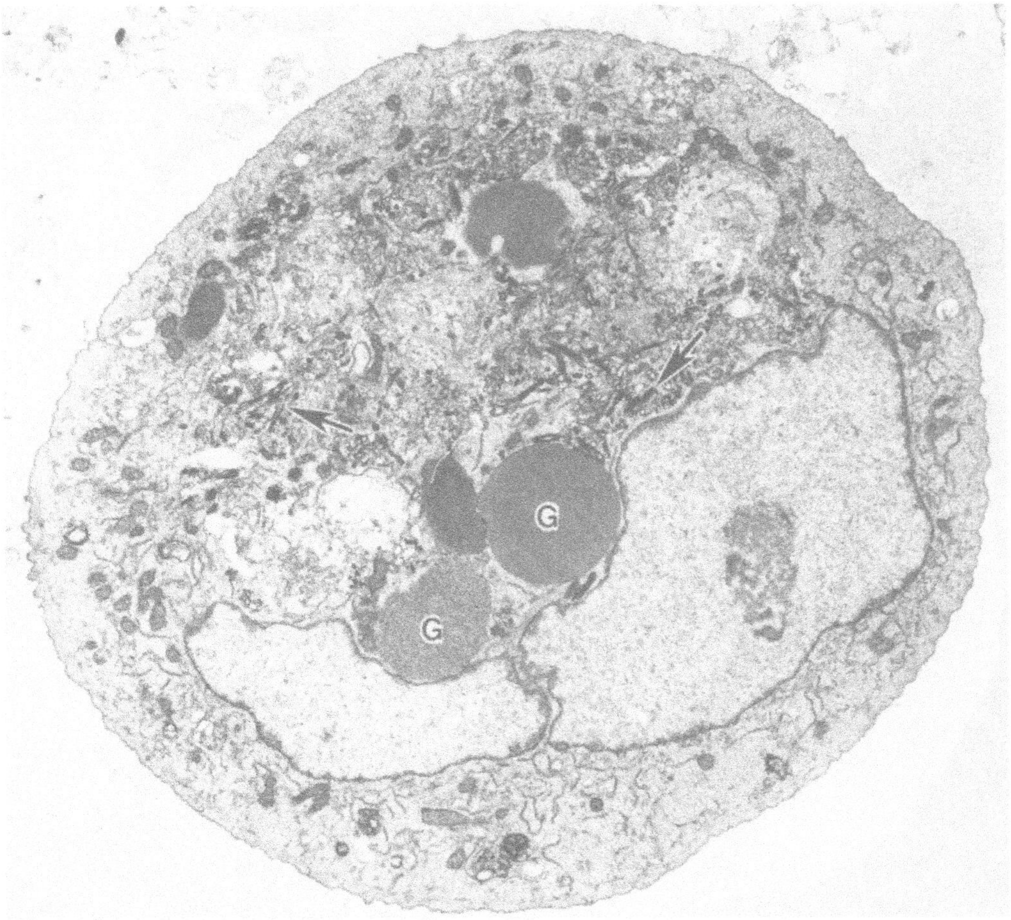

Figure 4. Paneth cells from a d 4 culture. Both secretory granules (G) and the distinctive inclusions (arrows) are present. (TEM, x9700)

Paneth cells. Transmission electron microscopy (TEM) was able to demonstrate the Paneth cells in our preparations. TEM, however, is time consuming and impractical for many types of studies. Nonetheless, it allows us to demonstrate the *in vitro* viable Paneth cells. The recent findings of trypsin immunoreactivity in human Paneth cells (12) and of intestinal phospholipase A2 immunoreactivity in rat Paneth cells (13) may offer a useful new approach. We are also interested in developing a monoclonal antibody specific for the rabbit Paneth cells.

The present work demonstrates that Paneth cells can be isolated from the intestine and remain viable for at least four days in tissue culture. Further purification of these cell populations will allow functional studies to be performed *in vitro*.

CONCLUSIONS

1. Chronically isolated ileal loops of rabbits show Paneth cells hyperplasia, increase in crypt depth, and villus atrophy. An assortment of viable cells can be harvested from this mucosa by trypsinization.

2. These trypsinized cells will attach and remain viable in tissue culture. Numerous cells can be identified as Paneth cells by transmission electron microscopic study of fresh trypsin harvest of d 4 culture.

ACKOWLEDGEMENTS

This study was supported in part by U.S. Army Medical Research Grant DAMD-17-80-C-0113. Presented, in part, at the 73rd Annual meeting of the International Academy of Pathology in San Francisco, CA, March, 1984.

REFERENCES

1. Genderen, H.V. and Engel, C., Enzymologia 5, 71, 1938.
2. Klein, S., Am. J. Anat. 5, 315, 1906.
3. Wheeler, E.J. and Wheeler, J.K., Abstract, Anat. Rec. 148, 350, 1964.
4. Speece, A.J., J. Histochem. Cytochem. 12, 384, 1964.
5. Ghoos, Y. and Vantrappen, G., Histochem. J. 3, 175, 1971.
6. Amano, T., Inai, S., Seki, Y., Kashiba, S., Fujikawa, K. and Nishimura, S., Med. J. Osaka, Univ. 4, 401, 1954.
7. Noller, E.C. and Hartsell, S.E., J. Bacteriol. 81, 482, 1961.
8. Erlandsen, S.L. and Chase, D.G., J. Ultrastruc. Res. 41, 296, 1972.
9. Erlandsen, S.L. and Chase, D.G., J. Ultrastruc. Res. 41, 319, 1972.
10. Keren, D.F., Elliott, H.L., Brown, G.D., Yardley, J.H., Gastroenterology 68, 83, 1975.
11. Sandow, M.J. and Whitehead, R., Gut 20, 420, 1979.
12. Bohe, M., Borgstrom, A., Lindstrom, C. and Ohlsson, K., Digestion 30, 271, 1984.
13. Senegas-Balas, F., Falas, D., Verger, R., Histochemistry 81, 581, 1984.

ANTIGEN-INDUCED GASTRIN RELEASE: AN IMMUNOLOGIC MECHANISM OF GASTRIC ANTRAL MUCOSA

H.-J. Krämling*, G. Enders, R.K. Teichmann*, T. Demmel,
R. Merkle and W. Brendel

Department of Surgery*, Institute of Surgical Research
Klinikum Grosshadern, Ludwig-Maximilians-University
Munich, West Germany

INTRODUCTION

Recent *in vivo* experiments have shown that the intragastral application of an antigen elicits a hormonal response of gastrin-cells in systemically immunized dogs (1). Further, there was a marked stimulation of antral blood flow and production of mucus. Several factors influence the activity of the stomach *in vivo*: vagus nerve, gut peptides, acid secretion, and intramural reflexes. An *in vitro* system (cell-suspension) should eliminate these factors and demonstrate the local mechanisms of antigen specific immunologic reaction of antral mucosa.

The purpose of this study was to show whether the immunologic stimulation of gastric functions, as shown by antigen specific gastrin release *in vivo*, is inducible in antral cell suspension and whether an early immunologic mediator like interleukin 1 is involved in this mechanism.

METHODS

Immunization

We used a synthetic antigen, 4-hydroxy-3-iodo-5-nitrophenylacetic acid (NIP) to avoid interference with known antigenic structures of protein sequences. Male Wistar-rats received 1 mg NIP-OVA (Ovalbumin) in 1 ml CFA (complete Freund adjuvant) i.p. initially. The animals were boosted weekly 3-4 times. For the experiments NIP was conjugated with human gamma globulin (HGG).

Preparation of cell suspension

Under ether anesthesia, stomaches of 4 rats were removed. Antral portions were everted to little sacs and filled with buffer (Hanks' balanced salt solution) containing pronase 7 mg/ml. After 4 incubation steps of 30 min each in Ca^{++}-, Mg^{++}-free buffer with EDTA (2 mMol/l) cells of the fourth step were separated, washed, counted (30-40 x 10^6 cells) and distributed into reaction tubes (1 x 10^6 cells). The substance to be tested was added to these tubes and after an incubation period of 15 min the supernatant was taken for the measurement of gastrin by radioimmunoassay.

Stimulating agent used was NIP, conjugated with human gammaglobulin (NIP-HGG - 100 µg/ml), which served as carrier protein to avoid interference with ovalbumin, used in immunization. An interleukin 1 preparation made from peritoneal macrophages of Wistar-rats was added in concentrations of 0.1 - 1 - 10 U/ml. Controls were: HGG (100 µg/ml), lipopolysaccharide (LPS) (100 µg/ml) and in nonimmunized rats NIP-HGG (100 µg/ml).

RESULTS

Viability of cells in suspension always exceeded 90% as determined by trypan blue exclusion. 10^6 cells of immunized animals produced considerable amounts of gastrin after incubation with the antigen. The gastrin response differed significantly from basal level: 142 $\pm$ 23 basal, 274 $\pm$ 60 pg/ml stimulated ($\pm$ SEM, n = 12, $p < 0.05$). This increase was antigen specific as shown by incubation of the cells with the carrier protein HGG alone and of cells from nonimmunized rats with NIP-HGG.

To test an early immune mediator we used various concentrations of an interleukin 1 preparation. A dose-dependent gastrin release from isolated antral cells was elicited. Even in a ten fold concentration, LPS, taken as a stimulant for the interleukin 1 preparation produced only a small and not significant release of gastrin.

Table 1. Dose-dependent gastrin release by stimulation with interleukin 1 in antral cell suspension

Interleukin 1 (U/ml)	Ø	0.1	1	10
Gastrin (pg/ml)	95 ± 26	226 ± 46[a]	792 ± 100[b]	1344 ± 226[b]

[a] $p < 0.05$
[b] $p < 0.001$

DISCUSSION

Using a clearly defined *in vitro* model of isolated antral cells from rats, an antigen-dependent gastrin response could be elicited. This confirms the *in vivo* effects of intragastral antigen application in immunized dogs. As histology of antral mucosa shows macrophages and other immunocompetent cells in the neighborhood of the crypts, interleukin 1 might serve as mediator. We found a dramatic increase of gastrin in a dose-dependent manner after stimulation with interleukin 1.

The secretion of gastrin in response to antigen and interleukin 1 gives evidence of a local immune mechanism in antral mucosa, which recognizes antigens and is linked functionally with the endocrine system.

REFERENCES

1. Teichmann, R.K., Andress, H.J., Gycha, S., Seifert, J., Brendel, W., Gastroenterology 84, 1333, 1983.

IMMUNOCYTOCHEMICAL MARKERS FOR HUMAN MILK MACROPHAGES AND EPITHELIAL CELLS

H. Liapis, M. Xanthou and H. Mandyla

B' Neonatal Intensive Care Unit of "Aghia Sophia"
Children's Hospital and Immunology Department of
1st Pediatric Clinic of Athens University
Athens, Greece

INTRODUCTION

Most of the cellular elements obtained from colostrum and early human milk are considered to be macrophages. A varying number of polymorphonuclear leukocytes and a small number of epithelial cells are also present. The morphologic distinction of epithelial cells within the macrophage population and routine staining is extremely difficult. A number of histochemical stains (nonspecific esterase, acid phosphatase, oil red, etc.) have been used in the past to further characterize the cellular population of human milk. Distinction, though, between the macrophages and the epithelial cells on a cytochemical basis has proved to be impossible (1).

In this study, we used four commercially available antisera to lysozyme, α_1-antitrypsin, keratin and α-lactalbumin in an indirect immunoperoxidase procedure to investigate the presence of the specific antigens on these cells. The existence of these antigens detected by immunostaining could help us to differentiate the human milk cell populations. In addition we could probably gain further information about the site of origin of these cells.

MATERIALS AND METHODS

We selected 20 samples of human milk. Fifteen of these were collected within the first week of lactation and the remaining five during the 3rd and 4th week.

The milk cells were obtained by centrifugation at 400 x g and subsequent washing with PBS. Samples of the cells were prepared by cytocentrifugation.

The cells were fixed in a H_2O_2-methanol solution for 5 min (Fixative: 50 ml 30% hydrogen peroxidase plus 200 ml methanol). This fixative was chosen to reduce the endogenous peroxidase activity. The cell pellet was circled with diamond pencil and the glass slides were stored in -20°C.

Four antisera used were purchased from Dakopatts (Glostrup, Denmark):

	(working dilution)
alpha-1-antitrypsin Cat No A012	1:50
lysozyme (muramidase) Cat No A099	1:50
keratin Cat No A575	1:100
alpha-lactalbumin Cat No A579	1:100

Dako's universal kit was used for the indirect immunoperoxidase procedure. The primary antibodies were incubated for 30 min. The slides were counterstained with Harris Hematoxylin (alcohol free) and mounted with glycerol. Paraffin-embedded tissues from normal tonsil, normal skin and fibrocystic disease of the breast were used as positive and negative controls. In addition, in each milk sample, one slide was used as negative control (the primary antibody was eliminated in order to be able to observe the amount of background staining). The immunoperoxidase slides (PAP) were contrasted to one stained with May Grünwald.

RESULTS

Alpha-1-antitrypsin and lysozyme marked 10-15% of cells with irregular, moderately condensed nuclei and with foamy abundant cytoplasm which contained numerous cytoplasmic vacuoles. These cells were considered to be macrophages. The staining ranged from moderate to strong within the same cell and between different cells. Some cells were stained diffusely and others only focally. Acellular material outside these cells stained weakly.

Alpha-1-antitrypsin and lysozyme also marked the majority of polymorphonuclear neutrophils in human milk.

Alpha-lactalbumin stained strongly and diffusely cells with round nuclei and fine chromatin which appear to be in clusters and have a moderate amount of cytoplasm. These cells were assumed to be breast epithelial cells. We were able to find 0-4% of these cells in the milk of the first week following lactation and up to 44% in the milk obtained during the third and fourth weeks.

Keratin marked (a) the skin keratinocytes characterized by small centrally located nucleus and abundant smooth cytoplasm and (b) the breast epithelial cells. The staining was strong and diffuse throughout these cells. All the immunoperoxidase slides had very little background staining.

DISCUSSION

Considerable information has been accumulated during the last years about the functional and metabolic differences that exist among human mononuclear phagocytes isolated from different anatomic sites. This heterogeneity may reflect the influence of environmental factors that stimulate circulating monocytes to differentiate in a distinctive manner, or may suggest the existence of predetermined subjects of macrophage precursors (2). Macrophage diversity at the membrane level is also being currently investigated by defining the expression of antigenic determinants on the surface of these cells (3). Regarding human milk macrophages, monoclonal antibodies hae been applied to distinguish them by Leyva-Cobian and Clemente (4). They found that the majority of these macrophages stain for the monocyte antigen OKM_1 (4). Furthermore, Taylor-Papadimitriou et al. (5) found monoclonal antibodies raised against the human fat globule to characterize the epithelial cells in the lactating breast. In order to further differentiate human milk cells we used antisera to lysozyme, α_1-antitrypsin, α-lactalbumin and keratin.

Lysozyme and α_1-antitrypsin are considered good histiocytic "markers". Lysozyme is found in the sinus histiocytes of lymph nodes while α_1-antitrypsin in histiocytes of lymph nodes and liver. In addition, lysozyme stains the monocytoid cells of the bone marrow. As such markers, they have been used in the characterization of histiocytic tumors (6,7).

We used these two markers in the human milk cell population in order to investigate probable differences in the presence of the two antigens. However, no differences were found. In addition, most of the cells presumed to be macrophages did not stain with either antisera. We assume that the negative staining indicates an absence of the corresponding antigens, however the absence of these antigens is not understood. To our knowledge, there is still a question of differences in the production of lysozyme by macrophages in different stages of maturation (8). It is possible that such differences exist and relate to the appearance of the specific antigens. The same probably applies for α_1-antitrypsin.

No conclusion about the origin of macrophages could be drawn using these two markers.

It is interesting that the majority of polymorphonuclear neutrophils in human milk stain with both lysozyme and α_1-antitrypsin. This knowledge is useful when trying to differentiate cell populations in human milk using immunocytochemical techniques.

Keratins are widely distributed in the tissues and, in general, characterize epithelial cells. The antiserum we used stained both the skin and ductal epithelial cells found in human milk.

The finding that α-lactalbumin stained specifically the epithelial cells in human milk supports the concept that epithelial cells in human milk mainly originate in the mammary gland.

Finally, regarding the differential counting of the epithelial cells and macrophages in human milk the use of the above mentioned immunocytochemical method helped us to differentiate them and actually see the nuclear and cytoplasmic differences described earlier (1).

CONCLUSIONS

The application of lysozyme, α_1-antitrypsin, keratin and α-lactalbumin antisera in the immunoperoxidase (PAP) technique in human milk samples, facilitates the differential counting of the morphologically similar cells (macrophages and epithelial cells). No conclusion is drawn about the origin of macrophages, while the hypothesis of breast origin of the epithelial cells gains support.

REFERENCES

1. Ho, F.C.S., Wong, R.L.C. and Lawton, J.W.M., Acta. Pediatr. Scand. 68, 389, 1979.
2. Bursuker, I. and Goldman, R., J. Reticuloendothelial Society 33, 207, 1983.
3. Bioundi, A., Rossing, T.H., Bennett, J. and Todd, R.F., J. Immunol. 132, 1237, 1984.
4. Leyva-Cobian, F. and Clemente, J., Immunol. Lett. 8, 249, 1984.
5. Taylor-Papadimitriou, J., Peterson, J.A., Arklie, J., Burchell, J., Ceriaki, R.L. and Bodmer, W.F., Int. J. Cancer 28, 1981.
6. Borowitz, M. and Croker, B., Am. J. Clin. Pathol. 74, 501, 1980.
7. Du Boulay, C.E.H., Am. J. Surg. Pathol. 6, 559, 1982.
8. Pitt, J., Pediatrics Suppl. 64, 745, 1979.

PLEOMORPHIC ADENOMAS CONTAIN A KERATIN-NEGATIVE POPULATION OF HLA-DR-POSITIVE DENDRITIC CELLS

P.S. Thrane, L.M. Sollid, H. Huitfeldt and P. Brandtzaeg

Laboratory for Immunohistochemistry and Immunopathology (LIIPAT), Institute of Pathology, Medical Faculty, Rikshospitalet, and Department of Oral Surgery and Oral Medicine, Dental Faculty, University of Oslo, Oslo, Norway

INTRODUCTION

It is controversial whether myoepithelial cells (MEC) are a major component of pleomorphic adenomas and contribute to their complex histological picture (1-8). MEC, with their stellate appearance and elongated processes have been classified as specialized epithelial cells on the basis of ultrastructural, histochemical and immunohistochemical studies (9). Pleomorphic adenomas have been extensively studied by both ultrastructural (1,14) and immunohistochemical methods (5,7,8); recent data indicate that the principal tumor cells are modified MEC (8,14).

MEC contain keratin (6,9), vimentin (5,6,8), myosin (4), actin (8), and S-100 protein (5,8,12). We have previously shown that an antiserum reacting with a 51 kD keratin polypeptide (keratin No. 14) detects selectively MEC in fetal and adult salivary glands (15,16). This keratin should, thus, serve as a marker for the tumor population of pleomorphic adenomas.

In fetal and adult salivary glands we observed a population of dendritic cells which were positive for HLA-DR determinants; these keratin-negative cells were often located like MEC but clearly represented a separate population. Our finding of numerous DR-positive dendritic cells in pleomorphic adenomas prompted us to study whether these cells were neoplastic MEC or, instead, represented a reactive population of histiocytic cells.

MATERIALS AND METHODS

Immunohistochemistry

Tumor specimens obtained from the parotid gland of 10 patients (7 women and 3 men; median age, 55.6 years; range, 35-75 years) were immediately fixed in 96% ethanol and processed for paraffin embedding (17). Serial sections were cut at 6 μm and incubated for 20 h with various pairs of primary antibody reagents (Tables 1 and 2). Specimens from 12 normal salivary glands served as controls and were processed and examined in the same way as the tumor specimens. A parallel specimen was in each case fixed in formalin for light microscopic evaluation and for immunohistochemical staining of S-100 protein.

The different monoclonal or polyclonal antibody reagents used are listed in Table 1 and the applied combinations appear in Table 2. A three-step immunofluorescence method (18) was used as well as peroxidase anti-peroxidase (PAP) (19) and immuno-alkaline phosphatase anti-alkaline phosphatase (APAAP) (20) methods.

Microscopy and photography

The Leitz Orthoplan microscope was equipped with an HBO 200 W lamp for rhodamine excitation and an XBO 150 W for fluorescein excitation. A Ploem-type vertical illuminator combined with interference filters was used for narrow-band excitation and selective filtration of red and green emission colors. PAP and APAAP staining was examined by conventional transmitted bright-field illumination.

Positive selection of DR-positive cells

One tumor specimen was cut into small pieces while kept in tissue culture medium and squeezed through a grid. Collagenase and deoxyribonuclease were added to obtain a suspension of dispersed cells. The cells were pelleted and magnetic polymer beads (kindly supplied by Dr. S. Funderud) conjugated with a monoclonal IgM antibody to HLA class II molecules were added. Thereafter the DR-positive cells were positively selected by a modification of the method described by Gaudernack et al. (22) and further characterized by APAAP staining.

Table 1. Polyclonal and monoclonal antibody reagents used for immunohistochemistry

Specificity	Dilution/working conc. (g/l)	Source (code)
HLA-DR determinants	1/20 (m)*	Becton Dickinson (a)
HLA-DR determinants	1/20 (m,s)	Dakopatts (b)
Broad keratin	1/100 (p)	Authors' lab. (R505) (c)
51 kD keratin (polypeptide) #14	1/200 (p)	D. Roop (d)
All cytokeratin polypeptides of most epithelial cell lines	1/100 (m,a)	Labsystems (PKK1) (e)
46-52 kD cytokeratin polypeptides	1/100 (m,a)	Labsystems (PKK2)
Vimentin intermediate filaments	1/100 (m,a)	Labsystems
Vimentin intermediate filaments	1/80 (m,a)	Amersham (f)
S-100 protein	1/340 (p)	Dakopatts (g)
Glial fibrillary acidic protein (GFAP)	1/100 (m,a)	Labsystems
Factor VIII-related antigen (endothelial cells)	1/350 (p)	Dakopatts (g)
Leukocyte common antigen (LCA)	1/20 (m,s)	Dakopatts (b)
CD1 (thymocytes & Langerhans' cells)	1/20 (m,a)	Becton Dickinson (Leu 6)
Follicular dendritic reticulum cells	1/20 (m,s)	Dakopatts (DRC1) (b)
L1 antigen	0.009 (pc)	Authors' lab. (h)

*monoclonal antibody (m); supernatant (s); ascites (a); polyclonal antiserum (p); polyclonal conjugate (pc)

(a) Becton Dickinson, Sunnyvale, CA; (b) Dakopatts, Glostrup, Denmark; (c) H.S. Huitfeldt and P. Brandtzaeg, Histochemistry 83, 381, 1985; (d) Kindly supplied by Dr. D. Roop, Laboratory of Cellular Carcinogenesis and Tumor Promotion, National Cancer Institute, Bethesda, MD; (e) Labsystems Oy, Helsinki, Finland; (f) Amersham International, Amersham, U.K.; (g) DAKO Corporation, Santa Barbara, CA; (h) Inge Dale et al., Am. J. Clin. Pathol. 84, 1, 24, 1985.

Table 2. Combinations of markers demonstrated by paired immunofluorescence

	Rhodamine label	Fluorescein label
1.	Broad keratin	HLA-DR
2.	51 kD keratin	HLA-DR
3.	Broad keratin	Vimentin
4.	S-100 protein	keatin PKK1
5.	S-100 protein	GFAP
6.	S-100 protein	Vimentin
7.	Factor VIII-related antigen	HLA-DR

RESULTS

Figure 1 summarizes the staining of different cell types in pleomorphic adenoma as compared with normal salivary gland, and some of the findings are demonstrated in Figure 2.

DISCUSSION

Immunohistochemical studies of pleomorphic adenomas have contributed to the understanding of this complex tumor. The finding of Kahn et al. (8) that more tumor cells were positive for S-100 protein than for cytokeratin or vimentin was confirmed in this study. Kahn et al. (8) proposed that only some MEC produced cytokeratin or vimentin intermediate filaments after neoplastic transformation. Our study indicated another possibility, namely that S-100 protein and vimentin are present both in MEC and in a separate but morphologically almost indistinguishable cell population. In most specimens we thus found a large population of HLA-DR-positive, keratin-negative dendritic cells that might represent a reactive population of dendritic histiocytic cells rather than being tumor cells. To our knowledge there exists only a case report considering dendritic cells in pleomorphic adenoma; some Langerhans' cells confined to squamouse epithelial areas were noted (21).

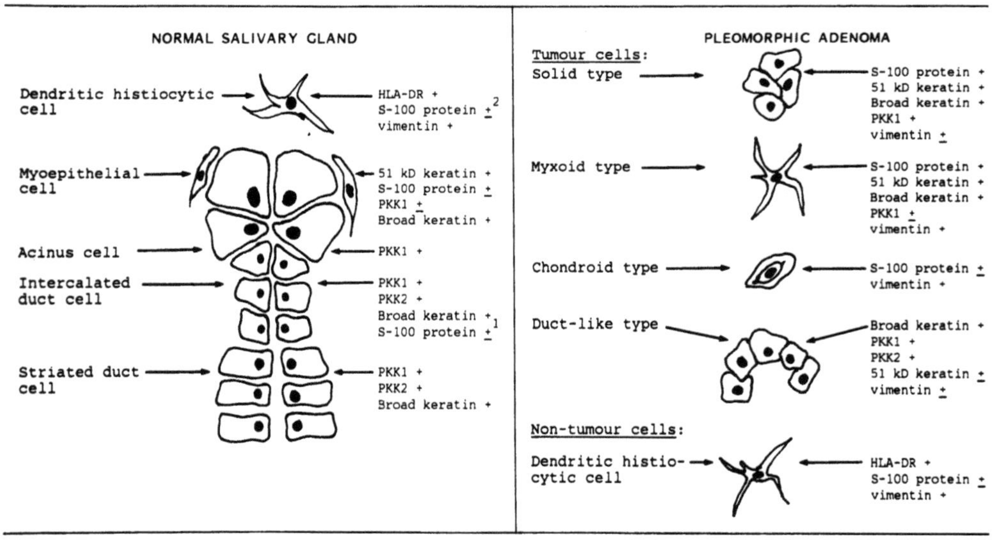

[1]Most cells positive (+)
[2]Occasional cells positive (±)

Figure 1. Staining response in pleomorphic adenoma as compared to normal salivary gland.

The DR-positive, keratin-negative dendritic cells were easily identified by paired immunofluorescence staining. They showed a distribution different from the Langerhans' cells found by David et al. (21) and did not stain with the Leu 6 antibody reacting with the CD1 marker of thymocytes and Langerhans' cells. The positively selected DR-expressing dendritic cells have so far been characterized incompletely, and a positive marker for human interdigitating reticulum cells is not yet available. The cells showed positivity for vimentin and S-100 protein but not for the myelomonocytic marker L1 (25).

S-100 protein is located in a wide variety of cells and tissues including cells of normal and neoplastic salivary glands (12,13). In our study, only MEC and some duct cells stained with antibody to S-100 protein in agreement with Crocker et al. (13) but contrasting a previous report of S-100 positivity in both acinic and duct cells (23). S-100 protein has been shown to be present in Langerhans' cells of the epidermidis, interdigitating reticulum cells of lymph node (24), and chondrocytes as well as in neoplastic epithelial cells of pleomorphic adenomas (12,13). This is in agreement with our observation that both the tumor cell population and the population of DR-positive dendritic histiocytic cells expressed this marker. The different immunoreactivity of the α- and β-subunits in S-100 protein-positive cells may prove to be helpful in an attempt to discriminate between various positive cell populations. Both interdigitating reticulum cells and Langerhans' cells show immunoreactivity for the β subunit. Monoclonal S-100 protein antibodies are now available.

Scattered cells in 8 out of the 10 specimens stained for GFAP as shown previously (12,23). The GFAP-positive cells coexpressed keratin and S-100 protein. They probably represented tumor cells that for some unknown reason produce filaments antigenically related to GFAP since we did not find any expression of GFAP in normal salivary glands. Coexpression of three different intermediate filaments have been shown in cultured human pleomorphic adenoma cells (11). Our study confirmed the observed coexpression of keratin and vimentin, and keratin and GFAP. We further demonstrated a complex coexpression pattern of S-100 protein and keratin, S-100 protein and vimentin, and S-100 protein and GFAP. Paired immunofluorescence staining was most useful in attempts to characterize this very complex tumor (Fig. 2).

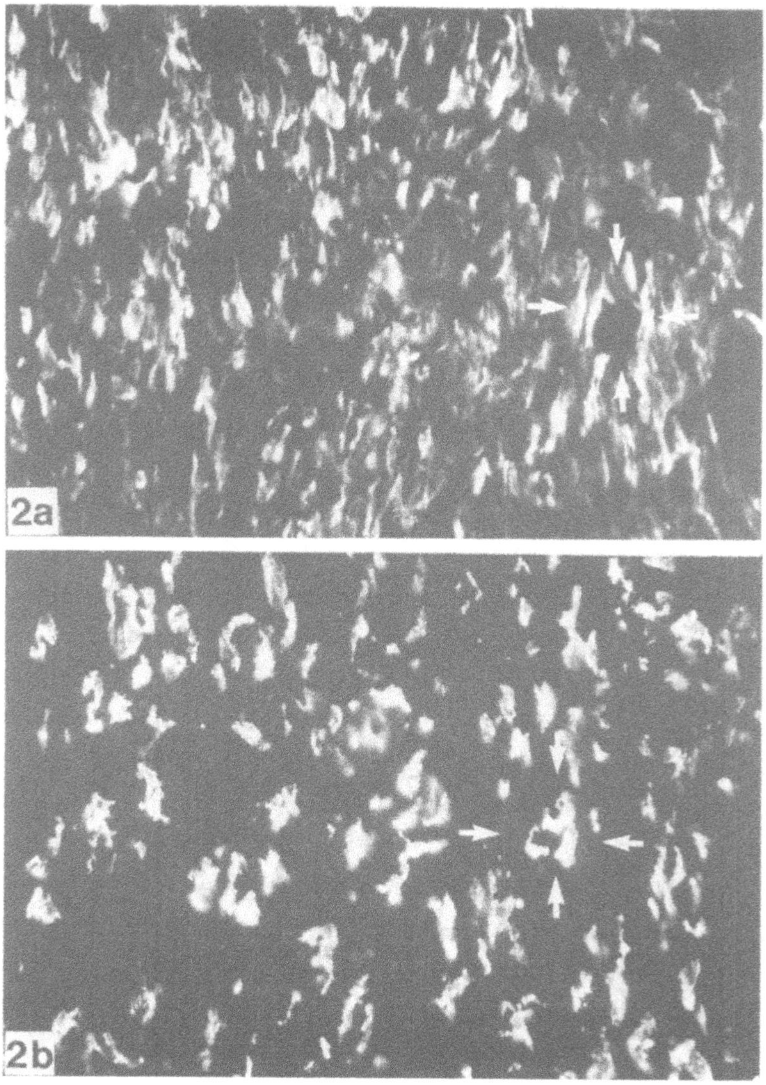

Figure 2. (a) Paired immunofluorescence staining of 51 kD keratin (No.14) and HLA-DR in pleomorphic adenomas. The keratin marker (a, rhodamine) identifies the tumor cells (arrows), whereas DR (b, fluorescein) is expressed by a separate population of dendritic cells and is absent in the tumor cells (x 200).

CONCLUSIONS

1. Myoepithelial cells or their immediate precursors most likely give rise to pleomorphic adenomas.

2. Pleomorphic adenomas often contain a substantial population of dendritic histiocytic cells which are positive for HLA-DR.

3. This cell population may represent antigen-presenting cells normally involved in immune regulation of salivary glands.

ACKNOWLEDGEMENTS

This work was supported by Anders Jahre's Fund, the Norwegian Cancer Society, Thorsted's Legacy and Knut and Liv Gards Fund. We thank Drs. Steinar Funderud and Frode Vartdal for kindly supplying the immunomagnetic beads.

REFERENCES

1. Dardick, I., van Nostrand, A.M.P., Jeans, M.T.D., Rippstein, P. and Edwards, V., Human Pathol. 14, 780, 1983.
2. Regezi, J.A. and Batsakis, J.G., Otolaryng. Clin. North Am. 10, 297, 1977.
3. Mills, S.E. and Cooper, P.H., Lab. Invest. 44, 6, 1981.
4. Palmer, R.M., Lucas, R.B., Knight, J. and Gusterson, B., J. Pathol. 146, 213, 1985.
5. Erlandson, R.A., Cardon-Cardo, C. and Higgins, P.J., Am. J. Surg. Pathol. 8, 803, 1984.
6. Krepler, R., Denk, H., Artlieb, U. and Moll, R., Differentiation 21, 191, 1982.
7. Korsrud, F.R. and Brandtzaeg, P., Virchows Arch. (Pathol. Anat.) 403, 291, 1984.
8. Kahn, H.J., Baumal, R., Marks, A., Dardick, I. and Nostrand, A.W.P.v., Arch. Pathol. Lab. Med. 109, 190, 1985.
9. Franke, W.W., Schmid, E., Freudenstein, C., Appelhans, B., Osborn, M., Weber, K. and Keenan, T.W., J. Cell. Biol. 84, 633, 1980.
10. Caselitz, J., Osborn, M., Wustrow, J., Seifert, G. and Weber, K., Path. Res. Pract. 175, 266, 1982.
11. Rozell, B., Stenman, G., Hansson, H.A., Dahl, D., Hansson, G.K. and Mark, J., Acta. Path. Microbiol. Immunol. Scand. 93, 335, 1985.
12. Nakazato, Y., Ishizeki, J., Takahashi, K., Yamaguchi, H., Kamei, T. and Mori, T., Lab. Invest. 46, 621, 1982.

13. Crocker, J., Jenkins, R., Campbell, J., Fuggle, W.J. and Shah, V.M., J. Pathol. 146, 115, 1985.

14. Palmer, R.M., Lucas, R.B. and Langdon, J.D., Histopathology 9, 1061, 1985.

15. Thrane, P.S., Brandtzaeg, P. and Huitfeldt, H., 6th Intl. Congress of Immunology, Toronto, Abstract 1.44.13, p. 57, 1986.

16. Thrane, P.S., Rognum, T.O., Huitfeldt, H. and Brandtzaeg, P., (this volume), 1987.

17. Brandtzaeg, P., Immunology 26, 1101, 1974.

18. Brandtzaeg, P. and Rognum, T.O., Histochem. J. 15, 655, 1983.

19. Sternberger, L.A., Hardy, P.H., Cuculis, J.J. and Meyer, H.G., J. Histochem. Cytochem. 18, 315, 1970.

20. Mason, D.Y., Techniques in Immunocytochemistry 3, 25-43, 1985.

21. David, R. and Buchner, A., J. Path. 131, 127, 1980.

22. Gaudernack, G., Leivestad, T., Ugelstad,J. and Thorsby, E., J. Immunol. Meth. 90, 179, 1986.

23. Nakazato, Y., Ishida, Y., Takahashi, K. and Suzuki, K., Virchows Arch. (Pathol. Anat.) 405, 299, 1985.

24. Rausch, E., Kaiserling, E. and Goods, M., Virchows Archs. (Cell. Pathol.) 25, 327, 1977.

25. Dale, I., Brandtzaeg, P., Fagerhol, M.K. and Scott, H., Am. J. Clin. Pathol. 84, 24, 1985.

DISCORDANCE BETWEEN IgA B CELL PRECURSORS AND THE SECRETION OF IgA ANTIBODY TO BACTERIAL POLYSACCHARIDES

C.G. Bell

Department of Microbiology and Immunology
University of Illinois, College of Medicine
Chicago, IL USA

INTRODUCTION

B cell precursors of IgA antibody forms cells (AFC) with specificity for antigenic determinants common in the mouse environment originate in Peyer's patches (PP) and migrate, via lymphatic ducts of the gut-associated lymphoid tissue (GALT) to mesenteric lymph nodes (MLN), and via the systemic circulation to distal mucosal secretory sites, to differentiate to IgA producing cells. It is thought that the commitment of B cell precursors to IgA production may be due to the effect of the PP microenvironment on the B cells (1,2), and the frequency of distribution of these precursors of IgA AFC show a relationship to the lymphoid tissue site in which the B cells differentiate (2-4). The mechanisms involved in the IgA cell cycle in the distal tissues and the signals triggering the differentiation of precursor B cells into IgA AFC remains less than clear. The regulation of IgA production by GALT T cells is well documented (2,5,6), and generation of IgA plaque-forming cells (PFC) to bacterial polysaccharides (Ps) is clearly T cell-dependent (TD) (2). However, the role of T cells in the IgA precursor cycle and the T cell contribution to IgA systemic antibody (Ab) to bacterial Ps have only been partly clarified (2,3,7,8).

Bacterial Ps, such as dextrans (dex) produced by Leuconostoc mesenteroides, cross-reacts with determinants present on a commensal Enterobacter cloacae common in the mouse environment, defined as type 2 antigens, and shares reactivity with Haemophilus influenzae type b (Hib) capsular Ps. These Ps are moderately immunogenic in young animals. The responses are not dependent on carrier-specific T helper (Th) cells: i.e., good IgM responses are seen in congenitally athymic, nude (nu/nu) mice and induce little, if any, memory (2,8,9). The mouse immune response to dex B-1355, which possess repeating ($1 \rightarrow 3$) and ($1 \rightarrow 6$) D-glucopyranosyl (αDGls) linkages (7,8), is controlled by structural genes that map to the variable (V) region λ_1 light (L) ($V_{\lambda 1}$) and to the V heavy (H) chain V_H and D, linked to the Igh-$1^{\underline{al}}$ allotype gene complex of the constant (C) region H chain. BALB/c, Igh-$1^{\underline{al}}$ allogroup mice are phenotypically high responders to the ($1 \rightarrow 3$), exhibit a λ_1-restricted PFC and serum Ab response predominantly related antigenically to the V_H idiotype (Id) shared (IdX) by BALB/c λ_1 plasmacytomas MOPC 104E and J-558 (8,10). C57Bl/6, Igh-$1^{\underline{b}}$ mice, exhibit a low restricted PFC and serum Ab response to the ($1 \rightarrow 3$) and a high κ response to the ($1 \rightarrow 6$). The V_HD Id defined mouse response to dex is IgM in early development and yields IgM > IgG3 PFC responses to thymus independent (TI) type 2 (TI-2) B-1355 antigen. However, IgM < IgA > IgG3 PFC responses occur to B-1355 conjugated to <u>Limulus polyphemus</u> hemocyanin (LPH) (TD) in late development (2,7,10). These responses provide a useful model for the study of the acquisition and development of the IgA isotype potential, in relation to the V_H and D Id, and for the effect of T cells in the IgA B cell response to Ps.

In this study, a dissection was made of the Igh isotype potential of B cell precursors from unprimed BALB/c (primary B), stimulated with B-1355 or B-1355-LPH in monofocal splenic fragment cultures. These studies were done with or without carrier-primed T cells, over 15 generations of limiting B cell dilution assays, permiting an analysis of the Ps and T cell requirements for Igh isotype expression.

METHODS

The frequency and profiles of B precursor repertoires specific for dex B-1355 were determined by limiting dilution, and adoptive transfer splenic focus assay (2,3,7,8). Briefly, cells taken from unprimed (primary B) or from B-1355-primed (secondary B), euthymic BALB/c mice of indicated ages, were enriched for B cells by affinity filtration or by treatment with specific monoclonal Ab (mAb) and complement (8) to deplete the Thy-1.2-positive and Lyt-1-positive cells. Enriched B cells were transferred intravenously (i.v.), alone or with 5 x 10^6 euthymic T cells into unprimed athymic, nude (nu/nu) or into LPH-primed, euthymic 1,600 rad ^{137}Cs irradiated BALB/c recipients. Sixteen hr after transfer, the nu/nu recipients were injected i.v. with 100 μg B-1355 (TI-2); the euthymic control mice were injected with phosphate-buffered saline (PBS). One hr later, 1 mm^3 fragments were prepared from the recipient spleen and cultured as individual monofocal organ cultures with B-1355 (TI-2) or B-1355-LPH (TD) for 3 days (d) and with antigen-free medium for 21 d in 93% O_2/7% CO_2 atmosphere. Culture supernatants collected at 3 d intervals from d 9 through d 21, were examined for anti-(1→3) dex Ab of the various isotypes by solid phase radioimmunoassay (sRIA) and enzyme-linked immunoassay (ELISA) (2,7,8). Briefly, supernatants (10-20 μl) in eight replicas were adsorbed on B-1355-BSA immunoadsorbent microtiter plates and bound Ab detected after reaction with monospecific anti-μ, -γ_1, -γ_{2a}, -γ_{2b}, -γ_3 and -α isotype-affinity purified rabbit anti-H chain Ab, followed by goat anti-rabbit Ig specific labeled Ab.

B cell precursors were considered (1→3)-responsive if over 10 or more progeny generations (2 to 3 consecutive supernatant collections) secreted Ab which bound to B-1355-BSA but not to B-512(F)-BSA immunoadsorbents ($P < 0.001$). Specificity was determined with dex B-1355 containing 35% (1→3)-, 45% (1→6)- and 10% 1,3,6-α DGls linkages and 5% nonreducing glucosyl end groups (NRE), and dex B-512(F), containing 90% (1→6) and 5% 1,3,6-α DGls linkages and 5% NRE (7,8). The frequency of responsive B cell precursors were calculated by regression analysis from the Poisson distribution relationship between the number of responding clonal cultures, using a 4% homing and cloning efficiency of the input cells in the recipient spleen. Significance in relation to background and controls was determined by Student's analysis of variance of independent groups (7,8). The (1→3)-binding Ab in supernatants were quantified by reference to standard curves obtained with reference myeloma proteins (MP) M 104E ($\mu\lambda_1$), J-558 ($\alpha\lambda_1$) and ($\gamma_3\lambda_1$) hybridomas (7,8) and the (1→6) dex-binding Ab by reference to (1→6) binding myeloma W-3129 (ακ). Total quantity of IgG2a, IgG2b and IgG3 isotypes were quantified by referenced to non-dex-binding reference myelomas J-606 (γ_3k), HOPC-1 ($\gamma_{2a}\lambda_1$) and M 141 (γ_{2b}k) (2,3,7,8). V_H and D IdI 104E and IdI J-558 were quantified by competitive sRIA and inhibition of ELISA by reference to the MP 104E and J-558 IdX and IdI (2,8).

PFC were enumerated from spleens of age-matched BALB/c mice 5 d after intraperitoneal (i.p.) immunization with B-1355 (100 μg) or 7 d after i.p. immunization with E. cloacae (10^8 formaldehyde-killed E. cloacae). Sheep red blood cells (SRBC) coated with oxidized B-1355 as indicators for quantification of the (1→3)-specific PFC, and SRBC coated with cyanogen-bromide activated B-512(F) as indicators for quantification of the (1→6)-specific PFC were used (2,7). Pre- and post-immunization sera were quantified for (1→3)-specific Ab by the sRIA and ELISA described (2,3,7,8).

RESULTS

The repertoire of antigen-binding structures encoded by H and L, κ and λ, Ig genes is generated early in B cell development from a limited repertoire of germline gene [V(D)J] segments. The Igh isotype repertoire is generated by a second Ig rearrangement occurring in the course of Ig class switching in activated B cells. Commitment to κ or λ expression is made early in the ontogeny of the B cell (Tables 1-3). The predominantly λ_1 B repertoire is expanded by B-1355 (TI-2) alone (Tables 1, 3-5), the λ_1 and κ by B-1355-LPH (TD) (Table 2); the (1→3)-responsive κ and the higher frequency of λ_1 and higher yields of released ab are all directly related to T cell help (Table 2 vs Table 1).

The dissection of the isotypes expressed during the 15 generations of B cell divisions in the monofoci showed sequential differentiation switches in the order of the genes encoded in the DNA, principally downstream $\mu>\gamma_3>\gamma_{2b}>\gamma_{2a}$, $\mu>\gamma_3$, and $\mu>\alpha$. B clones, whether λ_1 or κ generating IgM in monofoci stimulated with B-1355 or B-1355-LPH, also generated other isotypes and thus exhibited intraclonal switching (Tables 1,2,6). In the TI cultures with B-1355 the IgM>>>IgA and IgG3, IgG2b were minimally expressed; IgG2a was absent (Tables 1,6). In TD cultures with B-1355-LPH, there was a shift to expression of isotypes downstream from Cμ, the IgA being the predominant response. While multiple isotypes were delineated in monofoci with or without T cells, the higher frequency of IgM, IgA or IgM + other isotypes in cultures stimulated with B-1355-LPH clearly illustrates the effect of carrier-primed T cells in the Igh-C switching to IgA and IgG2a (Tables 2,6 vs. Table 1). Id analysis of the Igh isotypes in λ_1 monofoci indicated that the multiple isotypes originated from single B precursor clones (Table 6).

TABLE 1. Frequency of primary B precursors generating (1→3) dex-specific antibodies of various Igh isotypes in monofocal B or B + T splenic fragments stimulated with dextran B-1355.

Cells transferred (age-day)[a]	Frequency[c] of clonal precursors generating anti-(1→3) Ab per 10^6 B						% clones producing ng Ab/d/mf[d]		
	μ	γ3	γ1	γ2b	γ2a	α	0.5-2	2-5	>5
B (80)	1.4 ±0.3	0	0	0	0	0.2 ±0.1	58	40	2
B (80) + T[b]	2.1 ±0.2	0	0	0	0	0.3 ±0.1	41	52	7
B (155)	2.9 ±0.3	0.3 ±0.1	0	0.1 ±0.1	0	0.8 ±0.2	52	42	6
B (155) + T	4.7 ±0.4	0.6 ±0.3	0.1	0.9 ±0.2	0.1 ±0.1	1.1 ±0.2	39	51	10
B (≥360)	3.0 ±0.4	1.3 ±0.3	0	0.2 ±0.1	0	1.0 ±0.3	46	49	5
B (≥360) + T	4.5 ±0.4	2.5 ±0.6	0.1	1.2 ±0.2	0.2 ±0.1	3.1 ±0.2	38	50	12

[a]Limiting numbers of splenic cells taken from unprimed, euthymic BALB/c of indicated ages and enriched for B, were transferred i.v. alone or with the splenic T cells into unprimed, athymic, nude (nu/nu) 1,600 rad ^{157}Cs irradiated BALB/c recipients. 16 h after transfer, the recipients were injected i.v. with 100 μg B-1355 and 1 h later fragments were prepared from the recipient spleen and cultures with B-1355 or B-1355-LPH. Culture supernatants collected d 9 through 21 were quantified for (1→3) dex-binding Ab by sRIA and ELISA (2,7,8).

[b]Splenic T cells (~5 x 10^6) from unprimed, euthymic BALB/c or nu/+ BALB/c.

[c]Frequency of B precursors (1→3)-responsive d 9 through 21 were calculated by regression analysis, using a 4% homing and cloning efficiency of the input B cells in the recipient spleen (7,8). The mean and SEM values given for positive monofoci fragments (mf) from individual recipient spleen within the B or B + T groups.

[d]Quantification of (1→3)-specific Ab produced per d per monofocal fragment (mf), using (1→3)-specific reference λ_1 MP, M 104E (μ) and J-558 (α) and (1→6)-specific reference κ MP, W-3129 (α). The ratio of the λ_1:κ precursors responsive to B-1335 (TI-2) was ~15.0-16.3. The ratio of λ_1:λ_1 Id response precursors ~1.4-1.3.

TABLE 2. Age-dependent (1→3) potentially-responsive μ and α primary B precursors in monofocal splenic fragments stimulated with dextran B-1355-LPH.

					(1→3)-responsive B precursors				
					% clones producing ng Ab/d/mf		% clones producing ng Ab/d/mf[e]		
Donor B prec[a]	age (day)	T cell source	Freq[b]: 10^6B	Ratio λ_1:κ	μ^c +/μ^d	α^c +/α^d	0.5-2	2-5	>5
Sp	4	Sp	3.0	0.5	79/21	70/21	100	0	0
	10	Sp	8.5	0.7	80/30	61/25	85	15	0
	30	Sp	15.2	1.0	68/23	54/10	46	45	9
	80	Sp	23.4	1.1	49/18	50/29	30	50	20
	155	Sp	24.5	1.0	40/9	61/33	29	50	21
		PP	25.9	1.0	43/14	79/47	33	49	18
	≥360	Sp	27.9	1.0	49/8	81/49	18	45	37
GF[f] Sp	55	Sp	<1.0	1.0	0/100	0/0	100	0	0
	>150	PP	2.0	1.0	10/89	1/0	69	26	5
MLN	155	PP	20.4	1.3	49/21	57/39	44	52	4
	≥360	Sp	16.1	1.3	43/19	67/40	43	53	4
	530	MLN	18.9	1.0	42/18	84/40	39	53	8
PLN	≥360	Sp	<1.0	1.2	ND	ND	100	0	0
		PP	<1.0	1.3	ND	ND	100	0	0
PP	155	Sp	11.4	1.4	44/11	39/53	60	34	6
	155	PP	18.5	1.0	39/10	27/72	58	33	9
BM	150	PP	10.1	1.1	69/49	18/11	54	43	3
	≥360	PP	28.3	1.3	41/30	11/25	43	49	8

[a]Limiting numbers of spleen (Sp), mesenteric lymph node (MLN), axillary and inguinal peripheral lymph node (PLN), Peyer's patches (PP), and tibia and femur bone marrow (BM) cells taken from unprimed, conventional, euthymic BALB/c of indicated ages, and enriched for B, were transferred i.v. with Sp, PP or MLN enriched T cells (5×10^6) into LPH-primed euthymic, 1,600 rad irradiated BALB/c recipients. Fragments prepared from the recipient spleen 16 h after transfer were cultured with dex conjugated to LPH (B-1355-LPH). Culture supernatants collected d 9 through 21 were quantified for (1→3) dex-binding Ab of the various isotypes by sRIA and ELISA (2,7,8).

[b]The frequency of B precursors (1→3)-responsive d 9 through 21 were calculated by regression analysis and corrected for homing and cloning efficiency which is 4% of the donor injected B cells (7,8). The ratio of λ_1:λ_1 Id response Sp precursors was ~1.6-1.4.

[c]Supernatants positive for the indicated Igh isotype and for other Igh isotypes. Indicated values are for B clones producing more than one Igh isotype.

[d]Supernatants positive for the indicated Igh isotype only. Indicated values are for B clones producing single Igh isotype.

[e]Ab of various isotypes in supernatants were quantified by reference to standard curves obtained with precalibrated purified myelomas and hybridomas.

[f]Splenic (Sp) B cells taken from unprimed germfree (GF) euthymic BALB/c mice were transferred with Sp or PP T cells taken from LPH-primed, conventional, euthymic BALB/c.

DISCUSSION

The higher frequency of PP > MLN > Sp > BM > PLN precursors generating only IgA in the monofoci containing PP T cells than in the monofoci containing Sp T cells, illustrates the major contribution of PP B and T cells to the IgA precursor cycle (Table 2). In contrast, the higher frequency of IgA AFC in Sp > PP > MLN > BM PFC, following in vivo immunization (Table 4), despite the higher ratio of IgA to IgM AFC (PP > MLN > SP > BM PFC) (Tables 3 and 4), indicates that the PP was the major source of precursors of the IgA AFC. However, the spleen was the major site for terminal differentiation to IgA PFC. The generation of IgA PFC was strictly TD, was related to environmental stimuli and was absent in germfree mice (Tables 3 and 4). The relatively fewer IgM + IgA (~20%) double class PFC (Tables 3 and 4), than IgM + IgG (~70%) double class PFC (Table 3) together with the higher frequency of precursors producing IgA only in TD cultures with B-1355-LPH (Table 2), suggest that the dex-driven TD, terminal differentiation to IgA may involve more DNA rearrangements and less RNA splicing than the TI-2 dex-driven differentiation to IgG3. The low IgA $(1\rightarrow 3)$-specific serum Ab response, correlating neither with the frequency distribution of IgA primary B precursor potential $(1\rightarrow 3)$ response in monofoci (Table 5 vs. Tables 1, 2 and 6), nor with the dex-induced in vivo IgA PFC responses magnitudes (Tables 5 vs. Tables 3 and 4) corroborate the discordance between the mucosal and serum IgA Ab repertoire.

TABLE 3. Age-dependent μ, γ_3 and α, (1→3)-specific plaque-forming spleen cell responses by BALB/c immunized with dextran B-1355.

BALB/c spleen[a]	age (day)	PFC/10^6 spleen cells μ^b $\bar{X}^e \pm$ SEM	γ_3 [c] $\bar{X} \pm$ SEM	α^c $\bar{X} \pm$ SEM	$\mu + \gamma_3$ [d] $\bar{X} \pm$ SEM	$\mu + \alpha$ [d] $\bar{X} \pm$ SEM
euthymic	10	29 ± 10	0	ND	0	ND
	30	185 ± 39	2 ± 1	85 ± 15	8 ± 2	11 ± 4
	55	315 ± 59	2 ± 2	251 ± 52	11 ± 4	40 ± 20
	80	390 ± 48	6 ± 3	289 ± 65	16 ± 5	34 ± 21
	155	445 ± 68	31 ± 19	415 ± 49	121 ± 44	75 ± 42
	≥360	748 ± 79	135 ± 45	919 ± 82	681 ± 48	85 ± 21
	530	875 ± 49	229 ± 39	1059 ± 139	750 ± 60	101 ± 39
nude	80	299 ± 25	8 ± 2	0	10 ± 3	0
(nu/nu)	155	405 ± 51	37 ± 15	0	109 ± 21	0
reconsti-						
tuted[f]	80	395 ± 25	ND	117 ± 39	ND	31 ± 12
(nu/nu)	155	495 ± 31	ND	240 ± 41	ND	64 ± 18

[a]Day 10 BALB/c mice were injected i.p. with 50 μg dex B-1355 in PBS, d 30-530 BALB/c with 100 μg B-1355 in PBS. Congenitally athymic, nude (nu/nu) BALB/c mice were immunized after reconstitution with euthymic BALB/c thymocytes. Splenic PFC magnitudes were enumerated 5 d after immunization by a slide technique using sheep red blood cells (SRBC) coated with B-1355 or SRBC coated with B-512(F) as indicators (7,10).

[b]Six slide replicas containing splenocytes and B-1355-SRBC indicators (7,10) were assessed in parallel, 2 for direct μPFC, without developing Ab, and 2 each for indirect γ_3 and IgA PFC, with γ_3 and α class-specific antigen affinity purified Ab (2,7,10). Indicated values are for direct μ PFC.

[c]The γ_3 and IgA PFC were assessed in the presence and absence of anti-μ, class-specific Ab, added at concentrations inhibitory for the μ PFC. Indicated values are for PFC single class producers.

[d]Indicated values are for PFC double class producers.

[e]$\bar{X}$ = mean ± SEM. 5-8 mice/age group. ~90% of the PFC were of the λ_1 isotypes.

[f] ~5 x 10^7, d ~12 euthymic thymocytes.

PFC values for euthymic BALB/c mice immunized with E. cloacae were 359 (primary) and 2889 (hyperimmune secondary).

TABLE 4. Age-dependent μ and α, (1→3)-specific plaque-forming lymphoid cell responses by BALB/c immunized with dextran B-1355 or Enterobacter cloacae.

Donor	age	PFC/10^6 cells			
		μ[b]	α[b]	μ + α[c]	Ratio[d] of α:μ
cells[a]	(day)	$\bar{X}$[e] ± SEM	$\bar{X}$ ± SEM	$\bar{X}$ ± SEM	
Sp	30	185 ± 39	85 ± 15	11 ± 4	0.5 (0.5)
	80	390 ± 48	289 ± 65	34 ± 21	0.7 (0.8)
	155	445 ± 68	415 ± 49	75 ± 42	0.9 (1.1)
	155[f]	359 ± 71	295 ± 48	42 ± 21	0.8 (0.9)
	155[g]	2889 ± 215	1799 ± 312	212 ± 45	0.6 (0.7)
	≥360	748 ± 79	919 ± 82	85 ± 21	1.2 (1.3)
	530	875 ± 49	1059 ± 139	101 ± 39	1.2 (1.3)
Sp[h]	80	212 ± 17	42 ± 22	7 ± 7	0.2 (0.2)
MLN	30	3 ± 1	3 ± 2	0	1.0 (1.0)
	80	7 ± 2	19 ± 8	2 ± 2	2.7 (3.0)
	155	12 ± 3	29 ± 20	2 ± 2	2.4 (2.6)
	≥360	35 ± 10	131 ± 59	11 ± 4	3.7 (4.1)
	530	59 ± 18	279 ± 81	15 ± 8	4.7 (5.0)
PLN	155	0	0	0	
	≥360	10 ± 3	2 ± 1	0	0.2 (0.2)
	530	17 ± 3	3 ± 1	0	0.2 (0.2)
PP	155	5 ± 2	38 ± 11	1 ± 1	7.6 (7.8)
	≥360	17 ± 2	152 ± 31	6 ± 3	8.9 (9.3)
BM	155	40 ± 19	31 ± 10	3 ± 1	0.8 (0.9)
	≥360	41 ± 18	31 ± 14	8 ± 2	0.8 (1.0)

[a]Splenic (Sp), mesenteric lymph node (MLN), axillary and inguinal peripheral lymph node (PLN), Peyer's patches (PP) and tibia and femur bone marrow (BM) cells taken from 5 to 8 mice for each age group, 5 d after one i.p. injection with 100 μg B-1355 in PBS, or 7 d after one[f] or multiple[g] weekly injections with 10^8 formaldehyde-killed E. cloacae.

[b,c]Indicated values are for PFC single[b] and double[c] class producers.

[d]Outside parentheses ratios of PFC single class producers to direct μ PFC; inside parentheses ratios of PFC double class producers to direct μ PFC.

[e]$\bar{X}$ = mean ± SEM.

[f]One injection (primary) immunized.

[g]Multiple injections (secondary) hyperimmunized.

[h]Sp from germfree mice.

TABLE 5. Age-dependent μ, γ3 and α, (1→3)-specific serum antibody responses in dextran B-1355[a] or <u>Enterobacter cloacae</u>[b,c]-immunized, euthymic, nude (nu/nu) and thymocyte reconstituted nu/nu BALB/c mice.

BALB/c	age (day)	(1→3)-specific antibody[e] μg/ml μ	γ3	α	Ratio α:μ	α:γ3	γ3:μ	λ_1/λ_1Id
euthymic	30[a]	29 ± 14	0	1 ± 1	0.03	0	0	ND
	55[a]	145 ± 21	9 ± 3	10 ± 4	0.06	1.10	0.06	ND
	155[a]	196 ± 18	89 ± 24	27 ± 15	0.13	0.30	0.45	1.8
	≥360[a]	289 ± 12	142 ± 31	34 ± 10	0.12	0.24	0.43	1.5
	80[b]	192 ± 22	11 ± 5	11 ± 5	0.06	1.00	0.06	1.6
	80[c]	1851 ± 211	ND	ND	ND	ND	ND	1.9
nude	80[a]	75 ± 21	ND	0	0	ND	ND	ND
(nu/nu)	155[a]	99 ± 24	ND	0	0	ND	ND	ND
reconsti-								
tuted[d]	80[a]	114 ± 25	ND	12 ± 1	0.11	ND	ND	1.6
(nu/nu)	155[a]	167 ± 14	ND	17 ± 8	0.10	ND	ND	1.7
Germfree	80[a]	31 ± 14	ND	3 ± 3	0.16	ND	ND	ND

[a]BALB/c euthymic mice were pre-bled and injected i.p. with 100 μg B-1355 in PBS.

[b,c]BALB/c euthymic mice were injected i.p. with one[b] or multiple[c] weekly injections of 10^8 formaldehyde-killed <u>E. cloacae</u>.

[d]BALB/c nu/nu mice were reconsituted with 5 x 10^7, d 12 euthymic BALB/c thymocytes before immunization.

[e]Mice were bled from the retro-orbital plexus and the sera quantified for (1→3)-dex binding Ab by sRIA and ELISA. ~90% of the (1→3)-specific Ab were of the λ_1 isotype. The ratio of the λ_1: λ_1 Id (IdX ± IdI 104E and IdI J-558) is indicated.

TABLE 6. Coexpression of Igh isotypes in antibody generated by primary B precursors (1→3)-responsive in monofocal splenic fragments stimulated with dextran.

Cells transferred (age day)[a]	No. of Igh isotypes per mf[c]	% monofoci secreting (1→3)-specific Ab							
		μ	$\gamma 3$	$\gamma 1$	$\gamma 2b$	$\gamma 2a$	α	IdX	IdI
B(155)	1	80	0	0	14	0	4	91	51
	2	19	7	0	2	0	8	93	59
	3	2	1	0	0	0	1	89	63
	4	0	0	0	0	0	0		
B(155) + T[b]	1	10	2	1	2	0	45	83	57
	2	52	10	3	17	0	74	82	63
	3	10	2	0	3	6	6	75	68
	4	1	0	0	1	0	1	+	+

[a]Limiting numbers of B cells (2.5×10^6 - 5×10^6) alone or with 5×10^6 T cells were transferred i.v. to LPH-primed, 1,600 rad irradiated BALB/c recipients. 16 h after transfer fragments were prepared from the recipient spleen and cultured with B-1355 or B-1355-LPH.

[b]5×10^6 T cells. Irradiated recipients transferred with T cells only gave no positive foci, those transferred with B or with B+T are tabulated.

[c]Culture supernatants collected on d 7, 10 and 17 were quantified for (1→3)-binding Ab and dissected for λ_1, κ and Igh isotypes and for λ_1 Id profiles of Ab produced per monofocal fragment (mf), as described (see legends to Table 1 and 2). IdX and IdI profiles were analyzed by competitive sRIA (2,8).

REFERENCES

1. Gearhart, P.J. and Cebra, J.J., J. Exp. Med. 149, 216, 1979.
2. Bell, C.G., in The Secretory Immune System, Ann. N.Y. Acad. Sci. 409, 780, 1983.
3. Bell, C.G., Biochem. Soc. Trans. 11, 301, 1983.
4. Stohrer, R. and Kearney, J.F., J. Exp. Med. 158, 2081, 1983.
5. Elson, C.O., Heck, J.A. and Strober, W., J. Exp. Med. 149, 632, 1979.
6. Kiyono, H., McGhee, J.R., Mosteller, L.M., Eldridge, J.H., Koopman, W.J., Kearney, J.F. and Michalek, S.M., J. Exp. Med. 156, 1115, 1982.
7. Bell, C., Scand. J. Immunol. 15, 71, 1982.
8. Bell, C.G., Scand. J. Immunol. 18, 473, 1983.
9. R. Schneerson, Robbins, J.B., Parke Jr., J.C., Bell, C., Schlesselman, J.J., Sutton, A., Wang, Z., Schiftman, G., Karpas, A. and Shiloach, J., Infect. Immun. 52, 519, 1986.
10. Bell, C., Scand. J. Immunol. 9, 197, 1979.

CYTOTOXIC LYMPHOCYTES IN HUMAN INTESTINAL MUCOSA

F. Shanahan, M. Brogan, R. Nayersina and S. Targan

The Department of Medicine, U.C.L.A., Center for Health Sciences, Los Angeles, CA; and the Harbor/U.C.L.A. Inflammatory Bowel Disease Center, Los Angeles, CA USA

INTRODUCTION

Although cytotoxic lymphocytes have been well studied and characterized in the peripheral blood, the nature and function of these effector cells in human gut mucosa is still unclear. Previous studies have suggested that human intestinal lamina propria lymphocytes (LPL) exhibit mitogen induced cellular cytotoxicity and antibody-dependent cell-mediated cytotoxicity (ADCC) but that freshly isolated mucosal cells do not exhibit NK activity or exhibit it at very low levels (1-7). This is surprising since the intestinal mucosa is frequently affected by neoplastic, infectious and inflammatory diseases and is in apparent contrast with studies of the mucosal immune system in rodents where spontaneously cytotoxic cells are well represented (8,9). However, when isolated human colonic cells are cultured in the presence of interleukin-2 (IL-2) significant lytic activity is observed (lymphokine activated killers [LAK]) (10,11).

Since NK and LAK cells are heterogeneous (12-14) and their interrelationship is not clear, we have reevaluated human mucosal cell populations (a) to determine the existence of a cytolytically active subset of cells present in freshly isolated preparations, (b) to phenotype the cells responsible for the mucosal LAK phenomenon, and (c) to examine the relationship between mucosal cytotoxic cells and their peripheral blood counterparts.

MATERIALS AND METHODS

Peripheral blood lymphocytes obtained from normal donors were separated on Ficoll-Hypaque gradients (15) and were evaluated for NK markers (Leu-11 and NKH-1) by two-color immunofluorescence and flow cytometry. The intestinal specimens in this series of epxeriments were obtained from patients undergoing intestinal resection of carcinoma. Mucosa was taken from uninvolved areas. Lamina propria mononuclear cells were isolated by methods originally developed by Bull and Bookman (16) Adherent cells were depleted by incubation in plastic plates for 2 h and the LPL were then fractionated using a monoclonal antibody panning technique based on that described by Wysocki and Sato (17). Monoclonal antibodies to NKH-1, T11, T8 and T4 were obtained from Coulter Co. (Hialeah, FL) and anti-Leu-11 was obtained from Becton-Dickinson (Mountain View, CA). NKH-1 and Leu-11 are both NK-specific markers but unlike Leu-11, the NKH-1 antigen is not associated with surface Fc receptors for IgG. Cells were cultured in the presence and absence of recombinant interleukin 2 (IL-2, 10 U/ml) (Amgen Biologicals, Thousand Oaks, CA) for 3 days in RPMI 1640 supplemented with 10% fetal calf serum, L-glutamine, gentamycin and penicillin-streptomycin-fungizone (Irvine Scientific, Santa Ana, CA).

The cytotoxic activity of freshly isolated and cultured cells was assayed by 4 h chromium (^{51}Cr) release, as described elsewhere (14), using NK sensitive (K562) and NK resistant (Raji) target cells. Results are expressed in terms of lytic units which were calculated from a semilogarithmic curve plotting Ln effector cell number versus percent cytotoxicity. One lytic unit is the number of effector cells required to induce 30% ^{51}Cr release from 10^4 target cells.

RESULTS

Unfractionated freshly isolated LPL did not exhibit lytic activity against K562 targets even at effector to target ratios of up to 100 to 1. This was not due to inhibitory effects generated by the intestinal cell isolation procedure because when peripheral blood lymphocytes PBL were processed with the enzymatic digestion process no significant diminution in NK activity was observed in three separate experiments (data not shown).

Table 1

Phenotype	% of total lymphocytes[a]	
	Mucosa	Blood
NKH-1$^+$, Leu-11$^+$	0	7.3 $\pm$ 0.4 (62)
NKH-1$^-$, Leu-11$^+$	0	2.3 $\pm$ 0.2 (19.5)
NKH-1$^+$, Leu-11$^-$	2 (100)[b]	2.2 $\pm$ 0.1 (18.5)

[a](mean values $\pm$ S.E., n=12).

[b]The figures in parentheses represent the percentage of total NK cells.

NKH-1$^+$ cells represented 2% of the LPL population when examined by indirect immunofluorescence. As reported by others (10), LPL bearing the Leu-11 NK marker were not detectable. This is in contrast to the peripheral blood where NK cells represent a greater percentage of the total lymphocyte population and the majority of NK cells are Leu-11$^+$, NKH-1$^+$ (Table 1). The NK subpopulation of LPL was selectively studied by panning with the NKH-1$^+$ marker (Fig. 1). In contrast to unseparated LPL, the NKH-1 adherent fraction showed significant lytic activity which was evident at effector to target ratios of < 5 to 1 (Fig. 1).

The NKH-1 negative (NKH-1$^-$) fraction of LPL, although cytolytically inactive when freshly isolated, developed significant lytic activity (380 $\pm$ 55 lytic units/10^7 cells; mean $\pm$ S.D., n=5) when cultured in the presence of IL-2 (10 U/ml) for 3 days. Lysis of NK resistant targets such as Raji cells, a feature of peripheral blood LAK cells (18), was also exhibited by the cultured mucosal NKH-1$^-$ cells (data not shown). When the NKH1$^-$LPL

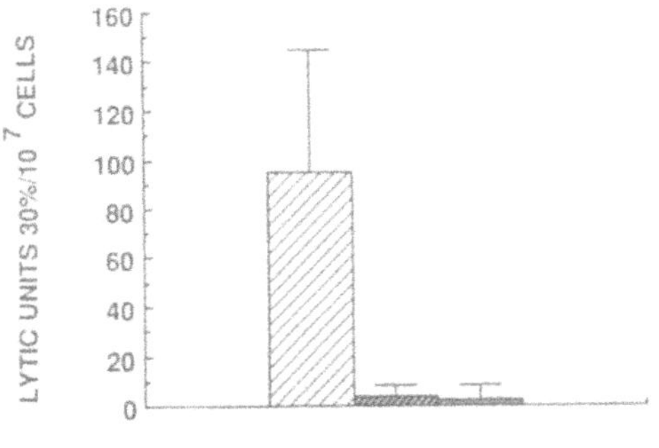

Figure 1. Comparison of the cytolytic activity of the NKH-1 fraction of freshly isolated LPL with that of unseparated LPL and NKH-1 depleted cells (mean $\pm$ S.D., n=5).

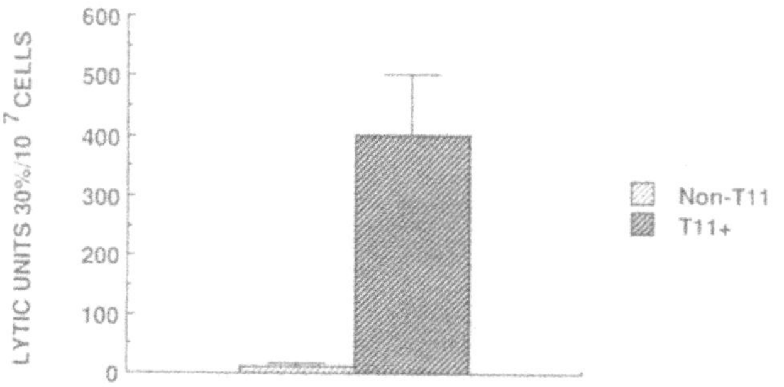

Figure 2. Mucosal LAK activity may be generated from $T11^+$ but not $T11^-$ precursor cells (mean ± S.D., n=3).

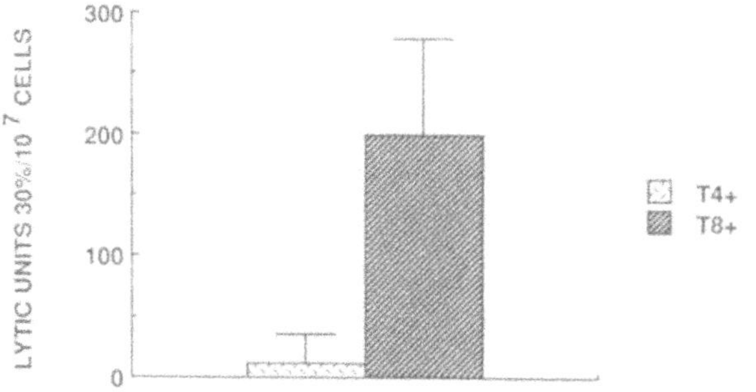

Figure 3. Mucosal LAK activity may be generated from T8 but not T4 precursor cells (mean ± S.D., n=5).

were further fractionated by panning using T11, T4 and T8 markers prior to culture, the mucosal LAK precursors were found to be $T11^+$, $T4^-$ and $T8^+$ (Figs. 2 ad 3).

DISCUSSION

The results demonstrate the heterogeneity of cytotoxic cells within the human intestinal mucosa and indicate major differences between mucosal and peripheral blood effector cells. We have identified a subset of human mucosal lymphocytes which exhibit significant NK activity when freshly isolated. The mucosal NK cells account for ≤2% of the total mucosal lymphocyte population and have an unusual phenotype ($NKH-1^+$, $Leu-11^-$). In the peripheral blood the $NKH-1^+$, $Leu-11^-$ subset represents a similar percentage of all lymphocytes. However, in contrast to the mucosa, the majority of peripheral blood NK cells are $NKH-1^+$ and $Leu-11^+$ (Table 1 and ref. 19).

The results also confirm the presence of a phenotypically distinct subpopulation of cells within human intestinal mucosa which become cytolytically active when cultured in the presence of IL-2 (10,11). These effector cells are NKH-1^- and, unlike the peripheral blood, where the major ity of LAK precursors are Leu-11^+ (20), the precursors of the mucosal LAK phenomenon are Leu-11^-.

The role of these killer cell populations in local defense mechanisms and in disease states is not clear. The paucity of NK cells within the intestinal mucosa relative to peripheral blood has suggested to some authors (7) that these effectors are probably not of importance in intestinal diseases while others (21,22) have argued that this is insufficient evidence for their dismissal as potentially important participants in the pathogenesis of intestinal disease. There is general agreement that the cell lines commonly used in assays of mucosal cytolytic activity may not be appropriate for the study of mucosal killer cell function. Other potential target cells including transformed and virally infected epithelial cells should be studied. Indeed, the potential importance of the intestinal epithelial cell in future investigations is underscored by the results of two studies (23,24) which indicated that under certain circumstances mucosal effector cells are capable of killing freshly isolated autologous epithelial cells. The development of techniques for the growth of intestinal epithelial cells in culture will considerably facilitate such studies since freshly isolated epithelial cells are technically difficult to work with (7,24). Finally, since NK cells may have an important immunoregulatory function (25), the possible effects of mucosal NK and LAK cells on other immunocytes including autologous immunoglobulin producing cells within the intestine should be considered.

CONCLUSIONS

At least two types of spontaneous cytotoxic cells exist among human intestinal lamina propria lymphocytes; (1) a small subset of cells (NKH-1^+, Leu-11^-) which are spontaneously cytotoxic when freshly isolated, and (2) lymphokine activated killer cells (T11^+, T8^+, T4^-, NKH-1^-, Leu-11^-) which acquire cytolytic activity during <u>in vitro</u> culture with IL-2. Both types of intestinal killer cells differ phenotypically from the majority of their counterparts in the peripheral blood. Thus, speculation about the role of cytotoxic cells in intestinal diseases should not be based on studies limited to peripheral blood effector cells.

ACKNOWLEDGEMENTS

This work was supported by the National Foundation for Ileitis and Colitis and the Harbor/U.C.L.A. Inflammatory Bowel Disease Research Center (U.S.P.H.S. grant AM 36200), and US PHS grant AM 27806.

REFERENCES

1. MacDermott, R.P., Franklin, G.O., Jenkins, K.M., Kodner, I.J., Nash, G.S. and Weinrieb, I.J., Gastroenterology 78, 47, 1980.
2. Bland, P.W., Britton, D.C., Richens, E.R. and Pledger, J.V., Gut 22, 744, 1981.
3. Falchuk, Z.M., Barnhard, E and Machado, I., Gut 22, 290, 1981.
4. Chiba, M., Bartnik, W., ReMine, S.G., Thayer, W.R. and Shorter, R.G., Gut 22, 177, 1981.
5. Gibson, P.R., Dow, E.L., Selby, W.S., Strickland, R.G. and Jewell, D.P., Clin. Exp. Immunol. 56, 438, 1984.
6. Beeken, W.L., Gundel, R.M., St. Andre-Ukena, S. and McAuliffe, T., Cancer 55, 1024, 1985.
7. James, S.P. and Strober, W., Gastroenterology 90, 235, 1986.
8. Tagliabue, A., Befus, A.D., Clark, D.A. and Bienenstock, J., J. Exp. Med. 155, 1785, 1982.
9. Nauss, K.M., Pavlina, T.M., Kumar, V. and Newberne, P.M., Gastroenterology 86, 468, 1984.
10. Fiocchi, C., Tubbs, R.R. and Youngman, K.R., Gastroenterology 88, 625, 1985.
11. Hogan, P.G., Hapel, A.J. and Doe, W.F., J. Immunol. 135, 1731, 1985.
12. Ortaldo, J.R. and Herberman, R.B., Ann. Rev. Immunol. 2, 359, 1984.
13. Burns, G.F., Triglia, T. and Werkmeister, J.A., J. Immunol. 133, 1656, 1984.
14. Shanahan, F., Brogan, M.D., Newman, W. and Targan, S., J. Immunol. 137, 723, 1986.
15. Boyum, A., Scand, J. Clin. Lab. Invest. (suppl 97) 21, 9, 1968.
16. Bull, D.M. and Bookman, M.A., J. Clin. Invest. 59, 966, 1977.
17. Wysocki, L.J. and Sato, V.L., Proc. Natl. Acad Sci. USA 75, 2844, 1978.
18. Grimm, E.A., Mazumder, A., Zhang, H.Z. and Rosenberg, S.A., J. Exp. Med. 155, 1823, 1982.
19. Lanier, L.L., Le, A.M., Civin, C.I., Loken, M.R. and Phillips, J.H., J. Immunol. 136, 4480, 1986.

20. Itoh, K., Tilden, A.B., Kumagai, K. and Balch, C.M., J. Immunol. 134, 802, 1985.
21. Gibson, P.R. and Jewell, D.P., Gastroenterology 90, 12, 1986.
22. Gibson, P.R., Gastroenterology 90, 1314, 1986.
23. Targan, S., Britvan, L., Kendal, R., Vimadalal, S. and Soll, A., Clin. Exp. Immunol. 54, 14, 1983.
24. Shorter, R.G., McGill, D.B., Bahn, R.C., Gastroenterology 86, 13, 1984.
25. Brieva, J.A., Targan, S. and Stevens, R.H., J. Immunol. 132, 611, 1984.

T CELL AND MONONUCLEAR PHAGOCYTE POPULATIONS OF THE HUMAN SMALL AND LARGE INTESTINE

L.K. Trejdosiewicz, G. Malizia, S. Badr-el-Din, C.J. Smart, D.J. Oakes, J. Southgate, P.D. Howdle, G. Janossy*, L.W. Poulter* and M.S. Losowsky

Departments of Medicine, University of Leeds, St. James's University Hospital, Leeds, U.K.; and *Academic Department of Immunology, Royal Free Hospital Medical School, London, U.K.

INTRODUCTION

Considering the diverse roles subsumed by the intestinal mucosal immune system, namely defense against potential luminal pathogens and maintenance of immune tolerance to dietary antigens, our knowledge of the local adaptations of immunocyte subpopulations remains sparse. In the past few years, the range of monoclonal antibodies to lymphocyte and mononuclear phagocyte (Mph) surface differentiation antigens has greatly increased. Such reagents, often shown capable of distinguishing between functional cell subpopulations, should therefore provide potent tools for the *in situ* analysis of the gut mucosal immune system.

Of particular interest are T lymphocytes, as they are both regulators and effectors of immune responses (1). Many questions remain unanswered concerning mucosal T cells, particularly about the possible role(s) of intraepithelial T cells, and the phenotypic identification of T cell subtypes identified to date only in functional assays (e.g., IgA-specific helper cells, Ig isotype switch cells, contrasuppressor cells) (2). Secondly, cells of the mononuclear phagocyte (Mph) series are known to be crucial accessory cells of immune system functioning (3). By morphological and histochemical criteria, these comprise at least two distinct lineages, namely poorly phagocytic, constitutively MHC class II^{+}, veiled, dendritic or interdigitating (ID) cells, thought to be mainly involved in antigen presentation to T and B cells (4), and strongly adherent, actively phagocytic macrophages (MØ), negative or weakly positive for class II antigens, thought to be mainly involved in scavenger functions (5,6). In functional assays, a further Mph type has been identified of regulatory function(s) (7), although the phenotype(s) of regulatory Mph remain to be identified unequivocally.

MATERIALS AND METHODS

Histologically normal tissues were obtained from patients with non-inflammatory conditions as peroral (jejunal) biopsies (n=25) colonoscopy biopsies (n=16) and resection material from diverticular disease or distal from colorectal carcinoma (n=14). Cryostat sections were double-labeled with combinations of monoclonal antibodies, one of IgG class and the other of IgM class (Table 1) with FITC- and TRITC-conjugated goat anti-mouse IgG and IgM (class specific) second layers, respectively (8). Granulocyte

Table 1. Monoclonal antibody panel

Antibody	Class	Antigen / Specificity and Distribution		
T cell :				
RFT1	IgG	67K	CD5 (T1)	pan T (95% peripheral T)
RFT2	IgG	40K	CD7 (T2)	T-blast
UCHT1	IgG	19-29K	CD3 (T3)	pan T (99% peripheral T)
Dako-T4	IgG	56-62K	CD4 (T4)	helper/inducer T, some Mph
RFT8	IgM	33K	CD8 (T8)	suppressor/cytotoxic T
RFT11	IgG	55K	CD2 (T11)	srbc receptor (T and some NK)
MBG6	IgM	120K	CD6 (T12)	pan mature T (95% peripheral T)
Leu 8	IgG			suppressor-inducers of CD4+ subset*
MHC class II :				
Dako-DR	IgG	28/33K		HLA-DR
RFDR1	IgG	28/33K		HLA-DQ
RFDR2	IgM	28/33K		HLA-DR
Activation/proliferation :				
Ki67	IgG			nuclei of dividing cells
OKT9	IgG			transferrin receptor
OKT10	IgG			"activated" lymphocytes, Mph, etc.
Tac	IgG			interleukin-2 (IL2) receptor
Mononuclear phagocyte :				
RFD1	IgG		interdigitating cells (± on some B cells)	
RFD2	IgG		monocytes, granulocytes (± on some T cells)	
RFD7	IgG		tissue macrophages	
Other :				
RFB4	IgG	135K	CD22	peripheral B cells
RFB6	IgG	140K	CD21	C3d receptor (B cells, FDr cells)
Leu 7	IgM			NK cells
Leu 11b	IgM			NK cells
H366	IgG			cytotoxic cells of CD8+ subset*

*Also positive on other T cell subsets, significance unknown.

crossreactivity was quenched with DAB (9). Histochemistry for adenosine triphosphatase (ATPase), acid phosphatase (ACP) and non-specific esterase (NSE) was performed as described (10,11).

RESULTS

T cell phenotypes

T cell populations occupied three distinct compartments: the epithelium, diffuse in the lamina propria and in lymphoid aggregates. Cells within each compartment had a distinctive distribution; essentially no NK cells were identifiable with Leu-7 or Leu-11.

Jejunal mucosa. Intraepithelial T cells (IEL) were numerous (Fig. 1). The dominant phenotype (70-90%) were $CD3^+CD8^+$ (suppressor/cytotoxic) cells, of which the majority (65-75%) were $CD5^-CD6^-$, and a substantial proportion (70-80%) were $CD7^+$ (Fig. 2). However, very few $CD8^+H366^+$ IEL were observed (Fig. 3), implying that the $CD8^+CD5^-CD6^-$ IEL cells are functional suppressor T cells. Only about 8-12% of the $CD4^+$ cells co-expressed CD7.

The diffuse lamina propria T cells (LPL) were 3:2 CD4:CD8. As for IEL, 65-75% of the $CD8^+$ cells were $CD5^-CD6^-$, although the overall percentage of $CD7^+$ cells was lower (30-40%). Of the $CD4^+$ (helper/inducer) subset, 80-90% were Leu-8^- (implying these cells are not suppressor-inducers), of which only 10-20% were also $CD7^+$. Essentially, no IEL or LPL expressed markers of activation (MHC class II, IL-2 receptor, transferrin receptor, OKT10).

Lymphoid aggregates were not observed in any of the samples of normal jejunum examined, although in coeliac disease, they were quite frequent, and consisted of aggregates of T cells (90-95% $CD4^+$, mainly $CD7^+$), of which 20-30% were class II^+ and about 5% were Tac^+. A substantial proportion (50-60%) were Leu-8^+ (suppressor-inducer).

Colonic mucosa. Numbers of IEL in colon (per unit length of epithelium) were 50-80% lower than in jejunum (cf. Figs. 1 and 5A) and unlike jejunal IEL, on average the CD4:CD8 ratio was virtually 1:1; although the spread was larger (33-80% $CD8^{+}$), and CD7 was expressed by roughly equal proportions of $CD4^{+}$ and $CD8^{+}$ cells. However, as in the small bowel, IEL $CD8^{+}$ cells in colon were mainly (about 60%) $CD5^{-}CD6^{-}$ (Fig. 4). Virtually all $CD8^{+}$ IEL were $H366^{-}$.

In the diffuse lamina propria, the CD4:CD8 ratio averaged approximately 5:2, and in contrast to jejunum, CD7 was expressed by $CD4^{+}$ cells to a slightly greater degree than by $CD8^{+}$ cells, although it was predominantly the $CD4^{+}CD7^{+}$ cells that were $CD6^{+}$ (Fig. 5). Again, as in jejunum, virtually all colonic $CD4^{+}$ LPL were $Leu\text{-}8^{-}$.

Lymphoid aggregates were distributed in colon well beneath the surface epithelium; isolated follicles (more frequent in histologically normal mucosa of cancer patients) had the typical CD4:CD8 distribution of lymph nodes in the germinal centers and mantle zone. T cell aggregates resembled closely those of normal jejunum, except they were more numerous.

Markers of activation. Outside the lymphoid aggregates and follicles, virtually no identifiable T cells expressed activation or proliferation markers (Class II, Tac, Ki67, OKT9, OKT10). Numerous $OKT10^{+}$ (but $CD6^{-}CD8^{-}$ and not corresponding to CD3) lymphocyte-like cells were observed in the lamina propria (never in the epithelium), and were excluded from the immediate sub-epithelial zone.

Interdigitating cells and macrophages

ID cells were $RFD1^{+}HLA^{-}DR^{+}ATPase^{+}NSE^{-}ACP^{-}lysozyme^{-}$ (Fig. 6; 10-13). MØ were of two basic phenotypes: type I were small regular $RFD2^{+}$, $ATPase^{\pm}$ cells (which were either $HLA\text{-}DR^{-}NSE^{\pm}ACP^{\pm}lysozyme^{-}$, or $HLA\text{-}DR^{+}NSE^{+}ACP^{+}lysozyme^{+}$, Fig. 7; 10-13), and type II larger polymorphic $RFD7^{+}HLA\text{-}DR^{+}ACP^{\pm}NSE^{-}lysozyme^{-}$ cells (Figs. 8-13). Other than follicular dendritic (FDr) cells in the germinal centers of lymphoid follicles, no Mph-like cells were positive for C3d receptor (CD21).

Jejunal mucosa. The ID cells accounted for some 20-30% of all Mph. They were found almost exclusively just beneath the epithelium, clustered towards tips of the villi, with interdigitating processes occasionally seen extending into the epithelium. Type I MØ were found scattered throughout the lamina propria, accounting for some 25% of all Mph. Of these, 90-95% were of the quiescent ($HLA\text{-}DR^{-}$) phenotype. Finally, about 50% of Mph were type III cells (Fig. 8).

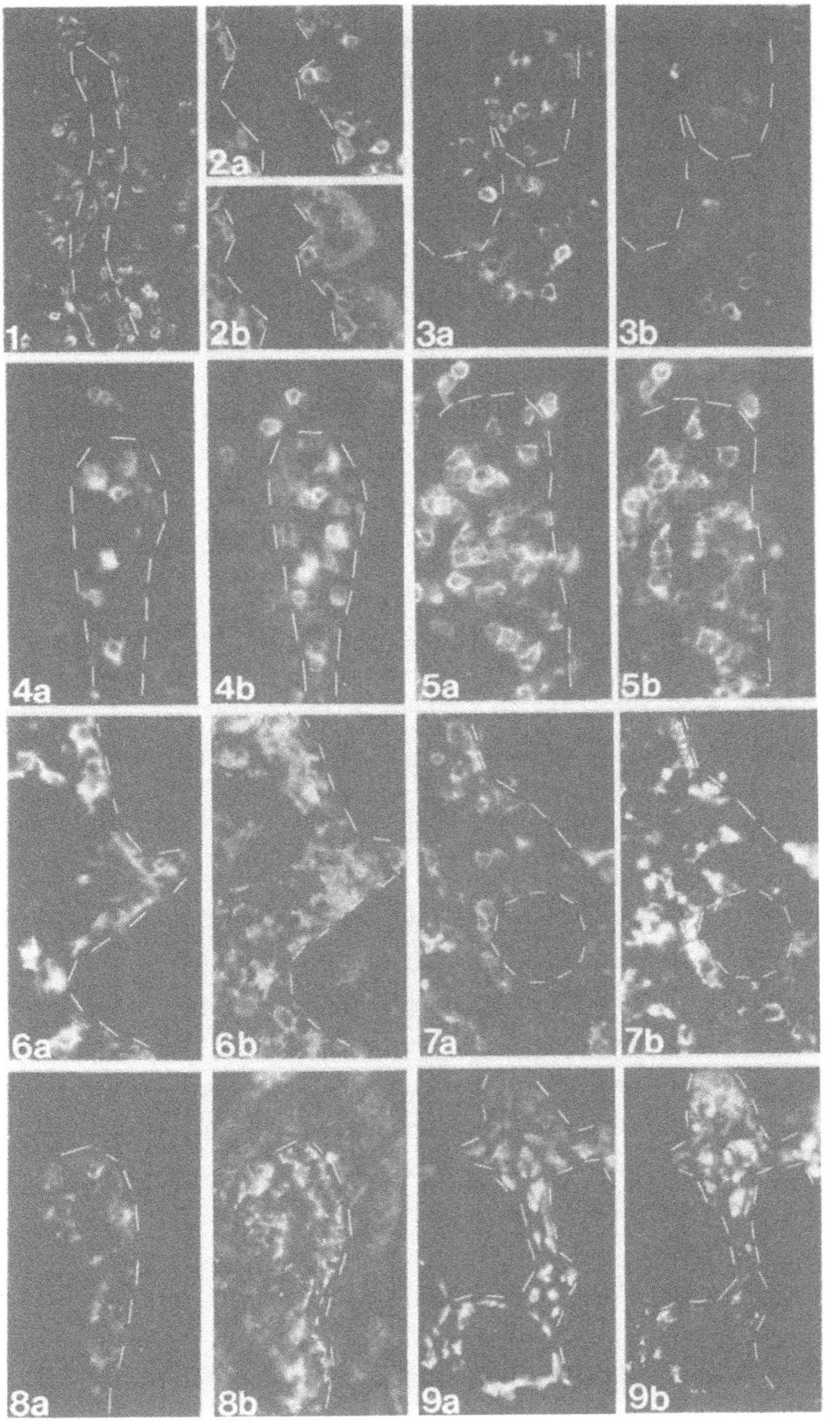

Figures 1-9. T Cells (1-5) and Mononuclear Phagocytes (6-9) of Intestinal Mucosae. Immunofluorescence labeling (paired where indicated a and b); dotted line follows basement membrane of epithelium in normal jejunum (1-3 and 8) and colon (4-7 and 9). Fig. 1: $CD3^+$ cells; Fig. 2: CD7 (a) and CD8 (b); Fig. 3: CD8 (a) and H366 (b); Fig. 4: CD5 (a) and CD8 (b); Fig. 5: CD3 (a) and CD6 (b); Fig. 6: $RFD1^+$ ID cells (a) and HLA-DR (b); Fig. 7: $RFD2^+$ type I MØ (a) and HLA-DR (b); Fig. 8: $RFD7^+$ type II MØ (a) and HLA-DR (b); Fig. 9: $RFD7^+$ type II MØ (a) and HLA-DR (b).

Colonic mucosa. Relative percentage distribution of ID cells was highly variable (even between ascending and descending colon), ranging from almost nil to 20-30% of all Mph (especially in histologically normal colon of patients with colorectal carcinoma). As in small bowel, they were found clustered just beneath the surface epithelium, with cytoplasmic processes extending through the basement membrane (Fig. 6).

Type I and type II MØ were distributed as about 30% and 55% of all Mph, respectively, found throughout the lamina propria; a rare $RFD2^+$ cell was sometimes found within the epithelial layer. Whereas, in the jejunum very few type I MØ were activated ($HLA\text{-}DR^+NSE^+ACP^+lysozyme^+$), in normal colon up to 40% of scattered lamina propria type I MØ were of this phenotype (Fig. 7). Moreover, clusters of ID and MØ cells were observed, containing mainly type I, $HLA\text{-}DR^+$MØ, with dispersed ID cells and type II MØ.

The type II MØ of the colon appeared to be distributed into 3 distinct zones (Fig. 9). The cells in the sub-surface epithelial zone were large and stellate, resembling the ID cells. In the deeper lamina propria glandular region, the type II MØ were more elongated, and often of crescentic shape. Finally, beneath the glandular zone, the type II cells were rounder, with short stellate processes.

Lymphoid aggregates and follicles. There was a characteristic distribution of Mph associated with lymphoid follicles (Figs. 14-17). Germinal centers, in addition to FDr cells identified with RFB6 antibody, contained distinct ID cells. Throughout the lymphocyte zones, type I MØ were observed evenly scattered, 40-50% being of the activated phenotype. Type II MØ were never found within lymphoid aggregates, they were invariably found surrounding aggregates as a shell of cells of crescentic morphology (Fig. 14) which were NSE^+ (Fig. 17).

Relationship to MHC class II expression

Normal jejunal epithelium was strongly positive for HLA-DQ both in villi and crypts (Fig. 10b). HLA-DR expression by enterocytes was weaker overall, and considerably weaker in the crypts (Fig. 8). By contrast, normal colonic epithelium was negative for class II antigens (Figs. 7-9).

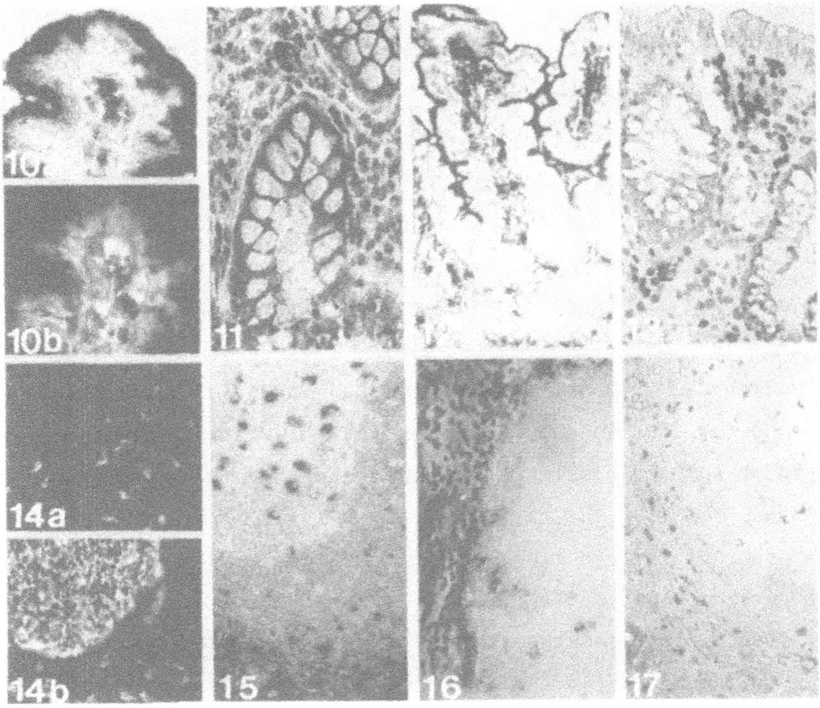

Figures 10-17. Mononuclear Phagocytes: Histochemistry (10-13) and Relationship to Lymphoid Follicles (14-17). ACP (10a) in combination with HLA-DR immunofluorescence (10b) in jejunum, compared with colon (Fig. 11); ATPase in jejunum (12) compared to colon (13); type II MØ surrounding lymphoid follicle of colon, immunofluorescence pair with RFD7 (14a) and HLA-DR (14b); distribution of ACP (15), ATPase (16) and NSE (17) cells in colonic lymphoid follicle.

DISCUSSION

These data show that the immunocyte populations of intestinal mucosa differ markedly in phenotype and disposition from cells of the peripheral circulation and lymphoid organs. Exactly how these adaptations reflect function remains to be elucidated, although several interesting speculations are now possible. However, it should be stressed that small and large bowel are exposed to quite different luminal conditions, and hence differences between the two organs probably reflect further functional adaptations to local microenvironments.

Intraepithelial cells have long been a puzzle, as they have yet to find a functional niche. We consistently found they were much more numerous in small bowel, compared to colon, suggesting they are involved in maintenance of immunosuppression to dietary antigens (i.e., oral tolerance), rather than in cytotoxic anti-luminal pathogen defenses. This is supported by our observations that in jejunum, the majority of IEL are $CD8^+$, but very few display the H366 marker of cytotoxic cells (12). Furthermore, the majority were $CD5^-$, further supporting this contention in view of the evidence that the CD5 molecule is involved in T helper functions (13). The strong expression of the CD7 T-blast antigen and absence of CD6 suggests these are active cells, of which we suggest the $CD8^+CD5^-$ subtype are committed suppressor cells (8), perhaps of an antigen-specific type. Our data also suggests there is a large pool of $T4^+$ lymphocytes which are resting ($CD6^+CD7^-$) $Leu\text{-}8^-$ helper cells in the lamina propria. It would be of considerable interest to see if this population were capable of functional activation during major antigen challenge, or in inflammatory bowel disease.

Mph populations were clearly divided into 3 subtypes. The ID cells, thought to be the principle effector cells in antigen presentation (4), were typically clustered beneath surface epithelium (presumably to process incoming antigens) and in lymphoid follicles. It is worth noting tht ID cells and $OKT10^+$ cells occupied mutually exclusive areas: the $OKT10^+$ cells being found only beneath the sub-epithelial ID cell zone and in the deeper lamina propria. The monocyte-like type I MØ show interesting variations between small and large bowel: a much higher percentage of these presumed scavenger MØ were activated in the colon, suggesting a higher degree of activity due to ingress of microbial material, and perhaps a role in antigen presentation by virtue of HLA-DR expression (14). However, perhaps the most interesting cells are the type II mature tissue MØ. In view of their disposition-related polymorphism, it could be argued that they are capable of functional diversity, e.g., antigen presentation; the characteristic crescentic NSE^+ type II MØ surrounding lymphoid aggregates and follicles suggest that this subtype represent regulatory cells, controlling lymphocyte traffic.

CONCLUSIONS

1. T cell and Mph subpopulations of small and large intestine occupy characteristic niches, and show distinct phenotypic distribution patterns.

2. These adaptations are presumably related to functional roles, some of which may be hinted at:

(a) IEL are suppressor cells involved in maintenance of oral tolerance;

(b) There is a large population of resting T helper cells in the LPL;

(c) Antigen-presenting cells are found in close association with surface epithelia and lymphoid follicles only:

(d) A higher degree of activation of scavenger MØ occurs in colon;

(e) Regulatory MØ might be identifiable phenotypically.

REFERENCES

1. Bolhuis, R.L.K., Gravekamp, C. and Van de Griend, R.J., Clinics Immunol. Allergy 6, 29, 1986.
2. Elson, C.O., Scand. J. Gastroenterol. 20(Suppl. 114), 1, 1985.
3. Unanue, E.R., Adv. Immunol. 31, 1, 1981.
4. Van Voorhis, W.C., Valinsky, J., Hoffman, E., Luban, J., Hair, L.S. and Steinman, R.N., J. Exp. Med. 158, 174, 1983.
5. Poulter, L.W., Clin. Exp. Immunol. 53, 513, 1983.
6. Fossum, S. and Ford, W.L., Histopathology 9, 469, 1985.
7. Unanue, E.R., Beller, D.I., Lu, C.Y. and Allen, P.M., J. Immunol. 132, 1, 1984.
8. Malizia, G., Trejdosiewicz, K.K., Wood, G.M., Howdle, P.D., Janossy, G. and Losowsky, M.S., Clin. Exp. Immunol. 60, 437, 1985.
9. Valnes, K. and Brandtzaeg, P., J. Histochem. Cytochem. 29, 515, 1981.
10. Poulter, L.W., Chilosi, M., Seymour, G.J., Hobbs, S. and Janossy, G., in Immunocytochemistry Today: Practical Application and Biology, (Edited by Polak, J. and Van Noorden, S.), p. 233, Wright Publishing, Bristol, 1983.
11. Selby, W.S., Poulter, L.W., Hobbs, S., Jewell, D.P. and Janossy, G., J. Clin. Pathol. 36, 379, 1983.
12. Al-Sakkaf, L., Pozzilli, P., Sensi, M., Irving, W.L. and Bottazzo, G.F., Clin. Exp. Immunol. 62, 594, 1985.
13. Thomas, Y., Glickman, E., De Martino, J., Wang, J., Goldstein, G. and Chess, L., J. Immunol. 133, 724, 1984.
14. Gonwa, T.A., Picker, L.J., Raff, H.V., Goyert, S.M., Silver, J. and Stabo, J.D., J. Immunol. 130, 706, 1983.

FUNCTIONAL AND PHENOTYPIC ANALYSIS OF LYMPHOCYTES ISOLATED FROM HUMAN INTESTINAL MUCOSA

C.J. Smart, J.E. Crabtree, R.V. Heatley, L.K. Trejdosiewicz and M.S. Losowsky

Department of Medicine
University of Leeds
St. James University Hospital
Leeds LS9 7TF, U.K.

INTRODUCTION

It is now well established that immunocytes in mucosal organs, including the gastrointestinal tract, form a relatively autonomous immune subsystem, with specialized adaptations appropriate for the particular microenvironment (1,2). The main regulatory cells of the immune system are T lymphocytes; however, little is known about T cell regulation at the gut mucosa. Previous studies on immunoglobulin (Ig) production of lamina propria lymphocytes (LPL) have shown IgA to be the dominant Ig isotype (3-5).

Inflammatory bowel diseases (IBD, Crohn's disease and ulcerative colitis) and coeliac disease, although of unknown pathogenesis, are thought to intimately involve the gut immune system. Mucosal Ig production in IBD has been shown to be grossly changed from normal (3,6), although the significance of this finding remains to be elucidated. Our aims were to study the immunoregulatory effects of mucosal and peripheral blood T cells on immunoglobulin secretion by non-T cells, as correlated with the phenotypic subset distribution.

MATERIALS AND METHODS

Mucosal biopsy specimens were taken from the duodenum (n=20) and colon (n=15) of patients with non-inflammatory conditions, as were peripheral blood samples. Resected macroscopically normal colonic specimens (2-5 g) were collected from 7 patients with colorectal tumors. Mononuclear cells were isolated from resected colonic specimens as described (7). After removal of the epithelium, lamina propria lymphocytes (LPL) were purified through a siliconized glass bead column (8) followed by double density barrier centrifugation (20% Percoll over Ficoll/Hypaque). Cell populations of less than 85% viability (assessed by dye exclusion) were discarded. Biopsy samples were processed as for the resected specimens, omitting the initial removal of the epithelial layer. Peripheral blood mononuclear cells (PBL) were isolated by Ficoll/Hypaque centrifugation; T cells (effectors) were separated from non-T (responder) cells by rosetting (9). Phenotypic analysis of cell populations was by double-label immunofluorescence (10) of cytospin preparations.

Cultures were established in 96-well microtiter plates in 200 µl RPMI 1640/HEPES + 10% FBS in duplicate or triplicate. For most assays, responder cells were used at 2×10^5 cells/ml with effector cells added at ratios from 1:1 to 10:1. Pokeweed mitogen (PWM, Sigma), where used, was at a final concentration of 1/100. After 6 days culture, supernatants were collected and stored at -70°C prior to assay. Ig contents were estimated by ELISA assay using alkaline-phosphatase conjugates of anti-IgG, IgM and IgA.

RESULTS

Cell yields were 1.13×10^4 ($\pm$ 1.08) and 6.2×10^3 ($\pm$ 8.3) cells/mg tissue for biopsies and resections, respectively; purity of isolated T cells (judged by immunofluorescence with T3 antibody) was > 90%.

Ig production by mucosal cells

IgA was the major immunoglobulin spontaneously secreted by mucosal cells, although production by colonic cells was higher than by duodenal cells, as was the ratio of IgA:IgM production (Table 1). Little IgG was produced by either cell population. Admixture of colonic T cells provided helper effects for Ig production in a dose-dependent fashion (Table 2); minimal levels of Ig were produced by the T-enriched cell population cultured alone. PWM did not significantly enhance production of any Ig isotype. Helper effects were also observed with admixed peripheral blood T cells on Ig production by autologous duodenal biopsy cells (Table 3).

Table 1. Spontaneous Ig secretion by isolated gut mucosal cell populations ($\mu g/10^6$ cells; mean $\pm$ SEM)

	IgG	IgA	IgM
Duodenum (n=20)	0.23 (0.07)	10.33[a] (2.4)	3.82 (0.83)
Colon (n=15)	0.38 (0.08)	31.23[a] (10.5)	2.26 (0.4)

[a]P < 0.002 (Mann-Whitney U-test).

Table 2. Ig secretion by colonic lamina propria lymphocytes ($\mu g/10^6$ responder cells; mean $\pm$ SEM) - T and non-T cell co-cultures

Ratio of	with PWM (n=3)			without PWM (n=7)		
T:non-T cells	IgG	IgA	IgM	IgG	IgA	IgM
0:1 (control)	1.30 (1.3)	13.8 (6.1)	3.20 (2.0)	0.29 (0.28)	11.2 (4.0)	2.0 (1.03)
1:1	1.28 (.95)	39.2 (23.5)	9.55 (6.55)	0.78 (.57)	55.87 (26.2)	3.54 (1.66)
2.5:1	2.84 (1.76)	127.5 (71.5)	20.6 (12.2)	2.12 (.95)	130.9 (88.6)	8.53 (5.47)
5:1	3.56[a] (2.45)	131.2[b] (60.1)	23.7[b] (19.3)	4.60[b] (1.42)	189.7[b] (63.5)	18.2[b] (9.71)

[a]P < 0.003 (Mann-Whitney U-test, relative to control).
[b]P < 0.001.

Table 3. Spontaneous secretion of Ig in co-cultures of isolated duodenal biopsy cells and peripheral blood T cells ($\mu g/10^6$ responder cells; mean $\pm$ SEM)

PBL-T:Mucosal Cell ratio (n=12)	IgG	IgA	IgM
0:1 (control)	0.23 (.07)	10.33 (2.4)	3.82 (.83)
1:1	0.1 (.05)	16.48 (4.62)	6.55 (1.6)
5:1	0.24 (0.1)	20.79 (5.32)	5.69 (.88)
10:1	0.29 (.09)	26.4[a] (6.05)	7.59[b] (1.74)

[a]P < 0.02.
[b]P < 0.05 relative to control (Mann-Whitney U-test).

Ig production by peripheral blood non-T cells

Ig production by PBL was PWM-dependent; with T to non-T cell ratios having a significant enhancing effect at ratios of up to 5:1. At ratios > 5:1 no further increases in Ig synthesis were seen, with reduced amounts being produced in the case of IgG (Table 4). IgA secretion by PBL responder cells was increased by co-culture with colonic lymphocytes in a non-PWM-dependent manner (PWM caused a small but consistent reduction). On the other hand, increased IgM production by co-cultures was further enhanced by PWM (Table 5).

Phenotypic analysis

No correlation was observed between the T4:T8 ratios and the secretion of Ig by isolated duodenal and colonic mucosal cell populations of individual patients. The T4:T8 ratios were higher in colonic lymphocytes (1.88:1) compared with duodenal lymphocytes (1.03:1), although both were lower than in PBL (2.24:1).

Table 4. T cell regulation of immunoglobulin secretion by peripheral blood lymphocytes (PBL) (expressed as $\mu g/10^6$ responder cells; mean $\pm$ SEM)

T:non-T PBL ratio		with PWM			without PWM		
		IgG	IgA	IgM	IgG	IgA	IgM
0:1 (control)	n=14	0.55 (0.17)	1.19 (0.34)	0.72 (0.19)	0.73 (0.23)	1.98 (0.54)	0.23 (0.09)
1:1	n=13	5.61 (0.84)	5.00 (0.86)	8.43 (2.23)	0.98 (0.26)	2.53 (0.67)	1.30 (0.48)
5:1	n=9	6.12[a] (0.58)	16.12[a] (5.85)	13.94[a] (3.12)	1.51 (0.50)	2.01 (0.45)	2.75 (1.03)
10:1	n=6	4.58 (0.73)	16.76 (7.47)	14.59 (2.94)	1.42 (0.64)	1.66 (0.69)	4.65 (1.53)

[a]$P < 0.002$ relative to control (Mann-Whitney U-test).

Table 5. Co-culture of gut mucosal and peripheral blood cells - regulatory effects (expressed as $\mu g/10^6$ responder cells; mean $\pm$ SEM)

Cell Population (n=14)		with PWM			without PWM		
		IgG	IgA	IgM	IgG	IgA	IgM
Peripheral blood non-T cells	(A)	.545 (.17)	1.19 (.34)	.715 (.19)	.735 (.23)	1.98 (.54)	.230 (.09)
Colonic mucosal lymphocytes	(B)	.590 (.37)	15.93 (4.17)	1.32 (.36)	.380 (.08)	21.80 (5.18)	2.26 (.44)
A+B (calculated)	(D)	1.135	17.12	2.035	1.115	23.78	2.49
Co-culture of A and B	(E)	2.21 (.64)	34.91 (7.64)	5.85 (2.18)	1.38 (.62)	61.79 (11.5)	3.13 (.81)
Helper index	(E/D)	1.95	2.04	2.88	1.24	2.60	1.26

DISCUSSION

Differences in the ratio of secreted IgA:IgM between the small and large bowel may reflect the differing antigenic challenge(s) encountered, with the former encountering food antigens and the latter predominantly microbial products. The lack of correlation between T4:T8 ratios in biopsy cell isolates and secretion of IgA and IgM would suggest that immunoregulatory T cell subpopulations are not just a function of subset phenotype, but may reflect varying activity of subpopulations such as contrasuppressor or isotype-specific helper cells. Variations in T4:T8 ratios between the small and large intestine possibly reflects the relatively much higher proportion of $T8^+$ (suppressor/cytotoxic) intraepithelial cells of the small intestine (see 11).

The relatively high spontaneous production of Ig by colonic non-T cells, compared with PBL, suggests that a higher percentage of mucosal B cells are functionally differentiated plasma cells, confirming the immunohistological studies of others (e.g. 14). Whereas lamina propria T cells had a marked helper effect on Ig production by colonic non-T cells, the suppressive effects at higher T to non-T cell ratios reported by others (12) were not observed. The reasons for this are unclear, but may be related to mucosal contrasuppressor cell activity (13).

IgA-specific helper cells (4) of the colon appeared to be unresponsive to PWM (a mitogen known to preferentially generate T helper cells), as judged by co-culture with non-T cells from either colon or peripheral blood. This observation argues that gut LPL IgA-specific T helper cells are already maximally stimulated; indeed the slight inhibition of IgA synthesis induced by PWM suggests that resting T suppressor cells are being recruited. Nevertheless, PWM did augment IgM production by PBL responder cells in the presence of colonic T cells. These data suggest that there are, in fact, two populations of Ig isotype-specific helper cells in the colon: IgA-specific T helper cells (which are already maximally stimulated), and IgM-specific T helpers (which are susceptible to further induction).

CONCLUSIONS

We suggest that two types of Ig isotype-specific T helper cells may exist in the colonic lamina propria:

(a) IgA-specific T helper cells (which are already highly stimulated);
(b) IgM-specific T helper cells (which can be further stimulated).

REFERENCES

1. Bienenstock, J., McDermott, M., Befus, D. and O'Neill, M., Adv. Exp. Med. Biol. 107, 53, 1978.
2. Elson, C.O., Scand. J. Gastroenterol. 20 (suppl. 114), 1, 1985.
3. Bookman, M.A. and Bull, D.M., Gastroenterol. 77, 503, 1979.
4. Elson, C.O., Weiserbs, D.B., Ealding, W. and Machelski, E., Ann. N.Y. Acad. Sci. 409, 230, 1983.
5. Drew. P.A., La Brooy, J.T. and Shearman, D.J.C., Gut 25, 649, 1984.
6. Fiocchi, C., Battisto, J.R. and Farmer, R.G., Dig. Dis. Sci. 26, 728, 1981.

7. Bull, D.M. and Bookman, M.A., J. Clin. Invest. 59, 966, 1977.
8. Rudzik, O. and Bienenstock, J., J. Lab. Invest. 30, 260, 1974.
9. Jondal, M., Holm, G. and Wigzell, H., J. Exp. Med. 136, 207, 1972.
10. Malizia, G., Trejdosiewicz, L.K., Wood, G.M., Howdle, P.D., Janossy, G. and Losowsky, M.S., Clin. Exp. Immunol. 60, 437, 1985.
11. Trejdosiewicz, L.K., Malizia, G., Badr-el-din, S., Smart, C.J., Oakes, D.J., Southgate, J., Howdle, P.D., Janossy, G., Poulter, L.W. and Losowsky, M.S. (this publication).
12. Clancy, R., Cripps, A., Chipchase, H., Gut 25, 47, 1984.
13. Green, D.R., Gold, J., St. Martin, S., Gershon, R. and Gershon, R.K., Proc. Natl. Acad. Sci. USA 79, 889, 1982.
14. Brandtzaeg, P., Valnes, K., Scott, H., Rognum, T.O., Bjerke, K. and Baklien, K., Scand. J. Gastroenterol. 20 (Suppl. 114), 17, 1985.

MONOCLONAL ANTIBODIES SPECIFIC FOR HUMAN AND RAT INTESTINAL LYMPHOCYTES

N. Cerf-Bensussan, A. Jarry*, N. Brousse*, B. Lisowska-Grospierre, C. Griscelli and D. Guy-Grand

INSERM U132, Hopital des Enfants Malades, 149, rue de Sevres, 75015 Paris, France; and *INSERM U239, Faculte de Medecine Xavier Bichat, 16, rue Henri Hucard 75018 Paris, France

INTRODUCTION

The nature of intraepithelial lymphocytes (IEL) present within the intestinal epithelium is intriguing. They differ from the lymphocytes present in lymphoid organs or in the lamina propria (LP) by their phenotypical characteristics. The majority express a surface marker associated with the cytotoxic/suppressor subset of T cells with a lesser number of cells coexpressing the pan T cell markers (1-7). In addition, 15 to 50% IEL contain intracytoplasmic granules rich in sulfated proteoglycans (8-10). The location of IEL in close contact with intraluminal antigens and epithelial cells suggests that they have an important function in local cell mediated immunity. In the mouse, it has been demonstrated that small subsets of IEL can exert some specific or non-specific cytotoxic functions (11-13). Yet, the function as well as the origin of the large subset of Thy-1^-, Lyt-2^+ granular IEL present in both normal and athymic mice remain unknown. Human intestinal IEL show many phenotypical similarities with rodents IEL (1,4,5,7). Yet, the various subsets of human IEL have not been defined precisely and little is known regarding their functional capabilities (5,10,14). Because of the peculiarities of IEL, we assumed that IEL might possess specific membrane antigen(s) against which monoclonal antibodies (mab) could be raised. These mab may be useful tools to define the function(s) or the differentiation pathway of IEL. We have previously described a mab directed to rat IEL (RGL-1). We report here that a mab with similar specificity has been obtained against human IEL (HML-1) and we discuss the possible role of a novel organ-specific membrane antigen defined by these mab.

MATERIALS AND METHODS

Human tissue specimens. Histologically normal small intestinal samples, 3 to 6 cm long, were obtained from patients aged 26 to 80 years undergoing intestinal surgery for colonic, gastric or pancreatic benign or malignant lesions. All other examined tissues were surgical or biopsy specimens obtained for diagnostical or therapeutic purposes whose examination revealed normal tissue or non-specific inflammatory lesions.

Animals. CD, Lewis and nude rats and BALB/c mice were obtained from Harlan Sprague Dawley Laboratories (Baltimore, MD) or from CNRS Breeding Laboratories (Orleans, France).

Lymphocyte suspensions were prepared as previously described (9,10,15).

Monoclonal antibodies. Production of HML-1 and RGL-1 were performed as previously described (15). Briefly, spleen cells of BALB/c mice immunized with 3 intraperitoneal injections of human or rat IEL (5-15 x 10^5), respectively, were fused with NS-1 myeloma cells according to Kohler and Milstein (16). Supernatants of hybridomas selected in aminopterin-containing medium were tested on frozen tissue sections of small intestine. Two hybridomas, HML-1 and RGL-1, that reacted with human and rat IEL, respectively, but neither with peripheral blood lymphocytes (PBL) nor with Peyer's patches lymphocytes (PPL) were thus obtained. They were subcloned twice and injected into pristane-primed mice to produce ascites. A series of mab directed to various lymphocyte subsets were used. They are summarized in Table 1.

Immunofluorescence technique for determination of surface markers or intracytoplasmic immunoglobulins (Ig), as well as procedures for immunoperoxidase staining of frozen tissue sections, immunoelectronmicroscopy and autoradiography have been previously described (4,10,15). Double staining of frozen tissue sections using peroxidase and alkaline phosphatase linked reagents will be described separately (17).

Labeling of IEL membranes with ^{125}I followed by sodium-dodecyl-sulfate polyacrylamide gel electrophoresis (SDS-PAGE) was performed as described (15).

Table 1. Monoclonal antibodies

	Specificity	CD	MW of Ag (Kd)	Ig Isotype
Anti-rat Mab				
3H3	T Cells	--	--	IgG1
OX8	T cytotoxic/suppressor	--	34 & 39	IgG1 (a)
W3/25	T helper	--	48 - 53	IgG1 (a)
Anti-human Mab				
T11	T cells (sheep erythrocyte receptor)	CD2	50	(b)
Leu 4	T cells (associated to the T cell receptor for antigen)	CD3	20 & 30	IgG1 (c)
T3				IgG2a(b)
Leu 3a+b	T helper	CD4	55	IgG1 (c)
Leu 1	T cells	CD5	67	IgG2a(c)
T8	T cytotoxic/suppressor	CD8	32 & 43	(b)
Leu 2a				IgG1 (c)
B1	Pan B cells	CD20	35	IgG1 (b)

[a]Seralab, Crawley Down, Sussex, UK.
[b]Immunotech, Marseille, France.
[c]Becton-Dickinson, Buc, France.

RESULTS

Studies of tissue sections and of isolated cells indicated that HML-1 and RGL-1 stained cells with similar distribution in human and rat tissues, respectively (Table 2). In the gastrointestinal tract, both antibodies labeled most IEL and numerous LPL. The highest number of positive cells was observed in the small intestine. Staining of cells isolated from the small intestine indicated that HML-1 labeled 94% human IEL and that RGL-1 revealed 91% rat IEL. RGL-1 stained 30-70% rat LPL. In humans, the percentage of positive cells among isolated LPL could not be determined accurately because of the unavoidable contamination of LP cell preparation by lymphoid follicles. This was indicated by the presence of over 30% $B1^+$ cells detected only in lymphoid follicles in tissue sections. However, double staining of tissue sections demonstrated that approximately 50% Leu 4^+ LPL stained with HML-1.

Table 2. Percentage of $HML-1^+$ and $RGL-1^+$ cells in human and rat lymphoid compartments, respectively

Organs	% $HML-1^+$ Cells (SD)	% $RGL-1^+$ Cells (SD)
Intestinal epithelium	93.8 (5.2)	91.0 (4.0)
LP	--	59.6 (17.0)
MLN	3.2 (1.1)	2.4 (1.2)
PP	--	2.6 (1.5)
Tonsils	4.5 (1.3)	--
PLN	--	0.5 (0.4)
Thymus	--	0
Bone marrow	0	0
Peripheral blood	0.4 (0.2)	0
Peripheral blood LGL	0.3	0.01

On the contrary, both antibodies labeled very few cells in the peripheral lymphoid tissues and blood. In the intestinal lymphoid follicles and Peyer's patches (PP), a few positive cells were observed in the T area. Rare positive cells were observed within the periarteriolar sheet and marginal zone of the spleen, in the medulla of the thymus and in the interfollicular area of the lymph nodes. Positive cells were more numerous in mesenteric lymph node (MLN) and human tonsils than in peripheral lymph nodes (PLN). Percentages of positive cells isolated from various lymphoid compartments are indicated in Table 2.

As already observed in rats with RGL-1 (15), the anti-human intestinal lymphocyte mab stained lymphocytes in other mucosae. HML-1 revealed numerous IEL in the ducts of the mammary gland. $HML-1^+$ cells were rare in normal uterus but they represented approximately 20% of the lymphocytes detected in between decidual cells of 20 week placentas.

Nature of $HML-1^+$ and $RGL-1^+$ cells in the intestinal mucosa

Percentages of isolated human and rat IEL that stained either with HML-1 and RGL-1 or with other known markers of IEL were compared (Table 3). As previously reported (15), RGL-1 stained all subsets of IEL in both normal and nude rats. In humans, a panel of mab directed to T cells allowed us to define at least 3 subsets of IEL, all of which stained with HML-1. Approximately 50% human IEL expressed CD2, CD3 and CD5 antigens and thus resembled normal peripheral blood (PB) T cells. A second subset of 30-45%

Table 3. Nature of HML-1$^+$ and RGL-1$^+$ IEL

	% Granular IEL$^+$ (SD)	monoclonal antibodies % (SD)					
		HML-1	CD8	CD4	CD5	CD2	CD3
Human IEL	21 (7)	94 (5)	77 (8)	9 (5)	54 (13)	81 (11)	88 (6)
		RGL-1	OX8	W3/25	3H3		
Rat IEL	44 (11)	91 (4)	77 (15)	20 (12)	45 (12)		

IEL, not observed in the PB, expressed CD3 and CD2 but not CD5 antigens. Both types of cells preferentially coexpressed the CD8 antigen associated with cytotoxic/suppressor function of T cells. Finally, a small albeit variable subset (3-18%) did not express any pan T cell antigens. On cytosmears stained with Giemsa, approximately 20% human IEL were granular lymphocytes. Immunofluorescence and phase contrast microscopy were used simultaneously to correlate the presence of intracytoplasmic granules and the expression of a given membrane marker. Only 10% IEL, likely those with the largest granules, contained granules detectable under phase contrast microscopy. Whereas 75% of these granular IEL did not express any T cell marker, even CD8, over 99% stained with HML-1. Thus, HML-1 labeled the small subset of granular IEL without T cell markers as well as the other subsets of IEL.

In rats, studies of isolated LP cells showed expression of RGL-1 by LPL of both helper and cytotoxic/suppressor phenotypes. In addition, a weak membrane staining was observed on a few IgA-containing large LP cells. In humans, the phenotype of HML-1$^+$ cells was studied in tissue sections using double staining techniques and immunoelectronmicroscopy. HML-1 stained approximately 50% CD3$^+$, almost all CD8$^+$, but only a minority of CD4$^+$ LP cells. Macrophages, granulocytes, mast cells and plasma cells were negative.

Nature of HML-1 and RGL-1^{+} lymphocytes in gut-associated lymphoid tissue (GALT)

Studies of both rat and human tissue sections indicated that many HML-1^{+} and RGL-1^{+} cells visible in MLN and human tonsils were large cells that resembled lymphoblasts. This was confirmed by applying simultaneously immunofluorescence and autoradiography to isolated MLN cells. As previously reported, RGL-1 stained 1-3% rat MLN but 56% large dividing cells that incorporated tritiated thymidine over a one hour incubation. Likewise, HML-1 labeled 2-5% human MLN total cells and 34-41% MLN blasts.

SDS-PAGE analysis of the molecules precipitated by HML-1 and RGL-1 from ^{125}I labeled IEL showed similar patterns of migration

HML-1 and RGL-1 precipitated 2 major components of approximately 100 and 130 Kd in both reducing and non-reducing conditions. A thinner band of 25 Kd was observed in human but not in rat immunoprecipitates. In addition, RGL-1 precipitated a minor band of 200 Kd.

DISCUSSION

Mab were raised against human and rat IEL that defined a novel organ-specific lymphocyte membrane antigen. Both mab were species specific but they labeled cells with similar distribution in each species, respectively. They revealed the majority of intestinal lymphocytes and many blast cells in the GALT. By contrast, they stained rare cells in all other lymphoid compartments with the exception of other mucosae. In addition, both antibodies precipitated membrane molecules of similar, although not identical, migration patterns. Because of the strict species-specificity of these antibodies, no cross-immunoprecipitation studies were attempted. Thus, further demonstration that these molecules belong to the same family will require more precise biochemical characterization such as biodimensional gel analysis or studies of biosynthesis or glycosylation.

The fact that RGL-1 and HML-1 defined similar differentiation antigens on rat and human lymphocytes, respectively, raises 2 main questions. The first one is the possible functional role of these molecules, if any. RGL-1 labeling of both intestinal lymphocytes and their immediate precursors circulating in MLN and thoracic duct lymph (15,18-20) suggested to us that this mab might reveal a membrane receptor involved in the migration of lymphocytes into the intestinal mucosa. Such receptors have been recently involved in the migration of lymphocytes into PLN and PP (reviewed in 21). Yet, the absence of the marker on most IgA-containing LP cells and on some LP T cells argued against this hypothesis. Moreover, in vivo treatment with RGL-1 failed to block efficiently the migration of ^{3}HTdR labeled MLN blasts into the intestinal mucosa of syngeneic recipients. A 20 day old rat was also treated during one month with 10 intravenous injections of RGL-1. This treatment failed to induce any significant decrease in the numbers of IEL revealed by RGL-1 or other mab (unpublished data). Yet, RGL-1 may recognize an epitope localized outside a possible site of interaction. Our current work is directed to obtain other mab directed to the same molecules but to different epitopes in order to test their blocking capabilities. However, the antigen defined by RGL-1 and HML-1 may have a different function, perhaps specific of mucosal lymphocytes. Such a function remains to be defined.

The second question to be considered is the nature of the mechanism that triggers the antigens expression. The fact that RGL-1 and HML-1 labeled weakly the blastic precursors of the intestinal lymphocytes in MLN, suggests that antigen expression is triggered at an early stage of differentiation. However, fluorescence labeling of mucosal lymphocytes, particularly of IEL, was much brighter than that of MLN blasts, suggesting that mature mucosal lymphocytes expressed more antigen. It is possible that a factor present in the intestinal microenvironment may reinforce antigen expression on mature cells. The progressive loss of the antigen defined by HML-1 in cultured human IEL (unpublished results) further suggests that a factor present in the intestinal microenvironment is necessary to maintain its expression. Yet, if this hypothesis is correct, the nature of the inducing factor remains to be elucidated.

CONCLUSIONS

Two species specific mab, HML-1 and RGL-1, obtained against human and rat IEL, respectively, show very similar reactivity. They label all subsets of IEL, approximately 50% LP T cells, many GALT lymphoblasts and some lymphocytes in other mucosae. On the contrary, they reveal rare cells in all other lymphoid compartments. Two main questions remain to be elucidated: the possible functional role of these antigens and the nature of the mechanism that triggers their expression.

REFERENCES

1. Selby, W.S., Janossy, G., Goldstein, G. and Jewell, D.P., Clin. Exp. Immunol. 44, 453, 1981.
2. Guy-Grand, D. an Vassalli, P., in Regulation of the Immune Response, 8th Intl. Convoc. Immunol., Amherst, N.Y., p 122, Karger, Basel, 1982.
3. Lyscom, N. and Brueton, M.J., Immunology 45, 775, 1982.
4. Cerf-Bensussan, N., Schneeberger, E.E. and Bhan, A.K., J. Immunol. 130, 2615, 1983.
5. Greenwood, J.H., Austin, L.L. and Dobbins III, W.O., Gastroenterology 85, 1023, 1983.
6. Schrader, J.W., Scollay, R. and Battye, F., J. Immunol. 130, 558, 1983.
7. Selby, W.S., Janossy, G., Bofill, M. and Jewell, D.P., Clin. Exp. Immunol. 52, 219, 1983.
8. Rudzik, O. and Bienenstock, J., Lab. Invest. 30, 260, 1974.
9. Guy-Grand, D., Griscelli, C. and Vassalli, P., J. Exp. Med. 148, 1661, 1978.
10. Cerf-Bensussan, N., Guy-Grand, D. and Griscelli, C., Gut 26, 81, 1985.
11. Tagliabue, A., Befus, A.D., Clark, D.A. and Bienenstock, J., J. Exp. Med. 155, 1785, 1982.
12. Carman, S.P., Ernst, P.B., Rosenthal, K.L., Clark, D.A., Befus, A.D. and Bienenstock, J., J. Immunol. 136, 1548, 1986.
13. Ernst, P.B., Carman, S.P., Clark, D.a., Rosenthal, K.L., Befus, A.D. and Bienenstock, J., J. Immunol. 136, 2121, 1986.
14. Chiba, M., Bartnik, W., ReMine, S.G., Thayer, W.R. and Shorter, R.G., Gut 22, 177, 1981.
15. Cerf-Bensussan, N., Guy-Grand, D., Lisowska-Grospierre, B., Griscelli, C. and Bhan, A.K., J. Immunol. 136, 76, 1986.
16. Kohler, G. and Milstein, C., Eur. J. Immunol. 6, 511, 1971.
17. Jarry, A., Brousse, N., Souque, A., Barge, J., Molas, G. and Potet, F. (submitted).
18. Gowans, J.L. and Knight, E.J., Proc. R. Soc. Lond. (Biol.) 159, 257, 1964.

19. Griscelli, C., Vassalli, P. and McCluskey, R.T., J. Exp. Med. 130, 1427, 1969.

20. Guy-Grand, D., Griscelli, C. and Vassalli, P., Eur. J. Immunol. 4, 435, 1974.

21. Gallatin, M., St. John, T.P., Siegelman, M., Reichert, R., Butcher, E.C. and Weissman, I.L., Cell. 44, 673, 1986.

ISOLATION AND CHARACTERIZATION OF RABBIT ILEAL LAMINA PROPRIA MONONUCLEAR CELLS

C.A. Hooper, R.H. Reid, T.G. Brewer and W.T. McCarthy

Department of Gastroenterology, Walter Reed Army Institute
of Research, Washington, D.C. USA

INTRODUCTION

Most antigens enter the host across a mucosal surface. Admitting nutrients, the surface that has the function of molecule uptake is the gastrointestinal alimentary canal. As molecules cross the mucosal surface of the gut, the molecules encounter the gut associated lymphoid tissue (GALT). Here antigens encounter either a primary or a secondary immune response. Antigen sampling takes place in the Peyer's patch, some antigens contact the intraepithelial lymphocytes, and the majority of the antigens first encounter immunocytes in the ileal lamina propria (LP) lymphoid cell layer.

Humoral and cell mediated immunity requires B cells, T cells, and antigen presenting cells. In rabbit GALT all of these cell types have been identified (1-5). In the rabbit appendix, sacculus rotundus, and Peyer's patch (GALT) organs, immunofluorescent staining of tissue sections revealed an organization that was similar among the tissues; B cells and T cells exist in domains separate from each other (2). Abundant IgA lymphoid cells reside in both human (6) and rabbit (4,5) LP.

RESULTS

Mononuclear cells were digested from Peyer's patch (PP) excised LP by collagenase (7). Ninety cm of ileum yielded 1.2 billion cells. Centrifugal elutriation separated the cells into two groups according to size. In the first 100 ml fraction, 600 million cells eluted which were very small, measuring 1.9 μm in diameter. Increasing the flow rate from 13 ml/min to 28 ml/min at 2180 RPM eluted the second 100 ml fraction containing 100 million cells. In young New Zealand white rabbits weighing less than 2 kg, the second fraction contained mostly larger cells measuring 3.5 μm in diameter. These larger cells were not observed in older rabbits.

This 1.9 μm small cell was found in large proportion in the spleen (SP), to a lesser extent in the PP and mesenteric lymph node (MLN), and not at all in the thymus (T). A medium size 2.8 μm cell was the major sized cell in the T, PP and MLN. It was also found in large proportion in the SP and was not found in the LP digest. The larger 3.5 μm cell was common in the spleen.

When the spleen cell population was sedimented over Ficoll-hypaque (FH), the small sized 1.9 μm cells settled to the bottom of the tube. This same sedimentation pattern occurred with the LP cells. Since the LP digest is comprised almost entirely of small dense cells, almost no cells were recovered at the FH interface.

By trypan blue dye exclusion, the small cells were 90% viable. When stained with eosin-methylene blue Leishman's stain, some of the cells contained metachromatic staining granules in their cytoplasm. Under light microscopy and electron microscopy, the small cells could be divided into two categories. One group contained cells having a large round nucleus and a thin perimeter of cytoplasm with very few mitochondria, while the other group could be characterized as having more cytoplasm due to an indented nucleus, and which contained many more mitochondria.

Esterase staining of the small cell population gave a 45% positive response. Morphologic epithelial cells responded positively to the esterase stain. Acid phosphatase gave the same 45% positive histochemical response. Immunofluorescent 9AE10 monoclonal anti-rabbit thymocyte antibody (8) stained 20% of the cells. An anti-rabbit immunoglobulin antibody stained $<$ 2% of the cells.

DISCUSSION

Cell morphology revealed by the Leishman's stain, a lack of esterase activity revealed by the esterase stain, and the lack of acid phosphatase activity showed the elutriated first fraction of small 1.9 μm LP cells to contain 55% lymphocytes. In addition to staining monocytes and macrophages, the esterase stain stained epithelial cells. Since the acid phosphatase stain, which does not stain epithelial cells (9), stained the same 45% proportion of cells as did the esterase stain, the elutriated fraction of small cells contained < 2% epithelial cells, and 45% monocytes and macrophages.

Metachromatic granules appear in intraepithelial lymphocytes and not in the LP (10). Tissue section staining showed these granules to be 0.2 to 1 μm in diameter (10), much larger than the granules observed from the Leishman's stain. When physical rubbing releases the cells, 25% of the lymphocytes contained intraepithelial lymphocyte granules (10). Since the EDTA incubation prior to the collagenase digestion removes and washes away the epithelial layer of cells (7), very few intraepithelial lymphocytes are recovered after the collagenase incubation.

Following the collagenase digestion and elutriation, less than 2% Ig staining lymphocytes were recovered from the LP. An abundance, however, of IgA lymphoid cells resides in both human (6), and rabbit (4,5) LP. Neither physical rubbing of the ileum to isolate lymphoid cells (10,11), nor collagenase digestion recovers a significant number of Ig bearing B cells.

According to the immunofluorescence stains, the small cell LP population contained 20% T cells, < 2% B cells, and a 35% population of non-T/non-B null lymphocytes. When physical rubbing of the ileum isolated the mononuclear cells (10), 70% of the lymphocytes were found to be null cells (11). At the base of each follicle in the rabbit appendix, the sacculus rotundus, and the Peyer's patch (GALT) organs resides a thin layer of small lymphocytes that are actively dividing (12) and that are non-T/non-B null lymphocytes (2). These follicle null cells morphologically resemble the null cells isolated from the rabbit LP.

By cell size and sedimentation properties, the dominant small 1.9 μm LP cells resemble the large proportion of similar size cells in the spleen, and the lesser number found in the MLN and in the PP. Larger cells found in other lymphoid organs are not found in the LP.

REFERENCES

1. Befus, A.D. and Bienenstock, J., in Animal Models of Immunological Processes (Edited by Hay, J.B.), p. 167, Academic Press, N.Y., 1982.
2. Sell, S., Raffel, C. and Scott, C.B., Developmental and Comparative Immunol. 4, 355, 1980.
3. Friedenstein, A. and Goncharenko, I., Nature 206, 1113, 1965.
4. Cebra, J.J., Craig, S.W. and Jones, P.P., Adv. Exp. Med. Biol. 45, 23, 1974.
5. Crandall, R.B., Cebra, J.J. and Crandall, C.A., Immunology 12, 147, 1967.
6. Crabbe, P.A., Carbonara, A.O. and Heremans, J.F., Lab. Invest. 14, 235, 1965.
7. Bull, D.M. and Bookman, M.A., J. Clin. Invest. 59, 966, 1977.
8. McNicholas, J.M., Raffeld, M., Loken, M.R., Reiter, H. and Knight, K.L., Mol. Immunol. 18, 815, 1981.
9. Morson, B.C. and Dawson, I.M.P., in Gastrointestinal Pathology, 2nd Ed., p. 219, Blackwell Scientific Publications, Oxford, 1979.
10. Rudzik, O. and Bienenstock, J., Lab. Invest. 30, 260, 1974.
11. Rudzik, O., Clancy, R.L., Perey, D.Y.E., Bienenstock, J. and Singal, D.P., J. Immunol. 114, 1, 1975.
12. Bienenstock, J., Johnston, N. and Perey, D.Y.E., Lab. Invest. 28, 693, 1973.

RABBIT ILEAL LAMINA PROPRIA (LP) LYMPHOCYTES GIVE POOR BLASTOGENIC RESPONSES TO KLH IMMUNIZATION AND CONCANAVALIN A MITOGENESIS

T.G. Brewer, R.H. Reid, C.A. Hooper and W.T. McCarthy

Department of Gastroenterology
Walter Reed Army Institute of Research
Washington, D.C. USA

INTRODUCTION

A clear understanding of oral immunization responses in animal models of infectious diarrhea is critical for development of effective vaccines against bacterial diarrhea. Work in this laboratory has demonstrated the feasibility of primary *in vitro* immunization of rabbit Peyer's patch (PP) antibody by RDEC-1 *E. coli* pilus protein (1) with detection of an antigen-specific antibody response (2). Our objective was to develop an *in vitro* microculture system to demonstrate a primary (T cell) proliferative response to Concanavalin A (Con A) mitogen stimulation and KLH immunization by lamina propria (LP) and Peyer's patch (PP) cells.

METHODS

Pathogen-free male New Zealand white rabbits (Hazelton-Dutchland, Denver, PA) aged 12-16 weeks were used for all experiments. Con A was obtained from Sigma (St. Louis, MO) and keyhole limpet hemocyanin (KLH) from Calbiochem Diagnostics (Behring, CA). The L11/135 and 9AE10 anti-rabbit T cell monoclonal antibody were derived from cell lines maintained at WRAIR. After rabbits were euthanized and distal 60 cm of ileum resected, (PP) were removed and bowel everted and washed in cold sterile saline. LP lymphocytes were extracted using a modification of the technique described by Bull and Bookman (3,4,5). Sequential washes and incubation steps with dithiothreital media, EDTA media and collagenase media were used to release LP cells. LP cells were then filtered through sterile gauze, concentrated in 2-3 ml media and then processed through a Beckman J2-21 counterflow centrifugation elutriator which separates cells by size and density. At an elutriation setting of 13 ml/min flow rate and 2,170 rpm, the first 100 ml media contained 90% of the total recoverable lymphocytes. Cell counts, viability and characterization were noted prior to placement of cells into culture. Spleen cells were prepared from spleen tissue extruded through a sterile mesh into cell culture media and treated with a 5 min wash in NH_4Cl lysing buffer to remove excess erythrocytes followed by three media washes. PP were washed in cold saline, extruded through fine sterile mesh into culture media and washed in 20% FCS media three times before being resuspended in cell culture media.

Cells were suspended in cell culture media to a final concentration of 3×10^5 cells/well on standard flat-bottomed 250 μl microtiter plates. All cell cultures were incubated at 37°C with 5% CO_2. Microtiter plates were prepared so that each treatment group had three to six replicate wells and there were appropriate blanks and non-immunized control wells included for each treatment. Primary immunization experiments were carried out by adding KLH (0, 10, 100 or 1000 ng/ml) or control media to cultures on day one followed by a KLH 'challenge dose' of either 2 μg/ml, 20 μg/ml, media or nothing to cells on day 7 and return to culture. Cells were then harvested 3 days after challenge and 18 hr after addition of 0.1 μCi ^3H CPM on dried glass fiber filter paper after harvest. For secondary immunization experiments, rabbits were immunized by gavage administration of 2 mg KLH or placebo after cimetidine pretreatment weekly for 3 weeks. Rabbits were sacrificed and cells isolated from culture after 5-6 weeks. Cells were cultured in the presence of KLH (2, 10, 50 μg/ml) or control media and harvested daily for days 1-9 after ^3H thymidine administration. Mitogen response was measured in cells cultured with Con A or control media for 72 hr with ^3H thymidine added 6 hr prior to harvest. Cell irradiation for lymphocyte neutralization was by use of a ^{60}Co source for a calculated dose of 2500 rads administered to cell suspensions prior to plating in culture. All data were transferred to VAX computer and statistical analyses carried out using Minitab for unpaired *t*-test, one way analysis of variance (ANOVA) and two way ANOVA with multiple pairwise comparisons between groups.

RESULTS

Results of primary immunization experiments for LP and SPL cells immunized with KLH are shown in Tables 1 and 2. There were no significant differences between any of the immunization or challenge groups of LP cells (Table 1). Responses by cultured SPL cells are shown in Table 2, however, the results show that significant differences ($p < 0.001$) between the response of the 2 μg and 20 μg KLH challenge dose groups compared to media and no-challenge groups by two-factor analysis of variance. These differences are independent of initial immunizing dose which has no apparent effect.

Since a primary immune proliferative response was not detectable in either LP or PP cells, a series of experiments were designed to evaluate mitogen responsiveness of LP, PP and SPL cells to Con A. Figure 1 shows the proliferative responses of cultured cells to Con A treatment compared

Table 1. LP Response to primary immunization

	Initial KLH Immunizing Dose (ng/ml)			
	1000	100	10	0
20 μg	405 + 699	122 + 78	148 + 133	94 + 19
2 μg	169 + 209	101 + 64	80 + 57	86 + 29
media	200 + 162	69 + 32	60 + 17	97 + 52
nothing	100 + 61	106 + 54	118 + 78	103 + 56

Mean+1SD; N=6; p-NS.

Table 2. SPL response to primary immunization

	Initial KLH Immunizing Dose (ng/ml)			
	1000	100	10	0
20 μg	2479 + 725	1996 + 1556	3424 + 1512	2540 + 1455
2 μg	1570 + 100	1213 + 508	1273 + 374	1058 + 1065
media	723 + 477	943 + 539	789 + 374	1257 + 1091
nothing	255 + 69	545 + 393	350 + 156	424 + 154

Mean+1SD; N=6; $p<0.001$.

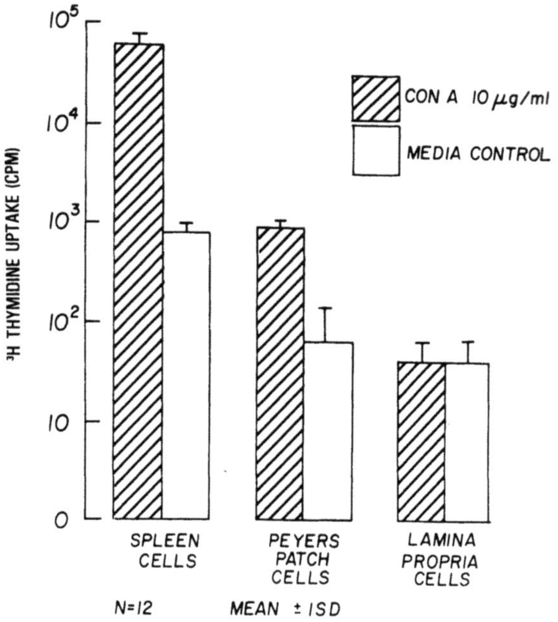

Figure 1. Concanavalin A stimulation. Proliferative response of cultured cells to Con A treatment compared to control treatment. A significant ($p < 0.01$) increase in response to Con A is noted for both SPL and PP cells but not for LP cells.

to control treatment. The complete absence of response by the LP fraction could not be explained by lack of T cells since immunofluorescent staining using both L11/135 and 9AE10 monoclonal anti-T cell antibodies showed that 20-25% were T lymphocytes. Figure 2 shows the results of Con A treated LP cells co-cultured with irradiated SPL cells in order to evaluate the possibility of inadequate accessory cell number in the elutriated LP fraction. Addition of SPL accessory cells in the irradiated fractions failed to improve the LP response to Con A and other add-back experiments in which SPL cells were co-cultured with differing concentrations of irradiated LP cell fractions in the presence of Con A failed to show any evidence of mitogen-induced suppressor activity (data not shown). Secondary immunization experiments revealed serial proliferative changes in (LP, PP and SPL) lymphocytes cultured from animals that had been orally immunized by KLH or by placebo. Daily proliferative responses by LP and PP cells cultured in the presence of 50 μg/ml KLH are shown in Figures 3 and 4. Note that there is no evidence of a significant early (less than 4 days) increased proliferative response by either cell type cultured from the immunized rabbits when cultured with KLH and compared to responses of control rabbit cells. In contrast, a significantly different ($p < 0.025$) serial proliferative blast transformation response can be noted in SPL cells cultured from an immunized rabbit and compared to control animal cells in Figure 5.

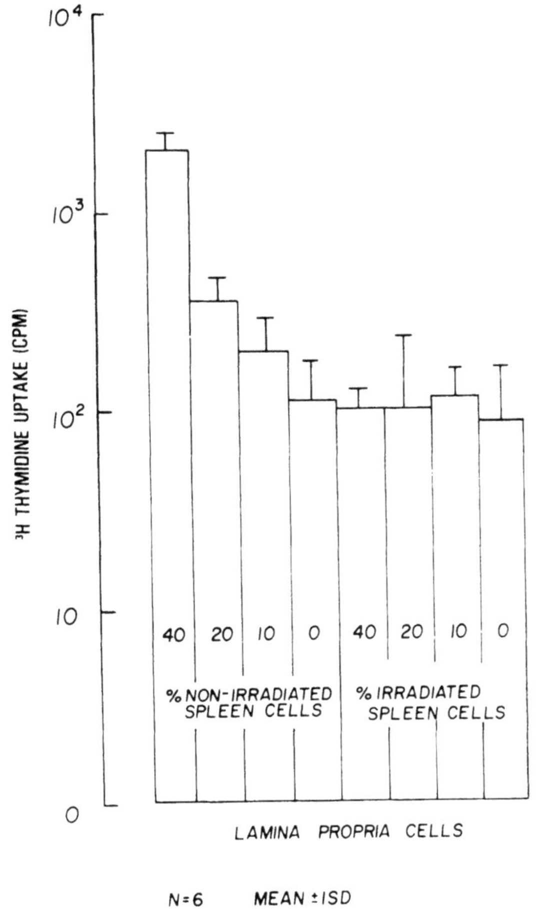

Figure 2. Lamina propria Con A response. Con A treated LP cells cocultured with 0% to 40% SPL cells which have been irradiated (right 4 bars) or not (left 4 bars). There is a progressive increase in response in the left bars corresponding to the increasing percentage of SPL cells indicating that LP cells are not suppressing SPL activity. Further, addition of SPL APC in the irradiated fractions failed to improve the LP response to Con A.

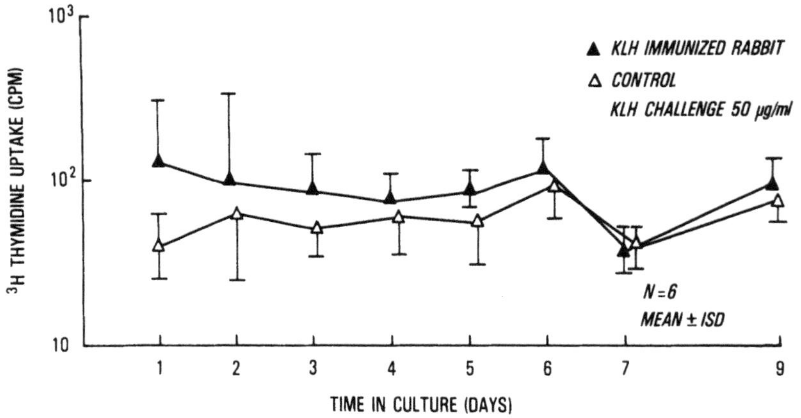

Figure 3. KLH induced response in cultured lamina propria cells. Serial proliferative responses of cultured LP cells from KLH immunized (▲) and unimmunized (△) rabbit culture in the presence of KLH (50 μg/ml). No significant differences over time were noted between proliferative responses of either animals' cells.

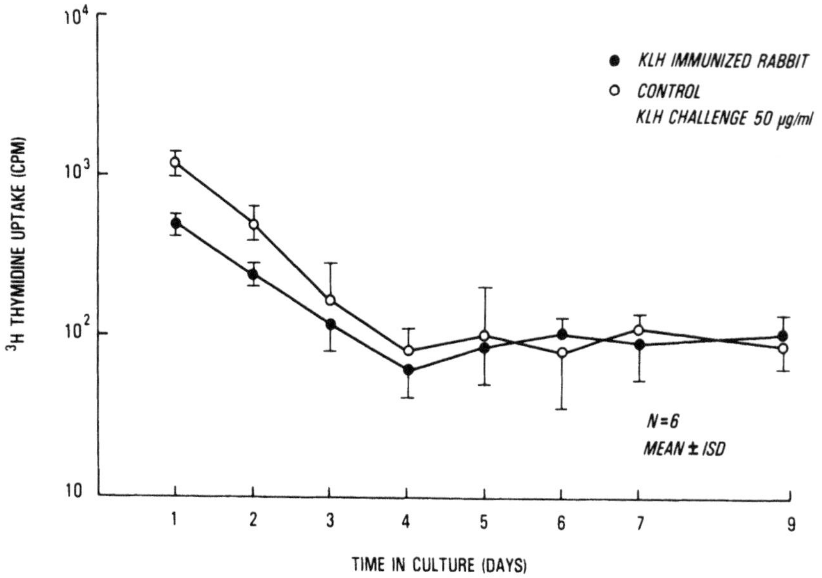

Figure 4. KLH induced response in cultured Peyer's patch cells. Serial proliferative responses of cultured PP cells from KLH immunized (●) and unimmunized animals (○). Although the difference between the two groups is significant at day 1 ($p < 0.05$), no other differences are noted over the 9 day culture period.

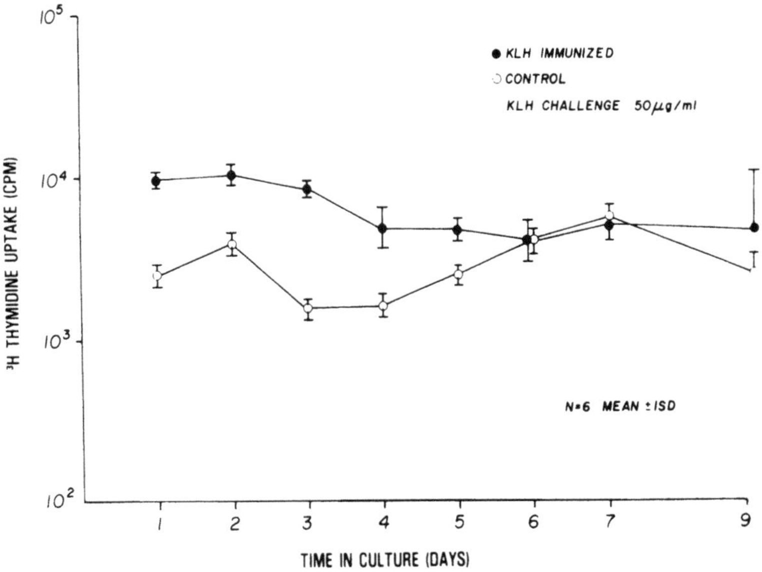

Figure 5. KLH induced response in cultured spleen cells. Serial proliferative response of cultured SPL cells to addition of KLH (50 μg/ml) to media. Note that SPL cells from immunized animals (●) have a significantly greater ($p < 0.025$) response to KLH during the first four days of culture compared to those from nonimmunized rabbit (○).

DISCUSSION

There is no evidence, from these data, of a demonstrable primary in vitro immunization response in either LP or PP cells in microculture. It is notable that these data do indicate a primary in vitro blast transformation response by SPL cells to KLH, and that a secondary proliferative response can also be noted in SPL cells (but not LP or PP cells) from orally immunized rabbits. The data here fail to support any clear-cut mechanism for the lack of an ileal lymphocyte response. Presence of T lymphocytes was confirmed by monoclonal antibody testing to be approximately 20-25% of cultured LP cell fractions and no suppressor activity was identified in Con A stimulated co-cultured cell systems (by either LP-SPL, PP-SPL or LP-PP combinations). Further, add-back of supplementary accessory cells by use of irradiated cell suspensions failed to improve mitogen or antigen related proliferative response of the ileal lymphocytes.

CONCLUSIONS

1. Isolated rabbit ileal LP lymphocytes give a poor blastogenic response to KLH immunization or Con A mitogenesis in in vitro microculture.

2. PP lymphocytes from the same animals show a positive mitogenic response to Con A but no proliferative blast response to KLH in a primary immunization microculture system. No secondary blast response was seen in PP cells isolated from orally immunized rabbits.

REFERENCES

1. Ulshen, M.H., in Attachment of Organisms to the Gut Mucosa, Vol. 1, (Edited by Boedeker, E.C.), p. 49, CRC Press, Boca Raton, FL, 1984.
2. Axelrod, D.A., Clin. Immun. Immunopathol. 37, 124, 1985.
3. Rudzik, O. and Bienenstock, J., Lab. Invest. 30, 260, 1974.
4. Bull, D.M. and Bookman, M.A., J. Clin. Invest. 59, 966, 1977.
5. Sanderson, R.J. and Bird, K.E., in Methods in Cell Biology, (Edited by Prescott, D.M.), p. 1409, Academic Press, New York, N.Y., 1977.

T CELL-DRIVEN APPEARANCE OF MONONUCLEAR CELLS, MAST CELLS AND GOBLET CELLS IN THE RESPIRATORY TRACT

S. Ahlstedt

Pharmacia Diagnostics AB, Uppsala, and the Department
of Clinical Immunology, University of Göthenburg
Göthenburg, Sweden

INTRODUCTION

Inflammatory reactions in the mucosal membranes are often mediated by antibodies of IgE and IgG isotypes. These antibodies work in concert with cells such as granulocytes, mononuclear cells, mast cells and goblet cells (1). The immunological regulation of the antibody formation by T cells and their products has been extensively studied and subsequently established (2). Whether similar regulation of the non-immunological cellular counterparts may occur is still an open question. During parasite infection experimental studies have provided evidence of a T cell triggering of the development of mast cells and goblet cells (3). We have been studying the appearance of cells in the airways of immunized rats and mice after inhalation of antigen.

Humoral and cell-mediated immunity after inhalation of protein antigens in rats and mice

Exposure of BNxWi/Fu rats and CBA/Ca mice to aerosolized ovalbumin (OA) during 2 wk periods triggered immune responses. Thus, a dose-response relationship was seen between antibodies of IgE, IgG and IgA isotypes in serum and bronchial washings on one hand, and the length of exposure on the other hand (4). The use of different doses of OA (0.001-1%) in the aerosol also affected the antibody formation. The highest aerosol concentration was most efficient in inducing IgE, IgG as well as IgA antibody levels in both bronchial washing and serum (5).

After aerosol exposure of rats, regional lymph node cells exhibited spontaneous proliferation in in vitro lymphoproliferation tests using ^{3}H-thymidine incorporation. Addition of syngenic spleen cells suppressed this spontaneous lymphoblastogenesis. Such mixtures of cells from regional lymph nodes and spleen could be stimulated to increased proliferation by addition of specific antigen and mitogen. The cells from regional lymph nodes alone showed less consistent increases after stimulation (5).

The humoral and cell-mediated immune responses in rats were accompanied by granuloma formation and increased numbers of mast cells and goblet cells in the lungs assessed after toluidine blue and hematoxylin-eosin staining (5). In unexposed controls, mast cells were mainly localized in connection with vessels. Some cells were also seen in the pleura. Occasional mast cells were scattered in connection with bronchioli, whereas no mast cells were seen in the alveolar interstitial tissue. In animals showing signs of pneumonitis, some mast cells were found in mononuclear cell accumulations around bronchioli. Few goblet cells were seen, which were preferentially localized in bronchi with a luminal diameter more than 1 mm.

In the lungs of rats exposed to OA aerosol, high numbers of mast cells were found in mononuclear cell accumulations around bronchioli, in the pleura, and in the interstitial tissue. The mast cell numbers decreased with time. In OA aerosol immunized animals a more widespread differentiation of goblet cells were found compared with that in control animals. In the immunized animals the lymphoid tissue could totally surround the bronchioli with a luminal diameter of 0.3-1.00 mm. The goblet cells were seen in the epithelium connected with the mononuclear cell accumulations. This inflammatory pattern was dependent on the OA aerosol concentration, the highest concentration inducing more inflammation reflected as increased numbers of mononuclear cells, mast cells and goblet cells (5).

Mucosal immune responses in mice after exposure to protein reactive haptens

Mice of BALB/c strain which were epicutaneously exposed to picrylchloride and oxazolone developed delayed hypersensitivity as assessed by earswelling after local challenge. Challenge in the lungs with the corresponding water-soluble derivative induced an accumulation of mononuclear cells around bronchioli and around blood and lymph capillaries. These mononuclear accumulations connected with bronchioli frequently contained increased numbers of mast cells. In epithelium associated with mononuclear cell accumulations, increased numbers of goblet cells were seen (Fig. 1).

Figure 1. Goblet cells in the epithelium associated with mononuclear cell accumulations in a lung from a mouse sensitized with PiCl and challenged intranasally with PSA.

Challenge with hapten conjugated proteins resulted in weaker inflammatory reactions in the lungs compared with the water-soluble protein reactive hapten (6). Untreated control animals sometimes showed discrete accumulations of 1-3 layers of mononuclear cells around vessels. Mast cells were sparse and goblet cells were occasionally seen.

Animals epicutaneously sensitized prior to aerosol immunization with hapten-conjugated carrier proteins exhibited enhanced local inflammatory responses in the lungs. This was particularly evident after prolonged exposure to aerosol for 2+2 weeks with a 4-week interval.

Both delayed hypersensitivity (7) and mononuclear and mast cell proliferation and differentiation (8) have been shown to be transferable with immune cells. In our model, such transfer of inflammation mediating immunity can also be achieved. With cells from sensitized animals, adequate challenge of the recipients resulted in delayed hypersensitivity both as earswelling and slightly increased numbers of mononuclear inflammatory cells in the lungs. After elimination in vivo of T helper cells with the GK 1.5 monoclonal antibody as assessed immunohistochemically on spleen specimens, the DTH reactivity was decreased as assessed as both earswelling reactions and development of mononuclear cells and goblet cells in the lungs (9).

It is also well established that delayed hypersensitivity reactivity can be suppressed by intravenous and oral administration of the protein

Table 1. Tolerance induction of DTH assessed in the lungs after i.v. administration of PSA, epicutaneous sensitization with PiCl and intranasal challenge with PSA

Group	n	Treatment	Accumulation of mononuclear cells diffuse around bronchioli	Mast cells around bronchioli	Epithelial mucous cell differentiation
A	3	PSA i.v. sensitization PiCl challenge PiCl, PSA	0	0	0.7
B	3	- sensitization PiCl challenge PiCl, PSA	1.3	1.0	1.3
C	3	- - challenge PiCl, PSA	0	1.0	0

Typical experiment of inflammatory reactions in mouse lung, mean histological score (6,10).

reactive hapten. Administration i.v. with neutralized picrylsulfonic acid consequently decreased the inflammations in the lungs reflected as the numbers of mononuclear cells and goblet cells after local challenge, whereas the mast cell numbers were less affected (Table 1).

Oral treatment with the PSA decreased the DTH assessed as earswelling, although the inflammations in the lungs after local challenge were very little affected (1). This may suggest that the mucosal immune system is differently regulated compared with the systemic one.

REFERENCES

1. Befus, D. and Bienenstock, J., Prog. Allergy 31, 76, 1982.
2. Ishizaka, K., Yodoi, J., Suemura, M. and Hirashima, M., Immunology Today 4, 192, 1983.
3. Miller, H.R.P., Nawa, Y. and Parish, C.R., Int. Archs. Allergy appl. Immun. 59, 281, 1979.
4. Ahlstedt, S., Björkstén, B., Nygren, H. and Smedegård, G., Immunology 48, 247, 1983.
5. Ahlstedt, S., Smedegård, G., Nygren, H. and Björkstén, B., Int. Archs. Allergy appl. Immun. 72, 71, 1983.
6. Enander, I., Ahlstedt, S., Nygren, H. and Björkstén, B., Int. Archs. Allergy appl. Immun. 72, 59, 1983.
7. Turk, J.L., Delayed Hypersensitivity, p. 1, North Holland, Amsterdam, 1975.
8. Haig, D.M., McKee, T.A., Jarrett, E.E.E., Woodburry, R. and Miller, H.R.P., Nature (London), 300 188, 1982.
9. Enander, I., Ulfgren, A., Nygren, H., Holmdahl, R., Klareskog, L. and Ahlstedt, S., Regulation of delayed hypersensitivity reaction in the lung reflected by mononuclear cells, mast cells and mucous cells appearing after T helper cell depletion and adoptive transfer, 1987 (submitted).
10. Enander, I., Nygren, H. and Ahlstedt, S., Immunological suppression of delayed hypersensitivity responses in lungs as reflected by numbers of mononuclear cells, mast cells and mucous cells, 1987 (submitted).

ANTIBACTERIAL ACTIVITY OF LYMPHOCYTES ARMED WITH IgA

A. Tagliabue, L. Nencioni, M. Romano, L. Villa,
M.T. De Magistris and D. Boraschi

Sclavo Research Center
Siena, Italy

INTRODUCTION

It is thought that IgA play a major role against bacterial and viral infections, particularly at the mucosal level. However, the mechanisms through which IgA express their activity are still a matter of debate. After the discovery of Fc receptors for IgA (Fcα) in different cellular subpopulations from experimental animals and humans, it was suggested that IgA might also drive mechansims of antibody-dependent cellular cytotoxicity (ADCC). To verify this hypothesis, we investigated whether murine lymphocytes from peripheral and gut associated lymphoid tissues (GALT) were capable of expressing IgA-ADCC against gram-negative bacterial targets. It was, in fact, observed that this activity can be expressed by cells from normal mice (1-5). Similar experiments were, therefore, performed employing human lymphocytes, and the results obtained demonstrated that IgA-ADCC also exists in humans (6-7). A summary of the results obtained so far is presented here, together with our most recent unpublished findings on this subject.

MATERIALS AND METHODS

The materials employed and the methods applied have been described previously in detail in both animals and in human studies (1-7). Since the antibacterial assay is of particular relevance in this study, a brief description of this method is hereafter reported.

Antibacterial assay

To test the direct cellular activity against bacteria, 10^4 bacteria were placed into 15 ml conical tubes (no. 24310, Corning Glass Works, Corning, NY) and centrifuged at 1300 x g for 10 min at 4°C. Lymphocytes from normal donors, patients and vaccinees were then added to the tubes which were centrifuged at 500 x g for 5 min at 4°C. In the same experiments, antibody-mediated cellular activity (ADCC) against bacteria was assessed by adding sera or purified antibodies from normal donors, before and after vaccination, to lymphocytes of unvaccinated donors. Sera and purified antibodies were employed at different concentrations below the agglutinating titer. To maintain the optimal proportion of reactants, the final volume of the mixture was limited to 0.3 ml, consisting of 0.1 ml of bacterial suspension, 0.1 ml of medium or antibodies, 0.1 ml of effector cells. The experimental and control tubes were incubated at 37°C for 2 h. At the end of the incubation period, the pellets were vigorously resuspended. After bringing the volume to 1 ml with complete cold medium, 1:30-diluted aliquots were plated on petri dishes containing tryptose agar. After overnight incubation, colony-forming units (CFU) were counted. Duplicate tubes were set up for each experimental group, and two petri dishes were prepared for each tube. The percentage of antibacterial activity was calculated as follows:

$$\% \text{ antibacterial activity} = 100 - 100 \times \frac{(\text{Number CFU of experimental tubes})}{(\text{Number CFU of control tubes without lymphocytes})}$$

RESULTS AND DISCUSSION

Murine, natural and IgA-mediated cellular activity against bacteria

Employing lymphocytes from different anatomical sites, including GALT, it was observed that gram-negative bacterial strains such as *S. typhimurium* and *Shigella- E. coli* hybrids are susceptible *in vitro* to natural as well as antibody-dependent antibacterial activity by murine lymphoid cells (1-3). It was of particular interest to note that antibacterial ADCC could be driven by IgA (2-3). Since secretory IgA armed lymphocytes from the gut epithelium, it was proposed that the capacity to drive ADCC may constitute an important local defense mechanism of this antibody isotype which is effective in preventing bacterial infections.

It was subsequently observed that the natural antibacterial activity is also a form of ADCC expressed by T lymphocytes of the L3T4 subset, armed by naturally pre-existing IgA (8).

Human IgA-driven cell-mediated activity against bacteria

Peripheral blood mononuclear cells from normal donors were tested for their antibacterial activity against *S. typhi* (7). It was found that a T lymphocyte with the phenotype reported in Table 1 is capable of expressing antibacterial activity (7). In this case, too, cellular immunity seemed to exert its action through an IgA-ADCC mechanism due to pre-existing IgA which are bound to the cell surface even in normal donors. This conclusion was reached, performing blocking experiments which consisted in pretreatments of the effector cells with $F(ab')_2$ fragments of IgG against human IgA or with intact IgA of unrelated specificity (7). These results provided the experimental basis for the hypothesis that also in humans, antibacterial ADCC driven by IgA may act as a defense mechanism in immunosurveillance.

To understand the relevance of this newly described immune response, IgA-ADCC was investigated in different physiopathological situations, and the results obtained are summarized below.

Deficient IgA-driven cell-mediated immunity against S. typhi in patients with LAS and AIDS

The observation that the effector cell of IgA-ADCC in normal donors is a $CD4^+$ lymphocyte, prompted us to investigate patients infected with

Table 1. Phenotype of the human effector cell of IgA driven ADCC against *S. typhi*

Positive	Negative
OKT3 (CD3)	OKT8 (CD8)
OKT4 (CD4)	5.9 (T subset)
OKT11 (CD2)	OKB7 (B cells)
Leu 8 (T subset)	OKM1 (CD11)
	AB8.28 (CD18)

The cell subset defined by the monoclonal antibody in parentheses.

HTLV III, which is thought to affect mainly CD4$^+$ lymphocytes. This study (performed in collaboration with G. Poli and A. Mantovani, Negri Institute, Milan and A. Lazzarin, Institute for Infectious Diseases, University of Milan, Milan, Italy) was of particular interest for two reasons. First, LAS and AIDS patients are increasingly reported to be affected by salmonellosis (9). Second, the effector cell of IgA-ADCC has recently been found to be a subset of CD4$^+$ lymphocytes bearing Leu 8 marker (unpublished observations). Indeed, the same T cell subpopulation was observed to be the main target of HTLV III infection (10).

When drug abusing HTLV III-positive patients with clinically confirmed LAS and AIDS were tested for _in vitro_ antibacterial activity against _S. typhi_, it was found that they were deficient for this immune mechanism which is present, on the contrary, in normal donors and symptom-free addicted donors negative for HTLV III (Table 2). Thus, it can be concluded that pathological deficiencies of the CD4$^+$, Leu 8$^+$ lymphoid subset results in the failure of IgA-ADCC expression. This might be at the origin of the increased susceptibility of LAS and AIDS patients to bacterial infections.

Increased IgA-driven cell-mediated immunity against S. typhi by oral vaccines

Another _in vivo_ model in humans that is useful to assess the role of IgA-ADCC against bacteria was offered by the new oral vaccine from the _S. typhi_ mutant strain Ty21a (10,11). Employing volunteers from a non-endemic area,

Table 2. Cell-mediated activity against _S. typhi_ in LAS and AIDS patients

Exp. group	No. of Donors	% antibacterial activity ± S.E.				HTLV III
		25[a]	50	100	200	
Normal	8	-16.7 ± 4.7	4.9 ± 7.0	22.5 ± 5.6	30.2 ± 1.5	-
Symptom-free drug abusers	5	ND	12.0 ± 6.9	18.6 ± 7.8	28.7 ± 8.4	-
LAS	9	-1.3 ± 6.4	-21.6 ± 7.4	-25.2 ± 9.3	-9.5 ± 11.4	+
AIDS	6	-20.6 ± 7.6	-8.8 ± 5.9	2.2 ± 7.7	ND	+

[a]Effector to target ratio. ND = not done.

we observed that the live oral vaccine is capable of increasing *in vitro* cellular immunity against *S. typhi* by T lymphocytes armed with IgA (7). It is likely that Ty2la vaccine increases IgA against *S. typhi* and that a potentiation of the humoral arm of ADCC results in a better protection against enteric infections. More details on these studies are provided in the paper by Nencioni et al. in this volume.

Ontogeny of cell-mediated immunity against S. typhi

In an attempt to better understand the origin of IgA-arming lymphocytes and what induces their specificity against bacteria, preliminary experiments were performed employing cord blood cells in the *in vitro* assay against *S. typhi*. It was found that at the cord blood level, cell-mediated activity is higher than in normal adults (Table 3), although it does not differ from that of the corresponding mother.

Since IgA are not present in cord blood, we analyzed the cause of the extremely high natural immunity against bacteria. Preliminary experiments showed that both monocytes and $T4^+$ lymphocytes armed by IgG are responsible for the increased activity, whereas the maternal cellular immunity against *S. typhi* is totally expressed as an IgA-ADCC mechanism.

Table 3. Cell mediated activity against *S. typhi* in cord blood

Exp. group	No. of donors	% antibacterial activity ± SE				
		6[a]	12	25	50	100
Peripheral blood from normal adults	20	-26.7±9.8	-24.1±9.0	0.9±1.8	4.1±3.6	13.8±3.5
Peripheral blood from mothers at delivery	11	7.0±2.2	6.3±1.4	10.9±4.0	31.8±6.0	48.6±5.6
Cord blood	11	6.1±2.6	11.9±5.4	23.9±7.1	31.4±6.6	49.0±8.9

[a]Effector to target ratio.

CONCLUSIONS

Even though further studies are necessary to clarify the biological relevance of IgA-ADCC, it can be concluded from the above mentioned results that this antibacterial mechanism may indeed be important for host defense to gram-negative bacterial infections.

REFERENCES

1. Nencioni, L., Villa, L., Boraschi, D., Berti, B. and Tagliabue, A., J. Immunol. 130, 903, 1983.
2. Tagliabue, A., Nencioni, L., Villa, L., Keren, D.F., Lowell, G.H. and Boraschi, D., Nature 306, 184, 1983.
3. Tagliabue, A., Boraschi, D., Villa, L., Keren, D.F., Lowell, G.H., Rappuoli, R. and Nencioni, L., J. Immunol. 133, 988, 1984.
4. Tagliabue, A., Nencioni, L., Villa, L. and Boraschi, D., Clin. Exp. Immunol. 56, 531, 1984.
5. Nencioni, L., Villa, L., Boraschi, D. and Tagliabue, A., Infect. Immun. 47, 534, 1985.
6. Tagliabue, A., Nencioni, L., Caffarena, A., Villa, L., Boraschi, D., Cazzola, G. and Cavalieri, S., Clin. Exp. Immunol. 62, 242, 1985.
7. Tagliabue, A., Villa, L., Boraschi, D., Peri, G., De Gori, V. and Nencioni, L., J. Immunol. 135, 4178, 1985.
8. Tagliabue, A., Villa, L., Sestini, P., Boraschi, D., De Magistris, M.T. and Nencioni, L., in Mucosal Immunity and Infection of Mucosal Surface, (Edited by Strober, W., McGhee, J. and Lamm, M.), in press.
9. Nicholson, J.K.A., McDougal, J.S., Spira, T.J., Cross, G.D., Jones, B.M. and Reinherz, E.L., J. Clin. Invest. 73, 191, 1984.
10. Profeta, S., Forrester, C., Eng, R.H.K., Liu, R., Johnson, E., Palinks, R. and Smith, S.M., Arch. Intern. Med. 145, 670, 1985.
11. Germanier, R and Fürer, E.J., Infect. Dis. 131, 553, 1975.
12. Wadhan, M.H., Serie, C., Cerisier, Y., Sallam, S. and Germanier, R., J. Infect. Dis. 145, 292, 1982.

ANTIBACTERIAL ACTIVITY AGAINST *STREPTOCOCCUS PNEUMONIAE* BY MOUSE LUNG LYMPHOCYTES

P. Sestini, L. Nencioni, L. Villa, D. Boraschi and
A. Tagliabue

The Institute of Respiratory Diseases, University of
Siena and the Sclavo Research Center, Siena, Italy

INTRODUCTION

Despite the presence of a relevant number of lymphoid cells in the lung, organized in follicles and lymphoid aggregates or free in the bronchial mucosa, submucosa, and in the alveolar fluid, the main function of these cells is still largely unknown (1,2). It has been suggested that they might belong to an immunological system common to other mucosae (MALT: mucosa associated lymphoid tissue) and that their main function is the production of immunoglobulins, mostly of the IgA class, which will be transported in secretions (3,4). Recently, however, it has been shown that lymphocytes from the gastrointestinal mucosa may be armed by specific IgA to express antibacterial activity against enteropathogenic organisms (5-7). Since lung lymphocytes (LL) were found to recognize bacterial antigens *in vitro* (8), and at the same time, to have cytotoxic activity against tumors (9), as also observed with lymphoid cells from other mucosal sites (10), it was of interest to investigate whether a population of LL could also exert antibacterial activity against a respiratory pathogen by means of a mechanism similar to those of other mucosal lymphocytes.

METHODS

Preparation of effector cells

To obtain LL, C3H/HeN mice were killed by exsanguination, the right ventricle was cannulated with a 26 gauge needle and the pulmonary circulation was perfused with PBS containing heparin to wash out the blood cells. The lungs were then removed, finely cut, and digested twice by incubation in culture medium containing 20 units/ml collagenase for 45 min at 37°C under continuous agitation. In order to obtain purified LL, adherent-phagocytic cells were removed by treatment with carbonyl iron powder and magnet. The resulting cell preparation consisted of $1 \pm 0.3 \times 10^6$ cells/mouse, composed of 90% lymphocytes. In depletion experiments, Thy 1.2, L3T4 and asialo GM1 (aGM1) positive cells were depleted by treating the effector population with antibodies and complement (C). Resident AMø (over 95% AMø) were obtained by bronchoalveolar lavage using medium containing 12 mM lidocaine (11). Peritoneal exudate cells (PEC) were obtained 15 hours after peritoneal injection of sterile thioglycollate broth and enriched with PMN by centrifugation on a Ficoll gradient.

Antibacterial antibodies

Monoclonal antibodies of the IgA class against phosphorylcholine (PC) from plasmacytoma S107 were employed for their capability of reacting with PC present on *S. pneumoniae* (12). Mouse IgA anti-*Salmonella tel aviv* from plasmacytoma MOPC 384 were also used to check specificity.

Antibacterial assay

A streptomycin-resistant strain of *S. pneumoniae* type 3 was obtained from our own bacterial collection. The bacteria were cultivated overnight and resuspended in RPMI 1640 supplemented with 10% heat-inactivated fetal bovine serum and streptomycin (assay medium). 10^4 bacteria were placed in 15 ml polystyrene conical tubes together with either appropriately diluted antibodies or medium, and were centrifuged at 1300 x g for 10 min at 4°C (5-7). The cell suspensions were then added to bacteria at different effector to target (E:T) ratios, and the tubes were again centrifuged at 500 x g for 5 min at 4°C to bring the cells in close contact with bacteria. The experimental and control tubes, which contained bacteria and medium or antibodies but no cells, were then incubated at 37°C for 2 h. At the end of the incubation period, the pellets were vigorously resuspended and appropriately diluted aliquots were plated on petri dishes containing BHI agar with 1% horse serum and 100 µg/ml streptomycin. After overnight incubation, colony-forming units (CFU) were counted. The percentage of antibacterial activity was expressed as number of CFU of experimental tubes/ number of CFU of control tubes without lymphocytes. Results were expressed as the mean of duplicate plates, the difference between duplicates never exceeding 10% of the mean. In blocking experiments, LL were incubated in ice for 1 h with affinity purified $F(ab')_2$ fragments from hyperimmune goat polyclonal anti-mouse IgA or anti-IgG and then washed in medium before the assay.

NK assay

NK assay was assessed as the ability to induce $Na_2{}^{51}CrO_4$ release from the YAC-1 tumor line used as target (10). The % specific cytotoxicity was calculated from the formula: (cpm release from cells during incubation - cpm spontaneous release)/(total cpm incorporated x 0.8 - cpm spontaneous release) x 100. Spontaneous release was usually between 6 and 12%.

RESULTS

Table 1 summarizes the results obtained in several separate experiments. The capability of lung cells to exert natural antibacterial (NA) activity in vitro against S. pneumoniae was first assessed in parallel with NK activity against YAC-1 tumor cells. Cells obtained by enzymatic digestion of lungs from normal mice were found to have detectable NA and NK activities. Both activities increased several fold after removal of phagocytic cells, thus suggesting that in both cases the effector cells might belong to a lymphoid subpopulation rather than to adherent/phagocytic cells. To further characterize the effectors of NA and NK activity at the lung level, depletion experiments were performed using monoclonal anti-Thy 1.2 or polyclonal anti-aGM1 antibodies and complement. Treatment with anti-aGM1 greatly decreased both the NA and the NK activities of LL; on the other hand, treatment with anti-Thy 1.2 drastically decreased the NA activity of LL against S. pneumoniae, but did not affect the NK activity of the same cells.

Since the effector cells of NA activity against enterobacteria found in human blood have been shown to be T cells with $CD4^+$ phenotype, depletion experiments were performed on mouse LL using GK 1.5 antibodies which recognize L3T4, an analogue of the human CD 4 antigen, on the surface of murine T lymphocytes (13). Treatment with anti-L3T4 antibodies and C, but not with antibody or C alone, caused a significant decrease of NA by LL, indicating that the effector cell belongs to a subset of mouse T lymphocytes with a phenotype similar to the human effector of antibacterial activity. Blocking experiments were then performed using affinity-purified anti-mouse IgA antibodies, in order to investigate whether the NA activity

Table 1. Effects of various treatments on NA and NK activities of LL

Treatment	NA	NK
C alone	unchanged	unchanged
anti-aGM1	unchanged	not determined
anti-aGM1 + C	decreased	unchanged
anti-Thy 1.2 + C	decreased	unchanged
anti-L3T4	unchanged	not determined
anti-L3T4 + C	decreased	not determined
anti-IgA	decreased	not determined
anti-IgG	unchanged	not determined
IgA anti-PC	increased	not determined
IgA anti-S. tel aviv	unchanged	not determined

Summary table of several different experiments. Results are referred to an E:T ratio of 1:100 and are expressed as M $\pm$ SE or as range of at least two separate experiments.

of LL against S. pneumoniae might also be due to an IgA-driven mechanism. Pretreatment of LL with anti-IgA but not with anti-IgG $F(ab')_2$ fragments resulted in the complete inhibition of their antibacterial activity. In addition, S107 antibodies (plasmacytoma-derived IgA with specificity against PC, a component of the outer wall of Gram-positive bacteria including S. pneumoniae, significantly increased the antibacterial activity of untreated LL and restored the antibacterial activity of anti-IgA treated cells. Thus, these results strongly suggest that NA activity is due to specific IgA naturally present in th LL surface and that, in addition to NA, an IgA driven ADCC mechanism may also be important at the lung level against pathogenic bacteria.

The above mentioned results clearly indicate that T lymphocytes are the only effector cells of NA activity, which is indeed mediated by an IgA-driven mechanism. However, receptors for IgA were also reported to be present on Mø and PMN (14,15). Therefore, we investigated whether IgA from S107 plasmacytoma could induce antibacterial activity in these cell populations by an IgA-ADCC mechanism. As expected, AMø and PEC were not capable of exerting NA activity, but they could be armed by IgA against S. pneumoniae (Fig. 1). This IgA-ADCC by AMø and PEC was specific, since an unrelated IgA (from MOPC 384 against Salmonella tel aviv) did not induce

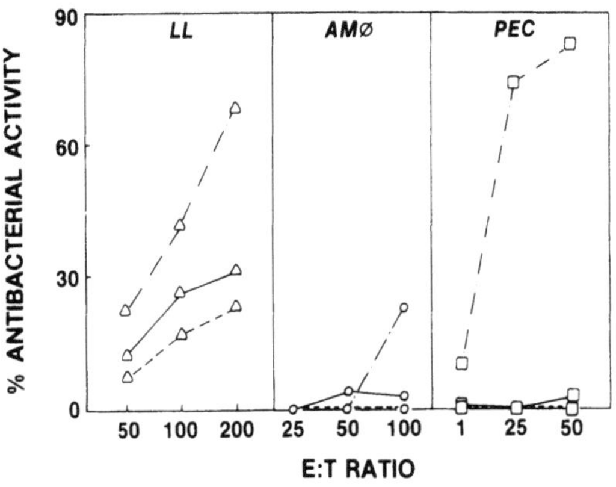

Figure 1. IgA-ADCC of mouse LL (△), resident AMϕ (O), and PEC (□) against S. pneumoniae. NA activity: (———); activity in the presence of S107 antibodies: (-.-.-.-); activity in the presence of MOPC 384 antibodies (----).

anti-S. pneumoniae activity. Since phagocytic cells were particularly effective after arming with specific IgA, experiments were performed to rule out the possibility that the enhancement of antibacterial activity previously observed in LL in the presence of S107 IgA might be due to the small number of AMϕ and PMN contaminating our LL preparations. However, treatment with anti-Thy 1.2 and C which was always effective in completely abolishing NA activity, greatly reduced the IgA-induced ADCC of LL (data not shown), thus indicating that all the NA activity and most of the S107-induced ADCC observed in LL was due to a population of T lymphocytes, though phagocytic cells could be also, in part, responsible for this latter activity.

DISCUSSION

Immunoglobulin of the IgA class are largely present in bronchial secretions (25) and are considered to play an important role in the defense of the lung against infections (16,17). The mechanism by which IgA exerts this protective activity, however, is not completely clear (16). In the last few years, however, receptors for the Fc portion of IgA (FcαR) have been demonstrated in lymphocytes, monocytes, alveolar macrophages and granulocytes in several species, and many activities of surface-bound IgA have been described including the ability to induce ADCC of human monocytes against bacteria (14), and to induce phagocytosis of bacteria by activated AMϕ (15). More recently, it has been shown that lymphocytes from the murine intestinal epithelium, Peyer's patches, mesenteric lymph nodes and spleen 5-7), as well as human blood lymphocytes (18), can exert IgA-ADCC in vitro against enteropathogenic bacteria. Our results further extend these observations, demonstrating that mouse LL can be armed by IgA against S. pneumoniae, a Gram-positive bacterium, and that unlike AMø, they seem to have preexisting antibodies on the cell surface which arm cells to express NA activity. The effector cell of NA activity of LL can be reasonably considered to be a lymphoid cell since this activity is increased after removal of phagocytic cells, is reduced by treatment with anti-Thy 1.2 and C, and in addition, PMN and resident AMø did not show direct NA activity. It is of interest that the effector of NA activity was found to have a $aGM1^+$ phenotype, since LL have been shown also to possess NK activity (9). Depletion experiments clearly demonstrated that the phenotype of the effector of antibacterial activity was Thy 1.2^+, $aGM1^+$, different from the Thy 1.2^- phenotype of the effector of NK activity (9), thus indicating that the two activities are expressed by different cell populations and possibly by different effector mechanisms. It is possible, however, that the two activities could be exerted by a different subset of LGL: it is of interest in this regard that recently a subset of human lymphocytes with the morphological characteristics of LGL and phenotypic markers of T cells has been described to be able to ingest and kill Gram-positive bacteria in vitro (19).

Analogy between the mechanisms of antibacterial activity of mouse LL and that of mouse intestinal and human blood lymphocytes was suggested by blocking experiments with anti-IgA antibodies and by the finding that the effector of NA activity among LL is a $L3T4^+$ lymphocyte. The fact that in analyses of different species, organs and bacteria, a subset of T lymphocytes with $L3T4^+$ or with the corresponding human $CD4^+$ phenotype typical of helper/inducer cells (18) has been found to be responsible for IgA-mediated NA activity might suggest that the effector of NA activity could also participate in the regulation of the local immune response. A subset of $Fc\alpha R^+$ T cells with isotype-specific helper activity on IgA synthesis have, in fact, been described in human blood (20). Whether the effector of NA activity also has similar regulatory functions at the mucosal level remains to be determined.

Though only LL seem to be responsible for NA activity against S. pneumoniae in the mouse lung, our data also confirm, as previously shown by others (14,15), that IgA can specifically arm resident AMø and PMN enriched exudate cells to kill bacteria. The reason why LL are able to exert IgA-mediated NA activity, whereas AMø acquire antibacterial activity only after addition of exogenous IgA, is unclear. One possibility is that LL might reside closer to the sites producing IgA, in the bronchial lymphoid follicles, and could have easier access to locally produced IgA, which in turn could cause an increase in their FcαR. Indeed it has been shown that exposure to IgA can increase the number of $Fc\alpha R^+$ lymphocytes *in vivo* and *in vitro* (21). If this is the case, LL could play an important role in the local defense against bacterial infections at the level of the bronchial mucosa, which is particularly exposed to contact with inhaled particles and bacteria, and where phagocytic cells are poorly represented (1). Recent studies in humans have shown protection from bronchial infection induced by an oral vaccine against *Haemophilus influenzae* (22), an immunization route which is known to increase IgA-driven cell-mediated antibacterial activity (23). This result could suggest a relationship *in vivo* between cell-mediated antibacterial activity and the mucosal immunological system at the lung level.

We have no information about the origin of IgA present on the LL surface in normal mice. It is of interest, in this regard, that IgA antibodies with a specificity for PC can mediate antibacterial activity in our system. Anti-PC antibodies of several classes, including IgA, are normally present in the serum of humans and several strains of mice, probably as a consequence of environmental exposure (24), and have been shown to be protective against experimental infection with several strains of *S. pneumoniae* *in vivo* (24). It thus, seems possible that serum derived anti-PC antibodies could be at least, in part, responsible for the NA activity, though the presence of IgA with different specificities cannot be excluded.

CONCLUSIONS

Taken together, our data suggest that IgA-ADCC by lymphocytes and phagocytic cells could constitute an important mechanism of defense of the lung mucosa against infection by *S. pneumoniae* and probably against other bacteria. Since similar mechanisms operate in different mucosal tissues (10-12), they also seem to suggest that IgA-induced, cell-mediated NA activity could be a common defense mechanism of the mucosal immune system.

REFERENCES

1. McDermott, M.R., Befus, A.D. and Bienenstock, J., Int. Rev. Exp. Pathol. 23, 47, 1982.
2. Clancy, R. and Bienenstock, J., J. Immunol. 112, 1997, 1974.
3. Weisz-Carrington, P., Roux, M.E., McWilliams, M., Phillips-Quagliata, J.M. and Lamm, M.E., J. Immunol. 123, 1705, 1979.
4. McDermott, M.R. and Bienenstock, J., J. Immunol. 124, 2536, 1980.
5. Tagliabue, A., Nencioni, L., Villa, L., Keren, D.F., Howell, G.H. and Boraschi, D., Nature 36, 184, 1983.
6. Nencioni, L., Villa, L., Boraschi, D., Berti, B. and Tagliabue, A., J. Immunol. 130, 903, 1983.
7. Tagliabue, A., Boraschi, D., Villa, L., Keren, D.F., Lowell, G.H., Rappuoli, R. and Nencioni, L., J. Immunol. 133, 988, 1984.
8. Clancy, R.L., Pucci, A., Jelihovsky, T. and Bye, P., Am Rev. Resp. Dis. 117, 513, 1978.
9. Stein-Streilein, J., Bennett, M., Mann, D. and Kumar, V., J. Immunol. 131, 2699, 1983.
10. Tagliabue, A., Befus, A.D., Clark, D.A. and Bienenstock, J., J. Exp. Med. 155, 1785, 1982.
11. Sestini, P., Bozelka, B.E., DeShazo, R.D. and Salvaggio, J.E., Cell. Immunol. 73, 264, 1982.
12. Leon, M.A. and Young, N.M., Biochemistry 10, 1424, 1971.
13. Dialynas, D.P., Quan, Z.S., Wall, K., Perres, H., Quintans, J., Loken, M., Pierraes, M. and Fitch, F., J. Immunol. 131, 2445, 1983.
14. Lowell, G.H., Smith, L.F., Griffis, J.McL. and Brandt, B.L., J. Exp. Med. 152, 452, 1980.
15. Richards, C.D. and Gauldie, J., Am. Rev. Resp. Dis. 32, 82, 1985.
16. Waldman, R.H. and Ganguly, R., J. Infect. Dis. 130, 419, 1974.
17. Chipps, B.E., Talamo, R.C. and Winkelstein, J.A., Chest 73, 519, 1978.
18. Tagliabue, A., Villa, L., Boraschi, D., Peri, G., De Gori, V., Nencioni, L., J. Immunol. 135, 4178, 1985.
19. Abo, T., Sugawara, S., Amenomori, A., et al., J. Immunol. 136, 3189, 1986.
20. Endoh, M., Sakai, H., Nomoto, Y., Tomino, Y. and Kaneshigi, H., J. Immunol. 127, 2613, 1981.
21. Yodoi, J., Adachi, M. and Masuda, T., J. Immunol. 128, 888, 1982.
22. Clancy, R., Cripps, A., Murree-Allen, K., Yeung, S. and Engel, M., Lancet 2, 1395, 1985.

23. Tagliabue, A., Nencioni, L., Caffarena, A., Villa, L., Boraschi, D., Cazzola, G. and Cavalieri, S., Clin. Exp. Immunol. 62, 2422, 1985.

24. Briles, D.E., Nahm, M., Schroer, K., Davie, J., Baker, P., Kearney, J. and Barletta, P., J. Exp. Med. 152, 694, 1981.

POTENTIATION OF RAT COLON INTRAEPITHELIAL LYMPHOCYTE (IEL) NATURAL KILLER (NK) ACTIVITY WITH INDOMETHACIN

D.S. Ross and T.R. Roy

Section of Surgical Oncology, Department of Surgery
Southern Illinois University School of Medicine
Springfield, IL USA

INTRODUCTION

Natural killer (NK) cells are thought to play a central role in host immunosurveillance against the development and dissemination of cancer (1-3). The role of gut associated lymphoid tissue (GALT) in anti-tumor host defense is not known. It is logical to assume that a malignancy developing within a specific organ would first encounter local immune elements. Rats treated with the colon carcinogens 1,2-Dimethylhydrazine have been widely used as a model of human colon carcinoma (4). In addition, this model is suitable for studying the immune response to large bowel cancer (5). The purpose of this study is to determine whether there is NK activity in rat colon intraepithelial lymphocytes (IEL) and whether treatment with the prostaglandin synthetase inhibitor, indomethacin, will enhance NK function.

MATERIALS AND METHODS

Ten to fifteen week old male Wistar/Furth rats, maintained on a pellet diet and water ad lib, were used in this study. With nembutal anesthesia, fresh colons were obtained and washed with sterile phosphate buffered saline (PBS). Intra-epithelial lymphocytes were obtained by disruption of the colonic epithelium as follows: the colons were incubated with 1.0 mM Dithiothreitol (DTT) at room temperature for 15 min. Following washing with PBS, the colons were incubated in 0.75 mM EDTA at 37°C for 90 min. The supernatant containing epithelial cells and lymphocytes was passed over a loosely packed nylon wool column to remove clumps and debris. The lymphoid cells were enriched on a discontinuous two-step percoll gradient (15/55%) by centrifugation at 400 g x 20 min at room temperature. The cells at the 15/55% interface were collected, washed in sterile PBS and counted with Turk's stain and trypan blue. The cells were incubated overnight at 37°C in a 5% CO_2 atmosphere in supplemented RPMI 1640 containing 1.0 mg/ml indomethacin or media alone. The following morning the cells were run in a 4 hour cytotoxicity assay against YAC-1 target cells radiolabeled with ^{51}Cr. In some experiments, peripheral blood lymphocytes and splenic lymphocytes, incubated with or without indomethacin, were run concurrently in NK assays. $\%^{51}Cr$ release was determined by the following formula:

$$\% \text{ Maximum } {}^{51}\text{Cr Release} = \frac{E - S}{T} \times 100$$

Where E = CPM of experimental sample; S = spontaneous CPM; T = total CPM. All assays were run in triplicate.

RESULTS

The result of NK assays using IEL incubated with or without indomethacin is shown in Figure 1. At an Effector:Target Ratio (E:T) of 25:1, the mean ($\pm$ SEM) ^{51}Cr release was 19.6 $\pm$ 7.3% for the indomethacin treated cells compared to 0% for the nontreated cells ($p < 0.05$ Student's non-paired *t* test). At an E:T ratio of 50:1 the mean % ^{51}Cr release for the indomethacin treated IEL was 24.6 $\pm$ 8% vs. 0.63 $\pm$ 0.48% for untreated IEL ($p < 0.01$). There were not enough viable cells in the preparation to allow higher E:T ratios. Table 1 shows the results of an assay of peripheral blood and splenic NK activity using lymphocytes that had been incubated with or without indomethacin. Radiolabeled YAC-1 cells were incubated alone with media containing indomethacin without effector cells and no ^{51}Cr release was observed.

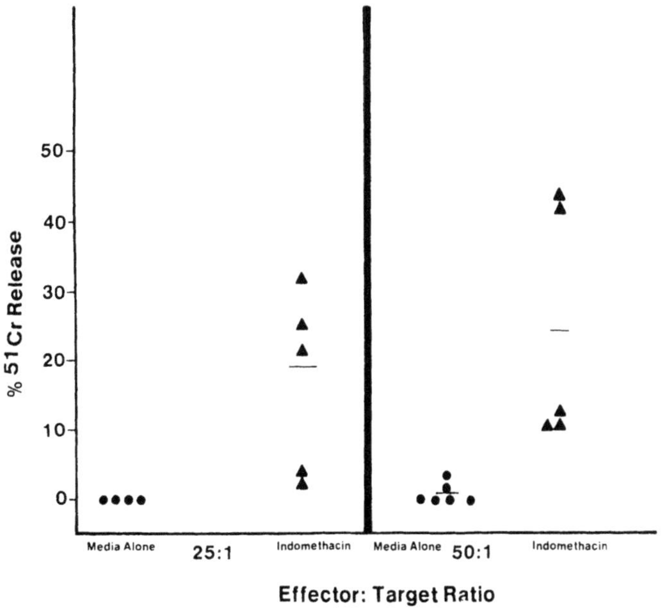

Figure 1. Comparison of rat colon IEL NK activity after overnight incubation with media alone (●), or media containing 1 mg/ml indomethacin (▲).

Table 1. Effect of Indomethacin on peripheral blood and splenic NK activity against YAC-1 target cells

	Effector:Target Ratio		
PBL	25:1	50:1	100:1
Media alone	11.7%[a]	19.1%	2.9%
Indomethacin	25.0%	27.5%	51.0%
Splenic lymphocytes			
Media alone	19.6%	12.9%	22.0%
Indomethacin	23.7%	32.9%	47.5%

[a]% ^{51}Cr Release.

DISCUSSION

Colon cancer, the second most common cause of cancer death in the United States, develops in an organ rich in lymphoid tissue. Whether GALT plays any role in host anti-tumor defense is not known. Bland et al. (6) and Vose et al. (7) have reported that lymphocytes isolated from the colons of patients with colon cancer exhibit negligible NK activity. Bland et al. (6) have suggested that prostaglandin E_2, produced locally by macrophages and/or tumor cells, may account for the observed immunosuppression. Pollard and Luckert (8) and Metzger et al. (9), utilizing the DMH rat model of human colon cancer have demonstrated that rats treated with indomethacin developed significantly fewer colon cancers than untreated controls. One possible explanation for their observation is that treatment with indomethacin enhanced the local anti-tumor immunity in the colon.

This study has shown that Wistar/Furth colon IEL exhibits negligible NK activity against YAC-1 target cells. Incubation with indomethacin resulted in enhanced NK function. IEL contains a mixed population of cell types and it is not clear which was enhanced by the indomethacin. The ability to stimulate anti-tumor immunity in gut associated lymphoid tissue may have important implications for the development of effective cancer immunotherapy.

ACKNOWLEDGEMENTS

The authors wish to acknowledge the expert manuscript preparation by Ms. Brenda Semon.

REFERENCES

1. Herberman, R.B. and Ortaldo, J.R., Science 214, 24, 1981.
2. Flannery, G.R. and Brooks, C.G., Int. J. Cancer 28, 747, 1981.
3. Wiltrout, R.H., Herberman, R.B., Zhang, S.R., Chirigos, M.A., Ortaldo, J.R., Green, K.M. and Talmadge, J.E., J. Immunol. 134, 4267, 1985.
4. Lamont, J.T. and O'Gorman, T.A., Gastroenterology 75, 1157, 1978.
5. Sjogen, H.O. and Steele, G., Jr., Cancer 36, 2469, 1975.

6. Bland, P.W., Britton, D.C., Richens, E.R. and Pledger, J.V., Gut 22, 744, 1981.
7. Vose, B.M., Gallagher, P., Moore, M. and Schofield, P.F., Br. J. Cancer 44, 846, 1981.
8. Pollard, M. and Luckert, P.H., Cancer Treat Rep. 64, 1323, 1980.
9. Metzger, U., Meier, J., Uhlschmid, G. and Weihe, H., Dis. Colon Rectum 27, 366, 1984.

NATURAL KILLER (NK) CELL ACTIVITY AGAINST ENTERIC MURINE CORONAVIRUS MEDIATED BY INTESTINAL LEUKOCYTES

P.S. Carman, P.B. Ernst, K.L. Rosenthal, D.A. Clark,
D.A. Befus and J. Bienenstock

McMaster University
Hamilton, Ontario, Canada

INTRODUCTION

Relatively little is known about local cell mediated immunity (CMI) in the gut and its role in resistance to enteric virus disease. Intraepithelial leukocytes (IEL), because of their location within the epithelium, may be involved in the defense of the gut mucosa against viruses. This study was initiated to assess the endogenous local CMI response of murine mucosal lymphocytes, especially IEL, to an enveloped enteric murine virus. The Yale strain of mouse hepatitis virus (MHV-Y) was chosen for these studies. MHV-Y causes diarrhea in infant mice (1) and has been shown to be highly tropic for the intestinal epithelium (2). It replicates in NCTC-1469 cells which have the $H\text{-}2^k$ phenotype (3).

IEL from conventional mice are heterogenous in phenotype and function. A large population of $Thy\text{-}1^-$, $Lyt\text{-}1^-$, $Lyt\text{-}2^+$ cells is present, but its function is unknown. Most of these $Lyt\text{-}2^+$ cells are granulated. They represent 45 to 55% of the total IEL population (4-7). Less than 15% of IEL have natural killer (NK) activity against YAC-1 tumor cells. The majority of these NK cells have the unusual NK cell phenotype $Thy\text{-}1^+$, $Lyt\text{-}1^-$, $Lyt\text{-}2^-$, $ASGM1^-$, $NK1^-$ (8). Unlike lymphocytes from the lamina propria (LPL), IEL do not bear surface immunoglobulin (5).

METHODS AND RESULTS

Cells from different compartments of the gut-associated lymphoid [IEL, LPL, Peyer's patch (PP) and mesenteric lymph node (MLN)] and spleen (SPL) cells were harvested (8,9) from inbred strains of mice. Because conventional mice were seropositive for MHV-Y, specific pathogen free (SPF) mice were used.

Since all previous IEL studies in our laboratory have used conventional mice, the distribution of surface antigen expression of IEL from conventional and SPF CBA/J mice were initially compared by flow cytometry (Table 1). Approximately 30% of IEL from conventional mice were Thy-1^+, Lyt-1^+, whereas 80% were Lyt-2^+, as has been previously reported (5). Although virtually all SPF-derived cells demonstrated the Ly-5 lymphocyte antigen, with few contaminating Ig^+ LPL evident, cells from SPF mice expressed less Thy-1^+, Lyt-1^+ and Lyt-2^+ antigens. This pattern of phenotypic expression by SPF mice is similar to that reported for nude mice (4) and most probably reflects limited antigen exposure for the gut in both groups.

Effector cells from CBA/J mice, syngeneic to the target cell and DBA/2 and A/J mice, allogeneic for the target cell, were assessed for their ability to lyse MHV-Y infected NCTC-1469 cells using standard chromium release assays. The data is expressed as lytic units per 10^6 effector cells (10). The lytic activity reported is virus-specific for it is the difference between virus-infected and uninfected targets. Cell populations harvested from these mice showed strong cytotoxic activity, especially IEL, for the MHV-Y infected target cell (Table 2). The lack of MHC restriction suggests that the cytotoxic cell is an NK cell.

Table 1. Phenotype of IEL from CBA/J mice determined by flow cytometry

	Thy-1.2	Lyt-1.1	Lyt-2.1	ASGM1	Ig^a	Ly-5
Conventional Mice	38.1±5.4	32.4±4.1	80.0±1.8	11.4±3.0	4.9±0.6	ND
SPF Mice	7.7±0.7	3.4±0.3	46.6±4.1	17.0±3.4	1.1±0.5	92.5±6.2

[a]Surface immunoglobulin.

Table 2. Specific cytotoxicity for MHV-Y infected target cells by different strains of SPF mice

Mouse Strain	IEL	LPL	PP	MLN	SPL
CBA/J (H-2^k)	21.9±1.2	3.3±1.6	4.1±0.8	0.9±0.4	2.3±0.3
DBA/2 (H-2^d)	14.2±0.7	ND	3.1±0.7	0.7±0.2	2.0±0.4
A/J (H-2^a)	4.4±1.4	ND	1.8±0.5	0.3±0.2	0.8±0.1

The lytic activity reported is the difference between virus-infected and uninfected targets calculated for each experiment and expressed as $LU_{20}/10^6$ cells; mean ± SEM.

Intraepithelial leukocytes and spleen cells harvested from SPF CBA/J (H-2^k) mice were assessed using in vitro ^{51}Cr release assays, for their ability to lyse the NK sensitive YAC-1 tumor cell line, syngeneic NCTC-1469 cells acutely infected with MHV-Y and NCTC-1469 cells infected with pichinde virus (PV), an enveloped but non-enterotropic arenavirus.

The MHV-Y NK cell appears not to be the same cell that lysis the classical murine NK target, YAC-1 tumor cells. In cytotoxicity assays (Table 3), effector cells from SPF mice showed low lytic activity to YAC-1 tumor targets. This ineffective YAC-1 tumor cell killing reflects the small numbers of Thy-1^+ cells in IEL preparation from SPF mice. This negligible cytotoxicity is in contrast to the pronounced ability of effector cells, especially IEL, to kill NCTC-1469 cells infected with MHV-Y. The cytotoxic cell appears to be "virus-specific" since it was not lytic for PV infected cells.

Table 3. Cell-mediated lysis of various target cells

Target	IEL	SPL
YAC-1	0.4 ± 0.0	1.0 ± 0.7
MHV-NCTC-1469	21.9 ± 1.2	2.3 ± 0.3
Pichinde-NCTC-1469	0.8 ± 0.8	0.4 ± 0.3

$LU_{20}/10^6$ cells; Mean ± SEM

Table 4. Phenotype of cytotoxic IEL from naive mice determined by complement-mediated lysis

Antisera + Complement	Percentage decrease in lysis
Thy 1.2	17
Lyt 1.1	0
Lyt 2.1	11.5
ASGM1	89

The phenotype of the IEL cytotoxic for MHV-Y infected NCTC-1469 cells was determined using in vitro complement-mediated lysis assays. The specific cytotoxicity of the IEL cells was reduced by 89% after treatment with anti-ASGM1 serum and complement (Table 4). Antisera to Thy-1, Lyt-1 and Lyt-2 antigens had little effect on the function of the lytic cells. This data suggests that the MHV-Y killer cell is an AsGM1$^+$ cell.

To confirm this observation, in vivo CBA/J mice were treated intravenously with anti-ASGM1 serum at levels previously reported to be effective for the elimination of AsGM1$^+$ cells in vivo (11), 24 hours prior to cell harvest. This in vivo treatment resulted in a 75% reduction in the in vitro lytic activity for MHV-Y infected target cells by IEL (Table 5), as well as an 83% reduction in the lytic activity by spleen cells. These experiments further define the MHV-Y killer cell, found in naive mice, as an AsGM1$^+$ NK cell.

Table 5. MHV-Y specific cytotoxicity following in vivo anti-ASGM1 sera

	IEL	SPL
CBA/J (H-2^k)		
Untreated	21.9 ± 1.2	2.3 ± 0.3
Treated with anti-ASGM1	5.5 ± 1.5	0.4 ± 0.3
% significant decrease in cytotoxicity	74.8%	82.6%

$LU_{20}/10^6$ cells; Mean ± SEM

CONCLUSION

The *in vitro* and *in vivo* results suggest that a subpopulation of the morphologically and functionally heterogenous IEL compartment is involved in the defense of the gut mucosa to enteric viruses. This population of cells has the phenotype $ASGM1^+$, $Thy\text{-}1^-$, $Lyt\text{-}1^-$, $Lyt\text{-}2^-$, but does not possess the target specificity of classic NK cells (12).

ACKNOWLEDGEMENT

This investigation was supported by the Medical Research Council of Canada.

REFERENCES

1. Barthold, S.W., Smith, A.L., Lord, P.F.S., Bhatt, P.N., Jacoby, R.O. and Main, A.J., Lab Anim. Sci. 32, 376, 1982.
2. Barthold, S.W. and Smith, A.L., Arch. Virol. 81, 103, 1984.
3. Van Loveren, H., Van Der Zeijst, A.M., De Weger, R.A., Van Basten, C., Pijpers, H., Hilgers, J. and Den Otter, W., J. Reticuloendothel. Soc. 29, 443, 1981.
4. Parrott, D.M.V., Mackenzie, S., Mowat, A. McI., Davies, M.D.J. and Micklem, H.S., Ann. N.Y. Acad. Sci. 409, 307, 1983.
5. Petit, A., Ernst, P.B., Befus, A.D., Clark, D.A., Rosenthal, K.L., Ishizaka, T. and Bienenstock, J., Eur. J. Immunol. 15, 211, 1985.
6. Schrader, J.W., Scollay, R. and Battye, F., J. Immunol. 130, 558, 1983.
7. Dillon, S.B. and Macdonald, T.T., Immunol. 52, 501, 1984.
8. Tagliabue, A., Befus, A.D., Clark, D.A. and Bienenstock, J., J. Exp. Med. 155, 1785, 1982.
9. Davies, M.D.J. and Parrott, D.M.V., Gut 22, 481, 1981.
10. Clark, D.A., Phillips, R.A. and Miller, R.G., Cell Immunol. 34, 25, 1977.
11. Habu, S.H., Fukui, H., Shimamura, K., Kasai, M., Nagai, Y., Okumura, K. and Tamaoki, N., J. Immunol. 127, 34, 1981.
12. Carman, P.S., Ernst, P.B., Rosenthal, K.L., Clark, D.A., Befus, A.D. and Bienenstock, J., J. Immunol. 136, 1548, 1986.

INHIBITION OF NATURAL KILLER (NK) ACTIVITY BY HUMAN COLOSTRAL AND SERUM IgA

K. Komiyama, I. Moro, S.S. Crago and J. Mestecky

Department of Microbiology, University of Alabama at Birmingham, Birmingham, AL USA; and Department of Pathology Nihon University School of Dentistry, Tokyo, Japan

INTRODUCTION

Natural killer (NK) cells are defined as effector cells with spontaneous cytotoxicity against tumor, virus-infected and undifferentiated normal cells. NK activity is closely associated with a subpopulation of lymphocytes, large granular lymphocytes (LGL), that contain azurophilic cytoplasmic granules. The NK cells show a characteristic organ distribution: they are numerous in peripheral blood and spleen, but relatively low numbers are found in lymph nodes, peritoneal cavity and bone marrow (1,2). Previous investigations have demonstrated that NK activity is influenced by various factors such as interferon, interleukin-2, hormones, suppressor cells, environmental factors and age. Recently, mucosal LGL have been isolated from the small intestines of humans, mice and rats (3-6). In the mouse and rat, mucosal LGL showed moderate levels of NK activity, while human mucosal LGL demonstrated low NK activity.

In our previous study (7), we demonstrated that $HNK-1^{+}$ cells present in colostrum displayed a low NK activity and exhibited characteristic morphological alterations. HNK-1 positive cells were also identified in inflamed human gingival tissues from patients with periodontal disease, but isolated gingival lymphocytes had a low cytotoxic activity against K562 target cells (8). In this study, we investigated the *in vitro* effect of cell free colostrum and IgA on NK activity of human peripheral blood mononuclear cells. Morphological changes in LGL cells after incubation with cell free colostrum and IgA were analyzed by electron microscopy. Furthermore, the ability of NK cells to bind IgA on the cell surface was examined using the immunocolloidal gold technique.

METHODS

A specific release cytotoxicity assay and K562 human erythroid cell were used as target cells. For morphological characterization, the HNK-1$^+$ or Leu-11$^+$ cells were isolated by the fluorescence activated cell sorter (7). These cells were incubated with S-IgA or p-IgA2 and then processed for EM study.

RESULTS AND DISCUSSION

Cell free colostrum revealed inhibition of NK activity in a dose dependent manner (0-100%). Purified p-IgA2 and S-IgA inhibited NK activity while IgG and IgM were not effective; other immunoglobulin preparations including p-IgA1, m-IgA1 F(ab), and Fc of IgA1 did not significantly inhibit NK mediated cell lysis (Fig. 1). However, these LGL still retained an ability to bind target cells. The minimum effective concentration of p-IgA2 that inhibited NK activity was 0.125 mg/ml, however, S-IgA was required in higher concentrations than p-IgA2 (0.5 mg/ml). Inhibition of NK activity with either p-IgA2 or S-IgA was partly recovered after incubation in IgA free medium for 24 hours. p-IgA2 (0.5 mg/ml) added together

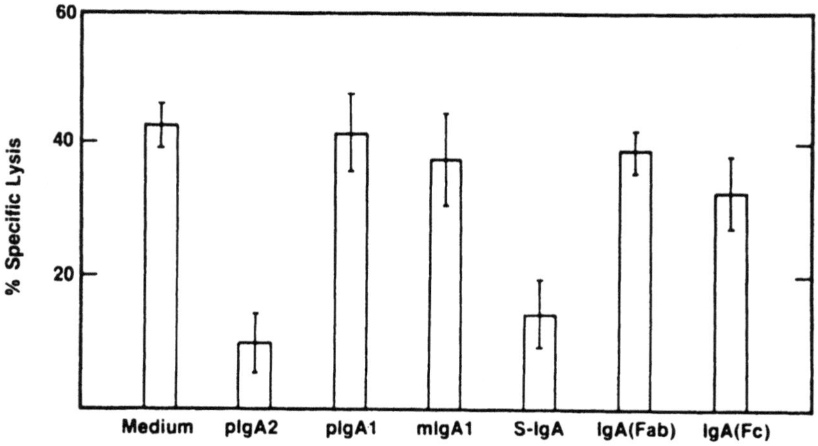

Figure 1. Inhibition of NK activity by IgA2, IgA1, F(ab')$_2$ and Fc fragments of IgA1 and S-IgA (0.5 mg/ml). E:T ratio was 20:1. Values represent the mean $\pm$ SD of four separate experiments.

with interferon-γ (200 U and 2000 U) during the preincubation period resulted in specific p-IgA2 inhibition of NK cell potentiation by interferon-γ.

Purified LGL (HNK-1^+ or Leu-11^+) with p-IgA2 or S-IgA incubation induced large vacuole formation in the cytoplasm which usually contained electron dense granular material. IgA bound to the cell surface was detected using goat $F(ab')_2$ anti-human IgA labeled immuno-colloidal gold (Fig. 2).

The present experiments have demonstrated that physiological concentrations of purified human IgA inhibited the NK activity of PBMC. This inhibitory activity was dependent on the molecular form of IgA, where p-IgA2 and S-IgA displayed strong inhibition, while p-IgA1 or m-IgA1 did not. The other classes of immunoglobulins tested (IgG and IgM) had no significant effect on NK activity. The reason for preferential inhibition of NK activity by p-IgA2 and S-IgA is unknown. However, this result should be considered with respect to the differences in the distribution of p-IgA and m-IgA and IgA1 and IgA2 subclasses in serum and external

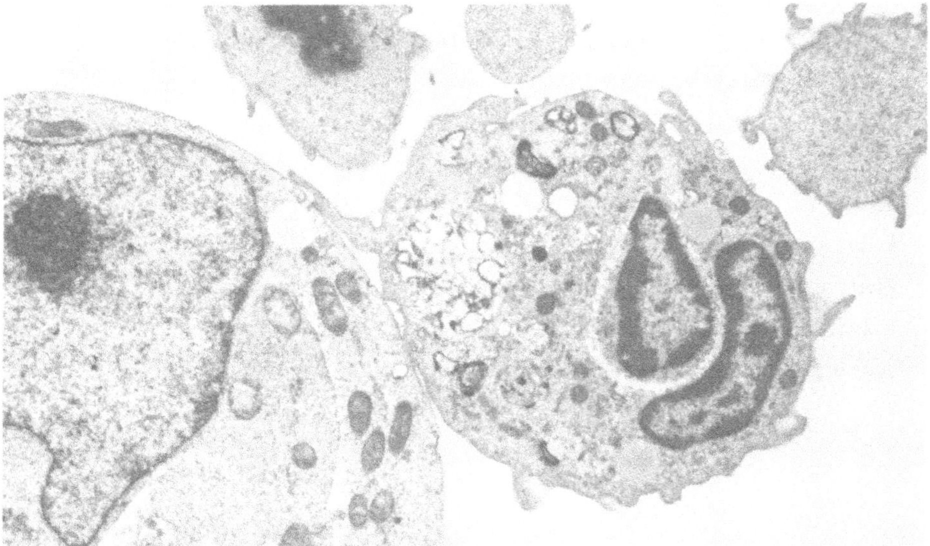

Figure 2. Electron microscopy showing LGL isolated from PBMC, precultured with pIgA for 12 h. Degranulation and numerous vacuoles are evident in the cytoplasm of pIgA2 treated cells. LGL retained binding ability to the K562T target cells.

secretions (9). IgA remained bound to the cell surface and morphological changes such as decreased numbers of granules and formation of cytoplasmic vacuoles that may have resulted in disruption of the intracytoplasmic vesicular transport of NK cytotoxic factors. In addition to differences in their primary structures, IgA1 and IgA2 exhibit different carbohydrate compositions (9) which may play a significant role in interaction with various cells, including NK cells.

REFERENCES

1. Ortaldo, J.R., Herberman, R.B., in Annual Review of Immunology, (Edited by William, P.E.), Vol. 2, pp. 359-394, Annual Reviews, Palo Alto, CA, 1984.
2. Reynolds, C.W., Timonen, T. and Herberman, R.B., J. Immunol. 127, 282, 1981.
3. Tagliabue, A., Luini, W., Soldateschi, D. and Boraschi, D., Eur. J. Immunol. 11, 919, 1981.
4. Tagliabue, A., Befus, D.A., Clark, D.A. and Bienenstock, J., J. Exp. Med 155, 1785, 1982.
5. Gibson, P.R., Verhaar, H.J.J., Selby, W.S. and Jewell, D.P., Clin. Exp. Immunol. 56, 445, 1984.
6. Shioda, Y., Nagura, H., Tsutsumi, Y., Shimamura, K. and Tamacki, N., Histochem. J. 16, 843, 1984.
7. Moro, I., Abo, T., Crago, S.S., Komiyama, K. and Mestecky, J., Cell. Immunol. 93, 467, 1985.
8. Komiyama, K., Hirsch, H.Z., Mestecky, J. and Moro, I., Fed. Proc. 45, 953 (Abstr. 4648), 1986.
9. Mestecky, J. and Russell, M.W., Mongr. Allergy 19, 277, 1986.

HSV-1 INFECTED ORAL EPITHELIAL CELLS ARE TARGETS FOR NATURAL KILLER CELLS

R.A. Lindemann, S.H. Golub and N.-H. Park

Sections of Oral Diagnosis, Oral Medicine, and Oral Pathology and Oral Biology, and the Dental Research Institute, UCLA School of Dentistry, Departments of Surgery/Oncology and Microbiology and Immunology, UCLA School of Medicine, Los Angeles, California USA

INTRODUCTION

Natural killer (NK) cells represent a ubiquitous subpopulation of large, granular lymphocytes with the ability to lyse certain tumor cells, virus-infected cells, and some normal cells without prior sensitization. Although they are often regarded as immune surveillance cells associated with restricting neoplastic growth, other important NK functions are now being explored, including their potential role in B cell regulation (1) and hematopoietic differentiation (2).

With regard to NK anti-viral activity, Santoli et al. (3) showed NK-mediated cytolysis of allogeneic fibroblasts infected with a variety of viral pathogens. They further suggested that interferon, which was induced during cytolysis, enhanced the cytotoxic efficiency of the NK mediators (4). In addition to fibroblasts, Bishop et al. (5) found that the human epithelial cell line WISH, when infected with herpes simplex virus type 1 (HSV-1), was a target for NK cells. Yasukawa and Zarling (6), using autologous B lymphoblastoid cell lines, reported that HSV-1 infected cells were lysed by autologous NK cells. These studies suggest an important role for NK cells in resistance to viral infection. The relationship between NK cells and virus-infected target cells is complex and probably involves many factors, including: (a) activation of interferon; (b) target cell protection by interferon; (c) target cell protection by viral control; and (d) interaction with appropriate surface antigens able to stimulate NK binding and lysis (7).

During the course of HSV-1 infection, glycoprotein antigens are inserted into the target cell surface (8). NK activity is related to the expression of HSV-1 glycoproteins (9) rather than the intact viral particles. Destruction of the virus is at the expense of the infected cells and local tissue damage may ensue. If the infected targets are epithelial cells, killing of targets would result in epithelial cell lysis and possible ulceration.

Resistance to viral infection and subsequent cytolysis may be a mechanism of recurrent local tissue destruction in the oral cavity. Cellular effector mechanisms of intraoral tissue damage are poorly understood. This is in large part due to the difficulty in isolating specific mucosal antigens as targets for cytotoxic lymphocytes. In oral diseases such as recurrent aphthous ulceration (RAU) and erosive Lichen planus where lymphocytic infiltrates are common, mucosal target structures have not been determined. Additionally, after tissue destruction occurs, presumably these specific antigens are eliminated, making studies of existing ulcers difficult to interpret reliably. The problem then becomes distinguishing effector cells causing lysis from cells responding to lytic products.

NK cells have been located in oral mucosa but their function has not been characterized. They have been detected in the pre-ulcerative and early ulcerative phases of RAU (10), but the impact of their presence was not defined. Interestingly, Greenspan et al. (11) had earlier also demonstrated a significant increase in antibody-dependent cellular cytotoxicity (mediated by Fc receptor cells including NK cells) in RAU subjects early in the disease. Prospective NK targets in oral mucosa may include epithelial cells transiently infected with a virus or dendritic cells modified during antigen presentation.

The purpose of this study was to determine if induced surface antigen determinants on epithelial cells render them susceptible to NK cytolysis. HSV-1, a common intraoral viral pathogen, was chosen because of its ability to rapidly fuse with epithelial cell membranes and display glycoprotein antigens when co-cultured. This study will test the hypothesis that transiently HSV-1 infected epithelial cells become targets for NK cytotoxicity.

MATERIALS AND METHODS

Cell preparation

PBL were prepared from heparinized normal human blood by Ficoll-hypaque (Pharmacia Fine Chemicals, Piscataway, NJ) density gradient centrifugation, and then were depleted of adherent cells by either plastic adherence or Sephadex G-10 column (Pharmacia) (12). Epithelial cells were scraped from the buccal mucosa of volunteers (without HSV-1 clinical history) by a tongue depressor, washed three times by centrifugation, and suspended in RPMI 1640 (Flow Laboratories, Inc., McLean, VA) with 10% human AB serum, 10 mM HEPES buffer, and antibiotics.

Separation of lymphocyte subpopulations

PBL were labelled with anti-Leu-11b monoclonal antibody (Becton-Dickinson, Mountain View, CA) for 35 min at 4°C. After washing twice, the cells were treated with a 1:5 dilution of rabbit complement with a low cytotoxicity for human lymphocytes (Cedarlane Lab., Ltd., Hornby, Ontario, Canada), for 1 h at 37°C and washed twice prior to use in assays.

L-leucine methyl ester treatment (LeuOMe)

LeuOMe (Sigma Chemical Co., St. Louis, MO) was prepared fresh for each experiment in RPMI 1640 Medium and the pH was adjusted to 7.4 with 1 N NaOH. PBL at 8×10^6 per ml were treated with 1/2:1 (v/v) concentration of LeuOMe in RPMI 1640 supplemented with 5% human AB serum, 10 mM HEPES buffer, and antibiotics at 37°C for 30 min, and then were washed three times by centrifugation.

Virus

HSV-1, F strain, was originally obtained from the American Type Culture Collection, Rockville, Maryland. The virus was propagated in Vero cell monolayers and the titer was adjusted to 1.0×10^7 plaque-forming units per milliliter (PFU/ml). The virus stock was stored at -80°C until used in the present study.

Viral treatment

Chromium labeled (described below) epithelial cells were inoculated with HSV-1 at an infectivity of 1 PFU per cell (one multiplicity of infection) for 1 h in a shaker water bath at 37°C. The cells were washed twice by centrifugation prior to assays.

Chromium-release assays

Target cells (1.0×10^6 epithelial cells in 1 ml RPMI 1640 with 10% fetal calf serum) were labeled with 250 μCi of sodium[^{51}Cr]chromate (Amersham International, Arlington Heights, IL) for 8 h at 37°C in a shaker water bath and were washed three times. Labeled target cells (5×10^3) were mixed with the indicated number of effector cells in round bottom microtiter plates containing 200 μl of RPMI 1640 with 10% human AB serum, and the microtiter plates were centrifuged at 50 x g for 4 min to initiate cell to cell contact. The plates were incubated for 4 h at 37°C in a humidified incubator with 5% CO_2. At the end of the assay, 100 μl of supernatant was harvested from each well and counted for [^{51}Cr] released from target cells. Cytotoxicity was defined as specific [^{51}Cr] released or [(experimental release-spontaneous release)/(maximal release-spontaneous release)] X 100%. Experimental release was the counts of chromium released from target cells caused by effector cells as measured by counts per min (cpm). Maximal release was the chromium released from target cells induced by 2% NP-40 detergent. Spontaneous release was the cpm by target cells incubated alone. Each assay was performed in quadruplicate.

Rosetting reagent

To determine the effectiveness of adherent cell removal by plastic adherence and Sephadex G-10 column, universal rosetting reagent, described elsewhere (13), binding to fluorescein diacetate stained adherent cells was counted under fluorescent UV microscope. Percentage of adherent cell rosettes was calculated by counting two hundred lymphocytes.

RESULTS

Cytotoxicity assays

The effect of PBL on untreated and HSV-1 infected epithelial cells was tested by performing short-term chromium release assays. Results in Table 1 show significant cytolytic activity remains after adherent cell removal only against HSV-1 infected target cells ($p = 0.03$, Student's *t* test). Adherent cell depleted PBL killed cells most effectively at a 50:1 effector to target ratio. Cytotoxicity decreased sharply at 25:1 and 12.5:1. Values are given for three effector target ratios when appropriate. The three data points were then converted into lytic units (14), defined as that number of cells required to cause a specified amount of target lysis (in this case 30%), and is usually expressed as LU/10^6. This method allows a more accurate comparison between lymphocyte donors.

Table 1. Lysis of human epithelial cells by autologous peripheral blood lymphocytes

		Untreated Ep. Cells		HSV-1 Infected Ep. Cells	
		% lysis	LU 30%[a]	% lysis	LU 30%
Unf.[b]	50:1	41		77	
	25:1	17	5	56	20
	12.5:1	02		36	
G-10[c]	50:1	<0		26	
	25:1	<0	0	05	3
	12.5:1	<0		<0	
Plastic[d]	50:1	<0		29	
	25:1	<0	0	01	3
	12.5:1	<0		<0	

[a]Lytic Units - Number of cells per 1 x 10^6 required to cause 30% target cell lysis.

[b]Unfractionated peripheral blood lymphocytes (PBL).

[c]PBL depleted of adherent cells by Sephadex G-10 column.

[d]PBL depleted of adherent cells by plastic adherence.

To test specificity of killing, PBL from one donor were tested against allogeneic infected and uninfected epithelial cells. At a 50:1 effector to target ratio, PBL were able to kill allogeneic HSV-1 infected cells only (24% cytotoxicity) (data not shown).

Untreated and HSV-1 infected cells were sensitive to lysis by unfractionated blood containing adherent cells. Both methods of adherent cell removal (plastic, G-10), however, were effective in eliminating these cells as determined by universal rosetting reagent.

Effects of LeuOMe treatment

PBL treated with LeuOMe, a lysosomotropic drug which has been shown to eliminate NK activity and most cells bearing NK markers (15) were not cytotoxic for either untreated or HSV-1 infected autologous epithelial cell targets (Table 2). The cytotoxic activity shown by PBL against allogeneic infected targets was also abrogated with LeuOMe treatment.

Table 2. Lysis of epithelial cells is due to NK cells

		Untreated Ep. Cells % lysis	HSV-1 Infected Ep. Cells % lysis
Anti-Leu-11b[a]	50:1	<0	04
+ C	25:1	<0	<0
	12.5:1	<0	<0
LeuOMe[b]	50:1	<0	<0

[a]PBL (adherent cell depleted) treated with anti-Leu-11b + complement.
[b]PBL treated with L-leucine methyl ester for 30 min.

Effects of anti-Leu-11b plus complement

The population of lymphocytes remaining after treatment with anti-Leu-11b monoclonal antibody plus complement was not cytotoxic for either infected or uninfected target cells (Table 2).

NK activity against K562 cells

To show that NK activity of subject blood was normal, PBL were tested against a standard NK sensitive target, the erythroleukemic cell K562 (16) in a 4 h assay. A normal profile of NK activity for the experimental subjects was recorded (data not shown).

DISCUSSION

Antiviral effector cells capable of lysing infected epithelial cells perform an important mucosal defense function. As a consequence of lysis, however, epithelial cells are destroyed during the lytic process. We have shown an *in vitro* mechanism for oral epithelial cell lysis mediated by NK cells. *In vivo*, NK cells have been detected prior to ulceration in recurrent aphthous ulceration subjects. Whether a viral antigen is present in RAU has not been established nor is it the intent of this paper to implicate viruses in mucosal ulcerative disease etiology. As a potential mechanism for mucosal cytolysis, however, NK lysis of altered targets should be considered.

Epithelial cells were taken from donors who were free from clinical signs of HSV-1 infection. Presumably, cytotoxic T cells (CTL's) could be responsible as effectors of lysis as well. This is not likely in subjects without a history of clinical HSV-1 infection because of the small possibility of sampling peripheral blood containing activated CTL clones against the virus. Most importantly, CTL's are HLA restricted and would preferentially lyse autologous cells. However, cells from subjects were able to lyse allogeneic epithelial cells infected by HSV-1.

As further evidence that NK cells were responsible for the lysis of HSV-1 infected cells, depletion studies with anti-Leu-11b monoclonal antibody were performed. Anti-Leu-11b reacts with the Fc receptor on PMN's and NK cells but not with the Fc receptor of monocytes/macrophages (17). NK cell activity as measured against a standard NK target, K562 cells, has been shown to be high in the Leu-11$^+$ fraction of PBL and almost completely undetectable in the Leu-11$^-$ fraction (18). In this study, PBL depleted of Leu-11b$^+$ cells were not cytotoxic against HSV-1 infected targets.

The primary mechanism by which NK cells kill involves direct binding to susceptible targets followed by the lytic process. However, NK cells may also lyse target cells by antibody-dependent cell-mediated cytotoxicity (ADCC). NK cell Fc receptors are capable of binding to antibody attached to targets which then results in lysis. Only small amounts of antibody are needed to trigger this system. While it is more likely that epithelial cell targets in this study were killed by direct NK binding to HSV-1 infected cells, ADCC cannot be completely ruled out. Two possible explanations exist that would allow ADCC to contribute to lysis in these experiments: (a) Antibody already bound to epithelial cells or HSV-1 determinants associated with epithelial cells could remain after collection of cells from donors. (b) B cells in peripheral blood were already primed to secrete antibody against HSV-1 antigens which could bind to NK effectors. If subjects had produced antibodies at the time of sampling, perhaps ADCC would be activated. However, all subjects were totally free from clinical HSV-1 symptoms which reduces the likelihood of ADCC involvement in this study.

A short viral infection time (1 h) for target cells was used to minimize the potential lytic effects of HSV-1 on the infected epithelial cells. The virus could not be responsible for epithelial cell lysis since a permissive

HSV infection requires more than 4-5 h (19). However, since HSV-1 is known to alter the cell membrane permeability during the early stage of lytic infection, it is possible that the increased ^{51}Cr release may be induced by the virus. To eliminate this possibility, we performed the same experiments with UV irradiated, inactivated HSV-1 from the same strain. Autologous adherent cell depleted PBL still lysed virus-infected epithelial cells only (29% cytotoxicity at 50:1 effector to target ratio). These data indicate that increased ^{51}Cr release is dependent on the change in the cell membrane, i.e., insertion of viral antigens into the target cell membrane.

Although macrophages have been reported to lyse HSV-1 infected cells (20), it is difficult to explain the high cytotoxicity from unfractionated blood against uninfected epithelial cells. Monocytes in these samples are apparently actively phagocytizing epithelial cells regardless of viral infection. The separation of epithelial cells from each other which occurs only *in vitro* may predispose them to phagocytosis, whereas *in vivo*, when they are contiguous, macrophages would be less likely to regard the cells as foreign. Fortunately, adherent cells were effectively removed, permitting analysis of non-adherent cell cytotoxicity. If monocyte contamination was responsible for cytotoxicity in depleted fractions, similar cytotoxicity would have been expected to be recorded against untreated targets.

NK cells have been shown to kill normal cells in some circumstances. We were interested in investigating the possibility that activated NK cells would lyse unaltered epithelial cells. Three day culture with 50 units per ml of recombinant interleukin 2 (Amgen, Thousand Oaks, CA) which is known to induce a lymphokine-activated killer cell (21) had no effect on the killing of normal targets (data not shown).

CONCLUSIONS

1. Oral epithelial cells infected by HSV-1 were lysed by adherent cell depleted PBL.

2. Evidence that NK cells mediated the lysis exists because:
   a. PBL were able to lyse allogeneic as well as autologous targets.
   b. When NK cells were depleted by the lysosomotropic drug L-leucine methyl ester, cytotoxicity against infected targets was abrogated.

c. Depletion of NK cells by the monoclonal antibody Leu-11b plus complement also eliminated cytotoxicity.

3. These findings suggest that NK cells initiate cell-mediated lysis of virus infected epithelial cells in the oral mucosa.

REFERENCES

1. James, K. and Ritchie, A.W.S., Immunol. Today 5, 193, 1984.
2. Hansson, M., Beran, M., Andersson, B. and Kiessling, R., J. Immunol. 129, 126, 1982.
3. Santoli, D., Trinchieri, G. and Lief, F., J. Immunol. 121, 526, 1978.
4. Santoli, D., Trinchieri, G., Koprowski, H., J. Immunol. 121, 532, 1978.
5. Bishop, G.A., Glorioso, J.C. and Schwartz, S.A., J. Immunol. 131, 1849, 1983.
6. Yasukawa, M. and Zarling, J.M., J. Immunol. 131, 2011, 1983.
7. Welsh, R.M., Jr. and Hallenbeck, L.A., J. Immunol. 124, 2491, 1980.
8. Baucke, R.B. and Spear, P.G., J. Virol. 32, 779, 1979.
9. Bishop, G.A., Glorioso, J.C. and Schwartz, S.A., J. Exp. Med. 157, 1544, 1983.
10. Savage, N.W., Seymour, G.J. and Kruger, B.J., Oral Surg., Oral Med., Oral Pathol. 60, 175, 1985.
11. Greenspan, J.S., Gadol, N., Olson, J.A. and Talal, N., Clin. Exp. Immunol. 44, 603, 1981.
12. Ly, I. and Mishell, R., J. Immunol. Methods 5, 239, 1974.
13. Karavodin, L.M. and Golub, S.H., J. Immunol. Methods 61, 293, 1983.
14. Pross, H.F., Baines, M.G., Rubin, P., Shragge, P. and Patterson, M.S., J. Clin. Immunol. 1, 51, 1981.
15. Shau, H. and Golub, S.H., J. Immunol. 134, 1136, 1985.
16. West, W.H., Cannon, G.B., Kay, H.D., Bonnard, G.D. and Herberman, R.B., J. Immunol. 118, 355, 1977.
17. Trinchiari, G. and Perussia, B., Lab. Invest. 50, 489, 1984.
18. Seki, H., Ueno, Y., Taga, K., Matsuda, A., Miyawaki, T. and Taniguchi, N., J. Immunol. 135, 2351, 1985.
19. Darlington, R.W. and Granoff, R., in The Herpes Viruses (Edited by Kaplan, A.S.), p. 94, Academic Press, New York and London, 1973.
20. Stanwick, T.L., Campbell, D.E. and Nahmias, A.J., Cell Immunol. 53, 413, 1980.
21. Grimm, E.A., Mazumder, A., Zhang, H.Z. and Rosenberg, S.A., J. Exp. Med. 155, 1823, 1982.

INVOLVEMENT OF HUMAN IMMUNODEFICIENCY VIRUS (HIV) IN GINGIVA OF PATIENTS WITH AIDS

M. Gornitsky and D. Pekovic

Dental Department, The Sir Mortimer B. Davis
Jewish Hospital, Montreal, Canada H3S 1Y9

INTRODUCTION

The acquired immune deficiency syndrome, "AIDS", is characterized by a reduction in the number and function of helper-inducer T cells, leading to severe immune suppression and allowing numerous opportunistic infections and neoplasms. Since the first reported case in July, 1982 (1), AIDS has achieved pandemic proportions, causing major health and socio-economic problems in several parts of the world. So far, AIDS remains an incurable disease which is fatal usually within three years.

The isolation of the "Human T-cell lymphotropic virus" type III (HTLV-III) (2,3) in the United States, and "Lymphadenopathy associated virus" (LAV) in France (4) from cells of patients, was the first indication that the etiology of the disease was related to a virus. These two isolates are currently considered as the same virus called "Human Immunodeficiency Virus" (HIV). Subsequent sero-epidemiological studies have shown the presence of HIV specific antibodies (Ab) in the serum of patients with AIDS and AIDS-related complex (ARC) and in the serum of individuals at risk for AIDS (5,6).

Recently, we identified viral antigens (Ag) in cells located in lymphatic and other organs and tissues, as well as in peripheral blood lymphocytes (PBL) and salivary lymphocytes from patients with AIDS (7-10). Some cells containing viral antigen displayed multinucleated giant forms, as well as immunoglobulins (Ig) and the C3 component of complement on its surfaces. These findings suggest involvement of the virus in cytopathic and immunopathogenic reactions in both target cells and tissues.

In 1984, Groopman and co-workers (11) had isolated the virus from saliva obtained from people with ARC and from healthy homosexual men at risk for AIDS. This and subsequent similar reports (10,12) have focused public and scientific attention on the role of HIV in the human oral cavity. We have noted the pathogenic potential of oral flora in immunocompromised AIDS patients with emphasis on alveolar bone resorption.

Within the last two years, we have studied 21 adult immunosuppressed patients at the Dental Department of The Sir Mortimer B. Davis - Jewish General Hospital. All patients were seropositive for HIV as demonstrated by Western blot technique (13) (12 had AIDS, 3 had ARC, 6 were asymptomatic). The patients displayed a variety of opportunistic diseases as shown in Table 1. All patients were submitted to a clinical assessment of the oral cavity, gingival pocket depth probe, examination of mobility of teeth and radiography using a orthopantometer 10 (Siemens). PBL from all patients, and marginal gingival biopsy samples from 12 AIDS patients were used in the search for HIV Ag by direct immunofluorescence (IF) (8,14). Twenty matched dental patients, without clinical symptoms of AIDS-related opportunistic diseases or seropositivity for HIV, served as controls. Autopsy samples of gingiva from two accident victims and biopsy samples from 5 HIV-seronegative periodontal patients were used as controls in the IF studies.

RESULTS

The general health status of the patients is summarized in Table 1. Briefly, 15 displayed leucopenia, 3 showed Kaposi's sarcoma (Fig. 1), 5 had Pneumocystis carinii pneumonia and 3 had tuberculosis. The incidence of opportunistic infections was higher in four patients with terminal AIDS, two of whom died at the end of the studies.

The health status of the oral cavity is summarized in Table 2. All AIDS and ARC patients displayed oral candidiasis located mainly on the buccal mucosa, tongue (Fig. 2), palate and floor of the mouth. Periodontal diseases were found in AIDS patients, ARC patients, and asymptomatic HIV seropositive subjects in 100%, 66.7%, 33.3%, respectively. Periodontal

Table 1. General health status of patients

Category of patients	Numbers	Patients displaying Leukopenia	HIV containing PBL	Skin Kaposi's sarcoma	*Pneumocystis carinii* pneumonia	Tuberculosis	Hemophilia
Initial AIDS	3	3	3	0	0	0	0
Advanced AIDS	5	5	5	1	1	1	1
Terminal AIDS	4	4	4	2	4	2	0
ARC	3	3	3	0	0	0	0
Seropositive	6	0	3	0	0	0	0
Control dental patients	20	0	0	0	0	0	0

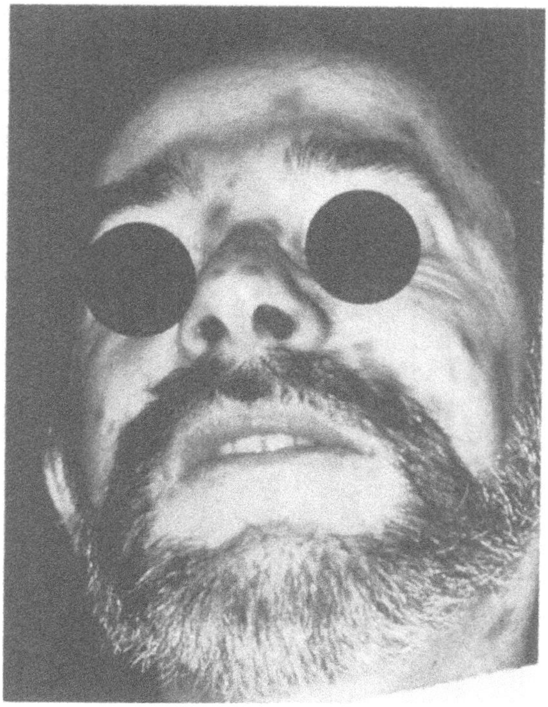

Figure 1. Numerous Kaposi's sarcoma lesions on face of patient with advanced AIDS.

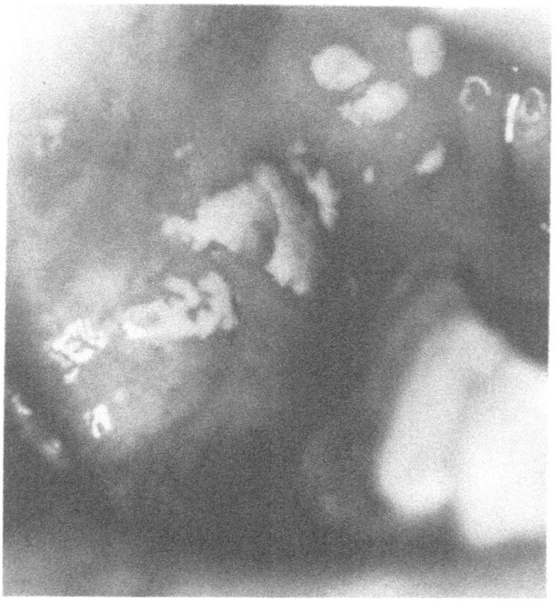

Figure 2. Oral candidiasis in patient with advanced AIDS. Infection is located on buccal mucosa.

Table 2. Health status in oral cavity

			Numbers of patients displaying:					
Category of patients	Numbers	Candi-diasis	Perio-dontal disease	Rapid severe alveolar bone resorption	Mobility of teeth	Peri-apical abscess	Dental caries	Hairy cell leukoplakia
Initial AIDS	3	3	1	0	1	0	0	0
Advanced AIDS	5	5	4	2	2	0	2	1
Terminal AIDS	4	4	4	4	4	4	4	0
ARC	3	1	1	0	0	0	0	0
Seropositive	6	0	1	0	0	0	2	0
Control dental patients	20	0	2	0	0	0	4	0

disease was characterized by redness, edema, bleeding to pressure at the marginal gingiva and the formation of gingival pockets. Along with the breakdown of marginal tissues, there was an extensive alveolar bone resorption (Fig. 3) leading to mobility of teeth and periapical abscess formation. The resorption could be positively correlated with the progression of AIDS. This was well illustrated by the absence of severe periodontal disease in 3 patients with initial AIDS and the rapid resorption in patients in the terminal stage of AIDS. The latter stages of the disease were also characterized by simultaneous involvement of teeth with caries. These patients also had oral Kaposi's sarcoma (Fig. 4) and one hairy cell leukoplakia (Fig. 5). Initial and/or slowly progressing forms of periodontal disease and dental caries were observed in 10 to 20 percent of control patients.

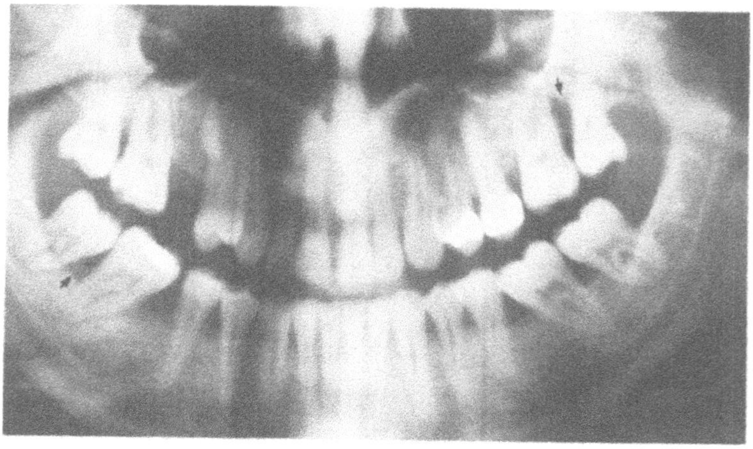

Figure 3. Severe alveolar bone resorption in advanced stage of AIDS. Note severe alveolar bone resorption (arrows).

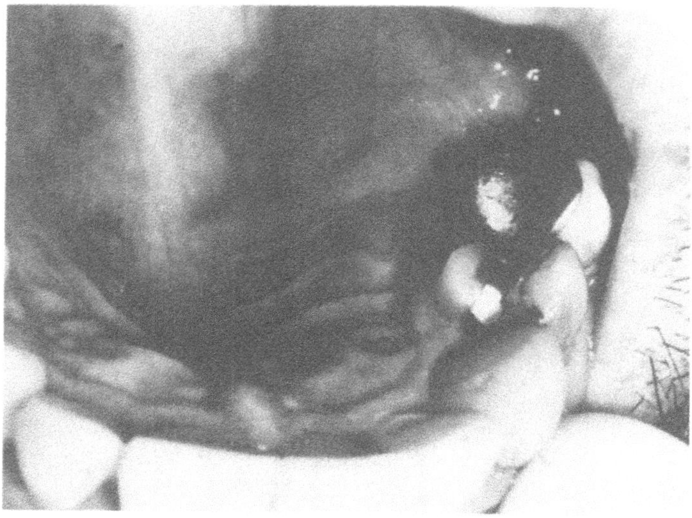

Figure 4. Oral Kaposi's sarcoma in patient with advanced AIDS.

Immunofluorescence studies of sections of gingival biopsy samples labeled with IgG against HIV or P24 monoclonal Ab yielded the demonstration of HIV-containing cells in crevicular epithelium of each sample (Fig. 6). Similarly, HIV containing PBL (Fig. 7) were found in all AIDS and ARC patients and in 50% of seropositive asymptomatic patients. No immunofluorescence was observed in sections of cells and tissues obtained from control subjects.

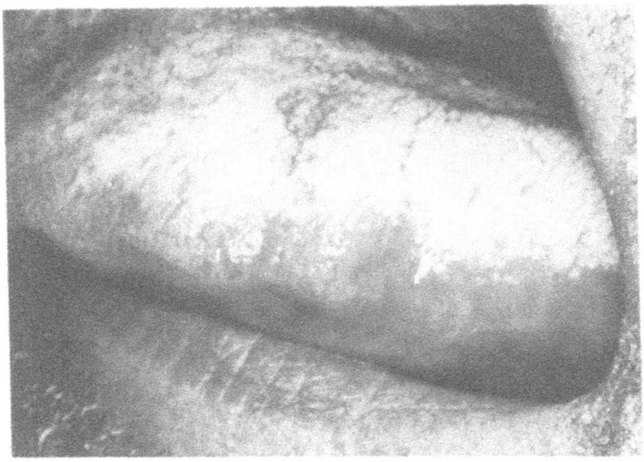

Figure 5. Hairy cell leukoplakia on tongue of patient in advanced stage of AIDS.

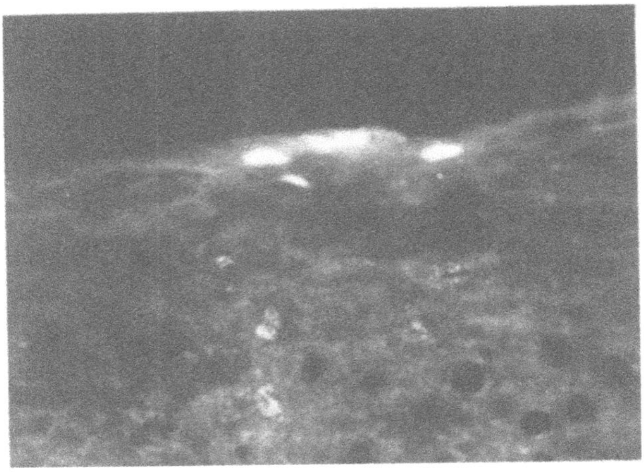

Figure 6. HIV in gingival epithelium of patient with initial AIDS. Section labeled with rhodamine conjugated IgG against HIV. (x250)

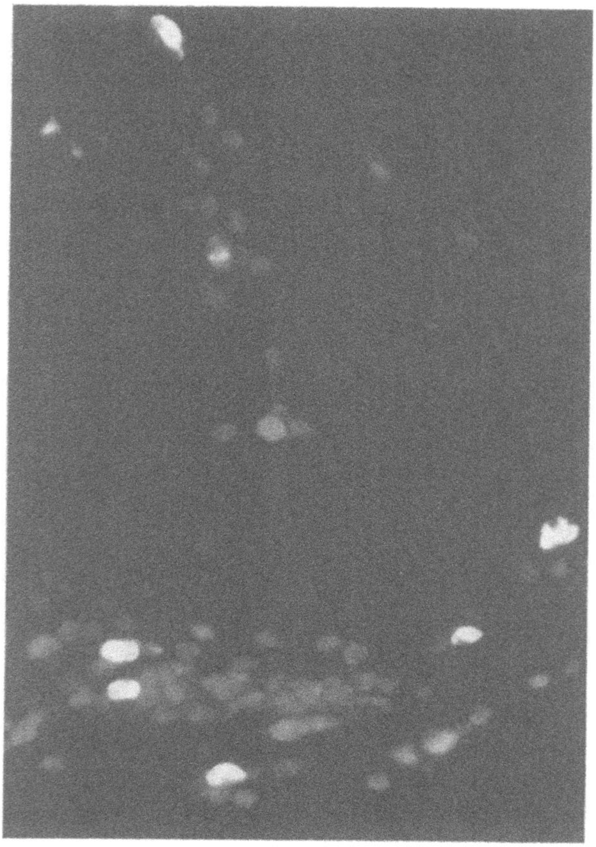

Figure 7. HIV in frozen sections of PBL of patient with advanced AIDS. HIV Ag labeled with P24 monoclonal antibodies. Note that some HIV containing cells display multinucleated form. (x250)

CONCLUSIONS

1. HIV is involved in cytolytic, cytopathic and hypersensitivity reactions in target PBL yielding a rapid lymphopenia and immunosuppression.

2. Virus-containing cells were found in gingiva.

3. Presence of HIV in gingiva can be associated with the absence of both local and systemic immunologic barriers allowing easier penetration of microorganisms and their Ag. Penetrated Ag activates osteoclasts with consequent alveolar bone resorption.

4. AIDS is an excellent condition for the illustration of the protective role of the immune system in the human oral cavity as well as for demonstration of the pathogenic capacity of the oral flora in the immunocompromised host.

REFERENCES

1. Center for Disease Control, A. NMWR 31, 65, 1982.
2. Popovic, M., Sarangadharan, M.G., Read, E. and Gallo, R.C., Science 224, 497, 1984.
3. Gallo, R.C., Salahuddin, S.Z., Popovic, M., Shearer, G.M., Kaplan, M., Haynes, B.F., Palicer, T.J., Bedfield, R., Oleske, J., Sarae, B., Foster, P. and Marcham, P.D., Science 224, 500, 1984.
4. Barre-Sinoussi, F., Chermann, J.C., Rey, F., Nuguyre, M.T., Chamaret, S., Gemst, J., Sanguet, C., Axler-Blin, C., Vezinet-Brun, F., Rousioux, C., Rosenbaum, N. and Montagnier, L., Science 220, 868, 1983.
5. Sarngadharan, M.G., Popovic, M., Bench, L., Schupbach, J. and Gallo, R.C., Science 224, 506, 1984.
6. Brun-Vezinet, F., Rousioux, C., Montagnier, L., Chamaret, S., Gruest, T., Barre-Sinoussi, F., Geroldi, D., Chermann, J.C., McCormick, J., Mitchell, S., Piot, P., Tarlman, H., Kapita Bila Mirlangu, Wobin, O., Mbendi, N., Mazebo, A., Kalambayi, K., Beidts, C., Desmyter, J., Reinsod, F.M. and Quinn, T.C., Science 226, 453, 1984.
7. Lapointe, N., Michaud, J., Pekovic, D.D., Chausseau, J.-P. and Dupuy, J.M., N. Engl. J. Med. 312, 1325, 1985.
8. Pekovic, D.D., Chausseau, J.P., Lapointe, N., Michaud, J., Garzon, S., Strykowski, H., Tsoukas, C., Gilmore, N., Goldman, H., Gornitsky, M., Popovic, M. and Dupuy, J.M., Arch. Virol. 91, 11, 1986.
9. Pekovic, D.D., Garzon, S., Strykowski, H., Ajdukovic, D., Gornitsky, M. and Dupuy, J.M., J. Virol. Meth. 13, 265, 1986.
10. Pekovic, D.D., Tsoukas, C., Ajdukovic, D., Lapointe, N., Michaud, J., Gilmore, N. and Gornitsky, M., Am. J. Med., 1987 (in press).
11. Groopman, J.E., Salahuddin, S.L. and Sarngadharan, M.G., Science 226, 449, 1984.
12. Ho, D.D., Byington, R.S. and Schooley, R.T., N. Engl. J. Med. 313, 1606, 1985.

13. Towbin, H., Staechelin, T. and Gordon, J., Proc. Natl. Acad Sci. USA 76, 4350, 1979.

14. Pekovic, D.D. and Fillery, E.D., J. Periodont. Res. 19, 329, 1984.

RFc ALPHA-BEARING CELLS AND IgA-MEDIATED PHAGOCYTOSIS IN THE MOUSE ORAL MUCOSA

J. Barbeau, J. Bourget and N. Deslauriers

Department de biochimie, faculte des sciences et genie
and groupe de recherche en ecologie buccale (GREB)
Ecole de medecine dentaire, Universite Laval,
Quebec, Canada G1K7P4

INTRODUCTION

IgA, the predominant immunoglobulin in the saliva, is the principal mediator of specific immunity in the oral cavity. Because IgA does not fix complement it is generally assumed that it is inefficient in acting directly as a bactericidal antibody (1). It is not excluded, however, that IgA can mediate bactericidal mechanisms by interaction with effector cells. Recently, receptors for the Fc portion of IgA have been demonstrated on different cell types (2-6). Moreover, some effector cells (lymphocytes, PMN, peripheral monocytes) were shown to kill bacteria via IgA-dependent mechanisms (7-10).

Indeed, such mechanisms may be involved at host parasite interfaces where IgA is the predominant isotype (11). In the oral cavity of BALB/c mice, natural salivary IgA antibodies were shown to display a characteristic pattern of antibacterial reactivities (12). If it could be demonstrated that IgA receptors are present on oral mucosal macrophages, it could be suggested that IgA may be involved in facilitating interactions between phagocytic cells and antibody-coated bacterial cells via RFc receptors, thus magnifying the antibacterial functions of salivary IgA.

We report here that a large portion of oral macrophages display IgA receptors and can be activated by IgA to bacterial ingestion and killing.

MATERIALS AND METHODS

Animals

BALB/c male mice, 18-24 weeks old, were obtained from Charles River Breeding Farms (St-Constant, Quebec).

Preparation of oral mucosal macrophages

The oral mucosa of 3-5 mice, including the cheeks and the soft palate, was dissected free of the underlying muscle tissue and cut into small fragments. After collagenase digestion (9 h, 37°C), cells were washed and incubated overnight in tissue culture chamber/slides (Lab-Tek, Miles Laboratories, Naperville, IL) in Iscove's medium supplemented with 20% inactivated fetal calf serum (FCS) and antibiotics (penicillin: 5000 IU/ml), streptomycin: 5000 μg/ml, gentamycin: 100 μg/ml and fungizone R: 250 μg/ml; Flow Laboratories, Missisauga, Ontario, Canada). Non-adherent cells were then removed by flooding the slides three times with warm Iscove's medium. The adherent cell population was typically greater than 90% macrophages (Fig. 1), of which 75-80% were viable (Barbeau et al., in preparation).

Collection of bile and sera

A pool of 10 BALB/c mice were used as a source of bile and serum. Mice were sacrificed by exsanguination and the blood collected in sterile

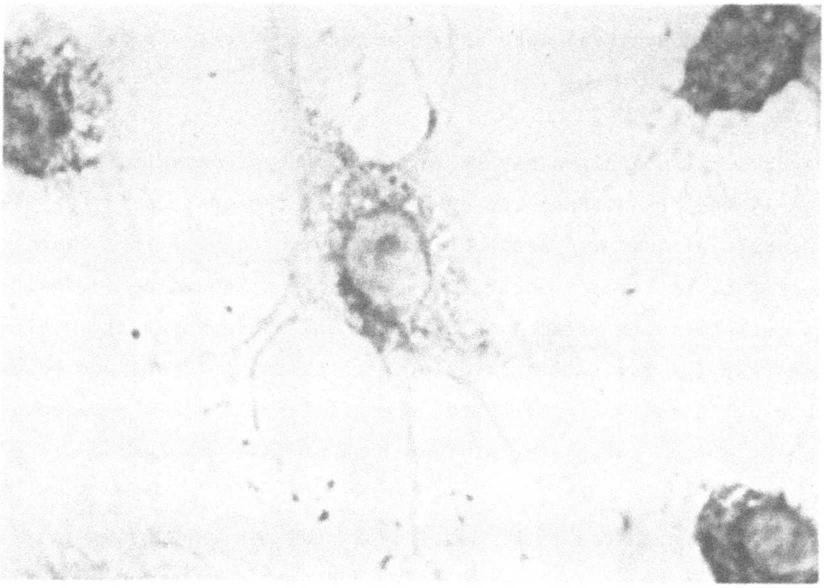

Figure 1. Oral mucosal macrophage; this picture shows the appearance of the cell. Adherent cells were characterized by nonspecific esterases, morphological criteria and adherent capacity after 18 h in culture. (x1000, Giemsa)

plastic petri dishes. Serum was recovered after overnight incubation at 4°C and residual blood cells removed by centrifugation (12,000 g, 3 min). Whole gall bladders were dissected and their contents expelled by centrifugation (12,000, 3 min). Quantitation of IgA and IgG in these samples was performed by ELISA (13).

Immunofluorescence

Direct immunofluorescence was performed with bile and serum samples on *Lactobacillus murinus* (*L. murinus*). Binding antibodies of the IgA and IgG isotypes were revealed by FITC-labeled mouse heavy chain alpha or gamma antibodies (Kirkegaard and Perry Lab, Inc.).

Preparation of bacteria

L. murinus was isolated by L. Trudel (of our group), from the oral cavity of a normal BALB/c mouse. This species represents about 37% of the oral indigenous flora in BALB/c mice (14). The bacteria were cultivated anaerobically overnight in tryptone soy broth (TSB) at 37°C. Before opsonization, the microorganisms were washed three times in Iscove's medium, resuspended, and diluted to 10^8 bacteria/ml in the same medium.

Opsonization

Natural secretory antibodies found in the bile, serum antibodies and specific IgA monoclonal antibodies were used to sensitize bacterial cells. Briefly, viable bacteria (10^8/ml) were incubated for 45 min at 37°C with bile (diluted 1/20 in Iscove's medium), with serum (diluted 1/10 in Iscove's medium), or with undiluted hybridoma supernatant (kindly provided by M. Oudghiri of our lab).

Demonstration of receptors for immunoglobulins on oral mucosal macrophages

10^9 fluorescent microspheres, 0.7 μ diameter (Covalent Technology, Ann Harbor, MI) were incubated with purified mouse IgG or purified mouse IgA (MOPC 315 myeloma protein, Bionetics, Willowdale, Ont.) at 2.5 mg/ml in EBSS. After 90 min, the particles were thoroughly washed in Earle's balanced salt solution (EBSS) and uncoated sites on microspheres were blocked with casein (0.4%). Washed particles were then incubated with adherent cells (2 to 4 x 10^8 beads/chamber) with gentle agitation. After 2 hours at 37°C, monolayers were carefully rinsed and slides observed with a fluorescent microscope. Cells showing more than 3 beads on their periphery were considered as positive. Control beads, coated with casein only, did not bind in significant numbers to these cells.

Phagocytic assay

Both sensitized and unsensitized, L. murinus (10^7/chamber) cells were incubated with monolayers for one hour at 37°C. Slides were then carefully rinsed, stained with acridine orange 1.25 mg/L (15), allowed to dry and then mounted in Eukitt. Cells showing at least one bacterium were considered as positive. Results were expressed as the percentage of positive cells among adherent macrophages. The distribution of positive cells having ingested from 1 to 3 bacteria, 4 to 6 bacteria and more than 7 bacteria, was also calculated. Phagocytic index were calculated as follows:

% phagocytosis X mean number of bacteria/macrophages (16)

RESULTS

Receptors for immunoglobulin on oral mucosal macrophages

Ig-coated fluorescent microspheres were used as an indicator system to investigate the presence of IgA and IgG receptors on murine macrophages (Fig. 2). The assay was set up with peritoneal adherent cells which showed optimal binding of IgG-coated beads (80-90% of the cell population, data not shown). Oral mucosal macrophages also displayed IgG receptors (Fig. 3), and a similar percentage (mean 33%) appear to bind IgA microspheres.

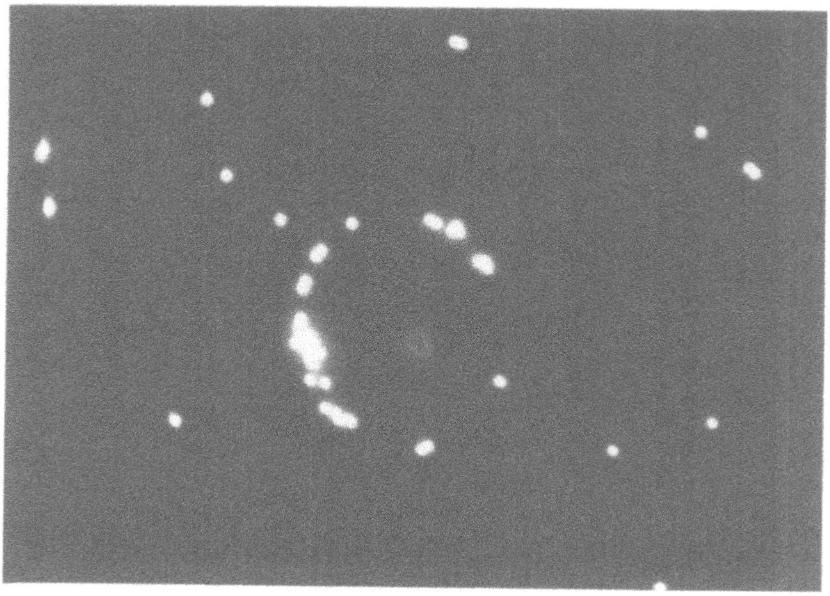

Figure 2. Demonstration of Ig receptors; a macrophage surrounded by IgG-coated microspheres. The cells are considered positive if > 3 microspheres are bound (x 1000).

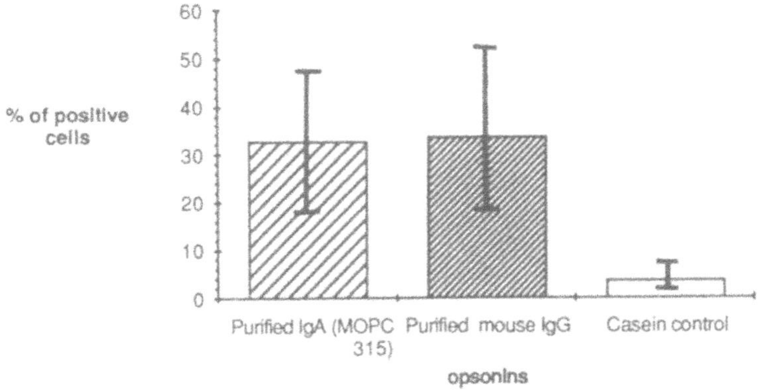

Figure 3. Incidence of FcR^+ cells among oral mucosal macrophages; adherent cells were incubated with IgA or IgG-coated microspheres and FcR^+ cells were enumerated by fluorescence microscopy.

The density of bound fluorescent particles was found to vary among these cells ranging from 3 to > 20 beads. Increasing the concentrations of immunoglobulins for the coating of microspheres or extending the incubation time with adherent cells did not significantly increase their specific binding. This suggests an intrinsic heterogeneity of oral macrophages with respect to their density of IgG and IgA receptors. In three similar experiments, each involving 3-5 mice, broad variations were also recorded in these determinations, IgA receptor-positive cells accounting for 18-47% of oral adherent cells, and IgG receptor-positive cells ranging from 18-52%. It thus appears that inter-individual variations can also be found in the incidence and distribution of cells bearing IgG and IgA receptors.

Bacterial ingestion and killing by oral mucosa macrophages

To evaluate potential effector functions of these receptors, we investigated the phagocytic capacity of oral mucosal macrophages. Target bacteria (*L. murinus*) were sensitized with specific IgG or IgA antibodies. Bile was used as a source of secretory (polymeric) antibodies (17,18) and serum as a source of monomeric IgA (19) and IgG antibodies. The presence of natural antibodies to surface determinants of *L. murinus* in these samples was confirmed by immunofluorescent staining. The phagocytic assay was also performed with specific monoclonal IgA (20). Present data (Fig. 4A and 4B) suggest that among phagocytic cells, opsonized bacteria are ingested in higher numbers than non-opsonized microorganisms. Moreover, a higher frequency of oral macrophages is activated to phagocytosis by antibody coated bacteria. Serum and bile antibodies are clearly the best opsonins

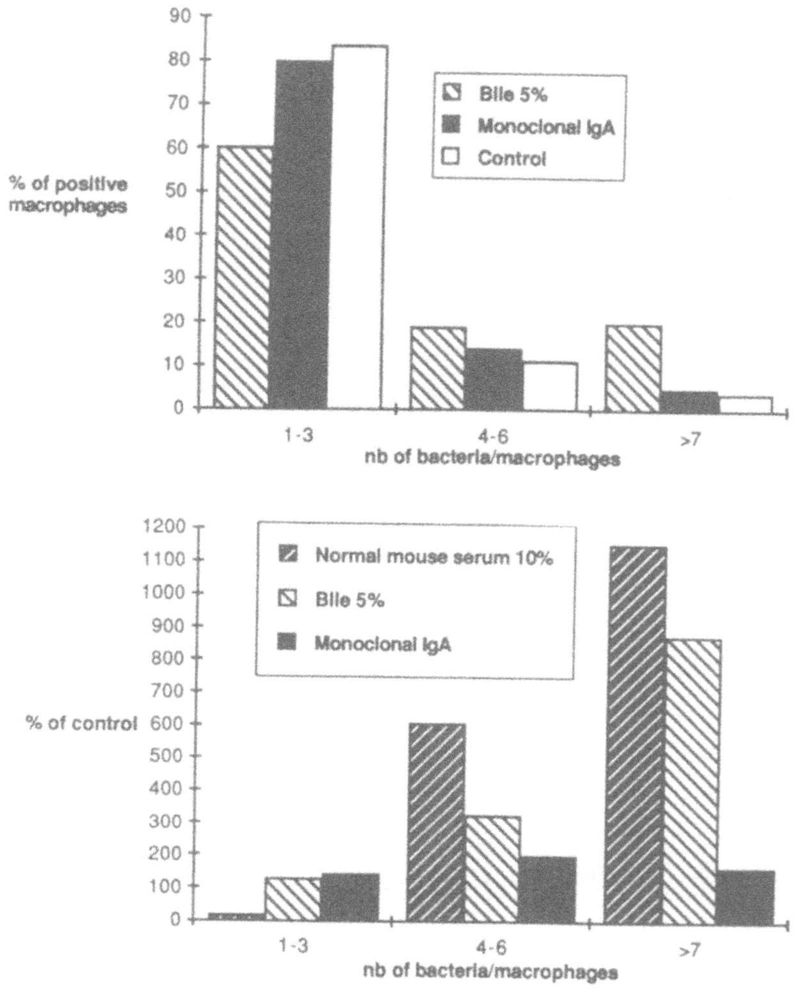

Figure 4. Phagocytic activity of mucosal macrophages; a murine oral bacterium, L. murinus was opsonized with secretory IgA (found in the bile), with normal serum, or with specific monoclonal IgA antibodies. After the phagocytic assay, positive cells were enumerated and the number of ingested bacteria was evaluated. Results are expressed as the percentage of positive cells among adherent macrophages; the distribution of cells having ingested 1 to 3 bacteria, 4 to 6 bacteria and more than 7 bacteria is presented on panel A. On panel B, results are expressed as % of the negative control (unsensitized bacteria).

for this process, whereas monoclonal IgA antibodies significantly, but minimally affected the phagocytic capacity of oral mucosal macrophages.

A close correlation was found between the frequency of IgA receptor bearing cells and the incidence of IgA-mediated antibacterial phagocytic activity (34%). Intracellular killing of target bacteria was demonstrated early after their ingestion by differential staining with acridine orange (Fig. 5).

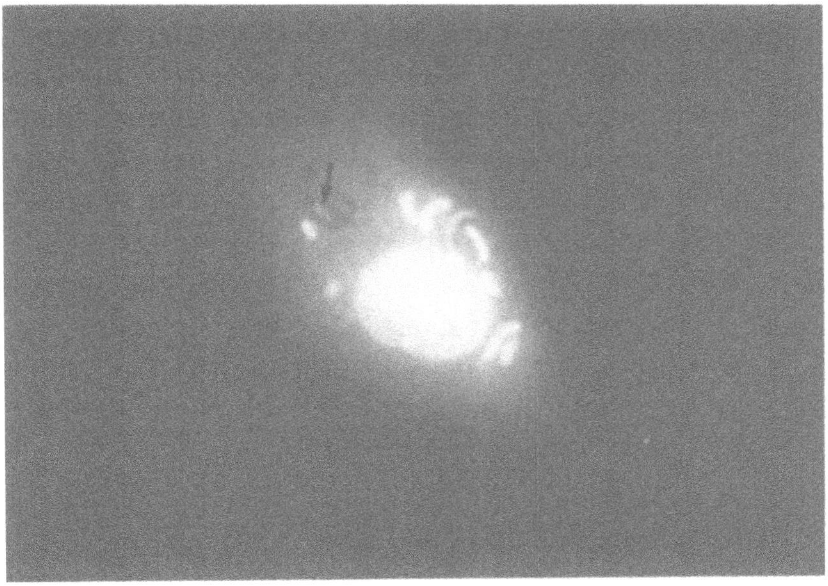

Figure 5. Acridine orange staining of a macrophage after interaction with opsonized L. murinus for 1 h at 37°C. All bacteria except one (arrow) were killed. Dead bacteria appeared red and living bacteria green (x1000).

DISCUSSION

Oral macrophages were isolated by enzymatic digestion of the mucosa and their Ig receptor status was investigated. Adherent cells of the oral mucosa were defined as macrophages following their characteristic morphology and the demonstration of nonspecific esterases. These cells were also shown to bind Ig-coated microspheres. A similar incidence of IgG and IgA-receptor bearing cells was found for oral mucosal macrophages. As double-labeling experiments were not performed, we cannot exclude a possible overlap between these two populations. Wide variations were observed in the binding capacity of oral macrophages. This heterogeneity may be due to the relative density of Fc receptors on these cells and/or to their affinity for IgA molecules. Since purified IgA and IgG were passively fixed to fluorescent beads, it is also possible that Fc presentation and molecular configuration were not optimal for a specific binding to occur with corresponding receptor. It is therefore possible, that the real proportion of Ig receptor-bearing cells was underestimated under our experimental conditions.

Functional studies of oral mucosal macrophages were conducted using a murine bacterium sensitized with specific antibodies. It appeared that the bacterial ingestion and killing capacity of these cells can be activated by IgA. Monoclonal IgA antibody-sensitized bacteria can induce phagocytosis in about 35% of oral macrophages. This percentage is in close correlation with the incidence of IgA receptor positive cells detected by the microsphere assay. Natural secretory antibodies found in the bile of our mice were shown to be better opsonins than MAbs for this process, promoting phagocytosis in about 42% of oral macrophages. This may indicate that the molecular form of IgA (monomeric-polymeric secretory) is critical for opsonizing capacity.

However, as small amounts of IgG were also present in the bile samples (Table 1), (IgA:IgG ratio = 112) we cannot state for the moment that sIgA alone is responsible for opsonization. Serum Igs with an inverse IgA:IgG ratio (0:4) are clearly the best opsonins for oral macrophages, 93% of these cells being able to phagocytize serum Ig-coated bacteria. With a high phagocytic index (369) this raises the interesting possibility of the additive or synergistic effect of both immunoglobulins in the phagocytic process. If we assume that only 18-52% of oral macrophages display receptors (Fig. 2), we can hypothesize that either serum antibodies can promote IgG and IgA dependent phagocytosis by distinct populations of Fc bearing cells, or that the presence of both isotypes on target bacteria can optimize phagocytosis, possibly via RFc alpha/gamma double bearing cells.

Table 1. Opsonizing capacity of serum, bile and monoclonal IgA

Opsonin source	IgA µg/ml	IgG µg/ml	% phagocytosis	# bacteria / macrophages (a)	P.I. (b)
Normal mouse serum 10%	100	700	93	7.3	369
Bile 5%	90	0.8	42	4.2	175
Monoclonal IgA	25	-	35	2.5	89
Control	-	-	23	2.3	53

[a]Mean number of bacteria/phagocytic macrophages.

[b]Phagocytic index; $\frac{\text{\% phagocytosis X mean \# bacteria}}{\text{\# phagocytic macrophages}}$

The presence of both IgA and IgG antibodies against oral bacteria in the murine saliva (21) would then be of functional relevance for these local processes. Present data suggest that complementary antibacterial functions of salivary IgA can be mediated via IgA-dependent phagocytosis. Current studies are aimed at characterizing the interactions between IgA and IgG in promoting immune phagocytosis by oral macrophages.

CONCLUSIONS

Oral mucosal macrophages were isolated and Ig-mediated adherence and phagocytosis were investigated.

These cells were shown to bind IgA-coated particles. A similar incidence of cells bound IgG-coated microspheres. Present data, therefore, suggest that oral macrophages normally express Ig receptor. It would be of great interest, though, to further characterize the specificity of this binding activity by blocking experiments to see if oral macrophages can simultaneously express both alpha and gamma receptor.

Functional studies of oral macrophages suggest that:

1. IgA can activate these cells to ingest and kill.

2. Secretory antibodies are better opsonins for these processes than monoclonal antibodies. However, as the bile contains low concentrations of IgG (IgA:IgG ratio = 112; Table 1), we cannot state that IgA alone is responsible for this opsonizing activity.

3. With an inverse IgA:IgG ratio (0.1) serum antibodies are also potent opsonins for oral macrophages.

Current research is aimed at characterizing these Ig-dependent mechanisms:

- Is the molecular form of IgA (monomeric-polymeric-secretory) critical for opsonizing capacity?
- What is the exact interaction between IgA and IgG in promoting immune phagocytosis by oral mucosal macrophages?

REFERENCES

1. Griffis, J.McL., Ann. N.Y. Acad. Sci. 409, 697, 1983.
2. Strober, W., Hague, N.E., Lum, L.G, Henkant, P.A., J. Immunol. 121, 240, 1978.
3. Lum, L.G., Muchmore, A.V., O'Connor, N., Strober, W. and Blaese, R.M., J. Immunol. 123, 714, 1979.
4. Lum, L.G., Muchmore, A.V., Keren, D., Decker, J., Koski, I., Strober, W. and Blaese, R.M., J. Immunol. 122, 65, 1979.
5. Fanger, M.W., Shen, L., Pugh, J. and Bernier, G.M., Proc. Natl. Acad. Sci. USA 77, 3640, 1980.
6. Gauldie, J., Richards, C. and Lamontagne, L., Mol. Immunol. 20, 1029, 1983.
7. Tagliabue, A., Boraschi, D., Villa, L., Keren, D.F., Lowell, G.H., Rappuoli, R. and Nencioni, L., J. Immunol. 133, 988, 1984.
8. Tagliabue, A., Nencioni, L., Villa, L., Keren, D.F., Lonell, G.H., Boraschi, D., Nature 306, 184, 1983.
9. Lowell, G.H., Smith, L.F., Griffiss, J.McL. and Brandt, B.L., J. Exp. Med. 152, 452, 1980.
10. Shen, L. and Fanger, M.W., Cell. Immunol. 59, 75, 1981.
11. Tomasi, T.B. and Bienenstock, J., Adv. Immunol. 9, 1, 1968.
12. Deslauriers, N., Seguin, J. and Trudel, L., Microbiol. Immunol., 1987, (in press).
13. Oudghiri, M. and Deslauriers, N., Eur. J. Immunol. 16, 281, 1986.
14. Trudel, L., St-Amand, L., Bareil, M., Cardinal, P. and Lavoie, M.C., Can. J. Microbiol. 32, 8, 1986.
15. Horn, W., Hansmann, C. and Federlin, K., J. Immunol. Methods 83, 233, 1985.
16. Richards, C.D. and Gauldie, J., Am. Rev. Respir. Dis. 132, 82, 1985.
17. Lemaitre-Coelho, I., Jackson, G.D.F., Vaerman, J.P., Eur. J. Immunol. 7, 588, 1977.
18. Hall, J., Orlans, E., Reynolds, J., Dean, C., Peppard, J., Gyure, L. and Hobbs, S., Int. Archs. Allerg. Appl. Immunol. 59, 75, 1979.
19. Kaartinen, M., Imir, T., Klockars, M., Sandhelm, M. and Makela, O., Scand. J. Immunol. 7, 229, 1978.
20. Oudghiri, M., Trudel, L. and Deslauriers, N., 1987 (This Issue).
21. Deslauriers, N., Oudghiri, M., Seguin, J. and Trudel, L., Immunol. Invest. 15, 1986.

IN VITRO EFFECTS OF IgA ON HUMAN POLYMORPHONUCLEAR LEUKOCYTES

Y. Sibille, D.L. Delacroix, W.W. Merrill, B. Chatelain
and J.-P. Vaerman

Experimental Medicine Unit (ICP) and University Hospital
Mont-Godinne, Catholic University of Louvain, Belgium;
and Pulmonary Section, Yale University, Medical School
New Haven, CT USA

INTRODUCTION

Receptors for immunoglobulin A (IgA) have been demonstrated on human polymorphonuclear leukocytes (PMN), monocytes and macrophages (1-3). However, little is known about the effector function of this Ig on human phagocytes. Recently, IgA was reported to have inhibitory effects on several effector functions of human PMN such as chemotaxis towards various chemoattractants (4), bactericidal activity (5), phagocytosis (5) and formyl-methionyl-leucyl-phenylalanine (FMLP)-stimulated chemiluminescence (6). However, these effects contrast with the increase of PMN cytotoxicity by IgA and with the absence of influence of IgA on Zymosan-induced chemiluminescence or on capping of PMN with fluorescent concanavalin A (7).

Therefore, we investigated the influence of concentration gradients of different forms of IgA on the mobility of human PMN and compared it to IgE, IgM and IgG.

MATERIALS AND METHODS

Human PMN

Human PMN were purified from venous blood by a one step Ficoll hypaque density gradient centrifugation (8). After two washes, the PMN were resuspended in 0.5% human serum albumin (HSA) in Hanks' solution with Ca^{++} and Mg^{++}.

Purification of Igs

Monoclonal (MC) IgA proteins were isolated from myeloma sera by a combination of repeated gel filtration on Ultragel AcA 22, preparative electrophoresis on Pevikon blocks and affinity chromatography (9). IgA characteristics are given in Table 1. MC IgM proteins were obtained by gel filtration followed by preparative zonal electrophoresis. Milk sIgA was obtained as previously reported (10). Polyclonal (PC) IgG was isolated from a large pool of normal serum by DEAE-cellulose chromatography and MC IgE as previously described (11). All Ig solutions were quantitated by light absorption at 280 nm and were dialyzed overnight against sterile HBSS and Millipore-filtered (0.2 μ) before concentration adjustment and addition to the

Table 1. Characterization of IgA proteins

No.	Major size	Origin	Subclass of IgA	L chain type	Size composition (percentages) Monomers	Dimers	Higher Polymers
1	Monomer	(Cle)[a]	IgA1	λ	95%	4%	0%
2	Dimer	(Del)[a]	IgA1	κ	9%	84%	7%
3	Monomer	(Gre)[a]	IgA2	λ	97%	3%	0%
4	Dimer	(Gre)[a]	IgA2	λ	9%	73%	18%
5	Monomer	(Mot)[a]	IgA1	κ	94%	6%	0%
6	Polymer	(Mot)[a]	IgA1	κ	3%	9%	88%
7	Monomer	Serum[b]	IgA1+IgA2	κ+λ	65%	28%	7%
8	Polymer	Milk[b]	IgA1+IgA2	κ+λ	0%	84%[c]	16%[c]

[a]IgA samples Nos. 1-6 are monoclonal, with abbreviated name of myeloma patient in parentheses.
[b]IgA samples Nos. 7 and 8 are polyclonal.
[c]Secretory IgA molecules, containing IgA-bound secretory component.

chemotactic chamber. Fcα and Fabα fragments were obtained by digestion of a MC mIgA_1 for 4 h at 37°C with an IgA_1-protease from Haemophilus influenzae (12). Digestion was verified by agarose gel electrophoresis and immunoelectrophoresis as described (12).

PMN chemotaxis

PMN chemotaxis was tested using a 48 well chemotaxis chamber (Neuroprobe®) and a 3 μm pore membrane (13). All Ig solutions contained 0.5% HSA in HBSS and spontaneous migration was tested with 0.5% HSA while maximal chemotaxis was obtained with 2 x 10^{-7} M FMLP. PMN were allowed to migrate through the membrane for 12 min at 37°C.

Data for a given Ig protein (R Ig) were expressed as percentage of maximal FMLP-induced chemotaxis according to the formula:

$$R\ Ig = \frac{X_{Ig} - X_{negative\ control}}{X_{FMLP\ 2 \times 10^{-7} M} - X_{negative\ control}}$$

Value X represent mean of 9 different high power microscopic fields (HPF).

RESULTS

Effect of MC IgA on PMN mobility

When added to 0.5% HSA in the lower compartment of the chemotaxis chamber, with PMN in 0.5% HSA in the upper part, all MC IgA proteins stimulated PMN mobility with a concentration dependent pattern (Fig. 1). At a concentration of 1.0 mg/ml, IgA induced 72.8 ± 9.1% (mean ± SD of six experiments) of the maximal neutrophil chemotaxis induced by FMLP, 47% ± 4.7% at 0.3 mg/ml and 22.0 ± 10.9% at 0.1 mg/ml without difference according to the size or subclass of IgA molecules. When PMN were resuspended in 0.5% HSA plus 0.3 mg/ml IgA and IgA was also present in the lower compartment of the chamber, the same mean PMN migration was observed as when PMN were in 0.5% HSA alone (Table 2).

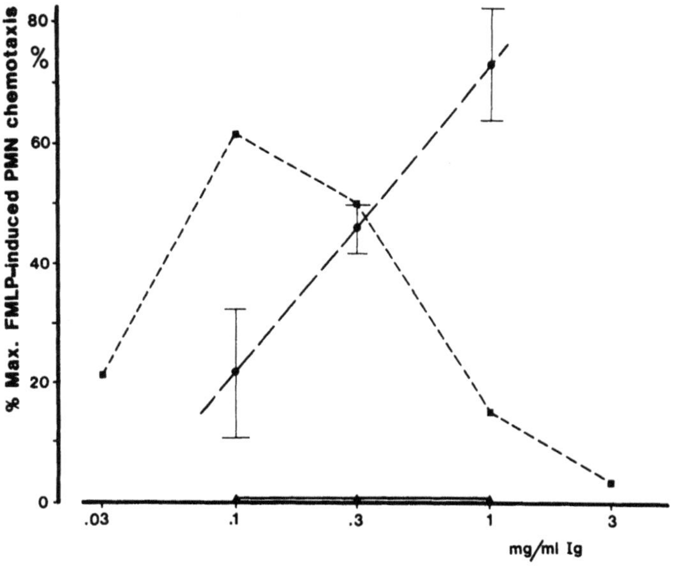

Figure 1. Influence of various concentrations of MC IgA (●---●; n=6), MC IgM (▲——▲; n=4) and PC IgG (■---■; n=2) on PMN migration. Data are expressed as mean percentages of maximal FMLP-induced (2×10^{-7} M) PMN chemotaxis. Vertical bars represent SD.

Effect of MC IgA on FMLP-induced chemotaxis

When MC m- and p-IgA (10 mg/ml) was added to the PMN (upper compartment), we observed a reduction of the maximal FMLP-induced chemotaxis to 44.5% of the control (for pIgA) and to 36% (for mIgA). When m- and p-IgA (0.3 mg/ml) were added to suboptimal concentrations of FMLP (10^{-9} M), we observed an increase of the FMLP-induced chemotaxis from 33% of the maximal (2×10^{-7} M) FMLP-induced chemotaxis to 84% (for the monomer) and 79% (for the dimer).

Effect of PC IgA and IgA fragments

Both serum and milk IgA increased PMN migration when placed in the bottom (85% and 52% of maximal FMLP-induced chemotaxis) or both compartments (43% for serum and 38% for milk IgA) of the chemotaxis chamber at 0.3 mg/ml. Two different Fcα preparations placed in the lower wells at 1.0 and 0.3 mg/ml induced an increased PMN migration to 86 ± 5% and 45 ± 3%,

Table 2. Effect of different concentrations of IgA in the bottom compartment and the addition of IgA (0.3 mg/ml) to PMN in the top compartment, on PMN mobility

Lower Compartment	Top Compartment (PMN)				
	0.5% HSA	MC m-IgA[a]	MC p-IgA[a]	PC serum[a] m-IgA	PC milk[a] d-IgA
0.5% HSA	0[b] (n=6)	0 (n=2)	0 (n=2)	ND[c]	ND
0.5% HSA+MC m-IgA or d-IgA					
at 1 mg/ml	72.8(n=6)	74.5(n=2)	60.0(n=2)	ND	ND
at 0.3 mg/ml	47.0(n=6)	52.0(n=2)	47.0(n=2)	ND	ND
at 0.1 mg/ml	22.0(n=6)	33.0(n=2)	23.0(n=2)	ND	ND
0.5% HSA+PC serum m-IgA at 0.3 mg/ml	85.0(n=2)	ND	ND	43.0(n=2)	ND
0.5% HSA+PC milk d-IgA at 0.3 mg/ml	52.0(n=2)	ND	ND	ND	38.0(n=2)

[a]All IgA samples in top compartment at 0.3 mg/ml.
[b]Data are mean values of experiments (N) and are expressed as percentages of maximal FMLP-induced chemotaxis.
[c]Not determined.

respectively, of the maximal FMLP-induced migration. When Fcα at 0.3 mg/ml was placed on both sides of the membrane, 45 ± 5% of the FMLP-induced chemotaxis was observed. In contrast, both Fabα samples at 1.0 and 0.3 mg/ml in the lower or both compartments had no effect on PMN migration.

Effect of PC IgG and MC IgM and IgE on PMN chemotaxis

PC IgG placed in the lower compartment induced PMN migration with maximal effect observed at low concentrations (0.1 mg/ml) (Fig. 1). When PC IgG was added to both compartments at 0.3 mg/ml, no migration was induced. None of the four MC IgM solutions nor MC IgE induced PMN migration at concentrations up to 3 mg/ml.

DISCUSSION

In the present report, we demonstrate a dual effect of IgA on PMN mobility: (a) IgA (both monomeric and polymeric forms) increase PMN random migration in a dose dependent manner; (b) IgA inhibits the maximal (2×10^{-7} M) FMLP-induced chemotaxis but increases the suboptimal (10^{-9} M) FMLP-induced chemotaxis).

The requirement of Fcα for this function is supported by the observation that Fcα but not Fabα, induces chemokinesis. IgM and IgE have no effect on PMN mobility while polyclonal IgG is chemotactic at low concentrations (0.1 mg/ml). Since the concentrations of IgA (0.1 to 3 mg/ml) are in the range of normal serum IgA and of the bronchial lining fluid, it is likely that *in vitro* chemokinetic effect of IgA occurs at concentrations observed *in vivo*, supporting its biological relevance. Thus, appropriate mobility of PMN phagocytes is believed to be an important part of the host defense mechanism, and the finding that physiological levels of IgA induce the *in vitro* chemokinesis of PMN may be important in IgA deficiencies, especially when associated with IgG subclass deficiencies.

REFERENCES

1. Fanger, M.W., Shen, L., Pugh, J. and Bernier, G.M., Proc. Natl. Acad. Sci. USA 77, 36, 1980.
2. Fanger, M.W., Pugh, J. and Bernier, G.M., Cell. Immunol. 60, 324, 1981.
3. Gauldie, J., Richards, C.D. and Lamontagne, L., Mol. Immunol. 20, 1029, 1983.
4. Van Epps and Williams, R.C., J. Exp. Med. 144, 1227, 1976.
5. Van Epps, D.E., Reed, K. and Williams, R.C., Cell. Immunol. 36, 363, 1978.
6. Van Epps, D.E. and Brown, S.L., Infect. Immun. 34, 864, 1981.
7. Shen, L. and Fanger, M.W., Cell. Immunol. 59, 75, 1981.
8. Ferrante, A. and Thong, Y.H., J. Immunol. Meth. 24, 389, 1978.
9. Delacroix, D.L., Meykens, R. and Vaerman, J.-P., Mol. Immunol. 19, 297, 1982.
10. Delacroix, D.L. and Vaerman, J.-P., J. Immunol. Meth. 40, 345, 1981.
11. Vaerman, J.-P., J. Lab. Clin. Immunol. 2, 343, 1979.
12. Kilian, M., Mestecky, J., Kulhavy, R., Tomana, M. and Butler, W.T., J. Immunol. 124, 2596, 1980.

13. Falk, W., Goodwin, R.H. and Leonard, E.J., J. Immunol. Meth. 33, 239, 1980.

PRESENCE OF FC RECEPTORS FOR IgA ON RAT ALVEOLAR MACROPHAGES BUT NOT PERITONEAL MACROPHAGES

Y. Sibille, B. Chatelain, Ph. Staquet, M. Rits and J.-P. Vaerman

Experimental Medicine Unit (ICP) and University Hospital of Mont-Godinne, Catholic University of Louvain, Belgium

INTRODUCTION

Different blood cells, including lymphocytes, polymorphonuclear leukocytes and monocytes, possess a receptor for the Fc portion of IgA (FcαR) on their surface (1-4). Recently, an FcαR has also been demonstrated on mouse alveolar marcrophages (AM) but not peritoneal macrophages (PM) (5), and the IgA-mediated phagocytosis correlated with the presence of FcαR (6). Despite early studies reporting the absence of FcαR on rat and human AM (7,8), up to 17% of human AM can ingest sIgA-opsonized *Pseudomonas* (9). Further, a possible role of AM has been suggested in a rat model of IgA-induced lung injury (10). Therefore, the present study was designed to assess by flow cytometry the issue of FcαR on rat AM and PM and to investigate whether the molecular size of IgA could influence its binding to the cells.

MATERIALS AND METHODS

Cells

Peritoneal and bronchoalveolar cells were obtained from male Wistar rats. The animals were sacrificed in a CO_2-filled chamber and the bronchoalveolar lavage (100 ml of sterile 0.9% saline in 10 ml aliquots) was performed via a cannula inserted into the trachea. Resting peritoneal cells were harvested from the same animals by injecting 30 ml of sterile 0.9% saline into the peritoneum and by immediately aspirating the peritoneal lavage fluid. Cells were washed twice and resuspended in RPMI 1640 supplemented with 5% heat inactivated fetal calf serum and kept on ice. Cells were counted and cytocentrifuged smears were stained by May-Grunwald-Giemsa for cell differential count, and macrophages were identified by esterase staining.

Protein preparations

Secretory IgA (sIgA) and free secretory component (FSC) were purified from rat bile (11). Monomeric, dimeric and polymeric forms of rat monoclonal IgA anti-DNP were produced as reported (12). Mouse monoclonal, monomeric and polymeric IgA anti-DNP were isolated from ascites of MOPC 315 mice by affinity chromatography on DNP-lysine-sepharose and gel filtration on Ultragel AcA 22. All IgA molecules were conjugated with fluorescein (FITC) and the final F/P ratio was between 1.1 and 1.7 (13). A mixture of FITC tri- and tetrameric MC rat IgA was incubated with rat FSC for 1 h at 37°C in a two-fold molar excess, resulting in FITC-MC sIgA, as demonstrated by immunoelectrophoresis. The FITC bovine serum albumin (BSA) with F/P = 5.5 was used as negative control.

Flow cytometry studies

100 µl of the cell suspension (5 x 10^5 cells/ml) were mixed with an equal volume of the different FITC-proteins at a final concentration of 100 µg/ml and maintained at 4°C for 1 h. The cells were then washed twice at 4°C and passed through an Epics C (Coulter®) flow cytometer at a flow rate of 1000 cells/sec. Cell bound fluorescence was determined by the change in fluorescence compared to the BSA control within the macrophage population.

RESULTS

Cell differentials

The differential cell counts of the bronchoalveolar and of the peritoneal lavage are given in Table 1. Macrophages represent over 95% of the alveolar cells while they account for only 65.7% of the peritoneal cells. Macrophages were further identified as esterase positive cells.

Table 1. Cell differentials

	Macrophages[a]	Lymphocytes	Eosinophils	Neutrophils	Mast Cells
Broncho-alveolar lavage (n=12)	95.3 ± 2.5[b]	3.8 ± 1.7	-	0.9 ± 1.1	-
Peritoneal lavage (n=7)	65.7 ± 5.4	2.6 ± 1.9	16.4 ± 3.6	2.2 ± 1.7	13.1 ± 4.9

[a]Data expressed in percent of 500 counted cells.
[b]Mean value ± standard deviations of n experiments.

Flow cytometry

AM and PM populations were cytometrically identified from the other cells by size and granular density and further studies were focused on those populations.

IgA binding

As illustrated in Figure 1, we observed an increase in IgA binding to AM proportional to the size of the IgA. Thus, MC monomeric IgA from rat and mouse did not bind to AM while dimeric MC IgA from both sources provided a minor binding (5.4% and 4.5%, respectively). In contrast, heavy MC polymeric IgA and polyclonal bile sIgA bound to 8.3% and 15.1% of AM, respectively. Furthermore, the complex formed with MC polymers of IgA and SC (MC tri- and tetrameric sIgA) increased the binding of the polymers to 11.4%. To evaluate whether IgA bound to AM through SC, we incubated the cells with FITC-SC and observed no binding.

Ninety percent FITC-sIgA binding to AM was prevented by adding non-fluorescent sIgA (3 mg/ml) 15 min prior to the FITC sIgA. To further demonstrate that the cell-bound fluorescence was bound to the AM, the fluorescent cells were sorted by the Epics and 100% of the cells were esterase positive and were morphologically identified as macrophages. Finally, none of the FITC-labeled IgA preparations nor FSC showed significant binding to PM.

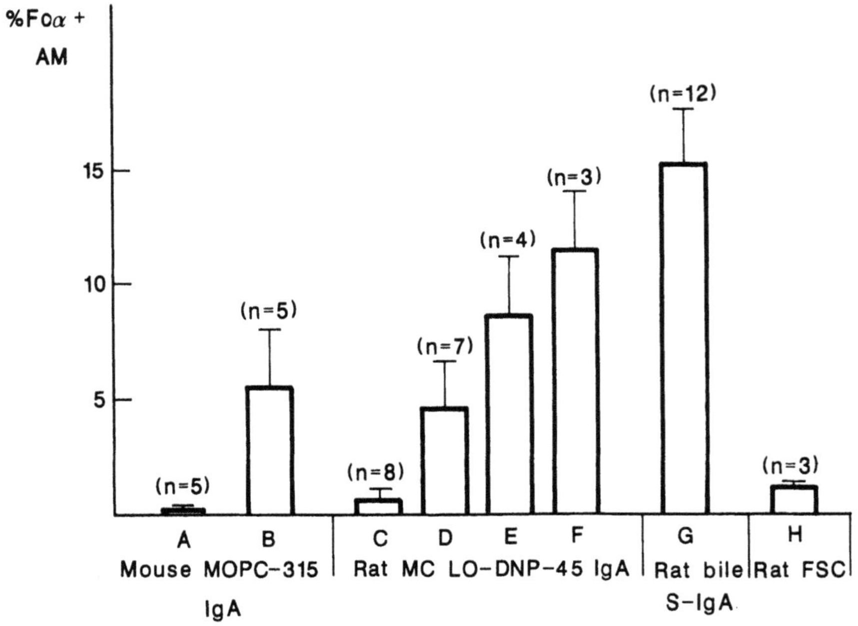

Figure 1. Percentage of AM binding different FITC-IgA preparations (0.1 mg/ml): (A) Mouse MC mIgA (F/P: 1.4); (B) Mouse MC pIgA (F/P: 1.3); (C) Rat MC mIgA (F/P: 1.3); (D) Rat MC dIgA (F/P: 1.7); (E) Rat MC tri- and tetrameric IgA (F/P: 1.1); (F) Rat MC tri- and tetrameric sIgA (F/P: 1.1); (G) Bile sIgA (F/P: 1.7); and (H) FITC-FSC (F/P: 2.2). The negative control is the cell bound fluorescence due to FITC-BSA (F/P: 5.5). Columns represent means and bars standard deviations.

DISCUSSION

The present study provides evidence for the presence of FcαR on the surface of rat AM, as reported for mouse AM (5). The presence of FcαR$^+$ AM was further supported by the inhibition of binding of FITC-IgA by non-fluorescent IgA and by sorting of the fluorescent cells representing 100% esterase positive cells with cytological characteristics of macrophages. A nonspecific internalization of IgA by macrophages was prevented by keeping the cells at 4°C during the experiment.

In contrast with other immune cells like lymphocytes, neutrophils or monocytes, only polymeric IgA bound significantly to AM. Thus, 15% of the AM bound polyclonal sIgA and 8% of the AM fixed tri- and tetrameric rat MC IgA, while only 5% of these cells bound dimeric MC IgA.

This may explain the difference between our work and previous reports suggesting the absence of FcαR on rat AM using monomeric or dimeric IgA (7). Methodological differences (in particular flow cytometry versus rosette formation) may also account for part of the discrepancies. The increase from 8 to 11% of $Fc\alpha R^+$ AM by complexing SC to polymeric MC IgA suggested a role for SC in the binding of IgA to AM. However, no receptor for FSC could be detected on the surface of AM. Whether SC increases the binding of IgA through a reinforcement of the stability of polymeric IgA and/or through a change of the molecular configuration of IgA remains to be elucidated.

As reported in mice, we could not detect FcαR on PM. Therefore, it is likely that the environment of the cells influences the expression of immunoglobulin receptors.

In this regard, a recent study reports that Kupffer cells, another type of phagocytic cells, bind equally monomeric and dimeric IgA (14). AM represent the majority of the cells of the alveoli and sIgA the second immunoglobulin of the alveolar lining fluid. Therefore, the demonstration of FcαR on rat AM further supports a role for these two immune components in host defense mechanisms.

ACKNOWLEDGEMENTS

This work was supported by grant 3.4504.70 from F.R.S.M., Brussels, Belgium.

REFERENCES

1. Lum, L.G., Muchmore, A.V., Keren, D., Decker, J., Koshi, I., Strober, W. and Blaese, R.M., J. Immunol. 122, 65, 1979.
2. Lum, L.G., Muchmore, A.V., O'Connor, W., Strober, W. and Blaese, R.M., J. Immunol. 123, 714, 1979.
3. Fanger, M.W., Pugh, J. and Bernier, G.M., Cell. Immunol. 60, 324, 1981.
4. Fanger, M.W., Shen, L., Pugh, J. and Bernier, G.M., Proc. Natl. Acad. Sci. USA 77, 3640, 1980.
5. Gauldie, J., Richards, C. and Lamontagne, L., Mol. Immunol. 20, 1029, 1983.
6. Richards, C.D. and Gauldie, J., Am. Rev. Respir. Dis. 132, 82, 195.
7. Boltz-Nitulescu, G., Bazin, H. and Spiegelberg, H.L., J. Exp. Med. 154, 374, 1981.

8. Reynolds, H.Y., Atkinson, J.P., Newball, H.H. and Frank, M.M., J. Immunol. 114, 1813, 1975.
9. Reynolds, H.Y., Kazmierowski, J.A., Newball, H.H., J. Clin. Invest. 56, 376, 1975.
10. Johnson, K.J., Wilson, B.S., Till, G.O. and Ward, P.A., J. Clin. Invest. 74, 358, 1984.
11. Acosta Altamirano, G., Barranco-Acosta, C., Van Roost, E. and Vaerman, J.-P., Mol. Immunol. 17, 1525, 1980.
12. Rits, M., Cormont, F., Bazin, H., Meykens, R. and Vaerman, J.-P., J. Immunol. Meth. 89, 81, 1986.
13. The, T.H., Conjugatie van fluoresceine isothiocyanaat aan antistoffen. Thesis, Aamstelstad Drukkerij, Amsterdam, 1967.
14. Sancho, J., Gonzalez, E. and Egido, J., Immunology 57, 37, 1986.

ENUMERATION, RECEPTOR EXPRESSION AND PHAGOCYTIC CAPABILITIES OF EOSINOPHILS OF HUMAN COLON MUCOSA

I. Northwood, C. Beliveau, D. Gump and W. Beeken

Department of Medicine, University of Vermont
Burlington, Vermont USA

INTRODUCTION

Eosinophils are present in normal human intestinal mucosa, where their main functions are presumably participation in hypersensitivity reactions and defense against helminthic infestations. However, these numbers are increased in inflammatory bowel disease (1) and other conditions (2) not normally associated with allergic states or paresitosis, and their role in these disorders is unknown. Therefore, we enumerated these cells in mucosal suspensions, measured their Fc and C3b receptors and assayed their phagocytic activity.

METHODS

Cell suspensions were obtained by EDTA-collagenase dissociation of histologically normal mucosa obtained from resections for colonic neoplasms (3). These suspensions were enriched for eosinophils by countercurrent centrifugation (4). Blood eosinophils were separated by gradient centrifugation after degranulation of neutrophils by use of FMLP (5,6). Stained cytocentrifuge preparations were examined for differential cell counts. Fcγ receptors were measured by flow cytometry after labeling of eosinophil-rich suspensions with human FITC-IgG. C3b receptors were determined by flow cytometry of cells doubly labeled with human C3b receptor monoclonal mouse antibody and FITC affinity purified $F(ab')_2$ goat anti-mouse Fcγ, IgG (7). Phagocytic assays were done at a 10:1 bacteria:phagocyte ratio with opsonized and nonopsonized *Escherichia coli* ON2 and eosinophil-rich suspensions incubated at 37°C for 30 min. Cells were examined microscopically for percent of cells ingesting bacteria and the number of bacteria per cell.

RESULTS

Results of eosinophil enrichment by countercurrent centrifugation of dissociated mucosal suspension are tabulated below.

		Eosin	Macro	Neutro	Lymphoid	Others
Collagenase dissociation n = 24	percent	8.5	7.5	1.2	71.8	9.7
	SEM	1.5	1.4	0.4	2.1	1.8
Countercurrent centrifugation n = 15	percent	43.0	21.5	3.1	30.7	0.7
	SEM	4.9	3.1	1.1	3.4	0.3

Eosinophil receptor expression is given in the following table.

		Gut	Blood
Fcγ	percent cells	91.8	90.6
	SEM	2.2	4.3
	n	7	4
C3b	percent cells	77.7	64.6
	SEM	4.9	4.2
	n	7	4

Mucosal eosinophil phagocytic activity is given below.

		Percent eosinophils ingesting bacteria	Number bacteria per eosinophil
Gut	mean	73.9	4.4
	SEM	5.8	0.8
	n	8	8

Blood eosinophils were not phagocytic in our assay.

CONCLUSIONS

Eosinophils are the most numerous phagocytes of normal colonic mucosa of persons with large bowel neoplasms. The large majority of these cells express Fcγ and C3b receptors, and are actively phagocytic for opsonized *E. coli* ON2. The role of these cells in this population is undefined.

REFERENCES

1. Sommers, S.C. and Korelitz, B.I., Am. J. Clin. Pathol. 63, 359, 1975.
2. Blackshaw, A.J. and Levison, D.A., J. Clin. Pathol. 39, 1, 1986.
3. Bull, D.M. and Bookman, M.A., J. Clin. Invest. 59, 966, 1977.
4. Beeken, W., Mieremet-Ooms, J. and Ginsel, L.A., J. Immunol. Meth. 73, 189, 1984.
5. Vadas, M.A., David, J.R. and Butterworth, A., J. Immunol. 122, 1228, 1979.
6. Roberts, R.L. and Gallin, J.I., Blood 65, 433, 1985.
7. Fearon, D.T. and Collins, L.A., J. Immunol. 130, 370, 1983.

COFACTOR REQUIREMENTS FOR EXPRESSION OF LACTOFERRIN BACTERICIDAL ACTIVITY ON ENTERIC BACTERIA

M.A. Motley and R.R. Arnold*

Department of Microbiology and Immunology, Morehouse School of Medicine, Atlanta, GA USA; and *Department of Oral Biology Emory University Dental Research Center, Atlanta, GA USA

INTRODUCTION

Lactoferrin (LF), is an iron-binding glycoprotein that is common to most mammalian excretions (1-3) and is a prominent component of the specific granule of neutrophilic leukocytes (4,5). It shares its distribution on mucosal surfaces with that of secretory IgA. Its high affinity binding in coordination with suitable anion has been well characterized (6-9). This ability to bind iron has been associated with a bacteriostatic deprivation of this essential nutrient (10-12). A variety of other biological activities have also been attributed to LF, including a direct bactericidal effect on a variety of bacteria (13,14). This killing mechanism is temperature and pH dependent and requires direct interaction of the LF with the bacterial cell surface (15). There are a variety of bacteria that are resistant to the bactericidal effects of purified LF binding including selected Gram-negative enteric bacteria (14). The resistance of these bacteria appears related, in part, to the impermeability of their outer cellular structures (16).

Recent studies from several laboratories have begun to investigate possible interactions between secretory antibodies and the innate defense proteins. It has been suggested that secretory IgA, as well as LF, may enhance the antimicrobial activity of lactoperoxidase (17). In addition, secretory IgA has been reported to enhance the activity of lysozyme and complement (18). Several investigators have examined the potentiation of the bacteriostatic effects of LF by secretory IgA (20-22). In contrast, early studies from this laboratory found that purified secretory IgA with antibody activity to Streptococcus mutans, can block LF killing of this microorganism (24). In the present study, selected strains of enteric bacteria were chosen on the basis of their resistance to the bactericidal activity of purified LF and on their differential sensitivity to serum. These studies suggest that there is a cofactor or cofactors in human colostrum that results in synergistic killing with iron-free LF of selected enteric bacteria.

MATERIALS AND METHODS

Lactoferrin preparations

Two forms of LF were employed in these studies for comparative purposes. Lactoferrin was purified to homogeneity by heparin-sepharose chromatography of human colostral whey collected from healthy volunteers (25). Briefly, whey was collected from pooled human colostrum or individual colostral samples by centrifugation at 10,000 g for 40 min. After adjusting the pH to 4.7 with 0.1 N HCl, the whey was heated at 40°C for 30 min and then centrifuged to remove casein. After dialysis against 0.05 M NaCl containing 5 mM veronal-HCl (pH 7.4), the whey was added to a heparin-sepharose column. The void volume, rich in secretory IgA, was collected and rerun on the heparin-sepharose column to assure removal of residual molecules with heparin affinity. Lactoferrin and other whey components retained on the column, were eluted with increasing gradients of sodium chloride. Lactoferrin elutes at approximately 0.6 M sodium chloride. This fraction was run over an antibody affinity column of rabbit IgG antibody to human LF coupled to sepharose and eluted using low pH buffer. Commercial human LF was obtained from Calbiochem (Lot number 903889). This LF preparation was found to contain approximately 70% LF. Secretory IgA, lysozyme, and lactalbumin were present as contaminating protein. The bound iron of both LF preparations was removed by dialysis against two changes in 100 volumes of 0.2 M acetic acid/sodium acetate buffer (pH 4.0) with 0.2 M NaH_2PO_4 and 0.04 M disodium ethylenediaminetetraacetate (EDTA) followed by exhaustive dialysis against deionized, distilled water.

Microorganisms

Salmonella typhimurium and its deep rough mutant SL1181 (26) were provided by Dr. Hiroshi Nikaido, University of California, Berkeley. Two clinical isolates of *Escherichia coli*, one isolate (strain 6) serum sensitive, the other (strain 2) serum resistant, were provided by Dr. Pinghui V. Liu, University of Louisville. Bacteria were maintained on triple sugar iron slants (Difco) at room temperature. For the bactericidal assays, bacteria were grown to early exponential phase (A_{660}nm = 0.2) in Todd-Hewitt broth. The bacteria were washed by centrifugation and diluted to a stock suspension containing approximately 10^7 colony forming units (CFU) per ml in 0.85% saline. Bactericidal assays were performed by resuspending 0.1 ml of the stock bacteria (10^6CFU) in 0.9 ml of appropriate concentration of test samples (colostral whey, lactoferrin, heparin void volume with or without LF) the bacterial suspensions were incubated at 37°C in plastic snap-cap tubes (Falcon, Bioquest). Aliquots (0.1 ml) were withdrawn at designated intervals, serially diluted, and plated in duplicate on trypticase soy agar (TSA). The TSA plates were incubated at 37°C for 24 hrs and colony counts determined. A reduction in colony counts of greater than half a log was considered indicative of bactericidal activity.

RESULTS

Serum sensitivity of E. coli strains

The two *E. coli* strains were incubated in fresh human colostrum at 37°C. Their growth was monitored by following the change in optical density at 660 nm and viability was determined by plating as described. *E. coli* 6 was readily killed by fresh serum, whereas *E. coli* 2 was capable of uninhibited growth in fresh human serum. Heating the serum at 56°C for 30 min removed the inhibitory effects on *E. coli* 6. This inhibitory effect was restored by the addition of dilute guinea pig serum (Cappel) as a source of complement. A total of ten serum samples from different individuals was tested against both strains of *E. coli* with identical results.

Sensitivity in milk whey samples

The whey from colostrum and milk samples from several different healthy donors, was tested individually for antibacterial activity against both *E. coli* 6 and *E. coli* 2 (Table 1). *E. coli* 2 was uneffected by any of the whey samples. *E. coli* 6 in contrast to its serum sensitivity, demonstrated a variable susceptibility to the various whey samples in different mothers. *E. coli* 6 was killed by selected samples of whey, but was not killed by others.

Table 1. Bactericidal activity[a] of individual colostral whey samples to the serum sensitive *Escherichia coli* 6

Subject number	Time (min) 0	120	$\log_{10}$ difference[c]
1	6.0[b]	6.8	+0.8
2	6.0	4.5	-1.5
3	6.0	5.2	-0.8
4	6.0	6.9	+0.9
5	6.0	6.8	+0.8
6	6.0	6.7	+0.7
7	6.0	6.6	+0.6
8	6.0	7.1	+1.1
9	6.0	4.3	-1.7
10	6.0	4.9	-1.1
saline control	6.0	6.0	0

[a]An aliquot (0.1 ml) containing 10^6 CFU of *E. coli* 6 was added to 0.9 ml of undiluted colostral whey and incubated at 37°C for 2 h.

[b]CFU/ml expressed as $\log_{10}$. Determined according to the text.

[c]The difference between the 2 h value of CFU and that of 0 time. A positive value is indicative of growth and a negative value of killing.

Lactoferrin bactericidal effects

The purified lactoferrin preparation at concentrations up to 0.5 mg/ml had no effect on the viability of either *E. coli* 2 or 6, or *S. typhimurium* LT2 or SL1181 (Table 2). The same preparation of LF demonstrated significant killing of *S. mutans* (NCTC 10449) and *Legionella pneumophila* (Knoxville strain) (27) under the same conditions at concentrations as low as 50 µg/ml. The commercial LF, in contrast, demonstrated potent activity against *E. coli* 6 and *S. typhimurium* SL1181 but had no effect on either *E. coli* 2 or *S. typhimurium* LT2. Molecular sieve filtration (100K molecular weight cutoff) resulted in a lack of bactericidal activity in either the retentate or the filtrate; however, when the retentate and filtrate were added together, the bactericidal activity was restored.

Table 2. Comparison of the bactericidal activity of heparin-affinity purified lactoferrin and commercial lactoferrin

Bacteria[a]	Log_{10} Difference[b]		
	Purified LF	Commercial LF	Saline
1. S. typhimurium LT2	0[c]	+0.1[c]	0
2. S. typhimurium SL1181	-0.2[c]	-2.2[c]	0
3. E. coli 2	+0.3[c]	+0.4[c]	0
4. E. coli 6	-0.2[c]	-1.4[c]	0
5. S. mutans NCTC 10449	<-4.2[c,d]	<-4.2[c,d]	0
6. L. pneumophila	<-4.2[c,d]	<-4.2[c,d]	0

[a]All bacterial strains were suspended in saline (10^6 CFU/ml) containing the appropriate concentration of the test LF preparation.

[b]See Table 1, $\log_{10}$ difference = -4.2 is the limit of detection.

[c]LF preparations at 0.5 mg of protein/ml.

[d]LF preparations at 100 µg of protein/ml.

Bactericidal whey samples and commercial LF were fractionated on heparin-sepharose and the void volume and LF were collected. None of the SIgA in the whey or the commercial LF was retained on heparin-sepharose, and thus SIgA was a principal component of the void volume. Neither the void volume nor the purified LF demonstrated bactericidal activity against any of the enteric bacterial strains tested. Purified LF was maintained at a constant concentration and increasing dilutions of void volume were added to the lactoferrin/bacterial suspensions and tested for bactericidal activity at 37°C after 2 h of incubation. As can be seen in Table 3, the heparin void volume resulted in synergistic bactericidal activity against both S. typhimurium SL1181 and E. coli 6. This synergistic bactericidal effect was maximal for E. coli 6 and S. typhimurium SL1181 at a void volume concentration of 0.5 and 0.25 mg/ml, respectively, with greater and lesser concentrations of the fraction causing less effective synergism. This may imply that either an optimal ratio of LF to void volume was necessary for maximum synergistic activity or that the void volume fraction contained both a LF inhibitor and a LF enhancer, which increased LF activity only after the inhibitor was sufficiently diluted.

Table 3. Bactericidal synergism between the heparin void volume (vv) from a bactericidal whey sample and purified LF[a]

Bacterial Strain							
	Log$_{10}$ Difference[c]						
(vv)[b]:	1.0	0.5	0.25	0.13	0.07	0.03	0
E. coli 6	-0.5	-3.0	-2.2	-2.4	-1.8	-0.3	-0.2
S. typhimurium SL1181	-0.2	-1.0	-1.9	-1.4	-1.0	-0.4	-0.2

[a]Bacteria (10^6 CFU/ml) were incubated at 37°C with a constant concentration of affinity purified LF (0.4 mg/ml) and with varying concentrations of the heparin void volume.

[b]Protein concentration of heparin void volume in mg/ml.

[c]See Table 1.

Anti-alpha chain antibody affinity chromatography

Bactericidal colostrum, commercial LF and the heparin void volume were absorbed with rabbit anti-human-alpha chain specific antibody (affinity purified) coupled to sepharose. This procedure removed all detectable IgA (less than 10 ng/ml) and eliminated any synergistic bactericidal activity. However, attempts to elute the synergistic component (low pH and chaotropes) failed, despite the fact that detectable SIgA with antibody activity could be recovered. The interpretation of these data could be complicated by the presence of SIgA antibody with LF-blocking activity (24).

DISCUSSION

These studies have demonstrated a marked difference between purified LF and commercially available LF in bactericidal activity against a deep rough mutant *S. typhimurium* and against a serum-sensitive *E. coli* strain. The commercial, iron-free preparation, was bactericidal against these organisms; whereas, heparin-sepharose purified LF had no detectable bactericidal effect. It has been previously noted in this laboratory, that the bactericidal activity of commercial LF preparations vary widely from one lot to another.

A principal contaminant associated with the SIgA-rich fraction, appears to be necessary for bactericidal expression against certain Gram-negative bacteria. This component alone has no bactericidal activity, however, it is capable of synergistic killing in the presence of purified iron-free LF. It was fortuitous that the lot of commercial LF used in most of these studies, contained a contaminant in an amount sufficient to allow bactericidal expression.

Secretory IgA enhancement of LF bacteriostatic activity had been reported (20-23). Enhanced bacteriostasis could be blocked by the addition of iron (20) or enterochelin (21). In addition, bacteriostasis could be blocked by adsorption of SIgA with live or heat-killed bacteria (22,28), although in one study, adsorption of milk had no effect on bacteriostatic activity (21). SIgA has been found to enhance LF bacteriostatic activity against enteropathogenic E. coli 0111, but not against commensal strains, and adsorption of these antibodies to 0-antigen blocked bacteriostatic activity (23), suggesting involvement of antibody specificity. The addition of colitose (3,6-dideoxy-galactose) abolished serum and LF-SIgA bacteriostatic activity against E. coli 0111 indicating that antibody specificity directed to the colitose unit of LPS was involved in enhancing bacteriostatic activity (29). However, a separate study has reported that bacteriostatic activity against E. coli was lost by adsorption of SIgA by not only the milk-sensitive E. coli strains, but also by milk-resistant strain as well as by certain members of the Enterobacteriaceae (28). Adsorption by unrelated bacteria such as staphylococci and streptococci did not effect this activity. These results suggested that the antibody involved had specificity for an antigen shared by several members of the Enterobacteriaceae and, therefore, probably was not directed at the O, H or K antigens.

Similarly, bacteriostatic activity resulting from the synergistic interaction of serum antibodies in transferrin has also been described (30-33). Antibody has been suggested to enhance the bacteriostatic activity of transferrin or lactoferrin by interfering with the iron-transport ability of bacteria (29,31,33). If research currently in progress verifies SIgA as a synergistic component in commercial lactoferrin preparations and in colostrum, this will be the first indication of SIgA enhancement of LF bactericidal activity. The involvement of SIgA as the synergistic cofactor with LF is suggested by its presence in active commercial preparations of LF. The SIgA contaminant in commercial LF contains antibody activity as detected by ELISA, indirect immunofluorescence and by microtiter agglutination (unpublished observations). Furthermore, specific SIgA antibodies may be involved since some, but not all colostral samples were capable of killing enteric bacteria. Specific SIgA antibodies that block LF bactericidal activity (24) may also be present as suggested by the fact that those SIgA-rich fractions that enhanced activity had to be diluted for optimal enhancement of bactericidal activity. Therefore, the presence or accessibility of a specific target antigen on the bacterial surface or even perhaps the ratio of LF-enhancing antibodies to LF-blocking antibodies bound on the bacterial surface may determine LF sensitivity.

CONCLUSIONS

1. There is a component in human colostral whey that is capable of synergistic killing with lactoferrin of selected enteric bacteria.

2. This bactericidal activity is expressed in some but not all colostral whey samples.

3. This synergistic factor is associated with the SIgA rich fraction of whey.

ACKNOWLEDGEMENT

This work was supported by U.S. P.H.S. grant R01-DE 06869 from the National Institutes of Health.

REFERENCES

1. Masson, D.Y. and Taylor, C.R., J. Clin. Pathol. 31, 316, 1978.
2. Masson, P.L. and Heremans, J.F., Prot. Biol. Fluids 14, 115, 1966.
3. Masson, P.L., Heremans, J.F. and Dive, C.H., Clin. Chem. Acta. 14, 735, 1966.
4. Leffell, M. and Spitznagel, J., Infect. Immun. 6, 761, 1972.
5. Masson, P.L., Heremans, J.F. and Schonne, T.E., J. Exp. Med. 130, 643, 1969.

6. Aisen, P., Aasa, R., Malmstrom, B.G. and Vanngard, T., J. Biol. Chem. 242, 2484, 1967.
7. Schade, A.L., Reinhart, R.W. and Levy, H., Arch. Biochem. 20, 170, 1949.
8. Aisen, P. and Leibman, A., Biochim. Biophys. Acta. 304, 797, 1973.
9. Bates, G.W. and Schlabach, M.R., FEBS Lett. 33, 289, 1973.
10. Oram, J.D. and Reiter, B., Biochim. Biophys. Acta. 170, 351, 1968.
11. Weinberg, E., Science 184, 952, 1974.
12. Bullen, J.J., Rogers, H.J. and Griffiths, E., Curr. Top. Microbiol. Immunol. 80, 1, 1978.
13. Arnold, R., Cole, M. and McGhee, J.R., Science 197, 263, 1977.
14. Arnold, R., Brewer, M. and Gauthier, J., Infect. Immun. 28, 893, 1980.
15. Arnold, R., Russell, J., Champion, W. and Gauthier, J., Infect. Immun. 32, 655, 1981.
16. Arnold, R., Russell, J., Champion, W., Brewer, M. and Gauthier, J., Infect. Immun. 35, 792, 1982.
17. Tenovuo, J., Moldoveanu, Z., Mestecky, J., Pruitt, K.M., and Rahemtulla, B.-M., J. Immunol. 128, 726, 1982.
18. Adinolfi, M., Glynn, A.A., Lindsay, M. and Milne, C.M., Immunology 10, 517, 1966.
19. Martinez, R.J. and Carroll, S.F., Infect. Immun. 28, 735, 1980.
20. Bullen, J., Rogers, H. and Leigh, L., Brit. Med. J. 1, 69, 1972.
21. Rogers, H. and Synge, C., Immunology 34, 19, 1978.
22. Spik, G., Cheron, A., Montreuil, J. and Dolby, J., Immunology 35, 663, 1978.
23. Stephens, S., Dolby, J., Montreuil, J. and Spik, G., Immunology 41, 597, 1980.
24. Arnold, R.R., Russell, J.E., Devine, S.M., Adamson, M. and Pruitt, K.M., in Cariology Today, (Edited by Guggenheim, B.), pp. 75-88, Basel, Karger Press, 1984.
25. Blackberg, L. and Hernell, O., FEBS Lett. 109, 180, 1980.
26. Smit, J., Kamio, Y. and Nikaido, H., J. Bacteriol. 124, 942, 1975.
27. Bortner, C.A., Miller, R.D. and Arnold, R.R., Infect. Immun. 51, 373, 1986.
28. Dolby, J. and Honour, P., J. Hgy. 83, 255, 1979.
29. Fitzgerald, S. and Rogers, H., Infect. Immun. 27, 302, 1980.
30. Bullen, J., Cushnie, G. and Rogers, H., Immunology 12, 303, 1967.
31. Bullen, J. and Rogers, H., Nature 224, 380, 1969.
32. Bullen, J., Rogers, H. and Lewin, J., Immunology 20, 391, 1971.
33. Rogers, H., Infect. Immun. 7, 445, 1967.

INTERACTION OF ANTISERA TO THE SECRETORY COMPONENT WITH FcαR

S.S. Crago, C.J. Word and T.B. Tomasi*

Department of Cell Biology, University of New Mexico, Albuquerque, New Mexico; and *Roswell Park Memorial Institute, Buffalo, New York USA

INTRODUCTION

The predominant immunoglobulin (Ig) in human external secretions is secretory IgA (SIgA) (1) which appears to be produced largely by IgA-containing plasma cells underlying the mucosal epithelium (1,2). IgA is unique in that two distinct receptors for the Fc portion of the molecule exist, the secretory component (SC) and the Fc receptor for IgA (FcαR) (3). SC is a glycoprotein associated with the epithelial cells lining mucosal surfaces (4), and functions both as a receptor for polymeric IgA and IgM and as a transport molecule in the translocation of Igs across secretory epithelium into exocrine fluids (4,5). The FcαR has been reported to be present on both B and T lymphocytes, monocytes and polymorphonuclear leukocytes (PMN) in a number of species (3). While the role of FcαR on these cells is not clear, there is evidence that T cells which express membrane-bound Fc receptors may regulate Ig production in an isotype-specific manner both _in vivo_ and _in vitro_. In some cases, this regulation is mediated via the release of soluble, isotype-specific Ig binding factors from FcR^+ T cells (3).

SC has been found to be a member of the super family of cell surface molecules which includes Ig, class I and class II major histocompatability antigens, β_2 microglobulin, Thy-1, the T4 antigen on helper T cells, the T8 antigen on suppressor T cells, the T cell receptor and several neuropeptides. Since SC and the FcαR both bind to the Fc portion of IgA, it is possible that these molecules are related and that the FcR falls into this superfamily of cell surface receptor molecules. To address this possibility, cells from the mouse and the human were examined for expression of FcαR and the ability of antisera to human and murine SC to interact with the receptor and block its ability to bind IgA.

MATERIALS AND METHODS

Murine tissue and cells

MOPC 315-bearing BALB/c mice were used in these studies since previous studies have shown that the high levels of circulating IgA associated with the presence of the tumor induce elevated expression of FcαR (3). Spleens were removed from 8-10 wk old BALB/c mice ten days after the injection of 1 x 10^6 MOPC 315 plasmacytoma cells, and teased into single cell suspensions. Red blood cells (RBC) were lysed and resultant cells were depleted of adherent cell populations by adherence to tissue cultures flasks. In some cases, cells were cultured overnight in RPMI 1640 supplemented with 10% fetal bovine serum (FBS), 2 mM L-glutamine, 100 units/ml penicillin, and 100 μg/ml streptomycin at 37°C in a humidified atmosphere of 7% CO_2 in air to allow for the disassociation of endogenous IgA from the FcαR. Lymphoid cells from the spleens of normal, age-matched BALB/c mice were used in control experiments. In some studies, the FS6 or SKK9.11 T cell hybridomas, the S49.ITB.2 or BW5147 T cell lymphomas are used. Somatic cell hybrids were also constructed in our laboratory between spleen cells from MOPC 315-bearing BALB/c mice (MSBW) or thymus cells from normal BALB/c mice (BTBW) and the BW5147 T cell fusion partner. Prior to fusion, spleen or thymus cells were allogenically stimulated in the presence of IL-2.

Isolation and culture of human cells

Peripheral blood was obtained from normal donors by venipuncture and mononuclear cells (PBMC) isolated on a ficoll Hypaque gradient (6). The mononuclear fraction was depleted of adherent cells by adherence to tissue culture plates. Purity of cell populations was ascertained by staining with reagents to detect B cells (B1, Coulter Diagnostics, Hialeah, FL), T cells (OKT3, Becton-Dickinson, Mountain View, CA) and monocytes (OKM1, Becton-Dickinson), and analyzing stained cells by flow cytometry. Washed, lymphocyte-enriched fractions were resuspended in RPMI 1640 with 2 mM L-glutamine, 100 units/ml penicillin, 100 μg/ml streptomycin and 10% FBS and processed for rosette or flow cytometric analyses.

The human monocytic cell line U937 and the promyelocytic cell line HL60 were maintained in RPMI 1640 supplemented as described above, and cultured at 37°C in a humidified atmosphere of 7% CO_2 in air. In experiments to induce expression of FcαR, cells were cultured for 48 hr in the presence of 500 units/ml recombinant γ-interferon (γIFN) (AmGen Biologicals, Thousand Oaks, CA).

Visualization of FcαR

Cells expressing FcαR were visualized by a rosetting technique according to the method of Hoover et al. (7). Murine lymphocyte-enriched populations or cell lines were incubated with MOPC 315 IgA (TNP-specific) and then allowed to form rosettes with TNP-derivitized sheep red blood cells (TNP-SRBC) (Colorado Serum Co., Denver, Co). In studies to determine the ability of various reagents to interact with the FcαR, cells were incubated with the reagent prior to incubation with MOPC 315 IgA. Initial studies determined optimal dilutions. Human cells expressing FcαR were visualized as described for murine cells, except that TNP-derivitized ox red blood cells (TNP-ORBC) (Colorado Serum Co., Denver, CO) rather than TNP-SRBC were used in the rosette assay.

Reagents

Antisera to murine SC were the kind gift of Dr. J.-P. Vaerman (Catholic University, Louvain, Belgium). This reagent was shown by immunodiffusion to react with a SIgA fraction from mouse bile, but not with MOPC 315 IgA. Anti-mouse SC was used at 10 $\mu l/10^6$ cells. Polyclonal antisera to human SC were obtained from commercial sources (Nordic Immunology, Leuven, Belgium; Dako Immunoglobulins, Copenhagen, Denmark; Miles Scientific, Naperville, IL), or were produced in this laboratory by immunization of rabbits with human SC and absorption of resultant antisera with human myeloma IgA. All anti-human SC reagents reacted with SIgA but not myeloma IgA by immunodiffusion. Antisera to human SC were used at 10 $\mu l/10^6$ cells. In some experiments, anti-human SC was absorbed with human myeloma IgA or with human SIgA prior to use. Monoclonal antisera to Thy 1.1, $H\text{-}2K^d$, Lyt-1 and Lyt-2 were produced in this laboratory and used at dilutions shown by immunofluorescence to give optimal staining of the appropriate cell type. OX3 (anti-rat Ia) was used at 10 $\mu l/10^6$ cells and was purchased from Sera-Lab, Sussex, UK. Anti-mouse IgA (α chain specific) was purchased from Sigma Chemical Co. (St. Louis, MO), monoclonal anti-human IgA (α1 and α2 chain specific) was purchased from Becton-Dickinson, fluorescein isothiocyanate (FITC)-labeled $F(ab')_2$ fragment of goat anti-mouse IgG was purchased from TAGO Diagnostics (Tilburg, The Netherlands) and FITC-labeled sheep anti-goat IgG was purchased from Cooper Biomedical (Malvern, PA). Human myeloma IgA1 or IgA2 were isolated from sera as previously described (8). Polyclonal human SIgA prepared from colostrum was obtained commercially (Calbiochem, La Jolla, CA). The MOPC 315 plasmacytoma was raised in BALB/c mice and IgA was purified from the ascites fluid as previously described (7). All IgA preparations were used at 300 μg/ml.

Fluorescence techniques

Cells to be examined for FcαR by flow cytometry were incubated with human myeloma IgA followed by monoclonal mouse anti-human IgA reagents. Cells were then incubated with the FITC-labeled $F(ab')_2$ fragment of goat anti-mouse IgG. Cells were analyzed on a Becton-Dickinson FACS III for fluorescence emission and low angle light scatter. Values reported have been corrected for non-specific, second-step fluorescence.

RESULTS

Expression of FcαR by murine T cell hybridomas, lymphomas and spleen cells

Initial studies determined the percent of $FcαR^+$ cells by rosetting techniques (Table 1). Spleens from MOPC 315-bearing BALB/c mice were found to have significantly more receptor-positive cells than those from age-matched, normal controls. The MSBW-1, MSBW-2, BTBW-1, FS6 and SKK9.11 T cell hybridomas and the BW5147 lymphoma were found to express significant levels of FcαR while S49.ITB.2 lacked FcαR and was used as a negative control in subsequent experiments. Specificity of receptors was confirmed by the ability of heterologous IgA (TEPC 15) (see below, Fig. 2) but not IgG (FLPC 21) or IgM (MOPC 104E) to block the formation of MOPC 315-mediated rosettes with TNP-SRBC.

Interaction of antisera to SC and other cell surface components with murine FcαR

To determine serological homology between the SC and FcαR, the MSBW-1 T cell hybridoma was incubated with various dilutions of anti-mouse SC prior to incubation with IgA. Initial studies indicated that anti-mouse SC inhibited the ability of IgA to insert into the FcαR at the optimal dilution of 10 $\mu l/10^6$ cells. Subsequent studies showed that anti-mouse

Table 1. FcαR expression on murine cells

Cells	% Rosette-forming cells[a]
MSBW-1	17
MSBW-2	22
BTBW-1	25
FS6	10
SKK9.11	13
BW5147	14
S49.ITB.2	1.6
normal BALB/c spleen	6
MOPC 315-bearing BALB/c spleen	17

[a]Cells incubated with 300 μg/ml MOPC 315 IgA and allowed to form rosettes with TNP-SRBC; $\geq$ 200 cells counted; only cells with $\geq$ 3 SRBC per cell were scored as positive.

SC also interacted with the FcαR on other murine T cell lines inhibiting the formation of IgA mediated rosettes by 55-97% (Fig. 1). A battery of polyclonal anti-human SC reagents were also examined for the ability to inhibit formation of MOPC 315 IgA-mediated rosettes. All anti-human SC antisera tested had significant inhibitory activity (56-84%) when tested with murine spleen cells and with two T cell hybridomas (Fig. 1). Because of the limited availability of anti-mouse SC reagents, anti-human SC reagents were used in subsequent studies.

To determine whether the inhibition of IgA-mediated rosette formation was a specific effect of antisera to SC or was seen with antisera to other cell surface components, MSBW-1, T cell hybrids and spleen cells from MOPC 315-bearing BALB/c mice were incubated with normal rabbit serum or with monoclonal antisera to murine Thy 1.1, H-2K^d, Lyt-1, Lyt-2 and rat Ia antigens prior to incubation with MOPC 315 IgA. Minimal or no inhibition was seen with any of these antisera (Fig. 2). In some experiments, cells were incubated with IgA proteins specific for antigens other than DNP and TNP (TEPC 15, dextran specific) prior to incubation with MOPC 315 IgA. Such preincubation reduced the percent of MOPC 315 IgA-mediated rosettes by 74%. To demonstrate that reactivity to the SC and not other, contaminating activity was responsible for the inhibition of rosette formation, one anti-human SC antiserum was absorbed with human myeloma IgA or with polyclonal human SIgA. After absorption with myeloma IgA, the antisera displayed strong reactivity with SC by immunodiffusion and inhibited the formation

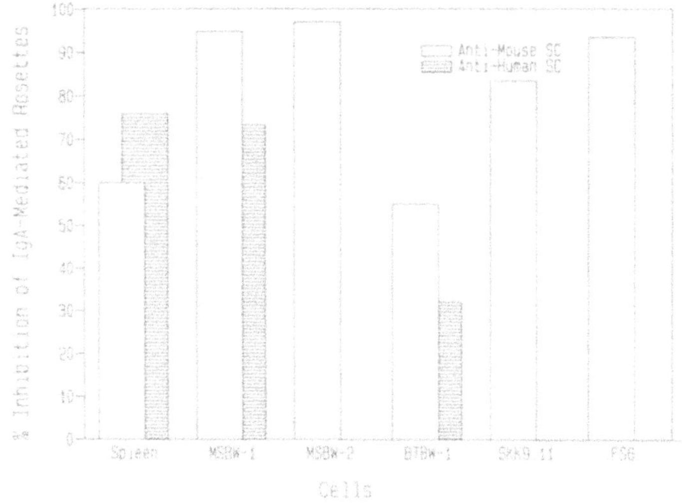

Figure 1. Interaction of anti-SC with FcαR. 2 x 10^6 T cell hybridomas or 2 x 10^6 cells from the spleen of a BALB/c mouse injected 10 days previously with 1 x 10^6 MOPC 315 plasmacytoma cells were incubated with rabbit anti-mouse SC or goat anti-human SC, followed by incubation with 300 μg/ml MOPC 315 IgA. The cells were then allowed to rosette with TNP-SRBC. $\geq$ 200 cells were counted and only cells with $\geq$ 3 SRBC bound were scored as positive. Percent inhibition was calculated by $(1 - \frac{\text{Experimental}}{\text{Control}}) \times 100\%$.

of IgA-mediated rosettes comparable to unabsorbed antisera (Fig. 2). Absorption with SIgA removed all reactivity for the SC, and inhibition of rosette formation was significantly reduced after these absorptions. These experiments further link the anti-SC activity with the inhibition of rosette formation.

Experiments were also undertaken to exclude the possibility that the anti-SC reagents were recognizing endogenous IgA associated with the $Fc\alpha R^+$ cells. Lymphoid-enriched spleen cells were incubated with polyclonal anti-mouse IgA prior to incubation with anti-SC and IgA. Preincubation with anti-mouse IgA had no significant effect on the inhibition of IgA-mediated rosettes by anti-SC, while anti-mouse IgA alone had no inhibitory activity on rosette formation (data not shown).

Inhibition of FcαR on human cell lines

The human cell lines U937 and HL60 were incubated for 48 h with or without γIFN and examined for expression of FcαR (Table 2). While neither cell line formed significant numbers of IgA-mediated rosettes in the

Figure 2. Interaction of antisera to T cell surface components with FcαR on murine cells. 2 x 10^6 MSBW-1 cells or cells from the spleen of a BALB/c mouse injected 10 days previously with 1 x 10^6 MOPC 315 plasmacytoma cells were incubated with antisera to various cell surface molecules followed by incubation incubation with 300 μg/ml MOPC 315 IgA and allowed to form rosettes with TNP-SRBC. Absorbed anti-SC 1 (absorbed a-SC 1) was absorbed with human myeloma IgA, and absorbed anti-SC 2 (absorbed a-SC 2) was absorbed with polyclonal human SIgA prior to addition to the cells. In some experiments, cells were incubated with heterologous IgA (TEPC 15) prior to incubation with MOPC 315 IgA. $\geq$ 200 cells were counted and only cells with $\geq$ 3 SRBC bound were scored as positive. Percent inhibition was calculated by $(1 - \frac{\text{Experimental}}{\text{Control}}) \times 100\%$.

absence of γIFN, incubation with γIFN induced expression of FcαR as detected by IgA-mediated rosettes. Anti-SC prevented the formation of IgA-mediated rosettes in γIFN-induced U937 cells by 64%.

Expression of FcαR on human peripheral blood lymphocytes (PBL)

Human PBL were examined by rosetting techniques and flow cytometry for the expression of FcαR (Table 3). 1.9 to 5.0 percent of the cells examined formed MOPC 315 IgA mediated rosettes, while 9.5-15.8 percent of cells bound human myeloma IgA as detected by fluorescence techniques. Anti-human SC reagents inhibited formation of IgA-mediated rosettes by a mean value of 63% (32%-87%).

DISCUSSION

The results outlined above indicate that antisera to human and mouse SC interact with the FcαR, thus inhibiting the binding of IgA to the receptor

Table 2. Induction of FcαR on human monocytic cell lines

	% Rosette-forming cells[a]			
Cell Line		−γIFN	+γIFN[b]	+γIFN + anti-SC[c]
U937		1%	55%	ND
		0	55%	ND
		2.4%	41%	26% (64)
	(mean)	1.1%	50%	
HL60		0	16%	
		0	11%	
		0	16%	
	(mean)	0	14.3%	

[a] Cells were incubated with 300 μg/ml MOPC 315 IgA and allowed to form rosettes with TNP-derivitized ORBC.
[b] Cells incubated with 500 units/ml recombinant γIFN for 48 h.
[c] Cells preincubated with 10 μg/10^6 cells of anti-human SC prior to sensitization with IgA; numbers in parentheses represent percent inhibition over control values.

and preventing the subsequent formation of rosettes. It is interesting that antisera to the human SC interacts with the FcαR on murine cells. In this regard, previous studies by other investigators have shown that SC from a variety of species interacts with human IgA (9), and that high molecular weight Ig from other species binds to human SC (9). In addition, there appears to exist species cross-reactivity in the interaction of IgA with the FcαR (3). These data suggest an interspecies conservation of the IgA binding sites for both the SC and the FcαR. Our finding that antisera against human and mouse SC recognize the murine FcαR, suggest that SC and FcαR are serologically related and may have some structural homology. Since the interaction of anti-SC with FcαR inhibits the subsequent binding of IgA to the receptor, a provocative supposition is that the proposed homologous region may be in or near the binding site for IgA. An alternative possibility is that the antisera to SC are interacting with a cell surface molecule other than the FcαR, and that the inhibition of rosette formation by anti-SC is due to steric hinderance. However, this seems unlikely, since inhibition by anti-SC is significantly greater than that observed with antisera to a number of other surface determinants present on murine T cells. This indicates that the anti-SC is not cross-reacting with any of the surface molecules examined thus far.

Table 3. Presence of FcαR on human peripheral blood cells

	% Rosette-forming cells		% Positive cells by fluorescence
Sample	IgA[a]	Anti-SC + IgA[b]	IgA
1	2.5	ND[c]	13.9
2	4.3	ND	10.2
3	3.4	ND	9.5
4	5.0	1.5 (70%)[d]	14.3
5	3.9	0.5 (87%)	13.6
6	1.9	1.3 (32%)	15.8

[a]Cells incubated with 300 μg/ml MOPC 315 IgA and allowed to form rosettes with TNP-ORBC (200 PBL counted).

[b]Cells incubated with 10 μg of polyclonal goat anti-human SC per 1 x 10^6 cells prior to incubation with IgA.

[c]Not done.

[d]Numbers in parentheses represent percent inhibition of rosette formation over control values.

The murine cells examined in these studies were T cell lymphoid lines, T cell hybridomas or splenic lymphocytes from MOPC 315-bearing mice. It has been shown that the IgA circulating in MOPC 315-bearing mice enhances the number of circulating and splenic T cells expressing FcαR (10). Thus, we assume that the majority of the rosette-forming cells are T cells. However, in the studies with human cells, monocytic or myelocytic cell lines and peripheral blood lymphocytes were examined for FcαR expression. Preliminary studies indicate that antisera to human SC also inhibit IgA-mediated rosette formation by these cells. This would suggest that the FcαR molecules on mouse and human T cells and human myeloid cells are also structurally related.

The protein and/or DNA sequence for many cell surface molecules involved in immunoregulation has been determined. Of these, the Ig heavy and light chain molecules, class I and II major histocompatibility antigens, β_2-microglobulin, Thy-1, T4 and T8 antigens, SC and the T cell receptor show substantial sequence and structural homologies and have been grouped into a supergene family. The suggested homology between SC and the FcαR predicts that the FcαR (and possibly FcR for other isotypes) belongs to this supergene family; in fact, recent analysis of the DNA sequence for the murine FcαR on monocytes supports this (11). The cross-reactivity of antisera to two distantly related molecules of this family is not without precedence, as an antiserum (OX3) to rat Ia antigens cross-reacts with rat IgE binding factors (12).

CONCLUSIONS

1. Antisera to mouse and human SC interact with FcαR on murine cells and inhibit insertion of IgA into the receptor and subsequent formation of IgA-mediated rosettes.

2. Antisera to other cell surface molecules do not appear to interact with FcαR.

3. Antisera to human SC interacts with the FcαR on human peripheral blood lymphocytes and inhibits insertion of IgA into the receptor and subsequent formation of IgA-mediated rosettes.

4. FcαR can be induced on the human cell lines U937 and HL60 by incubation with γ-interferon; anti-human SC interacts with FcαR on human monocytes to inhibit subsequent formation of IgA-mediated rosettes.

5. These findings suggest that FcαR has serological homology with SC and may be a member of the Ig supergene family.

ACKNOWLEDGEMENTS

We thank Joan Leyba and Patrick Martinez for technical assistance and Beverly Partin for her help in the preparation of this manuscript. Charlotte J. Word is a recipient of an American Cancer Society Junior Faculty Research Award and an American Heart Association Grant-in-Aid. Supported in part by NIH grant AM 31448 to Thomas B. Tomasi.

REFERENCES

1. Tomasi, T.B., Tan, E.M., Solomon, A. and Prendergast, R.A., J. Exp. Med. 121, 101, 1965.

2. Brandtzaeg, P., Clin. Exp. Immunol. 44, 221, 1981.

3. Word, C.J., Crago, S.S. and Tomasi, T.B., Ann. Rev. Microbiol. 40, 503, 1986.

4. Brandtzaeg, P., Ann. N.Y. Acad. Sci. 409, 353, 1983.

5. Crago, S.S., Kulhavy, R., Prince, S.J. and Mestecky, J., J. Exp. Med. 147, 1832, 1978.

6. Boyum, A., Scand. J. Clin. Invest. 21, 7, 1968.

7. Hoover, R.G., Dieckgraefe, B.K. and Lynch, R.G., J. Immunol. 127, 1560, 1981.

8. Mestecky, J., Hammack, W.J., Kulhavy, R., Wright, G.P. and Tomana, M., J. Lab. Clin. Med. 89, 919, 1977.

9. Underdown, B.J. and Socken, D.J., Adv. Exp. Med. Biol. 107, 503, 1978.

10. Gebel, H.M., Hoover, R.G., Lynch, R.G., J. Immunol. 123, 1110, 1979.

11. Ravetch, J.V., Luster, A.D., Weinshank, R., Kochan, J., Pavlovec, A., Portnoy, D.A., Hulmes, J., Pan, Y-C.E. and Unkeless, J., Science 234, 718, 1986.

12. Jardieu, P., Moore, K., Martens, C. and Ishizaka, K., J. Immunol. 135, 2727, 1985.

MAST CELL PLEOMORPHISM: PROPERTIES OF INTESTINAL MAST CELLS

M. Swieter, T.D.G. Lee, R.H. Stead, H. Fujimaki and D. Befus

Gastrointestinal Research Unit, University of Calgary, Calgary, Alberta, Canada; and The Department of Pathology, McMaster University, Hamilton, Ontario, Canada

INTRODUCTION

Consistent with their nearly ubiquitous distribution throughout the body, mast cells interact with a variety of cell types and react to numerous environmental stimuli. They can be activated by macrophage (1) and T cell factors (2), by complement fragments, as well as by IgE-allergen interactions. However, mast cells are involved in more than immediate hypersensitivity reactions because under appropriate conditions their mediators play a role in cell and organismal toxicity, immunoregulation, promotion of neovascularization and fibroblast proliferation (3). Moreover, mast cells and the nervous system appear to communicate with one another, an association that implies important physiological functions. For example, intimate contact between mast cells and nerves is common (i.e., 4,5), vagus nerve stimulation enhances antigen-induced histamine release (6); and neuropeptides and endorphins degranulate mast cells (7,8). Whether mast cells activate nerves and are, therefore, engaged in bidirectional interchanges is unclear.

The importance of microenvironmental controls on mast cell phenotype also remains to be elucidated. However, at least in the rat, mast cells at mucosal sites are histochemically, biochemically and pharmacologically pleomorphic (3,9). Consequently, efforts are now being made to define the bases (species, tissue, *in vivo*-derived or generated in culture) of mast cell heterogeneity and to initiate comparative functional studies of mast cells at different anatomical loci.

In this paper we will present results of investigations into the histochemical and functional bases of mast cell pleomorphism in rat and human gastrointestinal tracts, and outline some new approaches to study the biochemical and genetic basis of mast cell heterogeneity.

Rat intestinal mucosal mast cells

Mast cell pleomorphism, which has been most extensively studied in the rat, was carefully described by Enerback (10). His results established that among mast cells in tissues and organs in rats, those in the intestinal lamina propria required special fixation to be visualized. They could not be detected in tissues fixed in 10% neutral buffered formalin ("formalin-sensitive" intestinal mucosal mast cells), whereas most other mast cells, including those from the peritoneal cavity, were well preserved ("formalin-resistant" mast cells). More recently it has been found that intestinal mucosal mast cells are also smaller (9-13 μm) than peritoneal mast cells (18-30 μm), contain 10x less histamine and store large quantities (23 pg/cell) of a unique serine proteinase [rat mast cell protease II (RMCP II)] and a unique proteoglycan (chondroitin sulfate di-B; 11) in their granules (Table 1; 12). In contrast, peritoneal mast cells synthesize heparin as their predominant granule matrix proteoglycan and possess a subtype-specific endopeptidase [rat mast cell protease I (RMCP I); 13], that differs from RMCP II in amino acid sequence, number and placement of disulfide bonds and substrate specificity (14,15).

The two mast cell subtypes are also pharmacologically disparate (Table 1). Both cell types release histamine in response to antigen to which they were sensitized, to anti-IgE, or to the ionophores A23187, ionomycin and Br-X537A (16,17). In contrast, only substance P among neuropeptides tested is capable of activating intestinal mucosal mast cells, whereas dynorphin, alpha-neoendorphin, beta-endorphin, somatostatin, neurotensin, vasoactive intestinal polypeptide, bradykinin, and substance P are potent secretagogues for peritoneal mast cells (7,9). Similarly, bee venom peptide 401 and the well known peritoneal mast cell degranulator compound 48/80 are ineffective on intestinal mucosal mast cells (16).

The distinct responsiveness of the two mast cell subtypes extends to modulators of secretion. Phosphatidylserine is without effect on intestinal mucosal mast cells (16), although it potentiates mediator secretion by peritoneal mast cells up to 50%. By comparison, adenosine enhances histamine

Table 1. Characteristics of rat mast cell subtypes

	Mast cell source	
	Intestinal mucosa	Peritoneal cavity
Formalin sensitivity	sensitive	resistant
Diameter	13 μm	18 μm
Granule matrix		
Histamine content	1.5 pg	15 pg
Serine protease	RMCP II	RMCP I
Proteoglycan	chondroitin sulfate di-B	heparin
Secretagogues		
Anti-IgE, antigen	+	+
Ionophores	+	+
Neuropeptides (except substance P)	0	+
Substance P	+	+
Endorphins	0	+
Compound 48/80	0	+
Potentiators		
Phosphatidylserine	0	+
Adenosine	+	+
Antiallergics		
Disodium cromoglycate	0	-
Quercetin	-	-
Doxantrazole	-	-

+, stimulation or enhancement; -, inhibition; 0, no effect.

release by both mast cell subtypes (9). Subtype-specific differences likewise exist toward stabilizing compounds, known as antiallergic drugs. Quercetin (18) and doxantrazole (17) inhibit both mast cell subtypes, whereas disodium cromoglycate, theophylline and AH9679 are impotent against intestinal mucosal mast cells but inhibit mediator release by peritoneal mast cells.

Recently, it has become possible to obtain intestinal mast cell suspensions of >95% purity (12). The purified intestinal mast cells have an average diameter of 13 μm, histamine content of 1.5 pg per cell, and RMCP II content of 23 pg and are thus representative of mast cells in the initial isolated population as well as those *in vivo*. Enriched (65%) intestinal mucosal mast cells bear surface IgE receptors, but receptor number (36,000 per cell) and density (120 per square μm) are lower than on peritoneal mast cells (300,000 per cell and 280 per square μm, respectively; ref. 19). Investigations of the biochemical and molecular/genetic bases of heterogeneity can be initiated that should provide valuable insights into the mechanisms of differentiation and heterogeneity and bring experimental and clinical/therapeutic ramifications.

Human intestinal mast cells

As in the rat, at least two mast cell subtypes have been identified in human small and large intestines. Using classical mast cell fixation and staining protocols, formalin fixation-sensitive and formalin-resistant mast cells were found in the mucosa, submucosa and muscularis externa (20). The lamina propria was the most densely populated compartment where >75% of the mast cells had a fixation sensitivity analogous to the rat intestinal mucosal mast cell (formalin-sensitive). Immunohistochemical studies using monoclonal and polyclonal antibodies to the tryptase and chymotryptase enzymes found in human mast cells showed colocalization of the two enzymes in some mast cells, but only tryptase in others (21). Tryptase-positive cells predominated in the intestinal mucosa, whereas tryptase and chymotryptase combined-positive cells were more prevalent in skin and submucosal sites. Whether these protease distinctions correspond to histochemical subtypes of human mast cells remains to be established.

Human intestinal mast cells obtained by chemical, enzymatic and mechanical dispersion share certain features with human basophils and human lung mast cells. For example, the histamine content of intestinal mast cells or basophils is 1-2 pg and both cells release similar amounts of histamine in response to antigenic challenge (22), but sheep anti-human IgE induces maximal histamine release from human basophils over a greater concentration range than from intestinal mast cells. Pharmacologically, the human intestinal mast cell population resembles human lung mast cells (Table 2). This is particularly interesting because, like the intestine, the human lung contains two histochemically distinct mast cell subtypes (Shanahan, MacNiven, Bienenstock and Befus, unpublished), although until recently the existence of two mast cell subtypes in dispersed lung cell populations

Table 2. Effects of modulators of mediator release on mast cells from different sources

	Mast cell source		
	Human lung	Human Intestine	Rat Intestine
Secretagogues			
Compound 48/80	0	0	0
A23187	+	+	+
Human complement	?	+	+
Antiallergics			
Disodium cromoglycate	±	±	0
Theophylline	?	-	0
Salbutamol	-	-	?
Quercetin	?	-	-
Doxantrazole	?	-	-

+, stimulation or enhancement; -, inhibition; 0, no effect; ?, effect unknown.

has not been recognized. If these histochemically distinct mast cell subtypes are functionally distinct as in the rat, then existing data on properties of human lung mast cells will have to be reevaluated. Therefore, to define human mast cell properties methods to purify human intestinal mast cell subtypes are necessary.

New perspectives

We are developing methods to identify mast cell-specific and subtype-specific proteins to investigate the molecular mechanisms controlling mast cell pleomorphism. Toward this end, biochemical analysis and polyclonal and monoclonal antibodies to mast cell components will be essential. The rat peritoneal mast cell has been selected as the experimental mast cell model because it is easier to obtain and purify in large numbers than any other kind of *in vivo*-derived mast cell. Once appropriate techniques are available, comparisons with intestinal mucosal mast cells from rats and humans will be made.

SDS-PAGE analysis of mast cells. Using 5-20% linear gradient polyacrylamide gels (0.75 mm thick), 200,000 solubilized peritoneal mast cells can be separated into >30 bands under reducing conditions (using 2-mercapto-ethanol) when stained with silver (Fig. 1). The most prominent bands have molecular weights between 24,000 and about 40,000 daltons (24-40 kDa). The most abundant protein comigrates with purified RMCP I (kindly provided by Dr. R.G. Woodbury, University of Washington), at 26-29 kDa (consistent with previous estimates of RMCP I size; ref. 15,23). When fewer than 200,000 mast cells are loaded, major bands are sharper but there are fewer minor bands. When more than 200,000 cells are loaded, major bands are large, overlap with other bands and can distort the overall pattern of that lane and adjacent lanes without an appreciable increase in the number of minor bands. This major band distortion/minor band absence dichotomy occurs primarily because much of the total protein in mast cells resides in a few species of proteins, e.g., RMCP I is approximately 25% of the total.

Purified (12) rat intestinal mucosal mast cells can be separated by SDS-PAGE under reducing conditions into fewer stainable bands than peritoneal mast cells. The former lack the 24-40 kDa complex characteristic of peritoneal mast cells, but have two major polypeptides in that range (33 and 34 kDa) missing from peritoneal mast cells. The most prominent

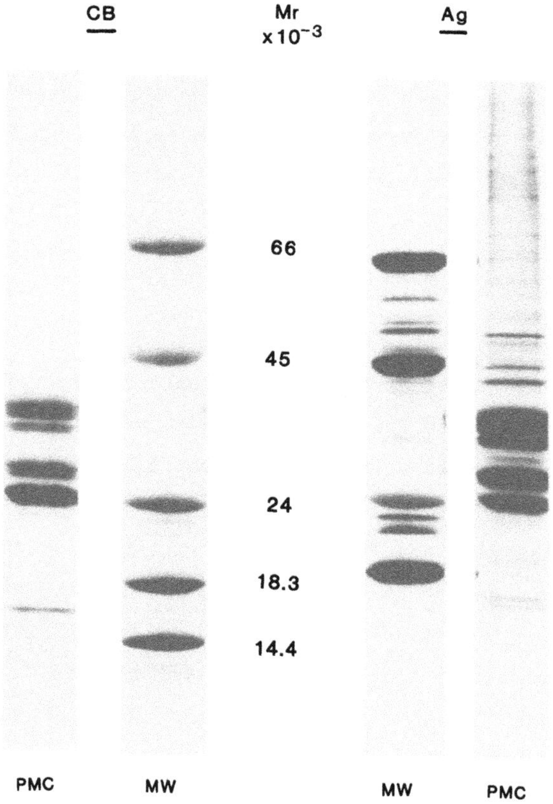

Figure 1. SDS-PAGE patterns run on 5-20% linear gradient gels (0.75 mm) of 200,000 whole peritoneal mast cells (PMC) and selected molecular weight markers (MW) stained with Coomassie blue (CB) or silver (Ag).

intestinal mucosal mast cell protein comigrates with affinity purified RMCP II (kindly provided by Dr. H.R.P. Miller, Moredun Research Institute, Scotland) which has a molecular weight of 25 kDa.

Subcellular fractionation of peritoneal mast cells. The relatively small number of bands we resolved from peritoneal and intestinal mucosal mast cells suggested that SDS-PAGE alone was not sufficient to detect many differences between mast cell subtypes. Hence, we devised a method for dividing peritoneal mast cells into granule, membrane and cytosolic fractions (Fig. 2). When coupled with SDS-PAGE, this method provides a powerful tool for comparing mast cell subtypes.

Electron microscopy revealed that the granule fraction contained only granules and that they appeared, for the most part, intact. The membrane fraction was primarily composed of membrane fragments, but some disrupted granule contents and mitochondria were present. Separation of the subcellular fractions by SDS-PAGE showed that the most abundant mast cell proteins (24-40 kDa) were localized to the granules, whereas most polypeptides with molecular weights above 40 kDa were found in the other two fractions. Of the three subcellular fractions, the cytosolic one was most

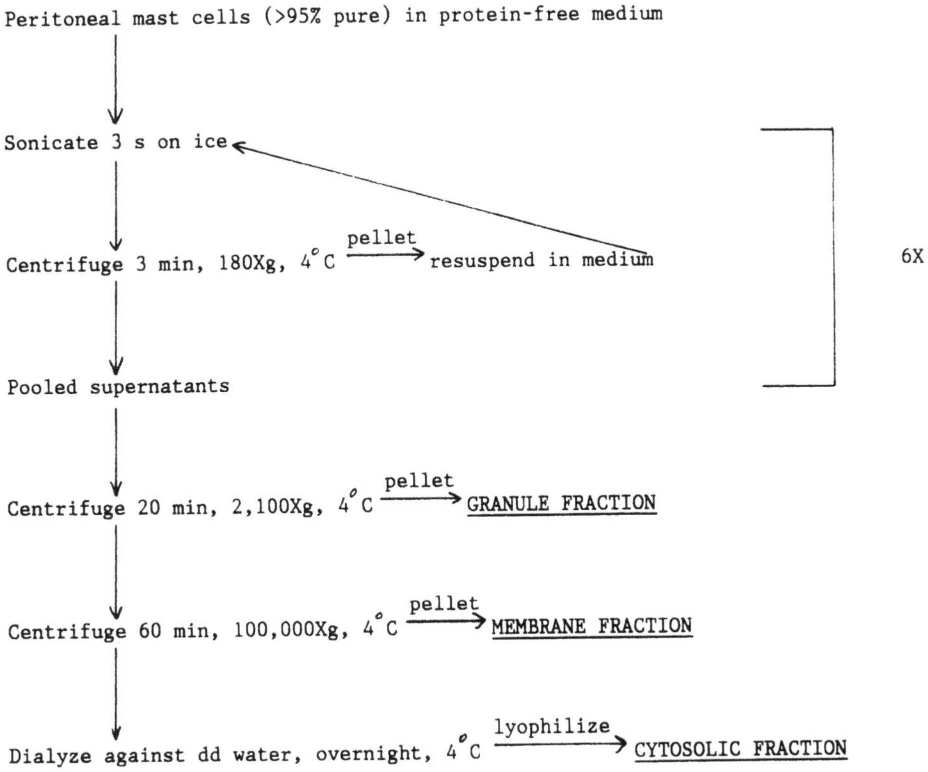

Figure 2. Subcellular fractionation scheme for peritoneal mast cells.

diverse, containing the largest number of bands. Interestingly, its most prominent component had an approximate molecular weight of 44 kDa, similar to actin which is thought to be involved in the degranulation process (24). Although there was some overlap in the distribution of components among the three fractions, we have demonstrated subcellular compartmentalization of mast cell proteins. Furthermore, because we had separated the granules from the rest of the cell, we were able to concentrate proteins in the other two fractions and increase the resolving power of SDS-PAGE on mast cells to the extent that >100 bands can now be visualized.

A polyclonal antiserum to mast cells. A mast cell-specific polyclonal rabbit serum has been developed by repeated immunization with purified rat peritoneal mast cells. Following adsorption with rat liver powder, its specificity for mast cells was demonstrated using peroxidase-antiperoxidase immunohistochemistry (33) combined with either alcian blue or toluidine blue as a mast cell counterstain. Furthermore, the antiserum was adsorbed with rat liver powder to reduce nonspecific reactivity. Strong, mast cell specific staining was seen in tissue sections of rat tongue (Fig. 3a) and in cytospin smears of rat peritoneal exudate cells with antiserum dilutions of 1:100. The antiserum also bound to mucosal mast cells in tissue sections of small intestine from N. brasiliensis-infected rats (Fig. 3b).

Immunoperoxidase staining of purified peritoneal and intestinal mucosal mast cell components electro-transferred to nitrocellulose from polyacrylamide gels (Western blot) with this serum reveals that RMCP I is strongly positive and cross-reacting RMCP II is weakly positive. Whether this cross-reactivity completely accounts for intestinal mucosal mast cell staining awaits further study. However, peritoneal mast cells contain other proteins (31 and 32 kDa) that are recognized by the antiserum and that are apparently absent from intestinal mucosal mast cells. Therefore, they are subtype-specific. Attempts will be made to use the antiserum to extract these polypeptides from mast cell granule homogenates and to characterize them further.

Monoclonal antibodies to mast cell components will complement the rabbit antiserum and provide the tools needed to obtain more information about the molecular and genetic controls of mast cell pleomorphism.

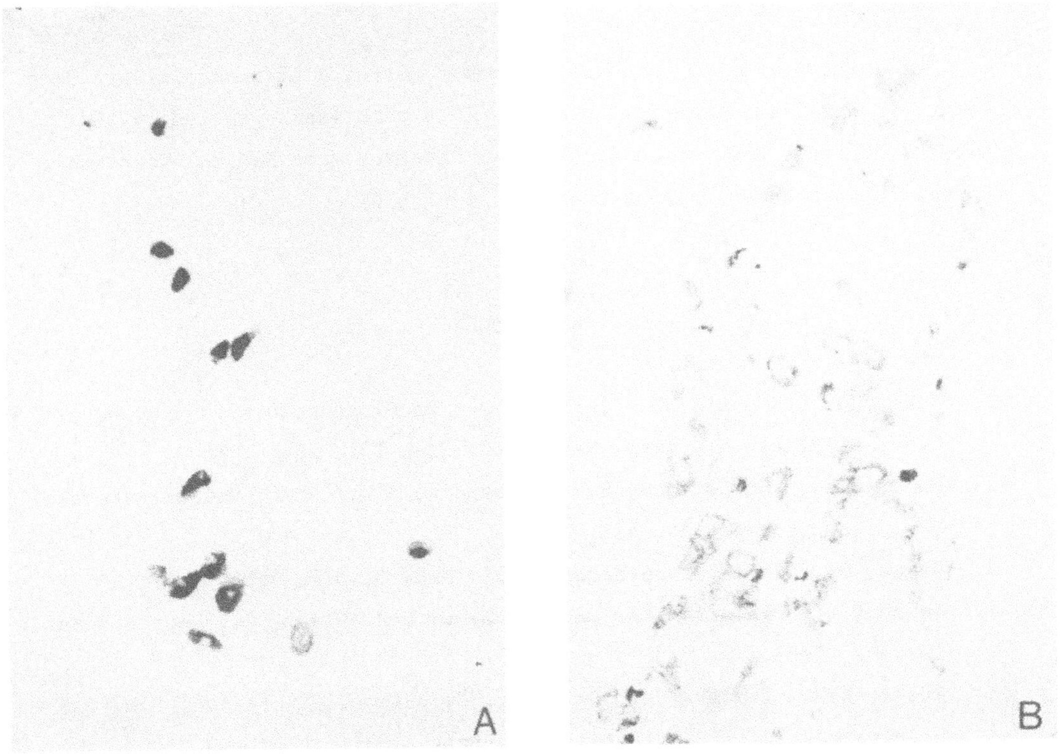

Figure 3. Peroxidase-antiperoxidase immunohistochemical demonstration of mast cell-specific antiserum. Primary antibody (1:100) is rabbit anti-rat mast cell serum produced in response to repeated injections of purified rat peritoneal mast cells. Mast cells in tissue sections of tongue (a) and small intestine (b) from rats infected with Nippostrongylus brasiliensis. Intestinal mucosal mast cells were counterstained with toluidine blue.

CONCLUSIONS

Recent advances in mast cell separation techniques (12,16) provide reason for excitement about work on mast cell pleomorphism. Because purified populations of both intestinal mucosal and peritoneal mast cells from rats are available, important issues about biochemical heterogeneity, mast cell proliferation, differentiation, activation, inhibition and desensitization are being addressed. Furthermore, the recent demonstration of immunohistochemical heterogeneity in human intestinal mast cell populations (21), coupled with the initial success in isolating these cells (22), provide impetus for further research. An improved understanding of mast cell function in mucosal pathology is forthcoming and thus improved therapeutic control of mast cells in disease processes may arise.

ACKNOWLEDGEMENTS

The authors wish to thank Connie Mowat, Carol Rimmer and Barbara Webb for their excellent technical skills. This work was supported by the Alberta Heritage Foundation for Medical Research, the Medical Research Council of Canada and Fisons Pharmaceuticals, UK.

REFERENCES

1. Schulman, E.S., Liu, M.C., Proud, D., MacGlashan, D.W., Lichtenstein, L.M. and Plaut, M., Amer. Rev. Resp. Dis. 131, 230, 1985.
2. Kops, S.K., Van Loveren, H., Rosenstein, R.W., Ptak, W. and Askenase, P.W., Lab. Invest. 50, 421, 1984.
3. Befus, D., J. Pediat. Gastroenterol. Nut. 5, 517, 1986.
4. Newson, B., Dahlstrom, A., Enerback, L. and Ahlman, H., Neuroscience 10, 565, 1983.
5. Stead, R.H., Tomioka, M., Quinonez, G., Simon, G., Felten, D.L. and Bienenstock, J., Proc. Natl. Acad. Sci., 1987 (in press).
6. Leff, A.R., Stimler, N.P., Munoz, N.M., Shioya, T., Tallet, J. and Dame, C., J. Immunol. 136, 1066, 1986.
7. Shanahan, F., Denburg, J.A., Fox, J., Bienenstock, J. and Befus, A.D., J. Immunol. 135, 1331, 1985.
8. Shanahan, F., Lee, T.D.G., Bienenstock, J. and Befus, A.D., J. Allergy Clin. Immunol. 74, 499, 1984.
9. Lee, T.D.G., Swieter, M., Bienenstock, J. and Befus, A.D., Clin. Immunol. Rev. 4, 143, 1985.
10. Enerback, L., in Mast Cell Differentiation and Heterogeneity, (Edited by Befus, A.D., Bienenstock, J. and Denburg, J.A.), p. 1, Raven Press, New York, 1986.
11. Stevens, R.L., Lee, T.D.G., Seldin, D.C., Austen, K.F., Befus, A.D. and Bienenstock, J., J. Immunol. 137, 291, 1986.
12. Lee, T.D.G., Shanahan, F., Miller, H.R.P., Bienenstock, J. and Befus, A.D., Immunology 55, 721, 1985.
13. Woodbury, R.G., Gruzenski, G.M. and Lagunoff, D., Proc. Natl. Acad. Sci. 75, 2785, 1978.
14. Woodbury, R.G. and Neurath, H., FEBS Lett. 114, 189, 1980.
15. Woodbury, R.G., Everitt, M.T. and Neurath, H., Method. Enzymol. 80, 45, 1981.
16. Befus, A.D., Pearce, F.L., Gauldie, J., Horsewood, P. and Bienenstock, J., J. Immunol. 128, 2475, 1982.

17. Pearce, F.L., Befus, A.D., Gauldie, J. and Bienenstock, J., J. Immunol. 128, 2481, 1982.

18. Pearce, F.L., Befus, A.D. and Bienenstock, J., J. Allergy Clin. Immunol. 73, 819, 1984.

19. Lee, T.D.G., Sterk, A., Ishizaka, T., Bienenstock, J. and Befus, A.D., Immunology 55, 363, 1985.

20. Befus, A.D., Goodacre, R., Dyck, N. and Bienenstock, J., Int. Arch. Allergy Appl. Immunol. 76, 232, 1985.

21. Irani, A.A., Schechter, N.M., Craig, S., DeBlois, G. and Schwartz, L.B., Proc. Nat. Acad. Sci. 83, 4464, 1986.

22. Befus, D., Dyck, N., Goodacre, R. and Bienenstock, J., J. Immunol., 1987 (in press).

23. Schwartz, L.B. and Austen, K.F., Prog. Allergy 34, 271, 1984.

24. Galli, S.J., Dvorak, A.M. and Dvorak, H.F., Prog. Allergy 34, 1, 1984.

25. Swieter, M., Lee, T.D.G., Stead, R.H. and Befus, D., Fed. Proc. 45, 388, 1986.

INTESTINAL MUCOSAL MAST CELLS IN RATS WITH GRAFT-VERSUS-HOST REACTION

A. Ferguson, A.G. Cummins, G.H. Munro, S. Gibson and H.R.P Miller

Gastrointestinal Unit, University of Edinburgh and Western General Hospital, Edinburgh EH4 2XU; and Moredun Research Institute, Edinburgh EH17 7JH; Scotland, UK

INTRODUCTION

In clinical practice, small intestinal mucosal damage with villus atrophy and crypt hyperplasia (enteropathy), occurs in association with immune reactions to alloantigens, parasites and dietary proteins. A similar, distinct pattern of mucosal pathology has been recognized in delayed type hypersensitivity reactions in animals, including mice, rats, pigs and calves. Experimental models used include allograft rejection, graft-versus-host reaction (GvHR), enteral challenge after immunization with protein antigen or contact sensitizing agent, and parasite infections. The features described in some or all of these situations are hyperplasia of the crypts of Lieberkuhn with or without shortening of the villi; an increase in the proportion of goblet cells; brush border enzyme deficiency; increased count of intraepithelial lymphocytes (IEL); an increased mitotic index of IEL; and expression of Ia antigen on crypt enterocytes (1).

In a detailed analysis of GvHR in neonatal mice, we also observed an increase in the count of mucosal mast cells (MMC) in the jejunal mucosa (2). This occurred later than changes in IEL and crypts, and the expansion of the MMC population was sustained for several weeks, after other pathological features had returned to normal. We have now undertaken a series of experiments, to further investigate the relationship between MMC and the intestinal mucosal damage characteristic of the GvHR. Since mast cells of the rat are more amenable to *in vivo* analysis than mouse mast cells (3) we have changed to this species. Studies were performed in F_1 hybrid rats in which GvHR was induced by injection of parental strain spleen cells. The regime used does not require prior irradiation of the host animals in order to induce GvHR, but since much of the literature on the subject has concerned irradiated hosts, we have also examined the GvHR in irradiated rats. The specific objectives were to document whether there is indeed an expansion of MMC in GvHR, and also, by measuring a specific granule protease in serum, to seek evidence of activation of MMC which, by leading to local release of mediators, could contribute to the enteropathy associated with GvHR.

Rat mast cell proteases

Rat mast cells are heterogeneous. MMC can be distinguished from connective tissue mast cells (CTMC) morphologically, by fixation characteristics and by their responses to secretagogues and anti-allergic compounds. In addition, these cell types differ in their granule proteases. Two rat mast cell proteases have been described, RMCPI and II. These enzymes, originally studied by Katanuma, Woodbury and colleagues (reviewed in 4), are biochemically very similar, having chymotrypsin-like substrate specificity, 75% amino acid sequence homology, and unusually basic iso-electric points. They are antigenically distinct by gel diffusion, and were reported to be present in different proportions in CTMC and MMC.

By applying fast protein liquid chromatography techniques we have improved the speed and efficacy of the purification procedures of RMCPI from CTMC and of RMCPII from MMC. A major distinguishing characteristic is the need for a high salt concentration to solubilize RMCPI. The present literature states that antibodies raised against one enzyme do not cross-react with the other (on agarose immunodiffusion), but that immunohistochemically, antibodies to either enzyme bind to both CTMC and MMC. We have investigated their antigenicity using the more sensitive technique of Western blotting, and have shown that there is indeed substantial cross-reactivity. This was eliminated by affinity chromatography cross-absorption, and when monospecific antibodies were used for immunolocalization, RMCPI was found to be present uniquely in CTMC and RMCPII in MMC (5,6).

The availability of affinity purified antibodies to the rat mast cell protease enzymes has recently allowed us to develop a very sensitive ELISA based on an antibody capture technique, in order to assay levels of RMCPII in serum (Huntley and Gibson, unpublished).

The systemic release of RMCPII enables it to be used as a specific marker for monitoring the secretory activity of MMC *in vivo*. For example, it is released into the blood circulation of rats primed with the intestinal nematode *Nippostrongylus brasiliensis* and challenged i.v. with worm antigen (7,8). As shown in Table 1, the amount of RMCPII in jejunal homogenates tends to parallel counts of MMC in the jejunum. Both are higher in *Nippostrongylus brasiliensis* primed rats than in naive animals; significant decreases occurred both in the number of MMC and jejunal concentrations of the protease as early as five minutes after i.v. challenge with parasite antigen. Furthermore, even with the relatively insensitive radial immunodiffusion technique, RMCPII was detected in the serum of rats five minutes after antigen challenge. With the recent development of a highly sensitive ELISA (Huntley and Gibson, unpublished) nanogram quantities of the protease can be detected in the serum of naive animals, as well as of *Nippostrongylus brasiliensis* primed rats.

In the present series of experiments, similar techniques have been used. Thus, counts of MMC and RMCPII content of jejunal homogenate have been used to quantitate MMC in the small bowel mucosa, and serum level of RMCPII has been assayed to seek evidence of activation of MMC in the course of the immune reaction.

Table 1. Mucosal mast cells, tissue and serum RMCPII in native and primed rats, and after i.v. challenge of primed rats with *N. brasiliensis* antigen (mean + SD) (data from references 7 and 8)

	MMC count (per VCU)	Tissue RMCPII[a] (μg/g)	Serum RMCPII[a] (μg/ml)	Serum RMCPII[b] (ng/ml)
Naive rats	10.1 + 0.8	796 + 111	0	200-400
Primed with *N. brasiliensis*				
a) i.v. saline	33.3 + 1.0	3180 + 137	0	1000-2000
b) i.v. antigen (1 hr before)	16.4 + 4	2184 + 289	121 + 27	

VCU - villus crypt unit.
[a]Radial immunodiffusion.
[b]Results in similar groups of animals using the recently developed, sensitive ELISA.

METHODS

Animals

Male DA rats and male DA x PVG^cF_1 animals were purchased from OLAC, Ltd., at 4 wk of age and used at 10 to 12 wk of age. Some of the rats were irradiated at a dose of 450 rads usig a 250 KV X-Ray source. Other animals were treated with Cyclosporin A (CyA, Sandimmun, Sandoz) sc on alternate days at a dose of 25 mg/kg body weight. GvHR was induced by injection of 1 x 10^8 parental strain spleen cells i.v. The spleen index (9) was used as a measure of the GvHR (this was positive in all experimental groups). The majority of animals were killed and examined at d 14 of the GvHR.

Measurements of intestinal mucosa

A stathmokinetic technique was used to determine the crypt cell production rate (CCPR). Each animal was injected with 1.0 mg/kg of vincristine i.p. and they were killed in groups of four, 30, 60, 90 and 120 min later. Using a microdissection method, villi and crypts were measured, metaphases per crypt were counted and the CCPR calculated (10).

Mucosal mast cell counts

Pieces of jejunum were fixed in 4% paraformaldehyde for six hr, and left in 70% ethanol for 24 hr before embedding. 5 μm sections were stained with Toluidine Blue and MMC counted with a calibrated square graticule and a x 100 oil immersion lens.

Quantitation of RMCPII in tissues

The technique was as previously described (11). Two to four cm lengths of jejunum were homogenized in three volumes of 0.15 M KCl and RMCPII measured by single radial immunodiffusion.

Qauntitation of RMCPII in serum

A direct ELISA method was used (Huntley and Gibson, unpublished). Titertek microtiter plates were coated with sheep IgG anti-RMCPII. RMCPII standards and serum samples (150 μl) in duplicate, were applied to the washed coated plates. After further incubation and washing, sheep $F(ab)_2$ anti-RMCPII peroxidase conjugate was added and the reaction product was developed as usual. The range of this test is 5-80 ng RMCPII per ml of sample.

EXPERIMENTS AND RESULTS

General features

As has been our experience with semi-allogeneic GvHR in unirradiated F_1 mice, rats with GvHR developed splenomegaly, but no clinical signs of graft-versus-host disease. In contrast, irradiated host animals appeared sickly and lost weight. No side effects of CyA were encountered and, as anticipated, GvHR did not occur in CyA treated rats.

Effect of prior irradiation on the enteropathy of GvHR

Measurements of villi, crypts and CCPR in control and GvHR animals on d 14 are illustrated in Figure 1. There was significant reduction in villus height in the unirradiated rats with GvHR, but other features of the intestinal architecture were identical to controls. On the other hand, rats which had been irradiated a few hours prior to the infusion of parental strain spleen cells had the characteristic crypt hyperplasia of moderately severe GvHR.

MMC in unirradiated rats with GvHR

Table 2 summarizes the information on MMC in the unirradiated rats, and includes data on rats treated with CyA. A significant increase in MMC count in GvHR animals was noted. Tissue levels of RMCPII tended to parallel the MMC counts but the differences were not statistically significant. Values for serum RMCPII in rats with GvHR were higher than controls (note that these are several orders of magnitude lower than the serum RMCPII levels found in rats with anaphylaxis) (8). Of considerable interest was the observation that serum RMCPII was almost undetectable in CyA treated animals. This observation has been confirmed in two further experiments, but its significance, and the relevance to the amelioration of GvHR by CyA, is uncertain.

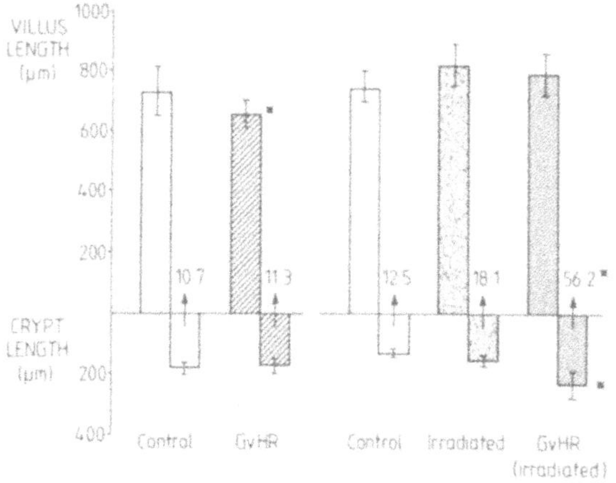

Figure 1. DAxPVG^{c} F1 rats: day 14 of GvHR. Measurements of jejunal villi, crypts and crypt cell production rate (⟶) in control rats, rats irradiated and reconsituted with isogeneic spleen cells 14 d previously, and rats with semi-allogeneic graft-versus-host reaction. * P < 0.01 compared to control.

Table 2. Mucosal mast cells and RMCPII in jejunal homogenate and in serum of rats with GvHR and controls, and the effects of treatment with Cyclosporin A (mean + SD)

	MMC count (per VCU)	Tissue RMCPII (µg/g)	Serum RMCPII (ng/ml)
Control Day 14	185 + 60	470 + 160	72 + 20
GvHR Day 14	278 + 82	620 + 270	103 + 20
CyA Day 14	146 + 45	430 + 180	11 + 4
GvHR + CyA Day 14	160 + 38	520 + 150	10 + 4

MMC in irradiated rats with GvHR

In this experiment, groups of rats were killed 7, 10 and 14 d after induction of GvHR, and the data in Figure 1, showing moderately severe enteropathy, was derived from the d 14 rats. In contrast to unirradiated animals,

Table 3. Mucosal mast cells and RMCPII in jejunal homogenate and serum of irradiated rats with GvHR (mean + SD)

	MMC count (per VCU)	Tissue RMCPII (µg/g)	Serum RMCPII (ng/ml)
Control	142 + 26	675 + 117	83 + 47
Irradiated, GvHR			
Day 7	2.62 + 2	0	17 + 7
Day 10	2.9 + 1.3	0	16 + 10
Day 14	0.7 + 1.2	0	59 + 29

the rats with GvHR had very few MMC and undetectable tissue RMCPII with the radial immunodiffusion assay used (Table 3). Furthermore, serum levels of protease were also lower than in controls. It would appear that irradiation profoundly depletes MMC, as has recently been reported by Levy et al. (12). The presence of crypt hyperplasia in the virtual absence of MMC indicates that, although mast cells may be implicated in DTH reactions in general, their presence and activation are not necessary to the evolution of the characteristic enteropathy of GvHR in the rat.

DISCUSSION

The results of experiments in unirradiated rats confirm our previous findings in neonatal mice, that there is an increase in the number of MMC in the jejunum during a GvHR. The protease, RMCPII, was an additional marker of MMC and the amounts of this enzyme in jejunal homogenates paralleled MMC counts. A raised serum level of RMCPII indicates increased activity of MMC in models of anaphylaxis (8) and of worm expulsion (13) but the rise of only 43% in serum RMCPII in these experiments, with values still in the nanogram range, suggest that serum levels of protease reflect the modest increase in the number of MMC in the small intestine during GvHR, and that these cells are not actively releasing their granule contents. On the other hand, the profound reduction in MMC counts and in tissue and serum RMCPII in irradiated rats confirms a recent report that in irradiated control rats as well as rats with GvHR, MMC virtually disappear for a week after irradiation (12).

There is now a substantial amount of evidence that lymphokines, secreted by helper T cells in the gut mucosa, can influence mitosis and differentiation of crypt enterocytes (1). It is probable that cytotoxic cells, immune complexes and mast cell products also contribute to immune-mediated enteropathy, but our recent results show that, although MMC may well play a role in the pathogenesis of intestinal inflammation in disease, the crypt hyperplasia (and other features such as Ia expression) of rat GvHR can evolve in the virtual absence of MMC.

CyA is an immunosuppressive agent that profoundly affects the T cell immune response. Among its actions are suppression of activation and proliferation of T lymphocytes and inhibition of delayed-type hypersensitivity reactions (14). CyA reduces the enteropathy associated with transplantation of the small intestine and of GvHR in experimental animals (15,16). In other work, we have found that CyA treatment leads to a gradual reduction in the number of MMC (and in intestinal RMCPII content), and to a rapid fall in serum RMCPII as described above. The mechanism of these effects may be via T cell suppression, since MMC proliferation is thymus dependent. Alternatively, CyA may have an antisecretory effect on MMC, or may interfere indirectly by inhibiting T cell promoted secretion. Corticosteroids are the only other class of drug known to reduce the number of MMC and tissue concentrations of RMCPII in the jejunum (17).

CONCLUSIONS

1. In rats with semi-allogeneic GvHR, there is expansion in the number of jejunal MMC.

2. Amounts of RMCPII in jejunal homogenate and in serum rises in parallel with the MMC counts, but the quantities are substantially lower than those in parasite infected rats.

3. Irradiation profoundly depletes MMC and even at 14 d, jejunal MMC are virtually undetectable.

4. Despite the virtual absence of MMC, rats with GvHR preceded by irradiation have a more severe enteropathy than unirradiated rats.

5. CyA not only prevents GvHR, including enteropathy, but also has a direct or indirect effect on mast cells, evidenced by a reduction in serum level of RMCPII.

ACKNOWLEDGEMENTS

This work has been supported by grants from the Wellcome Trust and Sandoz Pharmaceuticals. Dr. A.G. Cummins was the recipient of a Fellowship from the Association of Commonwealth Universities.

REFERENCES

1. Ferguson, A., in Immunopathology of the small intestine, (Edited by Marsh, M.N.), p. 225, Chichester, John Wiley and Co., Ltd., 1987.
2. Mowat, A.McI. and Ferguson, A., Gastroenterology 83, 417, 1982.
3. Miller, H.R.P., King, S.J., Gibson, S., Huntley, J.F., Newlands, G.F.J. and Woodbury, R.G., in Mast cell differentiation and heterogeneity, (Edited by Befus, D., Densburg, J. and Bienenstock, J), p. 239, Raven Press, New York, 1986.
4. Woodbury, R.G. and Neurath, H., Febs Letters 114, 189, 1980.
5. Gibson, S. and Miller, H.R.P., Immunology 58, 101, 1986.
6. Gibson, S. and Miller, H.R.P. (submitted).
7. King, S.J. and Miller, H.R.P., Immunology 51, 653, 1984.
8. King, S.J., Miller, H.R.P., Woodbury, R.G. and Newlands, G.F.J., Eur. J. Immunol. 16, 151, 1986.
9. Simonsen, M., Prog. Allergy 6, 349, 1962.
10. MacDonald, T.T. and Ferguson, A., Cell Tissue Kinet. 10, 301, 1977.
11. Woodbury, R.G. and Miller, H.R.P., Immunology 46, 487, 1982.
12. Levy, D.A., Wefald, A.F. and Beschorner, W.E., Int. Arch. Allergy Appl. Immunol. 77, 186, 1985.
13. Woodbury, R.G., Miller, H.R.P., Huntley, J.F., Newlands, G.F.J., Palliser, A.C. and Wakelin, D., Nature 312, 450, 1984.
14. Thomson, A.W., Whiting, P.H., Simpson, J.G., Agents and Actions, 15 306, 1984.
15. Kirkman, R.L., Lear, P.A., Madara, J.L. and Tilney, N.L., Surgery 96, 280, 1984.

16. van Bekkum, D.W., Knaan, S. and Zurcher, C., Transplant. Proc. 12, 278, 1980.

17. King, S.J., Miller, H.R.P., Newlands, G.F.J. and Woodbury, R.G., Proc. Natl. Acad. Sci. (USA) 82, 1214, 1985.

ATTEMPTS TO ENHANCE RNA SYNTHESIS AND ISOLATE mRNA FROM MAST CELLS

H. Fujimaki, T.D.G. Lee, M.G. Swieter, T. Morinaga*, T. Tamaoki* and A.D. Befus

Gastrointestinal Research Group, Department of Microbiology and Infectious Diseases and *Department of Medical Biochemistry, The University of Calgary, Calgary, Alberta, T2N 4N1, Canada

INTRODUCTION

With the development of isolation and purification techniques for mast cells from connective and mucosal tissues, histochemically, biochemically and functionally distinct mast cell subpopulations have been identified (1-6). However, there is little knowledge about the basis of mast cell heterogeneity. It could be due to differences in the stages of differentiation and development, or to microenvironmental influences which induce unique phenotypic expression. Moreover, histochemical and biochemical studies on peritoneal mast cells (PMC) in rats have shown that PMC are, themselves, heterogeneous populations (7,8), a problem which requires careful assessment of the use of the term "heterogeneity."

It is important to clarify the mechanisms responsible for mast cell heterogeneity because there are therapeutic implications and fundamental issues in cell differentiation. One approach to the analysis of mast cell heterogeneity is to investigate the character of mRNA in distinct mast cells.

Our aims in this study were: (1) to attempt to enhance RNA levels in mast cells for analysis of mast cell maturation and differentiation; and (2) to develop a method to isolate mRNA from mast cells for subsequent analysis. An underlying assumption in our studies is that newly differentiated mast cells and degranulated (activated) mast cells may have the greatest amounts of mRNA for isolation and study. Therefore, to develop procedures for isolation of large numbers of highly purified PMC with maximal amounts of mRNA (following activation), we have studied the changes of peritoneal mast cell numbers, RNA synthesis and histamine content after intraperitoneal (i.p.) injection of the mast cell activator, compound 48/80.

MATERIALS AND METHODS

Animals

Sprague-Dawley rats, 350-450 g, were purchased from Charles River Canada, Inc. Food and water were provided *ad libitum*.

In vivo injection of compound 48/80

Rats were singly injected i.p. with either 0.04 μg/g body weight compound 48/80 (Sigma Chemical Co., St. Louis, MO) in saline or saline alone (controls). The dose of compound 48/80 (0.04 μg) was reported to show 50% histamine release when injected i.p. (9). One day, 5 d, 10 d and 25 d later, rats were killed under ether anesthesia.

Procedure for PMC isolation and purification

PMC were isolated and purified by the methods described previously (6) using a discontinuous density gradient of Percoll (30/80%).

Histamine assay

Histamine content in mast cells was measured by radioenzymic assay (10).

Uptake of 3H-uridine to mast cells

One day before rats were killed, 3H-uridine, specific activity 29 Curies/m mol (Amersham), was given at 1.0 μCi/g body weight. Levels of radioactivity incorporated were measured by a Beckman LS 9800 beta counter on cells purified by Percoll gradient.

Isolation of mRNA

The procedure for isolation of mRNA from normal purified PMC was modified from Glisin's method (11). In brief, purified PMC in Hepes-buffered Locke's solution, pH 7.0, containing RNasin (1 unit/μl) were sonicated for 3 sec and then centrifuged at 180 g for 3 min to pellet intact cells. The cell pellet was resuspended in buffer and the sonication, pelleting and resuspension process repeated 5 additional times until no pellet remained. The supernatants were pooled and centrifuged at 16,000 g for 10 min to remove organelles. Following addition of CsCl (1 g/2.5 ml supernatant) to the supernatant, the mixture was layered onto a 1.2 ml cushion of 5.7 M CsCl buffered with 0.1 M EDTA, pH 7.5, and centrifuged at 140,000 g for 15 h at room temperature in a Beckman Spinco SW 50.1 rotor. The supernatant was removed and the pellet containing mast cell RNA was dissolved in 10 mM Tris-HCl buffer, pH 7.4, containing 5 mM EDTA, 1% SDS. The RNA suspension was mixed with phenol plus bentonite [to remove remaining carbohydrate and protein (12)]. The aqueous and organic phases were separated by centrifugation at 16,000 x g for 10 min and RNA in the aqueous phase was precipitated overnight in 2.2 volumes of ethanol with 0.3 M sodium acetate at -20°C. Precipitation of RNA was repeated at least twice. Isolation of poly (A)+ RNA by oligo(dT)-cellulose chromatography, agarose gel electrophoresis and *in vitro* translation by the use of rabbit reticulocyte lysate were performed by the method previously described (13).

RESULTS

Changes in mast cell numbers after compound 48/80 injection

In fractionation of normal peritoneal exudate cells (PEC) using 30% and 80% concentrations of Percoll, PEC were divided into two fractions of differing densities (30 - 80% interface and pellet). The pellet fraction contains >98% pure PMC, whereas the interface fraction contains other peritoneal cells and some less dense, presumably immature mast cells. After this fractionation of normal PEC, 69% (mean) of the total mast cells were in the pellet fraction and 31% at the interface (Fig. 1).

One day after injection of compound 48/80, mast cell numbers in the pellet fraction had markedly decreased and conversely those in the interface fraction had increased. Between d 5 and d 10, a gradual increase in mast cell numbers in the pellet fraction was observed, followed by a large increase between d 10 and d 25. By d 25 the numbers of mast cells in the interface and pellet fractions had recovered to control levels. The purity of mast cells in pellet fractions also decreased to 58% (d 1), 68% (d 5) and 91% (d 10) compared with control (98%). This decrease was due to contamination by macrophages and eosinophils.

Histamine content in mast cells after compound 48/80 injection

In normal rats, mast cells in the pellet fraction contained > 15 pg histamine per cell, but those in the interface fraction contained less histamine (5 pg/mast cell).

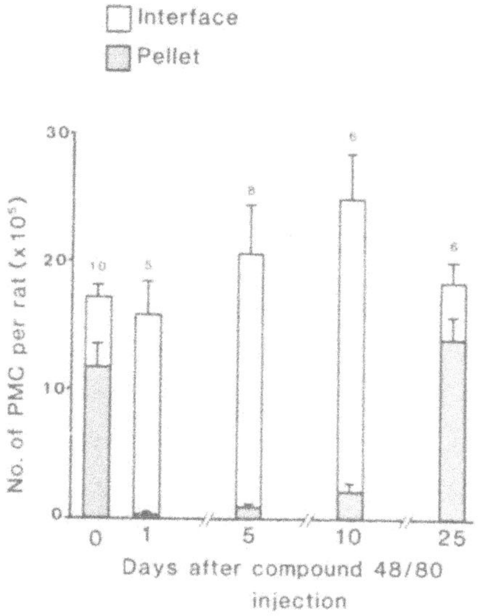

Figure 1. Rat mast cells in interface and pellet fractions collected by Percoll gradient after in vivo injection of compound 48/80. On top of the bars are the numbers of rats used. Each error bar represents standard error.

As a result of activation by compound 48/80, histamine content per mast cell decreased on d 1, d 5 and d 10 in the pellet fraction (Fig. 2). On d 25, after compound 48/80 injection, no difference in histamine content was seen in mast cells in the pellet fraction compared to control rats. Similar results were obtained in interface fractions. The percentage of the total histamine in the pellet fraction decreased to 15% - 18% on d 1, d 5 and d 10 compared to the control value of 94%. Total histamine content in the interface fraction slightly increased on d 5 and d 10 (7.11 μg and 10.27 μg as mean, respectively), but on d 1 and d 25 no difference was observed, compared to the control value (2.64 μg).

Thus, we established that in vivo compound 48/80 treatment stimulated mast cell degranulation and altered mast cell density. Accordingly, the numbers and purity of mast cells that could be recovered by density gradient centrifugation were reduced for at least the initial 10 days following treatment. This is important in efforts to get high numbers of recently activated mast cells for mRNA studies.

Uptake of ^{3}H-uridine by in vivo activated (compound 48/80) PMC

To investigate whether RNA levels in activated PMC are enhanced or not

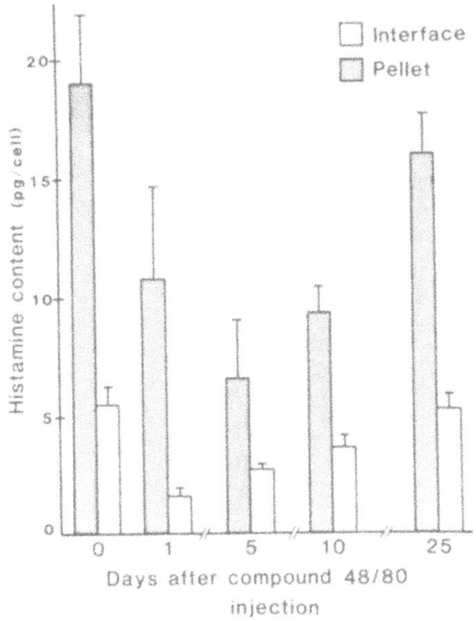

Figure 2. Histamine content (pg/mast cell) in interface and pellet fractions collected from Percoll gradient after *in vivo* injection of compound 48/80. Values are mean ± SE of 3-6 rats combined from two experiments.

when compared to those in normal PMC, RNA synthesis was measured by the uptake of ^{3}H-uridine given i.p. RNA synthesis in PMC of the pellet fraction was measured on d 5, d 10 and d 25 after *in vivo* compound 48/80 treatment. The radioactivity in the pellet fraction on d 5 (7333 ± 913 cpm/10^6 mast cells, mean ± SE) was increased compared to that of control (2947 ± 938 cpm/10^6 mast cells). However, the purity of mast cells in the pellet fraction was only 78% in the treated PMC, whereas it was 96% in control PMC. Whether or not this difference in ^{3}H-uridine incorporation can be attributed to enhanced RNA synthesis by activated PMC remains to be established by further experiments which contain *in vitro* labeling. Such experiments will require highly purified PMC following activation.

Isolation of mRNA from normal PMC

Firstly, we tried to isolate total RNA from normal PMC using guanidinium isothiocyanate plus CsCl centrifugation (13), but we could not get total RNA samples which showed clear ribosomal RNA bands (rRNA) after agarose gel electrophoresis. Because this was likely due to RNA contamination by granule-associated proteoglycans we sonicated the PMC to remove mast cell granules and then applied the granule free supernatant to CsCl gradient centrifugation. Moreover, RNA samples were extracted by phenol

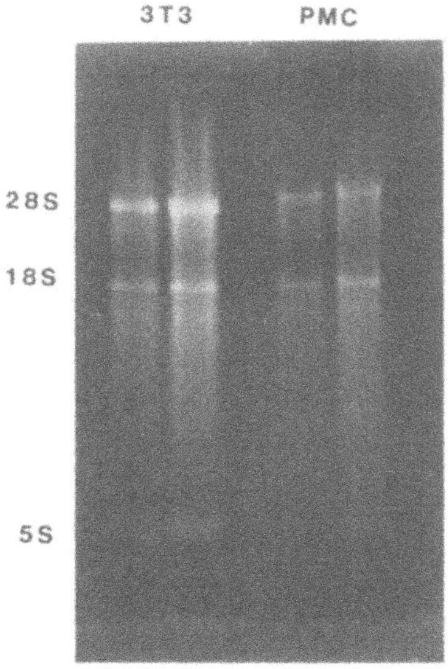

Figure 3. Agarose gel electrophoresis of total RNA isolated from 3T3 fibroblasts (left) and normal PMC (right). Applied RNA contents were 2.8 and 5.7 µg from 3T3, 2.7 and 5.4 µg from PMC. Electrophoresis using Tris-borate buffer was performed at 100V for 60 min and then stained by ethidium bromide. 28S, 18S and 5S rRNA bands are labeled.

and bentonite. By these procedures, we have isolated total RNA showing clear rRNA bands (Fig. 3). Poly (A)+RNA fractions were obtained by oligo (dT) cellulose chromatography (Table 1). Compared to total and poly $(A)^+$ RNA in 3T3 fibroblasts isolated by guanidinium-CsCl method, these levels of RNA from PMC are low. To investigate the activity of isolated mRNA, in vitro translation was performed and the result is shown in Figure 4.

Table 1. Amounts of RNA isolated from PMC and 3T3 fibroblast[a]

	Total RNA (µg)	$Poly(A)^+$ RNA (µg)
PMC	24[b] (18 - 27[d])	0.2[c] (0.1 - 0.3)
3T3	120 (105 - 142)	2.5 (1.9 - 3.1)

[a]RNA contents per 10^7 cells were shown. Mean OD 260/280 ratio is 1.8 and 1.6 in PMC and 3T3, respectively.

[b]Mean of three experiments.

[c]Mean of two experiments.

[d]The range of maximum and minimum values was shown in parenthesis.

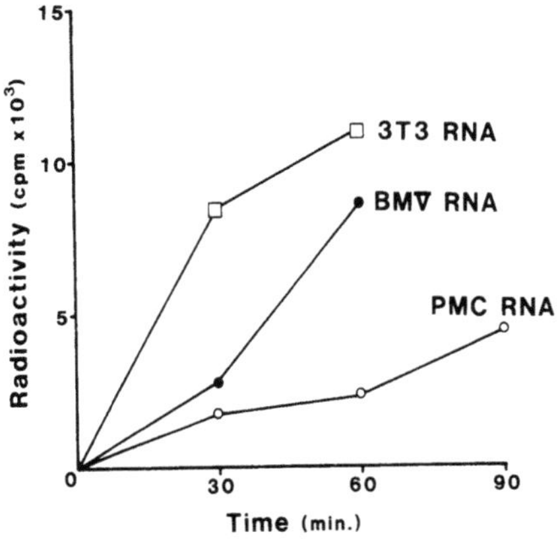

Figure 4. In vitro translation. Added RNA contents were 40 μg total RNA in both 3T3 fibroblasts and PMC, and 1 μg mRNA of Brome Mosaic Virus (BMV; positive control). After each incubation, TCA insoluble fractions in 2 μl of protein products were collected and radioactivity measured.

Time-dependent increases of radioactivity (35S-methionine) to newly translated proteins were observed using PMC and 3T3 fibroblast RNA. The amounts of protein translated from 3T3 RNA were greater than that from PMC RNA. Negative controls (-mRNA) showed < 300 cpm for 60 min incubation.

DISCUSSION

To elucidate the mechanisms responsible for distinct mast cell subpopulations, we investigated the enhancement of RNA synthesis in compound 48/80 activated PMC and isolated mRNA from normal purified PMC. In the experiment of uptake of ^{3}H-uridine by degranulated PMC, the purity of mast cells in pellet fraction was decreased on d 5 and 10 after compound 48/80 injection. Therefore, it is difficult to determine whether enhanced mRNA synthesis was attributable to activated mast cells.

Mast cell populations in the interface fraction following activation by compound 48/80 may contain degranulated (regranulating) mast cells as well as newly differentiating mast cells. Therefore, these cells may have higher levels of RNA synthesis than unstimulated mast cells. However, because of their lower densities they cannot be purified. Moreover, PMC collected on d 25 may differ from normal (non-activated) PMC and thus mRNA from these PMC must be compared with mRNA from normal PMC.

We have developed methods for isolation of mRNA from normal PMC. As shown in Table 1, the amounts of total cellular RNA and mRNA from PMC are considerably less than those from 3T3 fibroblasts. It is interesting that Enerbäck and Rundquist (14) reported that DNA content in the PMC population showed negative correlation to body weight in growing rats, although the total numbers of PMC increased in relation to body weight. In other words, the total PMC population in adult rats had less DNA than that of young rats, presumably because the proportion of PMC in S + G2 in young rats was about four fold greater than that in older rats. Similarly, our results show low amounts of RNA in PMC of normal adult rats. However, the amount of mRNA in activated (degranulated) or newly differentiated mast cells is expected to be higher than that in normal PMC. Hence, we are now investigating RNA synthesis in developing mast cells.

The characterization of mRNA in distinct mast cells will facilitate genetic and molecular investigations of different mast cell phenotypes. Our studies represent an initial step to understand the mechanisms underlying mast cell heterogeneity using such an approach.

CONCLUSIONS

We have investigated the optimum levels of purified PMC numbers and RNA synthesis in PMC following compound 48/80 injection. The numbers of purified PMC were reduced at least during the initial 10 days following activation. In vivo labeling studies revealed enhanced RNA synthesis in the pellet fraction on d 5 after compound 48/80 injection compared to normal PMC, but whether or not this difference can be attributed to activated PMC remains to be established. To estimate the amount of mRNA in normal PMC, we have developed a method for isolating mRNA. By the use of sonication and CsCl centrifugation, we can isolate active mRNA from normal PMC.

ACKNOWLEDGEMENT

This study was supported by Alberta Heritage Foundation for Medical Research, and Medical Research Council of Canada.

REFERENCES

1. Befus, A.D., Pearce, F.L., Gauldie, J., Horsewood, P. and Bienenstock, J., J. Immunol. 128, 2475, 1982.
2. Katz, H.R., Stevens, R.L. and Austen, K.F., J. Allergy Clin. Immunol. 76, 250, 1985.
3. Pearce, F.L., Befus, A.D., Gauldie, J. and Bienenstock, J., J. Immunol. 128, 2481, 1982.
4. Pearce, F.L., Befus, A.D. and Bienenstock, J., J. Allergy Clin. Immunol. 73, 819, 1984.
5. Lee, T.D.G., Sterk, A., Ishizaka, T., Bienenstock, J. and Befus, A.D., Immunology 55, 363, 1985.
6. Shanahan, F., Denburg, J.A., Fox, J., Bienenstock, J. and Befus, A.D., J. Immunol. 135, 1331, 1985.
7. Yong, L.C., Watkins, S. and Wilhelm, D.L., Pathology 7, 307, 1975.
8. Beaven, M.A., Aiken, D.L., Woldemussie, E. and Soll, A.H., J. Pharm. Exp. Therap. 224, 620, 1983.
9. Norrby, K., Virchows. Archiv. B. 38, 57, 1981.
10. Beaven, M.A., Jacobsen, S. and Horakova, Z., Clin. Chim. Acta. 37, 91, 1972.
11. Glisin, V., Crkvanjakov, R. and Byus, C., Biochemistry 13, 2633, 1974.
12. Singer, B. and Fraenkel-Conrat, H., Virology 14, 59, 1961.
13. Maniatis, T., Fritsch, E.F. and Sambrook, J., editors, Molecular Cloning - A Laboratory Manual, Cold Spring Harbor Laboratory.
14. Enerbäck, L. and Rundquist, I., Histochemistry 71, 521, 1981.

MUCOSAL MAST CELLS AND THE INTESTINAL EPITHELIUM

M.H. Perdue and D.G. Gall

Intestinal Disease Research Units
McMaster University, Hamilton, Ontario, and
University of Calgary, Calgary, Alberta, Canada

INTRODUCTION

Mast cell numbers in the mucosa of the small intestine are increased in a number of clinical and experimental conditions such as inflammatory bowel disease, intestinal infections (particularly parasitic infestations), celiac disease, graft-versus-host disease, and possibly in food allergy (1). These conditions may involve some degree of villus atrophy. Abnormalities of intestinal function which usually include diarrhea are prevalent. Are the functional changes related to the action of mast cell mediators? Our studies investigating the effects of mast cell mediators on the epithelium in anaphyactic rats suggest that they are.

Our early studies (2) showed that rats sensitized to ovalbumin respond *in vivo* to intraluminal antigen with decreased net absorption of water and electrolytes. Histamine levels in the mucosa and numbers of darkly staining mast cells in the lamina propria are reduced after antigen challenge suggesting a role for mast cell mediators. In addition, the transport abnormalities are prevented by doxantrazole (3), a compound which inhibits histamine release from both peritoneal mast cells and mucosal mast cells (4), but not by sodium cromoglycate, which has no protective effect on mucosal mast cells (4). The experiments to be described were performed to examine the immediate and more delayed effects of mast cell mediators on the intestinal epithelium. These studies were carried out *in vivo* and *in vitro*.

METHODS

Hooded Lister rats were sensitized by intraperitoneal injection of ovalbumin with aluminum hydroxide as adjuvant (5). Controls were sham-treated littermates. Fourteen days later, experimental rats had serum anti-ovalbumin IgE titers of at least 1:64; controls had no anti-ovalbumin antibodies. All studies were carried out at this stage after primary immunization.

In vitro experiments were performed by removing segments of jejunum from sensitized rats and examining transport parameters in flux chambers (6). In these chambers the intestine is cut into flat sheets each of which is mounted like a gasket between the two leucite chamber halves. The tissue is bathed on each side separately by warmed oxygenated Krebs buffer. The buffer on each side can be sampled and movement of labeled substances across the tissue can be determined. In addition, a current can be introduced across the tissue to eliminate the spontaneous potential current. This short-circuit current (Isc) is an indication of net ion movement across the tissue and can be monitored continuously via chart recorders. Using this approach, experiments were performed to determine the immediate effects of antigen challenge to tissue from sensitized rats. During a 30 min basal period the tissue was bathed with antigen-free buffer. Then ovalbumin, 100 μg/ml was added to the buffer. Additions were made to both sides of the tissue or to the mucosal side only. In addition, studies were conducted using tissue with or without a Peyer's patch. When a patch was present it occupied from one quarter to one third of the intestinal surface exposed in the chamber.

In vivo experiments were carried out using urethane-anaesthetized rats. Following a laparotomy the upper small intestine was perfused with isotonic electrolyte solution for 15 min to clear intraluminal contents. Two 10 cm segments of jejunum were tied off, beginning 5 cm distal to the ligament of Treitz and separated by a 5 cm segment. Ovalbumin, 100 μg/ml saline, was injected into one segment; saline alone was injected into the other. Injections were alternated between proximal and distal segments in successive animals. Four similar injections were conducted at hourly intervals. The intestine was returned to the abdominal cavity and the rat was maintained at 37°C during the experiment. After four hours, the segments were removed, rinsed in saline and blotted, separated and opened. A section was fixed and processed for histology. The contents of each segment were emptied into a small beaker and the lumen was washed with ice-cold saline containing protease inhibitor. These washings and contents were assayed for protein, DNA and sucrase (5). The mucosa was scraped from the underlying muscle layers, homogenized and assayed for histamine (2) as well as the above. Results from experimental sensitized rats were compared with controls.

RESULTS

In vitro experiments

During the basal period the net ion transport, as indicated by the Isc, was not different in control and sensitized rats. When antigen was added to both sides of the tissue, the Isc increased in tissue from sensitized rats but not in tissue from controls (Fig. 1A). This change was apparent by three minutes. Following the initial peak the Isc decreased somewhat but remained significantly greater than Isc in control tissue. Fluxes of Na^+ and Cl^- were performed to determine the driving force for the Isc changes. Antigen decreased the net absorption of Na and reversed net absorption of Cl to net secretion (Fig. 1B). In similar experiments, the antigen was placed only on the luminal side of the tissue. Two segments of tissue containing a Peyer's patch were compared with adjacent patch-free segments. Addition of antigen produced no immediate change in Isc. However, the Isc did increase after a lag period of approximately 30 min. There was no significant difference in either the lag time or the degree of increase in Isc between patch versus patch-free intestine (6).

In another series of experiments, several inhibitors provided information about reactions involved in producing the transport abnormalities. The tissue (with the external muscle removed for increased sensitivity) was pre-equilibrated for 10-20 min with the inhibitor in the buffer before the addition of antigen to the serosal side. The results are shown in Table 1. Doxantrazole at 10^{-3}M, a dose which completely abolished histamine release from isolated intestinal mucosal mast cells, completely prevented the rise in Isc in response to antigen in tissue from sensitized rats. Diphenhydramine, an H1 antagonist, at 10^{-4}M reduced the initial peak Isc response but had no significant effect on the sustained increase. At that dose, diphenhydramine blocked all changes due to added histamine. The neurotoxin, tetrodotoxin at 5×10^{-7}M, had no effect on the initial

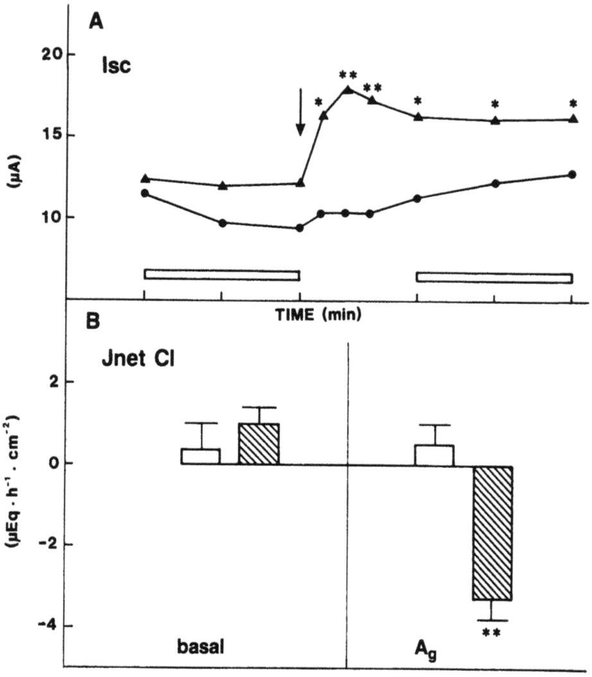

Figure 1. (A) The side effect of antigen (OVA, 100 µg/ml) added at arrow to both sides of jejunum from control (●) and sensitized (▲) rats. Values represent mean short-circuit current (Isc) in µA from 18 experiments. Isc rose significantly ($p < 0.01$) within 3 min (first point after antigen) and peaked ($p < 0.001$) at 6 min. The bars at the bottom represent 20 min periods during which samples were taken for Cl^- flux measurements (below). (B) Net flux of Cl^- across jejunum from control (open bars) and sensitized (hatched bars) rats in the basal state or after adding antigen. Values represent the mean ± SEM ($\mu Eq.h^{-1}.cm^{-2}$); results are from 9 experiments. Experiments were performed by adding $^{36}Cl^-$ as a tracer to either the luminal or antiluminal side of the tissue and taking samples from the opposite side at 10 min intervals. Fluxes were calculated by standard formula (6). The net flux is the numeric difference between the mucosal-to-serosal flux and the serosal-to-mucosal flux. Antigen caused a net secretion of Cl^- across tissue from sensitized rats ($p < 0.001$).

peak but reduced the sustained increase. This dose abolished changes in Isc due to endogenous neurotransmitters released by electrical transmural field stimulation.

In vivo experiments

In the control rats, antigen challenge for 4 h had no effect on any of the parameters measured. In the sensitized rats, decreased histamine levels in the mucosa were evident in the antigen-containing but not the saline segments (5). Mast cell degranulation was also suggested by reduced numbers of stained mast cells in the lamina propria of specifically fixed

Table 1. Effect of inhibitors on the response to antigen in sensitized rats

Tissue	n	ΔIsc / Isc_0 Initial	Sustained
Sensitized	16	2.56 ± 0.15	1.80 ± 0.10
+DOX	10	1.03 ± 0.06[b]	1.02 ± 0.04[b]
+DPH	12	2.05 ± 0.13[a]	1.69 ± 0.11
+TTX	6	2.43 ± 0.15	1.36 ± 0.09[a]

Results shown are the changes in short-circuit current (Isc) divided by the Isc during the basal period before the addition of antigen (Isc_0). The initial value is the peak change immediately after adding antigen (OVA, 100 μg/ml); the sustained value was measured 15 min later. All rats were sensitized. Concentrations were: doxantrazole (DOX) 10^{-3}M; diphenhydramine (DPH 10^{-4}M; tetrodotoxin (TTX) 5 x 10^{-7}M. Values are the mean ± SEM; (n) represents the number of tissue studied. [a]Indicates a significant difference $p < 0.05$; [b]$p < 0.005$ compared to results with no inhibitor added.

and stained sections. Analysis of the washings and contents of the segments revealed that antigen challenge for 4 h caused significant increases in protein, DNA and sucrase activity (Fig. 2). Examination of the histologic sections revealed detaching enterocytes from the tips of the villi only in the segments containing antigen from sensitized rats. Moreover, sloughed enterocytes with pycnotic nuclei covered the luminal surface (5).

DISCUSSION

Results from these experiments indicate that anaphylactic reactions in the small intestine can have profound effects on intestinal function. The *in vitro* experiments demonstrated that changes in ion transport take place within minutes following antigen presentation to both serosal and mucosal sides or to the serosal side only of the tissue. The rapidity of the response which occurred only in rats with high levels of anti-OVA IgE antibodies suggests an immediate hypersensitivity reaction. As in previous *in vivo* perfusion studies (3) the transport changes were prevented with the mast cell stabilizing agent, doxantrazole. Doxantrazole by itself did not affect ion transport. When antigen was presented only to

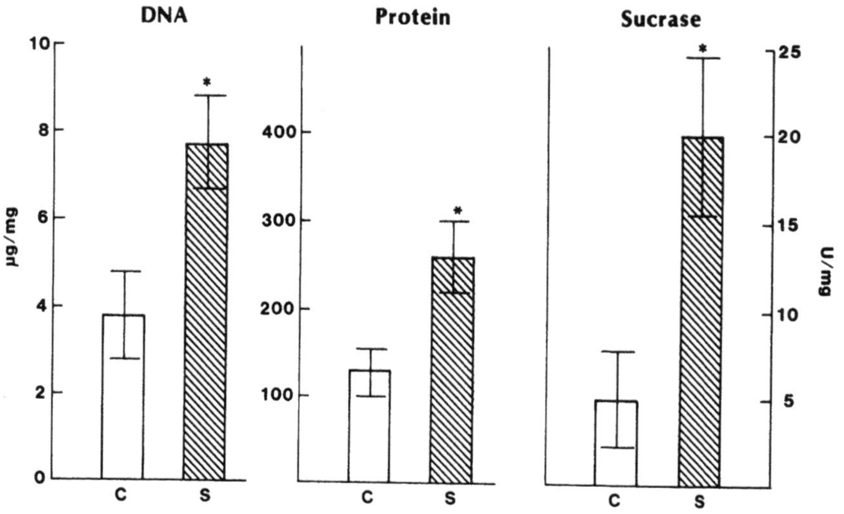

Figure 2. The effect of 4 h of antigen exposure (OVA, 100 µg/ml x 4) in ligated segments of small intestine in control (□) and sensitized (▨) rats. DNA, protein and sucrase activity were determined in luminal contents (5). Values are mean ± SEM; DNA and protein are expressed as µg/mg mucosal tissue protein. Sucrase activity is in units/mg mucosal tissue protein. * = $p < 0.025$; $n = 7$. Results from saline-injected segments in sensitized rats were similar to controls.

the mucosal side of the tissue no change occurred for at least 20 min. This lag time may represent the time required for the antigen to penetrate the epithelial barrier and reach mast cells in the lamina propria. The lag time and the response to antigen were similar regardless of the presence of a Peyer's patch. The pattern of the Isc and ion flux changes was typical of those seen in response to known secretagogues such as histamine, serotonin or arachidonic acid metabolites which are released or formed when mast cells degranulate (7). However, only a small component of the initial peak response was inhibited by the H1 antagonist, diphenhydramine, at a dose which abolished the response to exogenous histamine. The finding that tetrodotoxin inhibited the sustained part of the change in net ion transport suggests that a significant proportion of the response is due to an action on enteric nerves.

Results from the *in vivo* experiments demonstrated that longer exposure to antigen can have more deleterious effects on the intestinal epithelium. Destruction of the epithelium was demonstrated both biochemically and morphologically. Close examination of histologic sections showed peeling of enterocytes at the point of attachment to the basement membrane. These effects might also have been caused by mast cell events since the mucosal mast cell protease, RMCP II, which attacks type IV collagen in basement membrane, is released from stimulated mast cells during anaphyactic reactions (8). Our studies, however, do not rule out effects caused by other immune reactions, possibly due to mediators released from cells attracted to the site by mast cell chemotactic factors.

CONCLUSIONS

1. Intestinal anaphylactic reactions to a food antigen are complex and may consist of more than one phase.

2. The initial reaction which occurs within minutes is secretagogue-like, involving active secretion of Cl^- ions toward the luminal side of the tissue. This reaction appears to be the net result of direct and indirect effects of mast cell mediators acting on the epithelium.

3. Longer exposure to antigen may result in epithelial damage, which, if sustained could lead to villus atrophy.

ACKNOWLEDGEMENTS

These investigations were supported by the Medical Research Council of Canada.

REFERENCES

1. Bienenstock, J., Befus, A.D. and Denburg, J., in Mast Cell Heterogeneity (Edited by Befus, A.D., Bienenstock, J. and Denburg, J.), pp. 391, Raven Press, New York, 1986.
2. Perdue, M.H. and Gall, D.G., Gastroenterology 86, 391, 1984.
3. Perdue, M.H. and Gall, D.G., J. Allergy Clin. Immunol. 76, 498, 1985.
4. Pearce, F.L., Befus, A.D., Gauldie, J. and Bienenstock, J., J. Immunol. 128, 2481, 1982.
5. Perdue, M.H., Forstner, J.F., Roomi, N.W. and Gall, D.G., Am. J. Physiol. 247, G632, 1984.
6. Perdue, M.H. and Gall, D.G., Am. J. Physiol. 250, G427, 1986.

7. Marom, Z. and Casale, T.B., Ann. Allergy 50, 367, 1983.
8. Dunn, I.J., Buvet, A., Miller, H.J., Huntley, J.R., Gibson, S. and Gall, D.G., Gastroenterology 90, 1401, 1986.

INDUCTION OF PROLIFERATIVE AND DESTRUCTIVE GRAFT-VERSUS-HOST REACTIONS IN THE SMALL INTESTINE

M.V. Felstein and A.McI. Mowat

Department of Bacteriology and Immunology
University of Glasgow, Western Infirmary
Glasgow, G11 6NT Scotland U.K.

INTRODUCTION

Local cell mediated immunity (CMI) is a feature of certain intestinal diseases, including food sensitive enteropathies (FSE) and these disorders exhibit a similar pattern of villus atrophy, crypt hyperplasia and lymphocytic infiltration of the epithelium (1). Although the mucosal pathology shows both hyperplastic and destructive features, the underlying basis of the different changes is not fully understood.

Damage to the small intestine is also one of the major consequences of the CMI response found during a graft-versus-host response (GvHR). The advantage of experimental GvHR is that depending on the immunocompetence of the host, proliferative and destructive enteropathy can be induced separately or in sequence and the associated immune systems studied in parallel. In previous work, we have used the intestinal phase of GvHR in adult unirradiated F_1 mice as a model for the proliferative form of immune mediated enteropathy and have suggested that this is due to a local DTH reaction. However, other workers have shown that acute systemic GvHR may involve immunological factors which are different to those found in a proliferative GvHR.

Therefore, in this study, we have examined the intestinal phase of the GvHR in three different murine models each associated with either proliferative or destructive GvHR and have attempted to correlate the type of pathology with the effector mechanisms which are induced.

MATERIALS AND METHODS

Animals

CBA($H-2^k$) and (CBAxBALB/c)F_1($H-2^{kxd}$) mice were obtained from departmental stocks. Neonatal mice were used at 2 d old while adult mice were used at 6-8 wk of age in experiments using unirradiated hosts or were irradiated when aged 12-16 wk.

Induction of graft-versus-host reaction

Unirradiated (CBAxBALB/c)F_1 mice received 6 x 10^7 CBA spleen cells i.p., while irradiated adults received 950 rads and were reconstituted within 24 hr with 4 x 10^7 CBA spleen cells i.v. In 2 d old mice GvHR was induced with 1 x 10^7 CBA spleen cells i.p. Control mice received either medium alone (unirradiated and neonatal hosts) or 4 x 10^7 F_1 spleen cells i.v. (irradiated hosts).

Measurement of specific and non-specific cytotoxicity

Natural and specific cytotoxic activity of spleen cells were assayed against ^{51}Cr labeled YAC-1 and P815($H-2^d$) target cells, respectively, as described elsewhere (2,3).

Aliquots of spleen cells at 10^7/ml were mixed to a final volume of 200 μl, in microtiter plates, with target cells at 50:1 and 25:1 effector to target cell ratios. The percentage of lysis was determined as follows:

$$\% \text{ Cytotoxicity} = \frac{[\text{Experimental Release} - \text{Spontaneous Release}]}{[\text{Maximum Release} - \text{Spontaneous Release}]}$$

In natural killer (NK) experiments, normal thymocytes were used to obtain spontaneous release, while in cytotoxic T cell (CTL) experiments normal CBA spleen cells were used. In all experiments 10% Triton X (Sigma) was used to obtain maximum release.

Intraepithelial lymphocyte counts

Intraepithelial lymphocytes (IEL) were counted by the method of Ferguson and Murray (4), sections of jejunum taken 10 cm from the pylorus were stained with hematoxylin and eosin and the number of IEL expressed per 100 epithelial cells.

Assessment of mucosal architecture

Villus lengths, crypt lengths and crypt cell production rate were measured by microdissection of jejunum stained with Schiff Reagent (Difco) (5,6). Mice were killed at intervals after injecting 7.5 mg/kg colchicine i.p. to cause metaphase arrest in the crypts and the CCPR calculated from the linear regression slope of metaphase accumulation against time. Villus and crypt lengths were measured by micrometry and expressed as μm.

RESULTS

Progress of systemic GvHR in different models of GvHR

Adult (CBAxBALB/c)F_1 mice injected with 6 x 10^7 CBA spleen cells developed an entirely proliferative GvHR with no evidence of weight loss or clinically overt disease. The peak of the GvHR, assessed by splenomegaly occurred around d 12 after which the mice proceeded to a full recovery.

F_1 mice which received 4 x 10^7 CBA spleen cells after a lethal dose of irradiation developed an acute, lethal GvHR. The mice lost weight rapidly with clinical signs of GvHR appearing on d 4 and 5 and all animals were dead 6-7 days after cell transfer. All (CBAxBALB/c)F_1 mice given syngeneic spleen cells survived at least 100 days after irradiation.

When two day old (CBAxBALB/c)F_1 neonates were injected with 10^7 CBA spleen cells i.p., an acute GvHR developed which was associated with runting by d 8 and all the mice died within 21 d. Although marked splenomegaly is not a feature of this GvHR, maximum splenomegaly occurred about d 8-10.

Specific and non-specific cytotoxicity in different models of GvHR

During the GvHR, these mice developed a generalized increase in NK activity which corresponded with the development of the proliferative GvHR as assessed by splenomegaly. Splenic NK activity peaked around d 14 at 35-40% and then returned to normal levels, as the GvHR resolved. No specific cytotoxicity was found in any tissue at any time. Increased NK levels were also found in the gut after the same period. Controls levels of NK activity remained about 25% throughout.

In irradiated adult mice with GvHR, a transient increase in splenic NK activity occurred, which reached 10% by d 3, but then fell rapidly to zero. This fall coincided with the appearance of significant specific cytotoxicity, which rose from 2.7% on d 3 to 22.7% on d 4. The peak CTL activity occurred at the time when clinical disease first became apparent.

In neonatal mice, NK activity did not appear in controls until d 18. In contrast, neonatal mice with GvHR showed an early appearance in NK activity on d 5, but this rapidly disappeared and was absent by d 18, when control NK activity was developing. A high level of specific CTL was found in GvHR mice on d 11, after the early rise in NK activity.

Intestinal phase in different models of GvHR

Unirradiated adult $(CBAxBALB/c)F_1$ mice with GvHR induced 14 d before developed significant increases in crypt length and Crypt Cell Production Rate (CCPR). In this model, no evidence of villus damage was observed. These animals also had significant increases in IEL counts compared with controls, which again peaked on d 14. The increase in IEL count paralleled by the increased NK activity by isolated IEL during the GvHR and was maximal on d 14.

Irradiated mice with GvHR had significantly increased IEL counts by d 1 of the GvHR and this reached a maximum on d 3 (21.0 $\pm$ 3.76 vs. 9.61 $\pm$ 2.9 for controls) before falling toward control levels thereafter. The early increase in IEL count was accompanied by a marked rise in CCPR which also peaked on d 3 (42.9 $\pm$ 4.01 vs. 14.7 $\pm$ 3.26 for controls), but in this case, there was then an abrupt cessation of crypt cell turnover. Thus, the CCPR was unmeasurable on d 4 and was virtually nil by d 5. Villus atrophy was a marked feature of this model of GvHR, but did not become apparent until d 4, corresponding with the end of the proliferative phase and with the appearance of high levels of CTL and clinical runting.

Neonatal mice with GvHR induced on d 2, had marked crypt lengthening on d 9, reaching 162.5 $\pm$ 35 compared to control 80.5 $\pm$ 6 by d 15. At this stage, these mice had also developed significant villus atrophy compared with controls (414 $\pm$ 27 μm vs. 621 $\pm$ 30). Therefore, once again, the destructive phase of villus atrophy and runting was preceded by crypt hyperplasia.

DISCUSSION

The results confirm that the intestinal phase of GvHR produces a useful experimental means of studying the immunological basis of enteropathy associated with villus atrophy, crypt hyperplasia and lymphocytic infiltration of the epithelium. Nevertheless, the nature of the intestinal damage depends on the model of GvHR which is used. Thus, we have been able to produce either a proliferative enteropathy characterized by crypt hyperplasia, but without villus atrophy and CTL or a destructive enteropathy with both villus atrophy and marked CTL activity. However, this destructive pathology is also preceded by an early proliferative phase, highlighting the complexity of factors which determine immune mediated tissue damage.

An entirely proliferative GvHR occurred in unirradiated adult (CBAx BALB/c)F_1 mice which peaked at 2 wk and then proceeded to a full recovery (Table 1). This GvHR was associated with marked enhancement of NK activity both in lymphoid tissues and by IEL isolated from the small intestine, but no anti-host CTL were found. The changes in the gut reflected this proliferative response and were characterized by increases in IEL, CCPR and lengthening of the crypts. There was no evidence of damage to or shortening of the villi. All these changes occurred in parallel with the progress of the systemic GvHR and recently we have shown that the intestinal GvHR in unirradiated mice is due to recognition of I-A alloantigens by Lyt-2-donor T cells (7). Thus, we conclude that this proliferative enteropathy is due to release of lymphokines and recruitment of nonspecific effector cells by a local DTH reaction. That NK cells may be directly involved in this phenomenon is shown by the fact that depletion of host NK cells abolishes the proliferative enteropathy (unpublished observations).

Table 1. Intestinal and immunological features of different forms of GvHR

Hosts	Lethal Disease	Splenomegaly	Cytotoxicity NK	Cytotoxicity CTL	Intestinal Phase IEL	Intestinal Phase CCPR	Intestinal Phase Villus Atrophy
Adult, unirradiated	No	+++	↑↑	-	↑↑	↑↑	No
Adult, irradiated	Yes	±	Early ↑ Later ↓	↑↑	Early ↑	Early ↑↑↑ Later ↓	++
Neonatal	Yes	+	Early ↑	↑	↑	↑↑	+

Although the GvHR in unirradiated adult mice provided a suitable model of the proliferative changes found in FSE, it was important to find a model to investigate the destructive pathology which also typifies these disorders. The GvHR in irradiated F1 mice produced an acute, lethal disease which was associated with runting, villus atrophy and marked CTL activity and eventually resulted in mucosal necrosis. These destructive changes were preceded by a transient proliferative phase which was characterized by a large enhancement of NK activity and a corresponding increase in IEL counts and CCPR. At the same time, there is also an increase in crypt length, but no villus atrophy was present (Table 1).

The important finding from this experiment was that the onset of villus atrophy and CTL activity was associated with an abrupt loss of NK activity and cessation of crypt cell turnover (Table 1). Although these findings could be due to elimination of host NK cells and crypt stem cells by donor CTL, it is also possible that suppressor T cells mediate these inhibitory changes. This possibility is supported by studies of acute, systemic GvHR in unirradiated hosts (8,9) and by recent observations that active suppression of NK cell activity is present in irradiated mice with GvHR (unpublished observations).

These observations in irradiated mice are consistent with the idea that destructive enteropathy in an acute GvHR is due either to CTL or Ts. However, this model is limited by the rapid onset of clinical runting and severe enteropathy, which complicate examination of the immune mechanisms involved. This difficulty was partially overcome by using 2 d old neonates as hosts in GvHR. In these mice, runting did not begin until d 8 and the mice survived for up to 21 d. This model confirmed that villus atrophy was a feature of acute, lethal GvHR and that this was associated with specific CTL activity (Table 1). In addition, these changes were preceded by a proliferative phase of enhanced NK activity and increases in crypt length and CCPR. One interesting difference between neonatal and irradiated mice was that although NK activity was suppressed during the acute phase of GvHR, crypt hyperplasia was found throughout the GvHR in neonatal mice. We are currently investigating whether these differences reflect different immunological mechanisms or are merely due to more rapid evolution of disease in irradiated mice. Interestingly, these combined features of neonatal GvHR are most similar to those found in clinical FSE and this model may offer the greatest potential for studying these disorders experimentally.

These experiments in neonatal and irradiated mice show that the development of a destructive enteropathy in acute GvHR requires an early proliferative phase which is identical to that found in unirradiated adult mice (Table 1). This is consistent with the hypothesis that acute destructive GvHR is the consequence of a severe DTH reaction which is allowed to proceed in hosts which are immunocompromised by the fact that the intestinal phase of GvHR in both irradiated and neonatal mice (unpublished observations) is class II MHC restricted and we are currently studying the mechanisms which determine the development of such severe GvHR in these hosts.

In conclusion, we propose that a local DTH reaction is the critical event which produces enteropathy in GvHR and that this is also the mechanism for clinical FSE. The proliferative features of these disorders appear to be entirely due to soluble mediators, but villus atrophy also requires activation of a further population of effector cells, which may be CTL or Ts cells.

SUMMARY

We have used the intestinal phase of a GvHR to investigate the immunological basis of enteropathies associated with CMI. The nature of the damage depends on the model of GvHR used. Adult unirradiated (CBAxBALB/cF_1) mice with GvHR developed an entirely proliferative enteropathy characterized by crypt hyperplasia, increased numbers of IEL and enhanced NK cell activity, but there was no villus atrophy or CTL.

Although neonatal or irradiated adult (CBAxBALB/c)F_1 mice with GvHR developed a destructive enteropathy with marked villus atrophy and CTL activity, this also required an early proliferative phase identical to that found in unirradiated adult mice.

Thus, we propose that proliferative enteropathy in GvHR is due to soluble mediators released by a local DTH reaction but that villus atrophy also requires activation of a further population of effector cells, which may be CTL or suppressor T cells.

REFERENCES

1. Mowat, A.McI., in Local Immune Response of the Gut, CRC Press, 199, 1984.
2. Mowat, A.McI., Tait, R.C., Mackenzie, S., Davies, M.D.J. and Parrott, D.M.V., Clin. Exp. Immunol. 52, 19, 1983.
3. Davies, M.D.J. and Parrott, D.M.V., Clin. Exp. Immunol. 42, 273, 1980.
4. Ferguson, A. and Murray, D., Gut 12, 988, 1971.
5. Mowat, A.McI. and Ferguson, A., Transplantation 32, 238, 1981.
6. Mowat, A.McI. and Ferguson, A., Gastroenterology 83, 417, 1982.
7. Mowat, A.McI., Transplantation, 1987 (in press).
8. van Elven, E.H., Rolink, A.G., van der ween, F. and Gleichman, E., J. Exp. Med. 153, 1474, 1981.
9. Rolink, A.G., Radaszkiewixz, T., Pals, S.T., van der Meer, W.G.J and Gleichman, E., J. Exp. Med. 155, 1501, 1982.

GUT INJURY IN MOUSE GRAFT-VERSUS-HOST REACTION (GVHR)

D. Guy-Grand and P. Vassalli

Institut National de la Sante et de la Recherche Medicale
U 132 Hopital Necker-Enfants Malades 75730 Paris, France
and Department de Pathologie, Universite de Geneve
1211 Geneve 5, Switzerland

INTRODUCTION

The gut is one of the main targets of acute GVHR in man and the pathogenesis of the injury is poorly understood. Using various experimental models in mice we tried (1) to shed some light on the occurrence, nature and mechanism of lesions. Our observations led us to the conclusion that the basic situation responsible for intestinal tissue damage is the stimulation of the foreign "donor" T lymphocytes. T lymphocytes activated to proliferate under alloantigenic influence in Peyer's patches, reach the gut wall through the thoracic duct (2) and are further stimulated by contact with antigen. Release of T cell factors are probably mainly responsible for the acceleration of the epithelial renewal which is the most sensitive index of the epithelial damage.

MATERIALS AND METHODS

GVHR were elicited by injecting parental lymph node cells into F1 mice.

We varied (a) the nature of the host: normal (newborn or adult) or lethally irradiated (adult); (b) the injected parental T cells (mixed or subsets selected by a combination of panning and cytotoxicity procedures); (c) the nature of the antigenic stimulus: semi-congeneic with difference across class I MHC locus using B10A lymphocytes injected to (B10A-AQR)

Fl and with different across class I MHC locus using BIOT6R cells lymphocytes injected to (BIOT6R-AQR) Fl.

Newborn mice received 10^7 cells intraperitoneally, normal adult mice 10^8 cells intravenously in two equal dosages and irradiated mice the number of cells required to elicit the strongest GVHR without mortality 6 days after the injection (see below and Table 2).

Cell suspensions from mice with GVHR were obtained as described (1-3). Lamina propria cells represent mucosal lymphohematopoietic cells devoid of villous epithelium leukocytes (because epithelial cells contain radio-resistant host cells except in newborn mice) and are referred as gut lymphocytes.

Lymphocyte phenotype of mice with GVHR was studied after cell isolation or on tissue sections with fluorescent monoclonal antibodies. For studies of gut epithelial renewal, autoradiographies were performed on sections of duodenum 26 h after injection of 1 μCi 3HTdR/g body weight. We measured the extent of the labeling along the axis of the villi with an ocular micrometer.

Cytotoxicity and lymphokine release of gut lymphocytes were studied as described (1,3).

RESULTS

Gut alterations during GVHR

Whatever the intensity and the reason of the immuno-incompetence of the recipients of foreign lymphocytes, a strong GVHR induced across semi-allogenic differences (as assessed by the spleen weight and the rapidity of mortality), constant gut alterations are observed and the landmarks of the intestinal disease are (a) the infiltration of the gut mucosa by donor T cells and (b) epithelial damage.

The cell infiltration of the gut. Massive infiltration is seen since in lethally irradiated adult mice, more lymphocytes are isolated on day 6 from the wall of the small bowel, than from all the pooled lymphoid organs.

These T cells are of donor origin (as shown by the use of an anti-H2 allo-antiserum) except in unirradiated adult mice where host T cells, abundant before the induction of GVHR, may persist. On tissue sections, T cell infiltration predominates in the crypt area, the LP and the epithelium of the crypt, a localization in which lymphocytes are rare in normal mice.

This T cell infiltration in semiallogeneic recipients, consists in about 4/5 Lyt-2^+ and 1/5 L3T4^+ T lymphocytes. The capacity of both subsets to reach the gut and to elicit gut GVHR is confirmed by the possibility to induce GVHR with separate subsets. However, two points must be noted. First, in adult irradiated hosts, different cell numbers have to be used: in order not to cause death before day 6, it is necessary to inject three fold less L3T4^+ cells than Lyt-2^+ cells (Table 2) (the purity of the preparation is verified by the phenotype of the lymphocytes circulating in the thoracic duct and recovered from the gut). Second, with the L3T4^+ subset, the T cell infiltration is less severe but the epithelial lesions are as intense as with Lyt-2^+ subset or with total T cells (Table 2). In non-irradiated adult and newborn mice, injection of Lyt-2^+ parental cells also leads on day 12 to marked gut T cell infiltration. In contrast, with L3T4^+ cells, there is no detectable change in the adult gut while, in newborn mice, a minimal T cell infiltration is again associated with quite conspicuous lesions (Table 2).

The following questions can then be asked: What are the antigenic stimuli responsible for the gut GVHR? Can gut GVHR be observed in hosts differing from donor T cells only in class II or class I MHC antigens and in this case, what is the involvement of each of the two T cell subsets? In irradiated mice, gut GVHR can be observed across either class I or class II differences, but to elicit comparable GVHR, less parental T cells were required across class II than across class I MHC (Table 2). With differences across class II, an equal proportion of Lyt-2^+ and L3T4^+ lymphocytes are found in the gut. In GVHR across class I differences, gut T cell infiltrates consist predominantly of Lyt-2^+ cells. In the lymphoid organs of these mice, most of the cells are L3T4^+ across class II differences and most cells are Lyt-2^+ across class I differences (Table 1). The capacity of the two subsets to proliferate across class I or II differences and to reach the gut is evidenced by the possibility to induce GVHR with both separate subsets in both situations, provided a sufficient number of cells is injected. In newborn mice, with the identical amount of donor cells used, no GVHR gut lesions are seen across class I differences, while across class

II differences, injections of either total T cells or selected T cell subsets lead to a moderate gut T cell infiltration, but to intense intestinal lesions (Table 2).

The phenotype of the T subset infiltrating the gut mucosa also depends on the gut homing and circulating properties of the two subsets. Indeed, the two subsets of T blasts are different in their gut homing and circulating properties. The comparison of the composition of the proliferating lymphocytes in the Peyer's patches and in the other lymphoid organs, in the thoracic duct and in the gut shows that Lyt-2^+ blasts have less tendency to circulate in the thoracic duct than L3T4^+ blasts (Table 1). But transfer experiments performed with selected subsets show that Lyt-2^+ blasts migrate better into the gut (about 5 times more). These observations explain why, even in GVHR elicited across class II differences, in which L3T4^+ lymphocytes are preferentially stimulated, the gut T cell infiltration consists of both subsets.

Gut epithelial cell alterations. Acceleration of the epithelial renewal and appearance or increase of Ia molecules on the epithelium occur concomitantly with the infiltration of foreign T lymphocytes.

Renewal of the epithelium can be evaluated with precision using autoradiographic analysis after *in vivo* injection of 3HTdR. The crypts are the area of proliferation of the villous epithelial cells (only labeled 3 hours after 3HTdR injection) and the speed of epithelial renewal can be assessed by the extent of the villous labeling 26 hours after 3HTdR injection. The calculated index obtained comparing GVHR to control conditions is the most sensitive way to detect intestinal GVHR. In strong GVHR, hyperplasia of the crypts and shortening of the villi are evident and the indexes vary between 2 and 3 in adults and 3 and 9 in newborns. In milder GVHR, villi remain long but acceleration of the epithelial renewal is clearly indicated by indexes around 1.5 (Table 2).

Ia molecules are absent from epithelium of newborn mice before the seeding of T cells into the gut and appear in all cases of GVHR. In adult mice, the expression is increased, and this mainly occurs on the crypt epithelial cells.

Effect of GVHR on host cells of hematopoietic origin. These cells can be either destroyed or stimulated.

Lamina propria Ia + cells, numerous from birth (and radioresistant) become less numerous in strong GVHR. Decrease or even disappearance of IgA plasma cells is observed in strong acute GVHR of adult mice (IgA plasma cells are absent in newborn).

Although mast cells are infrequent in normal mice, precursors are detectable from birth (3) and may appear in newborn and adult nonirradiated mice with GVHR (Table 2). In addition, Thy-1^+, Lyt-2^+ intraepithelial lymphocytes which are numerous in adult mice but are normally absent in newborn mice may surprisingly appear in newborn mice (Table 2). Mast cells and Thy-1^+, Lyt-2^+ lymphocytes (of host origin as shown by the use of anti-H2 antibodies), mainly occur in GVHR elicited by L3T4^+ subsets or across class II differences.

Mechanisms of mucosal lesions

Gut infiltration by donor T lymphocytes is required for the elicitation of epithelial injury. This assertion is sustained by two experimental models. First, in adult lethally irradiated mice, 32 P polyvinylchloride strips were applied on the 4th day on each Peyer's patches. This selective irradiation prevents the accumulation of T cells into the gut on day 6 (but not their proliferation in lymphoid organs (2). This selective irradiation also prevents epithelial alterations, the index of acceleration is not increased. Secondly, in non-irradiated adult mice, the course of the disease varies with the nature of T lymphocytes used to elicit GVHR. When GVHR is elicited by selected subsets, most of the mice survive and donor T cells become undetectable in gut and spleen. When donor T cells have disappeared from the gut, this tissue returns to normal. Thus, all these experiments show a good correlation between T cell infiltration and epithelial lesions.

Gut epithelial injury is observed even when donor T lymphocytes eliciting the GVHR are syngeneic to the epithelium. In lethally irradiated mice bearing fetal gut grafts from both parents, syngeneic or allogeneic to the injected lymphocytes, acceleration of the epithelial renewal and induction of Ia molecules are identical in both grafts.

Donor T lymphocytes recovered from GVHR gut mucosa are specifically cytotoxic against host cells and are able to release lymphokines. The cytotoxicity is linked to the presence of Lyt-2^+ lymphocytes, is not

Table 1. T cell subsets in F1 lethally irradiated adult mice with GVHR elicited by total cells

	Recovered from	Total Lymphocytes Lyt2+	Total Lymphocytes L3T4+	Isolated Lymphocytes[a] Labeled cells among total cells	Rapidly dividing T blasts Lyt2	Rapidly dividing T blasts L3T4
semi-	gut[b]	81(±3.3)	16(±5)	19(±6)	83(±1.4)	16(±1)
allogeneic	TD	32.5(±6.0)	67(±5.8)	11(±1.9)	60(±5.3)	40(±4.3
GVHR	MLN	85	14	12	93	7
	PLN	77.5	22.5	16	88	12
semi-	gut[b]	64	18.5	8.2	83	14
congeneic	TD	32.5(±2.1)	71(±5.6)	23(±3.1)	52.5(±10)	46.5(±10)
GVHR across	MLN	82	13	17.5	96.6	5.6
cl.I MHC locus	PLN	76	15	12	91	9.4
semi-	gut[b]	42	50	10	49	48
congeneic	TD	15.7(±0.3)	87(±3.2)	16(±1.4)	20(±2.8)	79.5(±0.7)
GVHR across	MLN	26.5	68	12	40	59.5
cl.II MHC locus	PLN	27	68	12	32	68

[a] ^{3}HTdr labeled in 1 h *in vitro* incubation. (The residual lymphocytes from host origin are non-dividing cells).

[b] Gut lymphocytes are obtained from the LP and the crypt epithelial cells after removing of the villous epithelium (see methods). Isolated PP lymphocytes are often contaminated by epithelial cells and by lymphocytes of the adjacent gut because of their small size in GVHR thus, they are not accurately studied. On gut sections, however, the number of Lyt-2$^+$ and L3T4$^+$ PP lymphocytes correlates with that of PLN and MLN lymphocytes.

Table 2. Gut lesions in F1 lethally irradiated adult mice and in F1 newborn mice with GVHR

	Lymphocytes used to elicit GVHR x 10^6	T cell infiltr.	index epith. renewal	Ia on epith.	Mast cells[a]	IEL ratio Lyt2$^+$/Thy1^{+b}
I ADULTS						
Semi-allogeneic GVHR	Total 8	+++	2 - 3	+++		
	Lyt2$^+$ 12	+++	2 - 2	+++		
	L3T4$^+$ 4	++	2 - 3	+++		
Semi-congeneic GVHR across cl.I MHC locus	Total 20	++	2	+++		
	Lyt2 20	+	1.4	++		
	40	++	1.9	++		
	L3T4 20	+	1.7	+++		
GVHR across cl.II MHC locus	Total 10	+++	2 - 3	+++		
	Lyt2 20	++	1.3	+++		
	L3T4 6	+++	2 - 3	+++		
II NEWBORNS						
control mice d 10-14		0		0	0	-[c]
semi-allogeneic GVHR	Total 10	+++	3 - 6	+++	4	1
	Lyt2 10	+++	3 - 6	+++	2	1-2
	L3T4 10	+	1.5 - 4	++	12	2
Semi-congeneic GVHR across Class I MHC locus	Total or L3T4 10	0	1	0	0	0
GVHR across class II MHC locus	Total 10	+	3 - 4	+++	12	2
	Lyt2 10	+	3 - 4	+++	2	2
	L3T4 10	+	7 - 9	+++	23	2

[a]Per villous unit.

[b]Lyt-2$^+$ and Thy-1$^+$ cells numbers by fields on tissue sections in the epithelium. In normal adult mice the ratio is around 2.

[c]These cells are absent in normal mice before day 30-40.

demonstrable in mice whose GVHR has been elicited by L3T4 subsets and is abolished when anti-Lyt-2 antibody is added during the cytotoxic test. In contrast, interleukin release of IL-2, IL-3 and interferon is demonstrable after in vitro specific alloantigenic stimulation of the two subsets, gut T lymphocytes release little IL-2 and L3T4$^+$ lymphocytes are more efficient in IL-3 release.

DISCUSSION

Studies of various and complex models of GVHR demonstrate a basic pattern of gut lesions in GVHR and explain the involvement in these lesions of each population of parental T lymphocytes with respect to their functional properties and to the nature of the antigenic stimulation involved.

The three basic alterations found in the gut during GVHR are: (a) an infiltration of donor T lymphocytes predominant in the region of the crypts, but extending along the entire villi when GVHR is severe. This infiltration is the initial event in the associated lesion. Thus, after topical irradiation of Peyer's patches, which prevents the proliferation of precursors of gut T cells, without suppressing systemic GVHR (2), the gut wall is normal and in the course of GVHR, donor cell infiltration parallels gut injury; (b) an acceleration of the epithelial renewal, the most sensitive index of which is the extent of labeling of the epithelial cells along the villi axis as judged on autoradiographs of gut sections obtained one day after a pulse of ^{3}HTdR; (c) an increase of Ia expression of the epithelial cell membranes predominant within the crypts.

The following points will be discussed now:

(1) What is the subset composition of gut T lymphocytes in GVHR and what are the factors governing the degree of infiltration with each subset? In fully semi-allogeneic mice, as well as in hosts differing only at class I MHC locus, 4/5 of the donor T cells infiltrating the gut are Lyt-2$^+$, while in contrast, in hosts differing only at class II MHC locus and with gut injury of comparable intensity, gut T lymphocytes of donor origin are about evenly distributed between Lyt-2$^+$ and L3T4$^+$ cells. This relative importance of subset infiltration depends first on the extent of their proliferation in Peyer's patches (as in other lymphoid organs) and second on their properties of thoracic duct circulation and of gut homing. In

lymphoid organs, it is striking that differences at class II MHC locus preferentially stimulate donor L3T4 cells when compared to differences at class I MHC locus or to the semi-allogeneic situation. However, it must be noted that even in the case of antigenic differences restricted to class I or II MHC locus, both T cell subsets are induced to proliferate and selected subsets can proliferate in all situations. Thus, it appears that there is no absolute correlation between the surface phenotype of the parental T cells and their ability to be stimulated by class I or II MHC antigens but rather a preferential stimulation of $L3T4^+$ cells by class II and of $Lyt\text{-}2^+$ cells by class I MHC antigens. Nevertheless, the dose of cells required to induce gut injury varies with the antigenic stimulus and the subsets used. GVHR across full antigenic differences [including minor histoincompatibilities which preferentially stimulate $Lyt\text{-}2^+$ cells (4)] needs fewer cells than differences restricted to class I or II, and class II disparity is a more potent stimulator than class I. Furthermore, more Lyt-2 cells than $L3T4^+$ cells must be injected in order to induce GVHR in all combinations, a condition which probably is not always reached in other experiments (5,6). The capacity of both subsets to circulate and migrate in the gut are not identical. $L3T4^+$ blasts circulate sooner and better than $Lyt\text{-}2^+$ blasts. Indeed, when GVHR is elicited by total cells, there is always a higher proportion of $L3T4^+$ blasts in the thoracic duct than in the gut infiltrate and in the lymphoid organs. But the greater gut homing capacity of $Lyt\text{-}2^+$ blasts explain why, even when $L3T4^+$ blasts predominantly proliferate as across class II differences, a high proportion of $Lyt\text{-}2^+$ lymphocytes migrate into the gut.

(2) Are both subsets equally able to create gut damage? From comparison of the intensity of the T cell infiltration and of the epithelial alterations (as assessed by the index of epithelial renewal), it appears that $L3T4^+$ cells are very efficient in creating gut injury and also in stimulating host cells. It is evident in newborn mice with GVHR induced by $L3T4^+$ cells or across class II differences, with few $L3T4^+$ cells infiltrating the gut wall, the index of acceleration is very high and mast cells and $Lyt\text{-}2^+$ $Thy\text{-}1^-$ intraepithelial lymphocytes are conspicuous.

(3) What are the mechanisms of gut damage? Two lines of evidence suggest that cytotoxicity of donor cells against host cells cannot be an exclusive or even a major mechanism of epithelial injury. Indeed, a specific cytotoxic mechanism cannot be implicated in GVHR elicited by the $L3T4^+$ subset (which is not cytotoxic even when the target bears Ia molecules)

or in parental fetal gut graft borne by F1 and syngeneic with the parental cells used to elicit the GVHR, the injury of which is conspicuous (7,8). In that situation, the donor cells, when homing in the syngeneic graft (2), are probably stimulated by Ia^+ cells of the lamina propria which derive from the host bone marrow (9). These results suggest that lymphokines released by stimulated parental cells rather than direct specific cytotoxicity may be responsible for the epithelial lesions as proposed by McIntosh et al. (8). Both $Lyt\text{-}2^+$ and $L3T4^+$ are able to release comparable amounts of interferon which is likely to be responsible for the increased expression of Ia on the epithelium (10,11) and thus for further stimulation of donor cells. IL-3 release, responsible for the maturation of mast cell precursors in situ (3) is consistently higher with $L3T4^+$ cells than with $Lyt\text{-}2^+$ cells. Finally, the accelerated epithelial renewal is probably related also to the effect of some lymphokines, especially released by $L3T4^+$ cells. The nature of the lymphokines is unknown. It is not IL-3 alone, since experiments using <u>in vivo</u> perfusion of recombinant murine IL-3 (2) do not show modification of the epithelial renewal. Lymphokine release seems also responsible for the appearance of $Thy\text{-}1^-$, $Lyt\text{-}2^+$ intraepithelial lymphocytes of host origin. Nevertheless, the inducing factor in the appearance of characteristic granules of the gut mucosal lymphocytes appears to be the gut mucosal environment itself. Indeed, granules are observed in the donor T cells both of $Lyt\text{-}2^+$ or $L3T4^+$ nature (and not in lymphoid organs or thoracic duct lymphocytes) and in the peculiar $Lyt\text{-}2^+$ $Thy\text{-}1^-$ intraepithelial cells derived from the host whose thymic origin is unlikely, since similar cells are observed in nude mice.

CONCLUSIONS

1. In GVHR, three gut alterations are always associated, donor T cell infiltration, acceleration of the epithelial renewal and increased epithelial Ia expression. In addition, gut host cells may be either destroyed or stimulated.

2. T cell infiltration is the initial event, inducing the gut damage. Both $L3T4^+$ and $Lyt\text{-}2^+$ cells can infiltrate the gut wall. The extent of the infiltration by a given subset is dependent upon (a) the nature of the alloantigenic stimulation which governs the extent of each donor subset proliferation, (b) the capacity of the progenitors of each subsets to circulate in the thoracic duct and to home into the gut.

(3) The main mechanism of epithelial damage is not direct cytotoxicity but more probably lymphokine release. L3T4$^+$ cells are preferentially stimulated by class II MHC differences and are more efficient in inducing lesions.

REFERENCES

1. Guy-Grand, D. and Vassalli, P., J. Clin. Invest. 77, 1584, 1986.
2. Guy-Grand, D., Griscelli, C. and Vassalli, P., J. Exp. Med. 148, 1661, 1978.
3. Guy-Grand, D., Dy, M., Luffau, G. and Vassalli, P., J. Exp. Med. 160, 12, 1984.
4. Korngold, R. and Sprent, J., J. Exp. Med. 155, 872, 1982.
5 Piguet, P.-F., J. Immunol. 135, 1637, 1985.
6. Sprent, J., Schaefer, M., Lo, D. and Korngold, R., J. Exp. Med. 163, 998, 1986.
7. Elson, C.O., Reilly, R.W. and Rosenberg, E.H., Gastroenterology 72, 886, 1977.
8. McIntosh, A., Mowat, A. and Ferguson, A., Transplantation 32, 238, 1981.
9. Mayrhofer, G., Pugh, C.W. and Barclay, A.N., Eur. J. Immunol. 13, 112, 1984.
10. Barclay, A.N. and Mason, D.W., J. Exp. Med. 156, 1665, 1982.
11. Cerf-Bensussan, N., Quaroni, A., Kurnick, J.T. and Bhan, A.K., J. Immunol. 132, 2244, 1984.
12. Kindler, V., Thorens, B., de Kossodo, S., Allet, B., Eliason, J.F., Thatcher, D., Farber, N. and Vassalli, P., Proc. Natl. Acad. Sci. 83, 1001, 1986.

DEVELOPMENT OF INTESTINAL MUCOSAL BARRIER FUNCTION TO ANTIGENS AND BACTERIAL TOXINS

E.J. Israel and W.A. Walker

From the Combined Program in Pediatric Gastroenterology
Harvard Medical School, Children's Hospital and
Massachusetts General Hospital, Boston, MA

INTRODUCTION

During the past several years our laboratory has attempted to define factors that contribute to the mucosal barrier of the intestine against the uptake of pathologic quantities of antigens and microbial organisms and their enterotoxins. It has become apparent from these studies that numerous components contribute to the collective exclusion of these noxious substances within the gut. Table 1 lists the components of the mucosal barrier as we currently envision it. It consists of numerous luminal factors such as gastric acid and peptic enzymes to minimize bacterial/antigen penetration into the small intestine, and proteolytic pancreatic enzyme activity to decrease the protein antigen load to the mucosal surface. In addition to luminal factors, the mucosal surface, including the mucus layer, appears to be an important deterrent to the colonization of bacteria and to the attachment and uptake of foreign antigens. Finally, the unique secretory IgA antibody system is of major immunologic importance to the exclusion of antigens from the luminal surface (1,2).

More recently, our laboratory has become particularly interested in the microvillus membrane surface as a major factor in the attachment of antigens and bacterial toxin to enterocytes. We have hypothesized that the chemical composition of the microvillus membrane (MVM) helps to determine the interaction of antigens and toxins with the enterocyte and that in the immature animals and human newborns an incompletely developed MVM surface may in part account for an abnormal colonization of the gut and an enhanced antigen penetration that explains the increased incidence of

Table 1. Components of the mucosal barrier to intestinal pathogens, toxins and antigens

Intraluminal
Gastric Acidic/Peptic Activity
Pancreatic Proteolytic Activity
Mucosal Surface
Mucus Coat
Microvillus Integrity
Secretory Immunoglobulins (SIgA)

infectious and immunologic disease states commonly seen in this age group. This paper provides supportive evidence to help prove this hypothesis.

Development of the microvillus membrane surface

To study the importance of the MVM in intestinal barrier function, we have studied the composition and binding properties of this membrane developmentally (3-6). We have analyzed the biochemical composition of MVM and the contribution that this composition makes to the "organization" or "fluidity" of the membrane. In addition, we have measured the availability of glycoconjugates on the external surface and the potential importance of these carbohydrates to antigen/toxin attachment and penetration. Table 2 summarizes the actual studies done to compare the MVM of mature and immature animals.

Microvillus membrane composition. Since lipids make up a significant part of the membrane and may be responsible for the ease of antigen and toxin passage, the MVM lipid content was examined. We noted that a higher protein/lipid ratio existed in the adult compared to the neonatal enterocyte surface membrane, although the distribution of classes of lipid in the two groups were similar (3).

Microvillus membrane fluidity. The structural milieu of the membrane appears to influence the movement of antigen and toxins through the membrane, with a more fluid membrane environment allowing for greater penetration of these substances. The fluidity of the MVM of adult and infant

Table 2. Studies of MVM during development

1. Composition
2. Fluidity
3. Glycoconjugates
4. Toxin/Bacterial/Antigen Attachment

animals were therefore compared, using electron spin resonance spectroscopy. The spin label, 5 doxyl-stearic acid was incorporated into isolated membranes and its orientation in a magnetic spectrum was measured. There is an inverse relationship between the spectral distance and the membrane fluidity. In Figure 1, spectral differences at various temperatures are noted between intestinal MVM from adult and infant animals. It was noted that adult membrane has a higher order and has an abrupt change in the membrane characteristics with decreasing temperature at 37°C suggesting a shift in the membrane organizaton. In contrast, the MVM from neonates is more disorganized and there is no change in the organization as a function of temperature (Fig. 1) (3). This increase in fluidity in the newborn MVM may account for the increased ease of penetration of antigens and organisms through the neonatal gut surface.

Microvillus membrane glycoconjugates. We know from the literature that bacteria and toxins require certain sugars for attachment to occur (4). Figure 2 illustrates the importance of bacterial attachment to

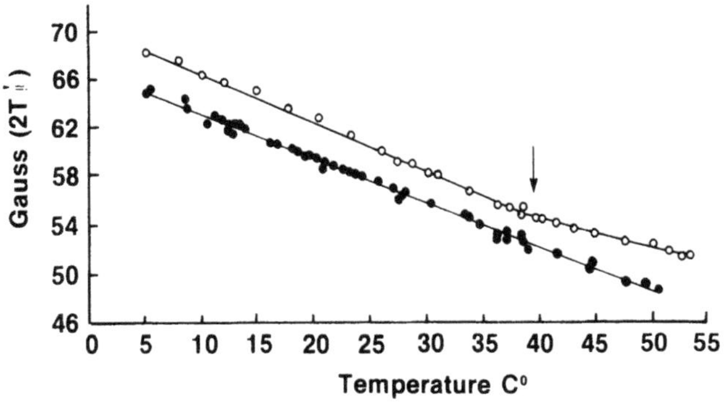

Figure 1. A representative curve for the temperature dependence of the hyperfine spliting parameter of 5-doxylstearic acid labeled adult (O) and newborn (●) microvillus membrane. The transition temperature for adult microvillus membrane is 39.6 $\pm$ 0.3°C, whereas there is no transition temperature for newborn microvillus membrane (Reproduced with permission from reference 3).

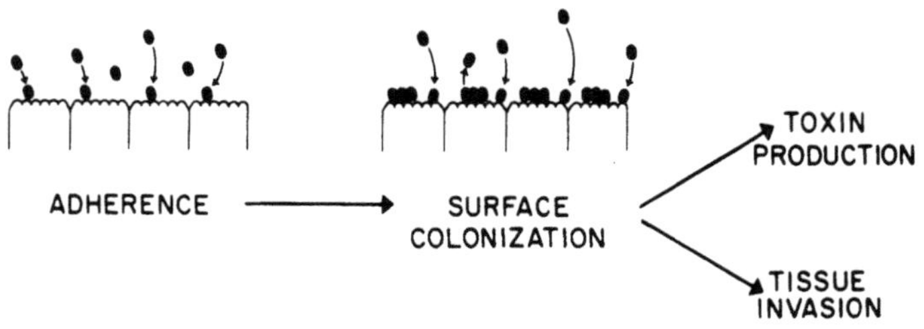

Figure 2. Diagrammatic representation of sequential steps in the pathogenesis of bacterial diarrhea. Bacteria must first adhere to the mucosal surface before surface colonization can occur. These steps are necessary for both toxin production resulting in toxigenic diarrhea or for tissue invasion resulting in inflammatory diarrhea. (Complements of C. Cheney and E. Boedeker, Walter Reed Institute of Research, Washington, DC).

colonization and to either toxin penetration or tissue invasion. The availability of glycoconjugates on the microvillus surface may, therefore, represent an important factor in the colonization and pathogenicity of bacteria within the gastrointestinal tract. Table 3 lists known associations between bacteria and toxins and intestinal glycoconjugates. Our hypothesis was that an increase in availability of certain glycoconjugates and a difference in membrane glycosylation of glycolipids or glycoproteins from the normal pattern shown in MVM could account for an increased attachment and penetration of these substances in the neonatal animal.

To examine the accessibility of carbohydrates on the side chains of glycoproteins and glycolipids in the microvillus membrane, we compared the binding of radiolabeled lectins to membrane preparations from neonatal and adult intestine (5). Standard lectins were used and their specfic carbohydrate moiety determined.

When radiolabeled concanavalin A agglutinin (Con A), which binds to glucose and mannose residues, was exposed to newborn and adult MVM preparations, more lectin bound to the adult MVM suggesting the increased availability of mannose and glucose. In contrast, when wheat germ agglutinin (WGA) lectin, which binds sialic acid and N-acetylglucosamine, was exposed to the MVM, more bound to the newborn preparation suggesting a striking increase in this glycoconjugate (Fig. 3A). Dolichos biflorus agglutinin (DBA), measuring N-acetylgalactosamine bound avidly to adult MVM preparations and not to newborn MVM preparations suggesting an absence of this

Table 3. Bacterial/Toxin receptors of the intestinal surface

Bacteria/Toxin		Carbohydrate Receptors
E. coli	--	mannose
V. cholerae	--	fucose
Clostridium toxin	--	N-acetylgalactosamine
Shigella toxin	--	N-acetylglucosamine

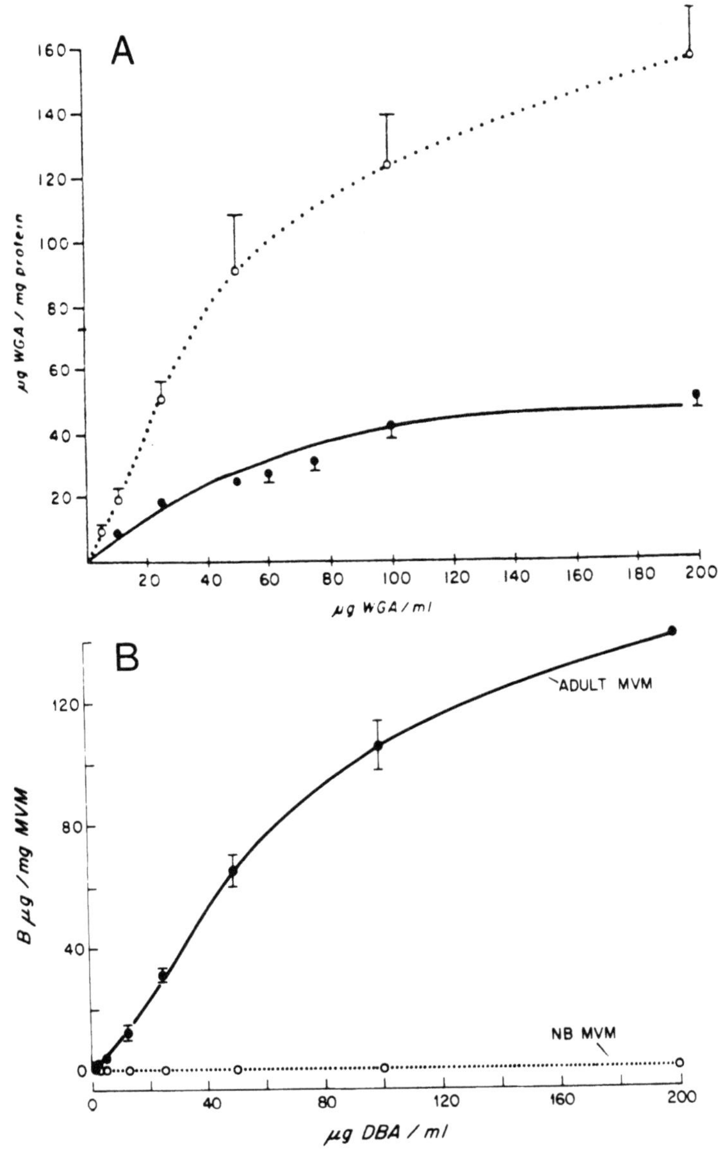

Figure 3. Availability of glycoconjugates in isolated microvillus membranes from adult and newborn rats. (A) When radiolabeled wheat germ agglutinin (^{125}I-WGA) was mixed with MVM preparations more WGA bound to newborn microvillus membranes (....) than to adult membranes (——) at various concentrations of WGA. (B) In contrast, when radiolabeled *Dolichos Biflorus* agglutinin (^{125}I-DBA) was mixed with MVM more bound to adult (——) membrane preparations than to newborn membranes (....) at various concentrations.

sugar moiety on the newborn enterocyte surface (Fig. 3B). In like manner, when Ulex europaeus agglutinin (UEA I) which is specific for fucose, was exposed to the MVM from newborn and adults, considerably greater quantities bound to adult preparations compared to newborns suggesting an absence of fucose in the newborn MVM.

To further examine glycosylation of glycolipids and proteins in the newborn, we measured the incorporation of radiolabeled sugars into isolated MVM preparations from newborn and adult animals. In these studies a striking difference between the two membrane preparations was noted. Very little fucose was incorporated into the newborn MVM preparation compared to adults (6).

Since our hypothesis was that immature glycosylation accounted for the difference in available sugars, we examined glycosyltransferases in the two age groups. When sialytransferase and sialic acid incorporation were measured as a function of age, we noted a striking increase of both during the newborn period and a rapid decline at the time of weaning. In contrast, when fucosyl transferase activity and fucose incorporation were measured as a function of age, the activity in newborn was at very low levels and increased at weaning (Fig. 4) (7).

Figure 5 depicts our interpretation of findings on glycoconjugates and glycosylation as a function of age. In mature MVM preparations, the normal glycosylation process operates and results in mature carbohydrate side chains on membrane glycolipids and proteins. In contrast to this, the newborn animal intestine has immature glycoslyation which provides differences in availability of glycoconjugates which may account for enhanced antigen/toxin binding and uptake.

Antigen/toxin binding to MVM

Antigen binding. How does the immaturity of the MVM surface composition in young animals relate to antigen attachment and uptake? In experiments done by Dr. Martin Stern in our laboratory (8), he showed that two common food antigens, beta-lactoglobulin (BLG) and bovine serum albumin (BSA) bound more avidly to the MVM surface of young animals than that of adults. Since we have shown that antigen attachment is directly correlated with its absorption (8), these studies suggest that increased antigen attachment in newborns may account for the enhanced uptake observed during this period (Fig. 6).

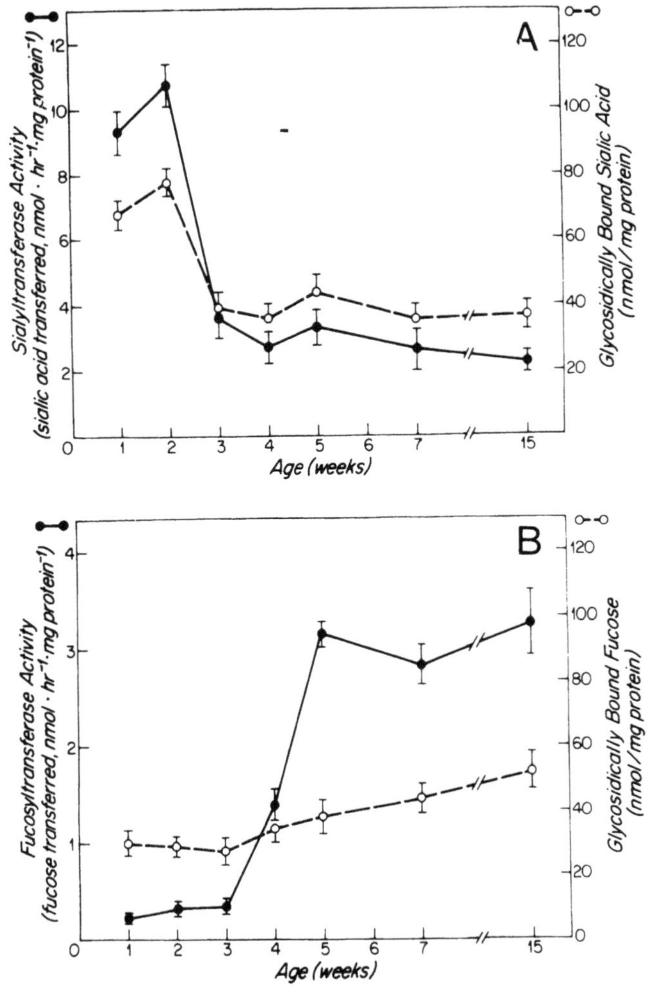

Figure 4. (A) Developmental pattern of the sialyltransferase actvity and the content of glycosidic-bond sialic acid in the membranous fraction (105,000 x g pellet) of mucosal cells of rat small intestine. Each point represents the mean S.E. of four mucosal membranous samples, prepared from a pool of three rat intestines per sample for the 1-3 week old and from a single rat intestine per sample for the 4-15 week old. (B) Developmental pattern of the fucosyltransferase activity and the content of glycosidic-bound fucose in the membranous fraction (105,000 x g pellet) of mucosal cells of rat small intestine. Each point represents the mean S.E. of four mucosal membrane samples, prepared from a pool of three rat intestines per sample, for the 1-3 week old and from a single rat intestine per sample for the 4-15 week old. (Reproduced with permission from reference (7).

Toxin binding. In additional studies, Dr Jean Bresson from our laboratory reported a greater binding of radiolabeled cholera toxin to the surface of young rabbits than to adults (9). Furthermore, he suggested that the binding of cholera toxin to MVM from young animals may involve more than one receptor as shown by the Scathard plot analysis on this slide (Fig. 7) (7). Since the binding of cholera toxin (CT) to its GM_1 glycolipid

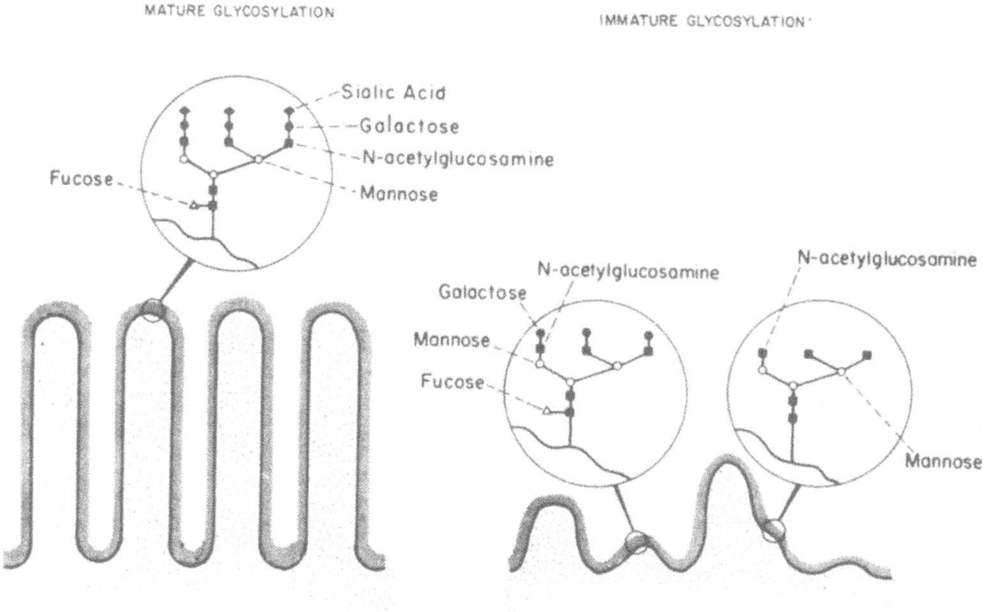

Figure 5. Diagrammatic representation of glycosylation of microvillus membrane glycoproteins and glycolipids in mature and immature animals. Because the addition of sugars to these molecules differs developmentally in the immature animal, the availability of glycoconjugates in MVM also differs. These differences in available glycoconjugates in MVM from mature and immature animals may explain the differences in binding of antigens and toxins to the intestinal surface.

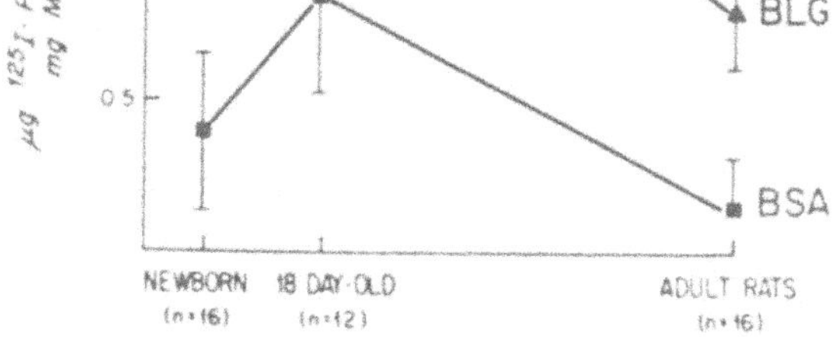

Figure 6. Binding of ^{125}I-BSA and BLG by jejunal MVM: effect of maturity. Numbers of experiments are given in parentheses. Means SD are shown. Protein concentration of BSA and BLG, 0.1 mg/ml; MVM protein concentration, 1.5 mg/ml. Differences in binding between immature and adult groups are significant ($p < 0.01$) for BSA binding in newborns versus adults, highly significant ($p < 0.001$) for both proteins in all the other groups. Differences in actual cpm/tube reflected the same changes (BSA, adults: 94 $\pm$ 99; newborns: 243 $\pm$ 162; 18 d old: 524 $\pm$ 193; BLG, adults: 431 $\pm$ 100; newborns: 763 $\pm$ 122; 18 d old: 990 $\pm$ 133). (Reproduced with permission from Ref. 8).

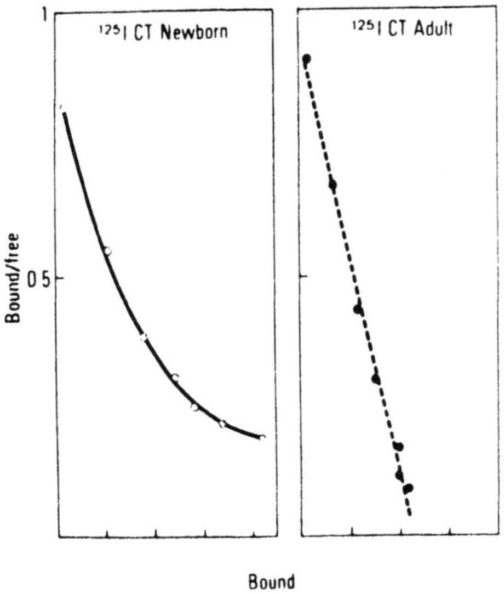

Figure 7. Scatchard plot analysis of ^{125}I-CT binding to newborn and adult MVM. Scatchard plot of adult data is consistent with a single class of receptor sites with Kd = 1.2 0.2 x 10^{-9} M. Analysis of newborn data suggests that additional binding might either be due to nonspecific binding or to additional receptor sites. (Reproduced with permission from Ref. 9).

receptor requires a specific carbohydrate side chain as shown by Holmgren et al. (10), we suggest that additional binding sites in newborns may be due to glycolipids with immature glycosylation and an increased availability of certain glycoconjugates. To summarize these results, we have shown that the composition and available glycoconjugates on the MVM surface of the immature intestine appear to be related to the increased attachment and penetration of intestinal antigens and toxin noted in this age group.

Growth factor modifications of MVM from newborns

Finally, having begun to relate immaturities in the enterocyte surface to antigen-toxin uptake, we briefly summarize our attempts to modify the MVM of newborns with growth factors. These growth factors include mother's colostrum or breast milk and two known modifiers of microvillus membrane, namely cortisone and thyroxin.

It is known from the literature that the early ingestion of colostrum or breast milk can alter the surface characteristics of the neonatal intestine. In preliminary studies using human colostrum, we have shown that the absorption of a common food antigen, BSA, can be decreased. The contribution of passive interference compared to an active stimulus of MVM structure and functional maturation in this system to account for the decrease attachment and absorption of BSA has not yet been worked out. However, the preliminary data in conjunction with observations made by others suggest that the implication of active MVM maturation to account for this observaton is a strong possibility. Using intrauterine injections of cortisone we can modify the fluidity (Table 4) and glycoconjugate attachment of lectins toward that pattern seen in adult MVM (11). In addition, intrauterine cortisone can reverse the sialotransferase and fucosyltransferase activity towards that noted in MVM preparations from mature animals. Finally, using thyroxin injections we can reduce the expression of Fc receptors and specific transport of homologous IgG in 15 day old rats and strikingly decrease the nonspecific uptake of BSA to that of post closure levels (12,13).

Table 4. Effect of maternal cortisone on order parameters of 5-Doxyl stearic acid labeled microvillous membrane (MVM)

MVM	S' (Order parameter)
Newborn	.679 ± .003 (6)[a]
Cortisone exposed	.706 ± .002 (6)[b]
Adult	.734 ± .002

[a]Mean ± standard error of the mean (number of preparations).

[b]$P<.001$ when cortisone exposed MVM were compared to newborn control MVM.

SUMMARY

In this paper, we have tried to provide evidence for the association between the microvillus membrane immaturity of young infants/animals and the enhanced attachment and uptake of intestinal antigens and toxins. Finally, we have reviewed observations that growth factors that alter the newborn MVM composition towards maturity may also affect the handling of antigens by the intestinal surface.

ACKNOWLEDGEMENTS

This work was supported in part by grants from the National Institutes of Health (AM 33506, HD 12437 and AM 37521).

REFERENCES

1. Walker, W.A., Clin. Gastroenterology 15, 1, 1986.
2. Udall, J.N. and Walker, in Immunopathology of the Small Intestine, (Edited by Marsh, M.N), p. 3, John Wiley and Sons Ltd, London, 1985.
3. Pang, K., Bresson, J.L. and Walker, W.A., Biochemistry Biophysics Acta. 727, 201, 1983.
4. Gemmell, C.G., J. Med. Microbiol. 217, 235, 1984.
5. Pang, K.Y., Bresson, J.L. and Walker, W.A., Develop. Biol. 114, 208, 1986.
6. Bresson, J.L., Hercovics, A. and Walker, W.A., Gastroenterology 82, 1025, 1982.
7. Chu, S.W. and Walker, Biochem. Biophys. Acta. 740, 170, 1986.
8. Stern, M., Pang, K.Y. and Walker, W.A., Pediatr. Res. 18, 1252, 1984.
9. Bresson, J.L., Pang, K.Y. and Walker, W.A., Pediatr. Res. 18, 984, 1984.
10. Holmgren, J., Nature 292, 413, 1981.
11. Pang, K.Y., et al., Am. J. Physiol. 249, G85, 1985.
12. Israel, E., Pang, K.Y., Harmatz, P. and Walker, W.A., Am. J. Physiol. 1987 (in press).
13. Israel, E.J., Pang, K.Y., Harmatz, P.R. and Walker, W.A., Ped. Res. 20, 189A, 1986.

ROLE OF LPS RESPONSIVENESS IN URINARY TRACT INFECTION

R. Shahin, L. Hagberg, I. Engberg and C. Svanborg-Eden

Department of Clinical Immunology
University of Goteborg
Goteborg, Sweden

INTRODUCTION

The inability of C3H/HeJ mice to respond to endotoxin (5,8,9) affects their susceptibility to infection with gram negative organisms such as *Klebsiella*, *Salmonella typhimurium* and *Escherichia coli* (2-4,7). Linkage of susceptibility to infection and the LPS defective phenotype has been inferred by genetic analysis (4). We have recently shown that C3H/HeJ mice have an increased susceptibility to *E. coli* kidney infection (1). Susceptibility was correlated with the lps^d gene, although strict linkage has not yet been proven.

Experimental urinary tract infection of C3H/HeJ mice with *E. coli* (1) affords a useful model system in which to study the role of effector mechanisms. The infection is local, rather than systemic and physiologic in that bacteria must penetrate a mucosal barrier prior to activating an inflammatory response. Cellular and soluble factors produced in response to infection can be monitored as excretion products in the urine. Infection of *E. coli* results in an inflammatory response in the kidneys (4). In this study, we have chosen to examine the relationship between bacterial persistence and white cell excretion in LPS responder and nonresponder C3H strain mice infected with *E. coli*.

MATERIALS AND METHODS

Mice

C3H/HeJ mice (original breeding stock, Jackson Laboratories, Bar Harbor, Maine) and C3H/HeN mice (original breeding stock, Charles River Laboratories, Margate, Kent, U.K.) were bred at the animal facilities, Department of Clinical Immunology, University of Gothenburg. Female mice, 8-12 weeks of age were used for the experiments.

Bacteria

E. coli strain Hu734, a *lac*$^-$ mutant of the wild type pyelonephritis strain GR12 (6) was used throughout these experiments. This strain is 075^+ $K5^+$ Hly^+, $ColV^+$ and expresses adhesins specific for mannose as well as for globoseries glycolipids. Additionally, one urinary isolate of *Staphylococcus saprophyticus* was used (2). *E. coli* Hu734, grown for 24 hours in Luria broth, were fixed by addition of formalin to a final concentration of 0.5%. Formalin fixed bacteria retained expression of both mannose and globoseries glycolipids specific adhesins.

Infection model

Mice were infected by depositing 0.05-0.1 ml of bacterial suspension, containing 10^9 bacteria per ml, in the bladder through a soft polyethylene catheter. At different times after infection, kidneys and bladders were removed, homogenized, diluted in sterile PBS and plated for viable counts.

White cell excretion

Urine was collected from individual mice prior to and at different times after infection by gentle compression of the mouse abdomen. Cells were enumerated using a hemocytometer chamber. Cytocentrifuge preparations for morphology were prepared, Giemsa stained, and inspected by light microscopy.

RESULTS

An inverse relationship between the urinary white cell concentration and number of viable bacteria was found in C3H/HeN and C3H/HeJ mice 24 hours after infection with *E. coli* Hu734. The number of *E. coli* was 2000-fold higher in the kidneys of C3H/HeJ mice (geometric mean of 6165.0) than in C3H/HeN mice (geometric mean of 36.3). The urinary white cell concentration was significantly higher in the C3H/HeN mice. No increase in leukocyte excretion over baseline levels was observed in C3H/HeN mice that received sterile PBS in the bladder. No significant difference was found in bacterial persistence in the bladders of the two mouse strains.

The urinary white cell excretion of C3H/HeJ and C3H/HeN mice at different times after infection with E. coli Hu734 is shown in Figure 1. In C3H/HeN mice, the increase in the number of urinary white cells excreted peaked around 24 hours after infection. A second peak was observed in these mice 5-6 days post infection. C3H/HeN mice that received sterile saline, showed no significant increase in urinary white cell excretion during the course of the experiment. In contrast to C3H/HeN mice, no significant increase in urinary white cell excretion was detected 24 hours after infection of C3H/HeJ mice. However, a peak occurred around 6 days post infection, similar to the second peak observed in C3H/HeN mice.

Giemsa stained cytocentrifuge preparations of urinary white cells, made daily during the first 10 days post infection, revealed that the urinary cell populations were composed almost exclusively of polymorphonuclear

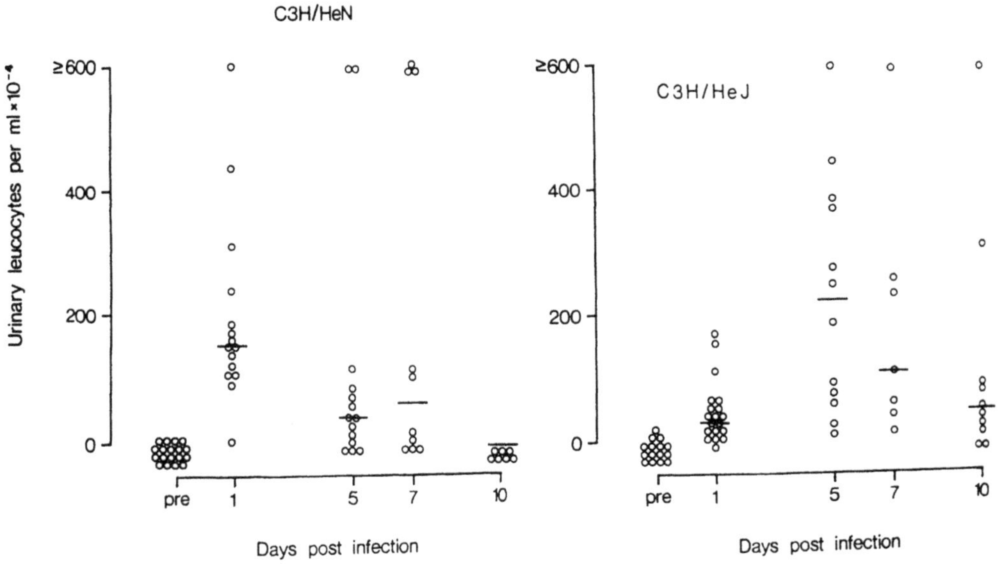

Figure 1. Time course of urinary leukocyte excretion after infection with E. coli Hu 734. Each point represents one mouse. Bars indicate geometric mean.

leukocytes. Paraffin sections of the kidneys from infected mice revealed a thin rim of inflammation around the renal pelvis in C3H/HeN mice, which was not observed in C3H/HeJ mice.

The difference between C3H/HeJ and C3H/HeN mice might obviously relate to their different ability to respond to endotoxin. The role of LPS in the induction of urinary white cell excretion was, thus, further investigated by analyzing the white cell response in mice infected with bacteria which lack LPS. After infection with S. saprophyticus, a gram positive organism, no increase in the urinary white cell concentration occurred in either C3H/HeN or C3H/HeJ mice, despite the recovery of significant numbers of gram-positive organisms from both kidneys and bladder.

The urinary white cell response was also compared between live and formalin-fixed bacteria. After inoculation with formalin fixed E. coli Hu734, which retained both mannose and globoside specific adhesins, increased urinary white cell secretion was observed in C3H/HeN mice. No significant increase in white cell excretion was observed in saline controls, or in C3H/HeJ mice that received formalin killed E. coli Hu734.

Urinary leukocyte excretion by C3H/HeN mice in response to either living or formalin killed E. coli was found to be dose dependent. Urinary white cell excretion above baseline was not consistently observed at doses below $5 \times 10^7 - 10^8$ bacteria per ml of inoculum. The lowest concentration giving a positive recovery from the kidneys of C3H/HeJ mice was 10 viable E. coli HU734. This bacterial inoculum was cleared from the kidneys of C3H/HeN mice.

CONCLUSIONS

These results suggest a relationship between LPS responsiveness and urinary leukocyte recruitment, as:

1. LPS responder mice showed a significant initial urinary leukocyte response and clearance of E. coli from the kidneys, both of which were lacking in LPS nonresponder mice.

2. Gram-positive infections did not activate urinary leukocyte excretion.

3. Infection with formalin killed *E. coli* also resulted in urinary leukocyte excretion.

Thus, experimental UTI in C3H/HeJ mice provides a tool to improve our understanding of the sequential activation by LPS of host defense mechanisms at the site of infection after a physiological challange.

REFERENCES

1. Hagberg, L., Engberg, I., Freter, R., Lam, J., Olling, S. and Svanborg-Eden, C., Infect. Immun. 40, 273, 1983.
2. Hagberg, L., Hull, R., Hull, S., McGhee, J.R., Michalek, S.M. and Svanborg-Eden, C., Infect. Immun. 46, 839, 1984.
3. Hagberg, L., Briles, D.E. and Svanborg-Eden, C., J. Immunol. 134, 4119, 1985.
4. O'Brien, A.D., Weinstein, D.A., Soliman, M.Y. and Rosenstreich, D.L., J. Immunol. 134, 2820, 1985.
5. Sultzer, B.M., Nature (London) 219, 1253, 1968.
6. Svanborg-Eden, C., Freter, R., Hagberg, L., Hull, R., Hull, S., Leffler, H. and Schoolnik, G., Nature 298, 560, 1982.
7. Vas, S.I., Roy, R.S. and Robson, H.G., Can. J. Microbiol. 19, 767, 1973.
8. Watson, J., Riblet, R. and Taylor, B.A., J. Immunol. 118, 2088, 1977.
9. Watson, J., Largen, M. and McAdam, K., J. Exp. Med. 147, 39, 1978.

A MODEL FOR LIPOPOLYSACCHARIDE-MEMBRANE INTERACTION

D.M. Jacobs and R.M. Price

Department of Microbiology
State University of New York at Buffalo
Buffalo, New York USA

INTRODUCTION

Lipopolysaccharide (LPS), a major component of the outer membrane of gram-negative bacteria, is a complex macromolecule both structurally and functionally (1). It induces metabolic and cellular changes mediating host defenses as well as pathogenesis (2,3). Unlike many macromolecules of biological importance, there is little data on the nature of the target cell structure with which LPS interacts. The structure of LPS and the importance of lipid A in biological activities has led to the assmuption that LPS interacts hydrophobically with the plasma membrane of target cells by edge attachment of LPS bilayers (4). However, since the prototype monomer of LPS is an amphiphile, LPS exists as bilayer or vesicular aggregates in solution, arrangements <u>without</u> edges (5). In addition, there is scant direct evidence in the literature that LPS interaction with cell membranes is hydrophobic. One recent paper examined fluorescence anisotropy of macrophages exposed to LPS using DPH; however, the time and temperature did not preclude the possibility that the measurements made reflected changes in internal membranes due to physiological activation by LPS (6). A few studies have demonstrated an interaction between LPS and phospholipid monolayer or bilayer films as detected by changes in surface pressure and surface potential (7,8). Interestingly, most of one study was carried out with alkali-treated LPS because this material was more efficient at mediating changes than the native material (7), but the relevance of these results is questionable since this material is biologically inactive (9). In other studies, vesicles prepared from LPS and various phospholipids were examined by NMR, ESR, fluorescence, and microelectrophoresis as models for bacterial outer membranes (10-14). LPS was found to affect the structural order of the hydrophobic portion of the bilayer, and interactions were dependent on charge and cation concentration.

A quite different concept of the basis of LPS-plasma membrane interaction has developed in cellular immunology. Within the lymphoid system, the major lymphocyte targets for LPS are bone marrow-derived lymphocytes (B cells) which are activated to DNA synthesis and immunoglobulin synthesis and secretion without the necessity for T cell help (15). The singular preference of LPS for B cells would suggest that these cells have a specific binding site or receptor for LPS. Attempts to demonstrate selectivity of binding using radiobinding techniques and mass cultures have yielded contradictory results (16-20). However, preferential binding to B cells has been demonstrated at the single cell level in this (21) and other laboratories (18,22). In addition, there are a few strains of mouse which are hyporesponsive to LPS in all its varied cellular and physiological manifestations (23,24), and one explanation for the clear genetic control (25) of this effect is the absence of a receptor for LPS. Coutinho and coworkers (26,27) have described an antiserum with the properties of an anti-LPS receptor antibody which detects a structure found on LPS responder lymphocytes but not on LPS hyporesponder lymphocytes, but their finding has not been confirmed (28). Differential binding of LPS to lymphocytes of responder and nonresponder mice has been demonstrated in only one (29) of several studies (17,19-22,30,31).

The existence of a "mitogen receptor" or "LPS receptor" has been proposed (32) and is a useful and consistent part of models of B cell activation and the lexicon of B cell membrane antigens (33). However, there is no direct evidence for the presence of a stereochemically specific plasma membrane receptor by which the ligand transduces a signal to a target cell, although there is some evidence consistent with this possibility, including the findings of our own laboratory. Some of our data did not fit comfortably into this straightforward explanation. We, therefore, proposed a model describing the initial interaction of LPS with intact murine lymphocytes as a two-step process (34). This paper is an extension and amplification of that model, describing the data which led to it and the characteristics of the two steps. The model goes some way to resolving the two different views and provides the basis for systemic examination of the process on a molecular level.

RESULTS

For several years, my laboratory has characterized the binding of LPS to murine lymphocytes in an effort to develop direct information on the nature of the binding site and the importance of LPS structural determinants which control the binding. We used a sensitive immunofluorescence technique and examined LPS binding to lymphocytes at the single cell level at 0° in the presence of azide to inhibit post-binding uptake (details of the method are in ref. 26). Preferential binding to spleen cells by comparison to thymus cells was demonstrated (Fig. 1). The tissue distribution of LPS^+ cells and their surface phenotype were determined by double labeling immunofluorescence. Most LPS^+ cells have the surface phenotype of mature B cells, but their distribution by age and in different lymphoid organs varies (21) (Table 1).

In addition, we have found that the LPS binding site moves laterally in the plane of the membrane into "caps" when cross-linked by ligand, and this is dependent on metabolic energy and a functional cytoskeleton. The LPS binding site is not identical to sIgM, sIgD or Ia as these surface structures do not co-cap with LPS (35). These results were all obtained when cells were incubated with relatively low concentrations of LPS, 20-30 ug/ml. At appreciably higher concentrations, selectivity in binding is obscured, and many more LPS^+ lymphocytes are detected. This observation indicates that there are two kinds of binding which appear as selective and non-selective under these conditions (Fig. 2).

Using immunofluorescence, we evaluated selective LPS binding in the presence of a variety of charged molecules and after different target cell treatments. Polymyxin B (PB), a cyclic peptide antibiotic which

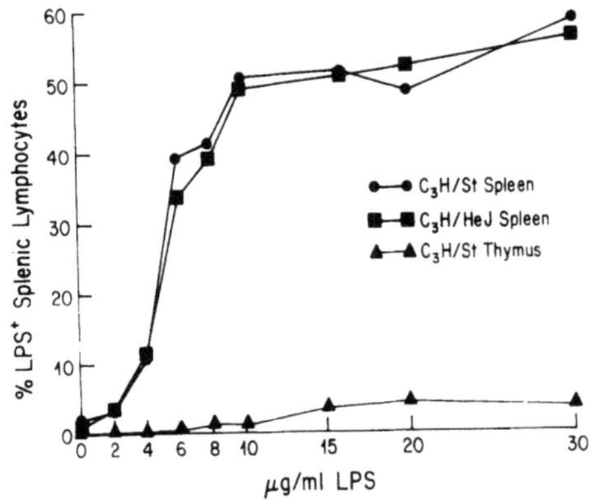

Figure 1. Fraction of LPS-binding lymphocytes in spleen and thymus of the indicated strains as detected by immunofluorescence.

Table 1. Phenotype and distribution of LPS-binding lymphocytes

Cell Source				
age	organ	$LPS^+\mu^+Ia^+\delta^+$	$LPS^+Thy1.2^+$	LPS^+ null
adult	spleen	40%	5%	5%
	PLN	11%	2%	0
	MLN	15%	3%	0
	PP	4%	0	0
1 day	spleen	0.2%	<0.08%	7.2%
6 day	spleen	1.2%	0.08%	11.4

Numbers given are the percentage of lymphocytes with the indicated markers as determined by double-labeling immunofluorescence. See ref. 21 for datails.

inhibits in vivo and in vitro activities of LPS (36-43), the cationic proteins egg white lysozyme and protamine chloride, and the anionic dextran sulfate inhibited LPS binding to murine lymphocytes. Pretreatment with proteolytic enzymes (pronase) abolished the capacity of lymphocytes to bind LPS (34). Inhibition by PB was less effective when added 30 min after initial time of incubation of LPS with cells at 0°, or when added at the initiation of incubation at 37°C. These results suggested that early LPS interaction with lymphocytes consists of two identifiable stages: 1) initial binding which depends on ionic interactions [with a protein(s)?], occurs efficiently in the cold and is inhibitable by PB and (2) subsequent interaction which occurs more slowly in the cold but rapidly at 37°C and is not inhibitable by PB (34) (Fig. 3).

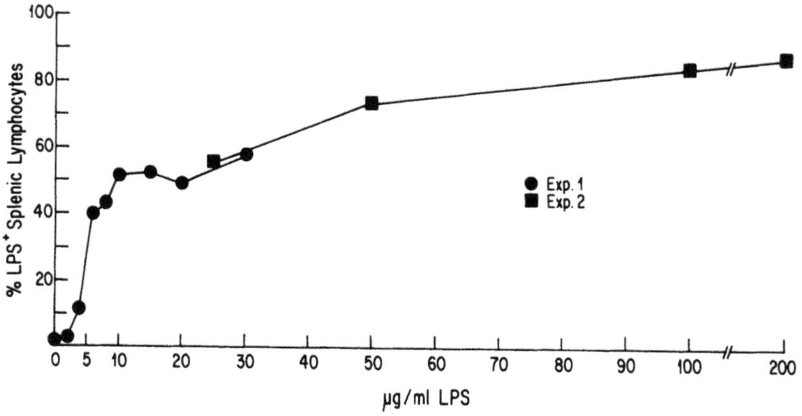

Figure 2. LPS-binding splenic lymphocytes at different concentrations of LPS.

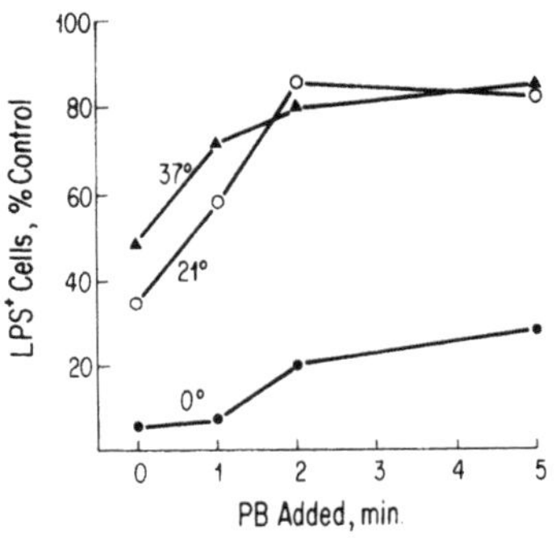

Figure 3. Time and temperature dependence of Polymyxin B inhibition of LPS binding to splenic lymphocytes.

Radiobinding experiments using high specific activity radiolabeled LPS also suggest two kinds of binding. The first is a nonspecific component which reaches equilibrium in 100 min. The second is revealed by subtracting radioactive LPS binding achieved in the presence of unlabeled LPS from that obtained in its absence; this reached equilibrium in 50 min and is by convention specific although it is only 25-45% of total binding (Rosenspire and Jacobs, submitted for publication).

Model of LPS interaction with cell membranes

On the basis of data previously described, we propose that the initial interaction of LPS with intact murine lymphocyte membranes occurs as a two-step process (34) in which each step has different characteristics and structural requirements. These two steps are equivalent to adherence and coalescence, and have certain characteristics.

Step 1 - Adherence	Step 2 - Coalescence
Ionic interactions	Hydrophobic interaction
Temperature independent	Temperature dependent
Inhibited by Polymyxin B	Not inhibited by Polymyxin B

Ionic interactions are involved in overcoming the electrostatic and hydration repulsion of the two aggregates of amphiphiles with hydrophilic surfaces so that adherence can occur. Adherence is followed by the rearrangement of phospholipids so that acyl chains of LPS subunits are integrated into the phospholipid bilayer. The two steps differ in their sensitivity to temperature changes and susceptibility to inhibition by Polymyxin

B. Many cells can bind LPS by this mechanism, and this binding is characterized as non-saturable and non-inhibitable and is detected at high doses of LPS.

In addition, some cells have membrane structures which facilitate this process. B lymphocytes have a structure(s) which is pronase-sensitive, presumably a protein, which facilitates ionic interactions characteristic of Step 1. The presence of this facilitator results in the appearance of binding with characteristics usually attributed to a specific receptor: detectable at low doses of LPS; saturable and inhibitable; selective for cells bearing the facilitator; and specifically inhibitable. We further propose that cell activation is a consequence of integration of the lipid A region of LPS with the lipid bilayer and not of LPS interaction with the facilitator site.

We have begun to test the validity of the model by evaluating the interaction of LPS with purified phospholipid vesicles. Small unilamellar vesicles of phosphatidylcholine containing the fluorescent probe, diphenylhexatriene, demonstrate changes of anisotropy upon interaction with LPS, evidence of perturbation of the hydrophobic region of the lipid vesicle (44) (Table 3).

LPS was titrated against the selected lipid concentration. From 0 to 50 μg/ml LPS, the changes in DPH anisotropy were indicative of a first-order interaction between LPS and the SUVs. At 100 μg/ml, however, the observed change in DPH anisotropy fell distinctly out of the pattern formed

Table 3. Changes in DPH anisotropy (r) induced by LPS interaction with SUVs at different LPS concentrations

	amount of LPS (μg/ml)					
	0	5	10	25	50	100
r (SUVs alone)	0.062	0.062	0.063	0.064	0.063	0.063
r (+ LPS)	0.062	0.065	0.070	0.073	0.074	0.089
% change in r	0	+5	+11	+14	+17	+41

SUV lipid 20 μM, reaction volume = 2 ml. T = 37°C. Anisotropies are the average of 2 separate determinations.

by the lower concentrations of LPS. The observed increase in DPH anisotropy could also be explained by a redistribution of DPH between the two available hydrophobic regions. Two different methods were used to rule out the transfer of DPH as an explanation for these results. In one, we used a system where DPH could not be transferred between aggregates. Egg PC vesicles containing DPH covalently bound to PC were reacted with LPS. In this system, LPS still produced an increase in DPH anisotropy. Further studies should determine whether the interaction in a model membrane occurs in a stepwise fashion with the same characteristics as the interaction with cells.

ACKNOWLEDGEMENTS

The research described was supported by U.S.P.H.S. grants AI 16915, AI 18506, NIH BRSG funds from SUNY/Buffalo and American Cancer Society Research Grant IM-141. Dr. Price is a recipient of a University at Buffalo Presidential Fellowship.

REFERENCES

1. Galanos, C., Luderitz, O., Rietschel, E.T. and Westpahl, O., Biochem. of Lipids II 14, 239, 1977.
2. Morrison, D.C. and Ryan, J.L., Adv. in Immunol. 28, 293, 1979.
3. Morrison, D.C. and Ulevitch, R.J., Am. J. Pathol. 93, 526, 1978.
4. Shands, J.W., Jr., in Bacterial Lipopolysaccharides, (Edited by Kass, E.H. and Wolff, S.M.), p. 189, The University of Chicago Press, Chicago and London, 1973.
5. Gingell, D. and Ginsberg, L., in Membrane Fusion, (Edited by Poste, G. and Nicholson, G.L.), p. 791, Elsevier/North-Holland Biomedical Press, Amsterdam, The Netherlands, 1978.
6. Larsen, N.E., Enelow, R.I., Simmons, E.R. and Sullivan, R., Biochim. Biophys. Acta. 815, 1, 1985.
7. Benedetto, D.A., Shands, J.W., Jr. and Shah, D.O., Biochim. Biophys. Acta. 298, 145, 1973.
8. Fried, V.A. and Rothfield, L.I., Biochim. Biophys. Acta. 514, 69, 1978.

9. Neter, E., Westphal, O., Luderitz, O., Gorzynski, E.A. and Eichenberger, E., J. Exp. Med. 76, 377, 1956.
10. Rottem, S., FEBS Lett 95, 121, 1978.
11. MacKay, A.L., Nichol, C.P., Weeks, G. and Davis, J.H., Biochim. Biophys. Acta 774, 181, 1984.
12. Onji, T. and Liu, M.-S., Biochim. Biophys. Acta. 558, 320, 1979.
13. Liu, M.-S., Onji, T. and Snelgrove, N.E., Biochim. Biophys. Acta. 710, 248, 1982.
14. Takeuchi, Y. and Nikaido, H., Biochemistry 20, 523, 1981.
15. Gery, I., Kruger, J. and Spiesel, S.Z., J. Immunol. 108, 1088, 1972.
16. Moller, G., Andersson, J., Pohlit, H. and Sjoberg, O., Clin. Exp. Immunol. 13, 89, 1973.
17. Symons, D.B.A. and Clarkson, C.A., Immunology 38, 503, 1979.
18. Bona, C., Juy, D., Truffa-Bachi, P. and Kaplan, G.J., J. Microscopie. Biol. Cell 25, 47, 1976.
19. Kabir, S. and Rosenstreich, D.L., Infect. Immun. 15, 156, 1977.
20. Zimmerman, D.H., Gregory, S. and Kern, M., J. Immunol. 119, 1018, 1977.
21. Jacobs, D.M. and Eldridge, J.H., Proc. Soc. Exp. Biol. Med. 175, 458, 1984.
22. Gregory, S.H., Zimmerman, D.H. and Kern, M., J. Immunol. 125, 102, 1980.
23. Sultzer, B.M., Nature 219, 1253, 1968.
24. Coutinho, A., Forni, L., Melchers, F. and Watanabe, T., Eur. J. Immunol. 7, 325, 1977.
25. Watson, J. and Riblet, R., J. Exp. Med. 140, 1147, 1974.
26. Forni, L. and Coutinho, A., Eur. J. Immunol. 8, 56, 1978.
27. Coutinho, A., Forni, L. and Watanabe, T., Eur. J. Immunol. 8, 63, 1978.
28. Watson, J., Kelly, K. and Whitlock, C., in Microbiology 1980, (Edited by Schlesinger, D.), p. 4, ASM, Washington, D.C., 1980.
29. Nygren, H., Dahlen, G. and Moller, G., Scand. J. Immunol. 10, 555, 1979.
30. Watson, J. and Riblet, R., J. Immunol. 114, 1462, 1975.
31. Sultzer, B.M., Infect. Immun. 5, 107, 1972.
32. Moller, G., Transplant. Rev. 23, 49, 1975.
33. Levitt, D. and Cooper, M.D., in Basic and Clinical Immunology, (Edited by Stites, D.P., Stobo, J.D., Fudenberg, H.H. and Wells, J.V.), p. 79, Lange Medical Publications, Los Altos, CA, 1984.

34. Jacobs, D.M., Rev. Infect. Dis. 6, 501, 1984.
35. Swartzwelder, F. and Jacobs, D.M., Rev. Infect. Dis. 6, 578, 1984.
36. Rifkind, D., J. Bacteriol. 93, 1463, 1967.
37. Rifkind, D. and Palmer, J.D., J. Bacteriol. 92, 815, 1966.
38. Bader, J. and Teuber, M., Z. Naturforsch 28, 422, 1973.
39. Corrigan, J.J., Jr. and Kiernat, J.F., Pediat. Res. 13, 48, 1979.
40. Issekutz, A.C. and Biggar, W.D., J. Lab. Clin. Med. 92, 873, 1978.
41. Palmer, J.D. and Rifkind, D., Surg. Gynecol. Obstet. 138, 755, 1974.
42. Jacobs, D.M. and Morrison, D.C., J. Immunol. 118, 21, 1977.
43. Morrison, D.C. and Jacobs, D.M., Immunochemistry 13, 813, 1976.
44. Price, R.M. and Jacobs, D.M., Biochem. Biophys. Acta., 859, 26, 1986.

PULMONARY CELLULAR REACTIONS TO *SCHISTOSOMA MANSONI* SCHISTOSOMULA IN NORMAL AND VACCINATED MICE

J.E. Crabtree and R.A. Wilson

Department of Medicine, St. James University Hospital, Leeds LS9 7TF, England; and Department of Biology, University of York, York YO1 5DD, United Kingdom

INTRODUCTION

Mice vaccinated with radiation-attenuated *Schistosoma mansoni* cercariae develop significant resistance to challenge infections (1,2). The resistance generated is both species specific (3) and dependent on a functional B and T cell system (4). Elucidation of the effector mechanisms of protective immunity has been complicated by the complex migratory pathway of the parasite, which involves passage through the pulmonary capillaries (5). *In vitro* studies have shown that newly transformed (skin) schistosomula are susceptible to a variety of immune effector mechanisms involving antibody, complement and leucocytes. Later developmental stages are refractory (reviewed in ref. 6). *In vivo*, however, there is little morphological evidence of skin attrition of challenge parasites in vaccinated mice (7,8). Moreover, a recent autoradiographic tracking study using ^{75}Selenomethionine-labeled parasites has shown the lungs to be the major site of challenge elimination (9). This suggests that mucosal immune responses might have a significant role in vaccine-induced resistance. To investigate the effector mechanisms involved in immunity, we have undertaken a histopathological and ultrastructural examination of pulmonary cellular responses to schistosomula in normal and vaccinated mice.

METHODS

C57BL/6 mice were vaccinated percutaneously via the abdomen with 300 cercariae, attenuated with 20 krad gamma radiation from a ^{60}Co source.

Nine weeks later vaccinated mice and age-matched controls were infected percutaneously via their flanks with 450-500 ^{75}Se-labeled cercariae. On days 7 to 31 post-infection the lungs were fixed and processed for transmission electron microscopy as previously described (5). Isotopically labeled parasites were used to facilitate the location of schistosomula in lung tissue (10). Differential counts of polymorphonuclear and mononuclear cells were undertaken from semithin 1 μm sections stained with 1% toluidine blue.

Six vaccinated mice and 6 control mice were challenged with 215 cercariae. The worm burdens assessed by portal perfusion at 5 wk post-challenge showed that the vaccinated mice were 73.5% resistant.

RESULTS

Cellular responses in normal mice

Intravascular schistosomula generated no inflammatory reactions (Table 1). From day 11 an increasing percentage of schistosomula were located in the alveoli (Table 2) and cellular accumulations were evident both in the region of vascular damage and associated with alveolar parasites.

Table 1. Dimensions of cellular foci (μm) around intravascular and intra-alveolar schistosomula (values are mean ± S.E.M.)

	Intravascular	Intra-alveolar
Normal Mice (n = 52)		
Day 11	0	291 ± 127
Day 13	0	295 ± 175
Day 17	0	506 ± 77
Day 20	0	404 ± 49
Day 24	0	550 ± 71
Vaccinated Mice (n = 84)		
Day 7	84 ± 21	
Day 11	231 ± 43	280 ± 70
Day 13	237 ± 33	361 ± 39
Day 17	180 ± 33	423 ± 57
Day 20	105 ± 35	396 ± 53
Day 24	202 ± 29	465 ± 58

Table 2. Percentage of observed lung schistosomula located in alveoli with time post-infection

	Normal mice (n=52)	Vaccinated mice (n=84)
Day 7	0	0
Day 11	25	12
Day 13	42	40
Day 17	50	44
>Day 20	80	64

Foci around alveolar parasites measured up to 743 μm. Cellular infiltrates on day 11 consisted of roughly equal proportions of polymorphonuclear and mononuclear cells (mainly macrophages) (Table 3). The polymorphonuclear population was mixed containing neutrophils and eosinophils (Fig. 1). By day 20, foci contained significantly more mononuclear cells ($p < 0.01$), some of which were lymphocytic. From day 17, multinucleated giant cells were evident and hyperplasia of the bronchus-associated lymphoid tissue was observed.

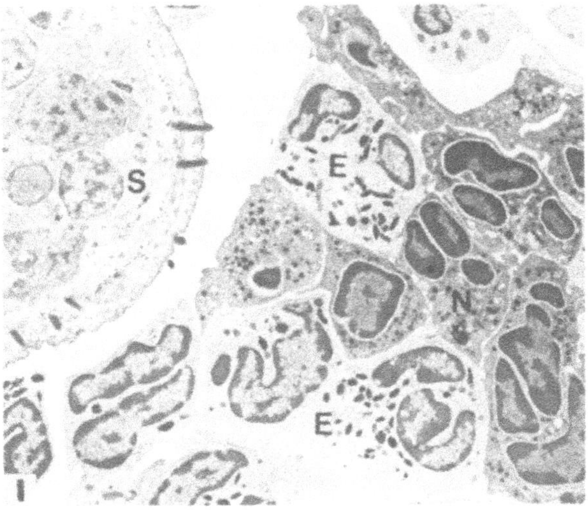

Figure 1. Normal mouse lung. Eosinophil (E) and neutrophil (N) infiltrate adjacent to day 13 alveolar schistosomulum (S). (x4600)

Table 3. Percentage mononuclear cells (lymphocytes and macrophages) within foci of normal and vaccinated mice. (Values are mean % $\pm$ S.E.M. of total, where total = mononuclear and polymorphonuclear).

	Normal mice (n=20)	Vaccinated mice (n=32)
Day 7	-	90 $\pm$ 3.9
Day 11	53 $\pm$ 6.3	87 $\pm$ 1.3
Day 13	60 $\pm$ 1.4	85 $\pm$ 2.8
Day 17	68 $\pm$ 6.7	92 $\pm$ 1.2
>Day 20	73 $\pm$ 2.4	92 $\pm$ 1.7

Cellular responses to challenge schistosomula in vaccinated mice

In contrast to the controls, in vaccinated mice there was a marked cellular response to intravascular schistosomula (Table 1). Early responses (day 7) consisted of diffuse perivascular infiltrates of mononuclear cells (macrophages and lymphocytes) in the alveoli (Fig. 2). Infiltrating cells enlarged the interstitium, separating the alveolar epithelium from the vascular endothelium, and "collagen" like material was deposited in the interstitium (Fig. 2). By day 11, foci around intravascular parasites extended over several alveoli and often contained giant cells and epithelioid macrophages. The blood-air barrier was largely disrupted but despite close apposition of leucocytes and parasites there was no evidence of cytotoxic damage to the schistosomula. The cellular composition of the foci in vaccinated mice was significantly more mononuclear than in normal mice (Table 3) (Days 11 & 17 $p < 0.05$; Days 13 & 20 $p < 0.001$). Unusual electron-dense, membrane bound, elongate inclusions were observed both in alveolar macrophages and giant cells (Fig. 3).

Late stage reactions often contained fibrin-like material and very occasionally plasma cell infiltration was evident (Fig. 4), suggesting some limited local antibody production.

DISCUSSION

In normal mice, pulmonary inflammation was only generated in response to alveolar schistosomula. The initial mixed leucocyte reactions were

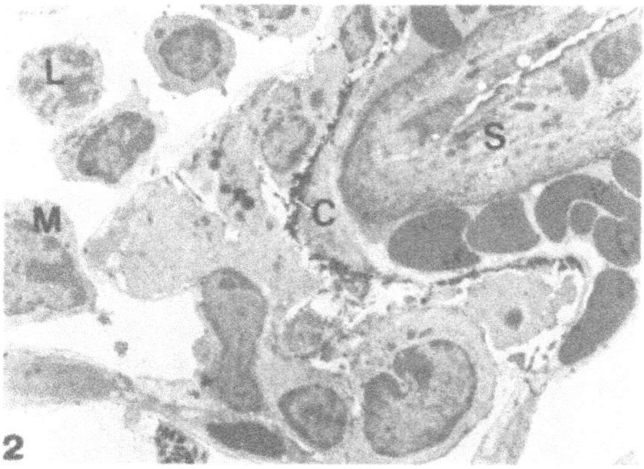

Figure 2. Lymphocytes (L) and macrophages (M) in alveoli adjacent to intravascular day 7 challenge schistosomulum (S) in vaccinated mouse. Note thickened interstitium and 'collagen' deposition. (x3000)

presumably a consequence of the tissue damage associated with entry of the parasites into the alveoli.

In vaccinated mice there were clear differences in both the timing and composition of the pulmonary cellular responses to schistosomula. Challenge parasites located within the pulmonary vasculature stimulated an early anamnestic mononuclear response. The infiltration of mononuclear cells into the interstitium adjacent to intravascular parasites resulted in erosion of the alveolar epithelium and eventual disruption of the vascular endothelium. The inflammation and localized pathological changes in the vasculature, therefore, effectively terminated the migration of schistosomula in the lungs. There was no evidence that the cellular infiltrates were cytotoxic to the parasites. *In vitro* tests have similarly shown lung schistosomula to be resistant to cytocidal killing (11).

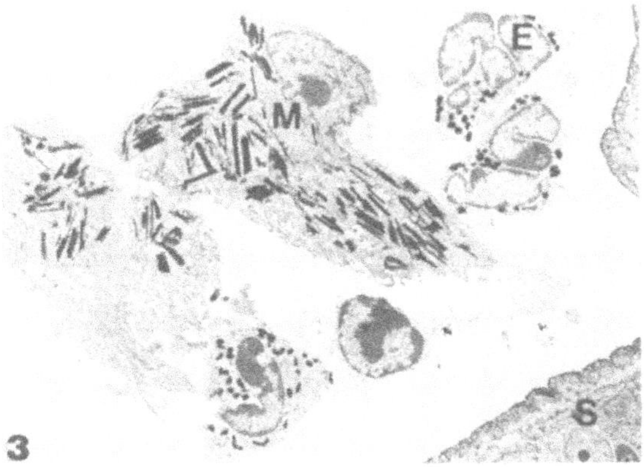

Figure 3. Alveolar macrophages (M) and eosinophils (E) near day 13 challenge schistosomulum (S) in vaccinated mouse. Note electron-dense, elongate inclusions in macrophages. (x3300)

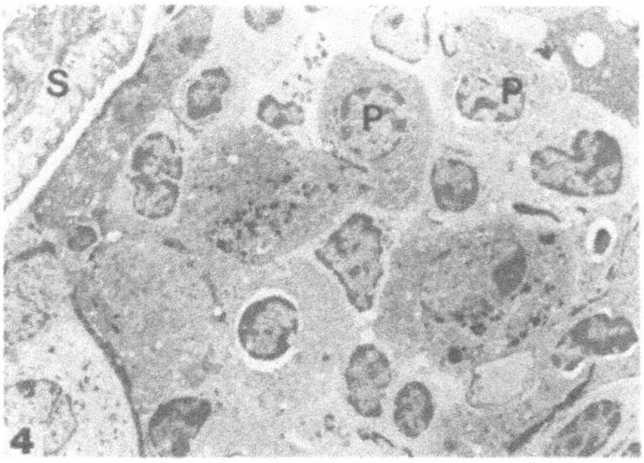

Figure 4. Plasma cells (P) in focal reaction around day 24 challenge schistosomulum (S) in vaccinated mouse lung. (x3250)

The pulmonary cellular reactions to challenge schistosomula have a number of features in common with delayed-type hypersensitivity responses. This implies that the lung phase resistance may be T cell rather than antibody mediated. Other studies have similarly concluded that cellular responses are an important component of the mechanism of resistance in vaccinated mice (12,13).

CONCLUSIONS

1. Normal mice - Pulmonary inflammation is generated only by alveolar parasites, initially in response to tissue damage.

2. Vaccinated mice - Mononuclear pulmonary inflammation by impeding the passage of challenge schistosomula through the capillaries, terminated migration in the lungs and generated the observed resistance.

ACKNOWLEDGEMENT

This study was carried out with financial support from the Medical Research Council.

REFERENCES

1. Minard, P., Dean, D.A., Jacobson, R.H., Vannier, W.E. and Murrell, K.D., Am. J. Trop. Med. Hyg. 27, 76, 1978.
2. Bickle, Q.D., Taylor, M.C., Doenhoff, M.J. and Nelson, G.S., Parasitology 79, 209, 1979.
3. Bickle, Q.D., Andrews, B.J., Doenhoff, M.J., Ford, M.J. and Taylor, M.C., Parasitology 90, 301, 1985.
4. Sher, A., Hieny, S., James, S.L. and Asofsky, R., J. Immunol. 128, 1880, 1982.
5. Crabtree, J.E. and Wilson, R.A., Parasitology 92, 343, 1986.
6. Smithers, S.R. and Doenhoff, M.J., in Immunology of Parasite Infections (Edited by Cohen, S. and Warren, K), p. 527, Blackwell Scientific Publications, Oxford, 1982.
7. Mastin, A., Bickle, Q.D. and Wilson, R.A., Parasitology 87, 87, 1983.
8. von Lichtenberg, F., Correa-Oliveira, R. and Sher, A., Am. J. Trop. Med. Hyg. 34, 96, 1985.
9. Wilson, R.A., Coulson, P. and Dixon, B., Parasitology 92, 101, 1986.
10. Crabtree, J.E. and Wilson, R.A., J. Helminth. 60, 75, 1986.
11. Sher, A., James, S.L., Simpson, A.J.G., Lazdins, J.K. and Meltzer, M.S., J. Immunol. 128, 1880, 1982.
12. James, S.L. and Sher, A., Parasite Immunol. 5, 567, 1983.
13. James, S.L., Natovitz, P.C., Farrar, W.L. and Leonard, E.J., Infect. Immun. 44, 569, 1984.

THE ROLE OF ANTIGEN PROCESSING AND SUPPRESSOR T CELLS IN IMMUNE RESPONSES TO DIETARY PROTEINS IN MICE

A.McI. Mowat, A.G. Lamont, S. Strobel* and S. Mackenzie

Department of Bacteriology and Immunology, Western Infirmary, Glasgow; and *Department of Immunology, Institute of Child Health, Guilford Street London, U.K.

INTRODUCTION

Enteropathies which are associated with immunological hypersensitivity to dietary protein antigens are rare, probably because feeding proteins to naive animals normally results in systemic tolerance. Therefore, investigating the mechanisms underlying the induction of oral tolerance in experimental animals should help clarify the pathogenesis of clinical food sensitive enteropathy (FSE).

Suppressor T cells are implicated in many forms of immunological tolerance and several workers have identified suppressor T cells (Ts) in mice with systemic tolerance after feeding ovalbumin (OVA) (1-3). In initial studies, we showed that treating mice with cyclophosphamide (CY) not only prevented tolerance of systemic delayed type hypersensitivity (DTH) in mice fed OVA but also allowed a pathological DTH response to develop in the intestine and we concluded that this was due to depletion of Ts (4,5). However, others could not prevent the induction of oral tolerance with CY despite proving that depletion of Ts did occur (6). In addition, CY is a potent pharmacological agent with a wide range of actions, including an ability to damage the intestine. Therefore, CY may not be an ideal means of investigating the role of Ts in immunity to dietary antigens. In the present work, we have attepted to confirm the role of Ts in regulating immunity to dietary OVA by treating mice with 2'-deoxyguanosine, an agent with a selective effect on Ts, but without any harmful effects on the small intestine (7,8).

One further aspect of our study was to examine some of the factors underlying the induction and expression of Ts activity after feeding antigen. We have shown previously that stimulation of the reticuloendothelial system prevents oral tolerance to OVA (9) while recent evidence suggests that activation of Ts by parenteral administration of antigen involves specialized antigen presenting cells (APC) and is regulated by products of the I-J locus (10). Therefore, we have examined the role of APC in the induction of oral tolerance to OVA and have investigated whether I-J$^+$ cells play a part in determining the immunological consequences of feeding OVA. In these studies, we have concentrated on modulation of systemic DTH in OVA fed mice, as previous studies have shown that this was the most accurate pointer to the pathogenesis of FSE.

MATERIALS AND METHODS

Mice

All mice were bred in the Department of Bacteriology and Immunology, Western Infirmary, Glasgow and maintained on an OVA-free diet.

Anti-I-J^k alloantiserum

B10.A3R mice were immunized weekly with 2 x 10^7 B10.A5R spleen cells i.p. and bled after 16 wk.

Antigens

OVA (Fraction V, Sigma) was dissolved in distilled water for feeding. Heat aggregated OVA was prepared by heating a 2% solution for 1 h at 70°C and was stored at -20°C before using to assess systemic DTH.

Induction of oral tolerance

Mice were fed 25 mg OVA 7-14 d before intradermal immunization with 100 ug OVA in Complete Freund's Adjuvant (CFA-Bacto H37Ra, Difco, Ltd.). 21 d later, mice were assessed for systemic DTH by measuring the increment in footpad thickness 24 h after intradermal challenge with 100 ug aggregated OVA.

Prevention of oral tolerance

To inhibit the induction of Ts, BALB/c mice were given 1 mg 2'-deoxyguanosine (Sigma) i.p. daily for 10 d between feeding and immunizing. For depletion of I-J^+ cells, CBA mice were treated with 0.2 ml of 1:10 anti-I-J^k alloantiserum i.v. on days 1-, 0 and +1 and fed OVA on d 0. To activate the reticuloendothelial system, BALB/c mice received either 2 mg oestradiol (Paynes & Byrne, Ltd.) s.c. 3 d before feeding OVA, or were given 50 μg lipopolysaccahride (LPS (E. coli 011:B4 Sigma) i.v. 3 h after feeding OVA or received 50 μg muramyl dipeptide (MDP; Sigma) i.p. at the time of feeding. To induce a graft-versus-host reaction (GvHR), adult F1 hybrid mice were injected with 6 x 10^7 parental spleen cells i.p. and fed OVA 12 d later.

Induction of suppressor T cells

Mice were fed 20 mg OVA and 7 d later, 10^8 viable spleen cells were transferred i.v. into syngeneic recipients which were then immunized immediately with OVA in CFA. Recipients were assessed for systemic DTH, 3 wk after immunization.

Phagocytic activity in RES

Mice were injected with 16 mg/kg colloidal carbon i.v. and bled at intervals of 1-15 min thereafter. Blood was analyzed on a spectrophotometer at OD_{700} and carbon clearance (K_{16}) calculated from the linear regression slope.

Assay for antigen presenting cell activity

APC activity was assessed as described previously (11). Briefly, OVA-primed lymph node T cells were purified on nylon wool and treated with monoclonal anti-Ia plus complement, before culture for 5 days in the presence of 20% spleen adherent cells (SAC) and 500 μg/ml OVA. Cultures containing 2 x 10^5 T cells in 100 μl were pulsed with ^{14}C-thymidine, 18 h befor harvesting cell bound DNA.

RESULTS

Effect of 2'deoxyguanosine on oral tolerance to OVA

Control mice fed OVA and injected daily with saline had significantly suppressed systemic delayed-type hypersensitivity (DTH) responses compared with unfed controls (Fig. 1: 89% suppression $p < 0.025$), but mice treated with 2'deoxyguanosine (dGuo) had DTH responses with were similar to unfed controls (35% suppression pNS). dGuo itself had no effect on the DTH response of control mice.

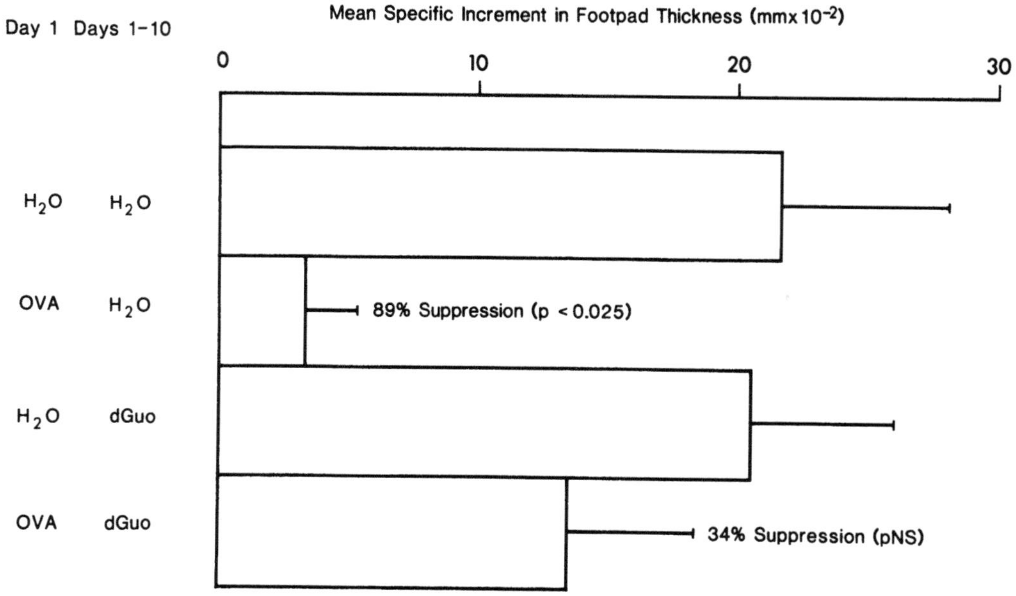

Figure 1. Effects of 2'-deoxyguanosine on oral tolerance to OVA. Systemic DTH responses in mice treated with 1 mg dGuo daily and fed OVA 10 days before immunizing with OVA/CFA. Results shown are mean OVA-specific increments in footpad thickness 24 h after intradermal challenge with OVA + 1 standard deviation (s.d.) for 6-8 mice/group.

Depletion of suppressor T cells by dGuo

As dGuo prevented the induction of oral tolerance, we investigated whether dGuo was acting by eliminating Ts. Spleen cells from mice fed OVA produced significant suppression of DTH responses in syngeneic recipients (Fig. 2: 57% suppression $p < 0.005$), but this was abolished if spleen cell donors were treated with dGuo daily for the period between feeding and spleen cell transfer. The suppressor cells were also depleted by treatment with anti-Thy 1.2 + complement (data not shown). Thus, dGuo both prevented induction of systemic tolerance and eliminated generation of Ts in mice fed OVA.

Effect of anti-I-J^k treatment on oral tolerance to OVA

We next examined the role of I-J^+ cells in the induction of oral tolerance to OVA. CBA mice fed OVA and injected with saline had significantly suppressed systemic DTH responses compared with controls (Fig. 3: 107% suppression $p < 0.001$) and this was abolished if mice received 3 injections of anti-I-J^k around the time of feeding OVA (18% suppression pNS). Thus, an I-J^+ cell is involved in the induction of oral tolerance to OVA.

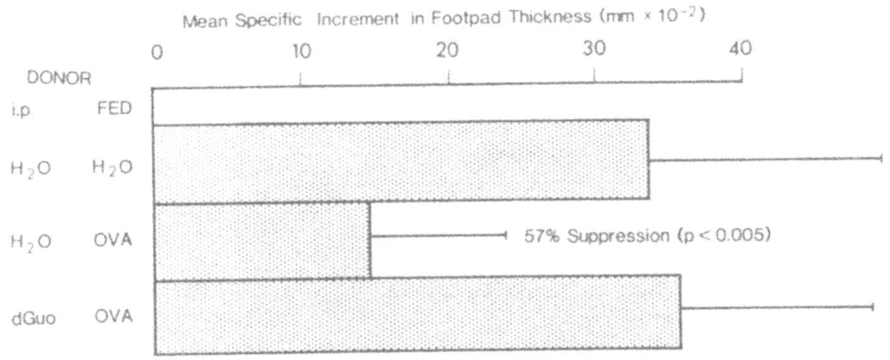

Figure 2. Effect of dGuo on induction of Ts by feeding OVA. Systemic DTH responses in recipients of spleen cells from donor mice fed OVA and treated with dGuo. Results shown are mean OVA-specific increments in footpad thickness + 1 standard deviation for 10-12 mice/group.

<u>Effects of activating the RES on oral tolerance to OVA</u>

In the next set of experiments, we examined the effects of agents which activate the RES on immunity to fed OVA. Initial experiments showed that 2 mg oestradiol given 3 d before feeding OVA prevented the tolerance of systemic DTH found in control mice fed OVA (9). Subsequently, we found that i.p. administration of 50 µg muramyl dipeptide at the time of feeding OVA also prevented the induction of tolerance (12), whereas 50 µg LPS had no effect on the tolerance of DTH (13).

<u>Effects of graft-versus-host reaction on oral tolerance to OVA</u>

Induction of GvHR is also known to activate the RES (6) and the GvHR provided the opportunity to modulate RES activity under defined genetic conditions.

In initial experiments, we showed that 12 d after induction of a GvHR with 6×10^7 CBA spleen cells, $(CBAxBALB/c)F_1$ mice were partially resistant to the induction of systemic tolerance by feeding OVA and had a generalized enhancement of systemic immune responsiveness (11). We went on to examine the nature of the genetic incompatibility which was required for a GvHR to prevent the induction of tolerance.

F_1 hybrids were bred from congenic parents differing only at specified MHC loci and a GvHR was induced in adult mice with spleen cells from one parental strain. As shown in Fig. 4, when control mice of these strains

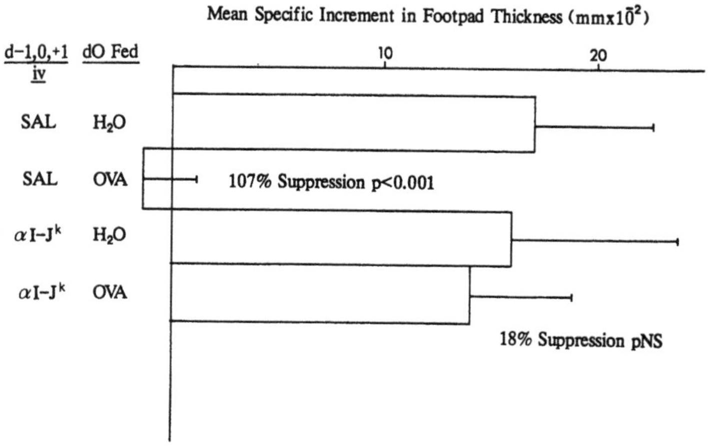

Figure 3. Effect of anti-I-J^k on oral tolerance to OVA. Systemic DTH responses in CBA mice given anti-I-J^k or saline i.v. around the time of feeding OVA, 14 d before immunization with OVA/CFA. Results shown are mean OVA-specific increments in footpad thickness + 1 s.d. for 6-8 mice/group.

were fed OVA, all developed excellent tolerance of their systemic DTH responses compared with unfed controls (60-98% suppression). When GvHR mice were fed OVA, 12 d after spleen cell transfer, there was significant inhibition of tolerance induction if the GvHR was induced across the entire H-2 complex (B10xB10.BR) across the Ia region (A.THxA.TL) or across H-2K+I-A (B10xB10.A4R). In contrast, a GvHR induced across H-2K (B10.AxB10.AQR) or H-2D (B10.BR.xB10.AKM) had no significant effect on induction of tolerance, while an incompatibility at the I-J locus (B10.A3RxB10.A5R) produced significantly enhanced tolerance in GvHR. Thus, incompatibility at I-A is alone sufficient and necessary for the inhibition of tolerance of systemic DTH during a GvHR.

Correlation of antigen presenting cell activity and oral tolerance

Of the agents which prevented the induction of oral tolerance by a putative effect on the RES, only oestradiol enhanced the clearance of colloidal carbon by the RES, while LPS had no effect on either oral tolerance or on clearance of colloidal carbon (Fig. 5). In view of the fact that the ability of GvHR to prevent tolerance was restricted by the I-A locus, we examined whether the inhibition of tolerance by oestradiol, MDP and GvHR correlated with an enhancement of APC activity.

Adherent spleen cells from control mice, mice treated with oestradiol, MDP, LPS or from mice with GvHR, were pulsed with OVA and used to stimulate

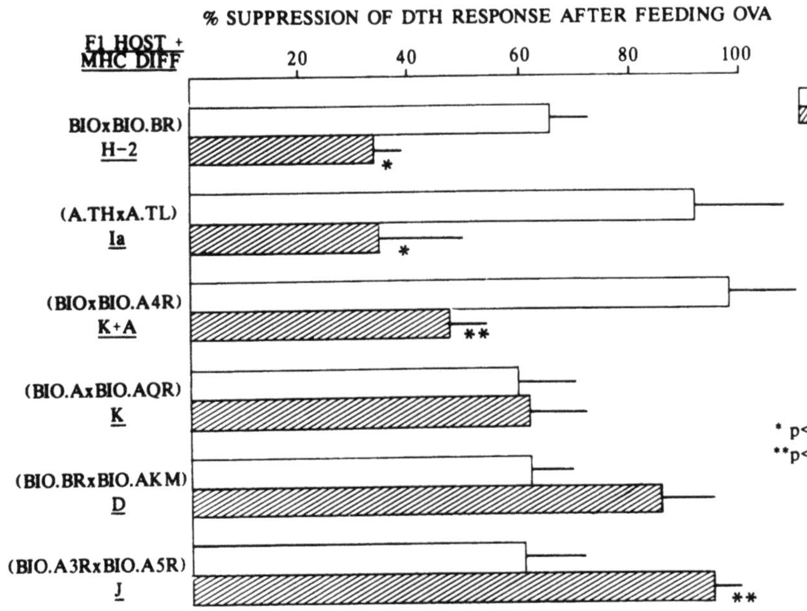

Figure 4. Genetic restriction of the inhibition of oral tolerance by GvHR. A GvHR was induced across different MHC loci 12 d before feeding OVA and mice were immunized 14 d after feeding. Results shown are mean % suppression of systemic DTH responses in OVA fed control or GvHR mice compared with responses in appropriate controls for 5-8 mice/group.

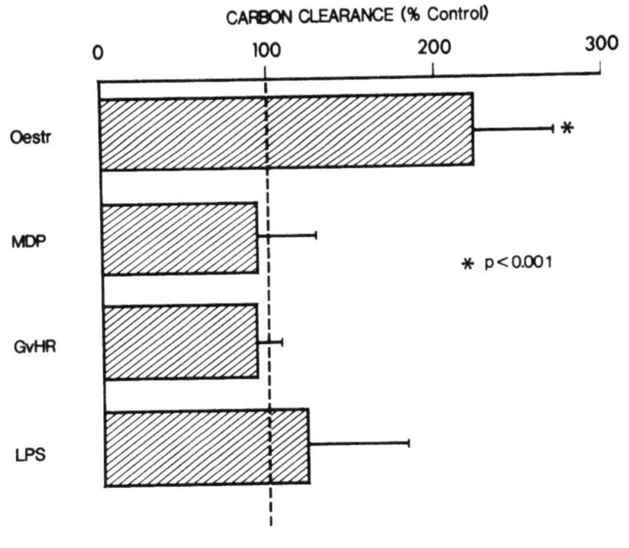

Figure 5. Effects of RES activating agents on phagocytic activity of RES. Clearance of colloidal carbon (K_{16}) was assessed 3 d after oestradiol, 1 d after MDP or LPS or on d 7 of the GvHR and results are expressed as mean % of carbon clearance found in appropriate controls + 1 s.d. for 6 mice/group.

OVA-specific T cells *in vitro*. In each case, control SAC allowed T cells to respond to OVA, but this APC activity was significantly enhanced in mice given oestradiol or MDP and on d 7 of a GvHR (Fig. 6). In contrast, SAC from LPS-treated mice were less able to stimulate T cells than control SAC.

Effect of activating APC on generation of Ts

In the final experiments, we examined whether activation of APC was associated with depletion of Ts. Mice were treated with oestradiol 3 d before feeding OVA and, 7 d later, spleen cells were transferred to normal recipients. Spleen cells from normal mice fed OVA produced moderate, but significant suppression of systemic DTH (Fig. 7: 40% suppression $p < 0.05$) compared with recipients of normal spleen cells. Oestrogen-treated spleen cells had no effect on systemic DTH responses, while oestrogen treatment of OVA fed mice abrogated transfer of suppression by spleen cells.

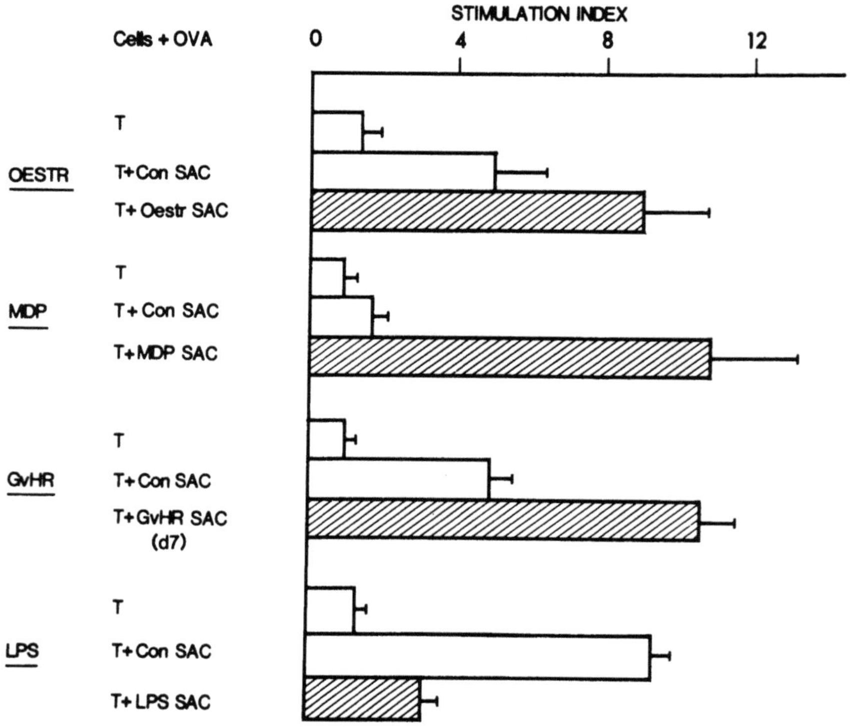

Figure 6. Effects of RES activating agents on APC activity. Adherent spleen cells were taken from mice 3 d after oestradiol, 1 d after MDP or LPS or on day 7 of the GvHR and compared with control SAC for their ability to stimulate OVA-specific T cells in presence of OVA. Results were expressed as a Stimulation Index, calculated from the response of T cells cultured without OVA and are means + 1 s.d. for triplicate assays.

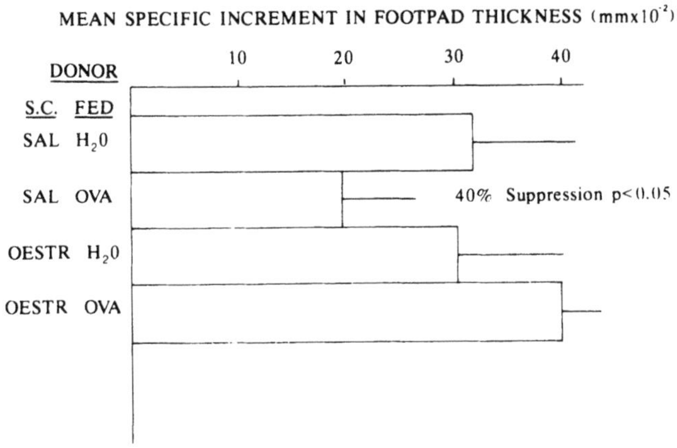

Figure 7. Effects of oestradiol on generation of Ts by feeding OVA. Systemic DTH responses in recipients of spleen cells from donors fed OVA and treated with oestradiol. Results shown are mean OVA-specific increments in footpad thickness + 1 s.d. for 5-8 mice/group.

DISCUSSION

We have shown here that the tolerance of systemic DTH in mice fed OVA can be prevented by depleting Ts with 2'-deoxyguanosine, by in vivo removal of I-J$^+$ cells or by agents which activate the APC functions of the RES. These results support the hypothesis that oral tolerance for systemic DTH reflects an interaction between populations of Ts and APC, either or both of which may carry-I-J coded markers.

Ts are frequently found in mice fed OVA (1-3) and our finding that treatment of mice with dGuo prevented the induction of oral tolerance confirms and extends our previous report that CY also inhibited systemic tolerance to fed OVA (5). In these experiments with CY, we did not examine Ts function directly and the interpretation was complicated by the potentially harmful effect of CY on the intestine. dGuo is unlikely to damage the intestine and, within the immune system, as we confirmed, has a selective effect on Ts (7,8).

This study is the first to demonstrate that induction of oral tolerance requires an I-J$^+$ cell in vivo. In several models of systemic tolerance associated with Ts, these Ts are often I-J$^+$ and treatment of mice with anti-I-J in vivo prevents the induction of tolerance (10,14) Furthermore, there is now considerable evidence that generation of Ts in vivo requires one or more populations of I-J$^+$ APC for presentation of antigen or of antigen-specific suppressor factors to different Ts in the suppressor cell cascade (11). Thus, the ability of anti-I-J^k to prevent the induction of oral tolerance to OVA could be due to depletion of these I-J$^+$ APC or may reflect the presence of Ts which are themselves I-J$^+$.

The potential importance of APC in oral tolerance was emphasized by experiments which examined the effect of a GvHR on oral tolerance. In the first of these studies, we confirmed that a GvHR induced by a full MHC incompatibility abrogated oral tolerance for systemic DTH (11) and showed that disparity at the I-A locus was alone sufficient and necessary for this to occur. Although this genetic restriction is identical to that required for intestinal pathology in adult mice with GvHR (15), the time course of interference with tolerance does not correlate with the evolution of intestinal GvHR (11). In addition, preliminary results indicate that the ability of a GvHR to enhance APC function is also I-A restricted. Thus, we propose that interference with tolerance induction is one further manifestation of an I-A restricted allogeneic effect of GvHR on accessory cells (16). Interestingly, an incompatibility at the I-J locus appeared to increase susceptibility to oral tolerance induction, confirming the negative allogeneic effect of an I-J-restricted GvHR (15,16) and underlining the possible role of I-J products in oral tolerance.

In addition to these effects of GvHR, we have shown previously that tolerance of systemic DTH is prevented when the RES is activated with oestrogen and MDP. We found here that, of these protocols, only oestradiol enhanced the phagocytic activity of the RES, but MDP, oestradiol and GvHR all produced significant enhancement of APC activity. In contrast, although LPS interferes with the induction of tolerance for systemic antibody responses (13), it has no effect on the tolerance of DTH responses and did not enhance APC activity. Thus, we conclude that enhancement of APC activity is a potent means of modulating immunity to dietary proteins and that DTH responses are particularly susceptible to this form of immunoregulation. Systemic DTH is also much more readily suppressed by Ts from OVA-fed mice (5,6,17) and, in this study, we found that oestradiol not only enhanced APC activity, but also prevented the generation of Ts. As there is no evidence that oestradiol has a direct effect on Ts, this result suggests that inhibition of oral tolerance due to activation of APC is due to bypassing of Ts induction. This could occur either because more fed antigen is now available on APC to activate T_H or T_{DTH} efficiently, or because there is a shift in the balance between different populations of APC required to activate T_H and Ts. This latter possibility has been suggested as an explanation for the finding that the level of APC activity determines Ts-dependent immune responsiveness to lysozyme in mice (18) and we are currently studing the relationship between APC and Ts in OVA fed mice in more detail.

The important practical implication from our study is that preventing oral tolerance with CY, dGuo, MDP or oestradiol also allows an active, local DTH response to be induced in the intestine on oral challenge with OVA (4,9,12,19). As this local DTH response produces mucosal alterations which are qualitatively similar to those found in FSE, we suggest that FSE may arise as a result of a breakdown in oral tolerance to dietary proteins and that this is due to genetically determined defects in the function of Ts and/or APC.

SUMMARY

We have examined the role of Ts cells and APC in regulating the tolerance of systemic DTH in mice fed OVA. Oral tolerance to OVA was prevented by eliminating Ts with dGuo and by treating mice with anti-I-J antiserum. In addition, activating the reticuloendothelial system (RES) with oestradiol, muramyl dipeptide (MDP) or GvHR prevented the induction of tolerance. Further studies showed that prevention of oral tolerance correlated with the ability to enhance APC activity and that oestradiol also abrogated the induction of Ts after feeding OVA.

Our results show that the tolerance of systemic DTH in mice fed OVA reflects complex interactions between APC and Ts and suggest that defects in these regulatory events may be responsible for clinical food sensitive enteropathy.

ACKNOWLEDGEMENTS

This work was supported by MRC Grant G8513090.

REFERENCES

1. Ngan, J. and Kind, L.S., J. Immunol. 120, 861, 1978.
2. Miller, S.D. and Hanson, D.G., J. Immunol. 123, 2344, 1979.
3. Challacombe, S.J. and Tomasi, T.B., J. Exp. Med. 152, 1459, 1980.
4. Mowat, A.McI. and Ferguson, A., Clin. Exp. Immunol. 43, 574, 1981.
5. Mowat, A.McI., Strobel, S., Drummond, H.E. and Ferguson, A., Immunology 45, 105, 1982.
6. Hanson, D.G. and Miller, S.D., J. Immunol. 128, 2378, 1982.
7. Carson, D.A., Kaye, J. and Seegmiller, J.E., Proc. Natl. Acad. Sci. 74, 5677, 1977.
8. Bril, H., Van Den Akker, Th.W., Molendijk-Lok, B.D., Bianchi, A.T.J. and Benner, R., J. Immunol. 132, 599, 1984.
9. Mowat, A.McI. and Parrott, D.M.V., Immunology 50, 547, 1983.
10. Dorf, M.E. and Benacerraf, B., Immunol. Rev. 2, 127, 1984.
11. Strobel, S., Mowat, A.McI. and Ferguson, A., Immunology 56, 57, 1985.
12. Strobel, S. and Ferguson, A., Gut 27, 829, 1986.
13. Mowat, A.McI., Thomas, M.J. and Parrott, D.M.V., Immunology 58, 677, 1986.
14. Pierres, M., Germain, R.N., Dorf, M.E. and Benacerraf, B., J. Exp. Med. S14, 656, 1978.
15. Mowat, A.McI., Borland, A. and Parrott, D.M.V., Transplantation 41, 192, 1986.
16. Zinkernagel, R.M., Immunogenetics 10, 373, 1980.
17. Richman, L.K., Chiller, J.M., Brown, W.R., Hanson, D.G. and Vaz, N.M., J. Immunol. 121, 2429, 1978.
18. Sadegh-Nasseri, S., Dessi, V. and Sercarz, E.E., Eur. J. Immunol. 16, 486, 1986.
19. Mowat, A.McI., Immunology 58, 179, 1986.

ORAL TOLERANCE INDUCED BY GUT-PROCESSED ANTIGEN

M.G. Bruce and A. Ferguson

Gastro-Intestinal Unit, University of
Edinburgh and Western General Hospital
Edinburgh EH4 2XU, Scotland, UK

INTRODUCTION

Different mechanisms operate to produce the suppression of humoral and cellular immune responses after feeding protein antigen to mice (1). In experiments designed to examine the role of the gut in "processing" of fed antigen, (ovalbumin, OVA), we found that serum collected one hour after feeding and administered intraperitoneally into naive recipients transferred tolerance for CMI but not for antibody responses (2). We postulated that in the time between feeding and collection of serum, OVA had been processed by the gut, and converted from immunogenic into tolerogenic forms. Further experiments are now reported, in which we have investigated the relevance of systemic as opposed to gut antigen processing by using a biological filtration experiment similar to that used by others in the investigation of macrophage function (3,4). We attempted to mimic physicochemical alteration to the native protein by injecting mice with a range of doses of native, deaggregated and urea-denatured OVA. The relevance of epitopes recognized by anti-OVA antibody has been studied by immunoabsorption of tolerogenic serum and, finally, the size of the tolerogen has been estimated by transfer of fractions of serum, separated on the basis of molecular weight.

MATERIALS AND METHODS

Animals. Female BDF_1 mice aged 6-8 weeks were used in all experiments. There were four to six animals per group apart from serum donors where 20 mice were used.

Antigens. Ovalbumin (Grade V; Sigma) was used. Deaggregated OVA was prepared by centrifugation at 100,000 g for 3 h (5). The method of Chesnut et al. (6) was used to prepare urea-denatured OVA.

Assessment of systemic immunity. All mice were immunized in the right hind footpad with 100 μg OVA in complete Freund's adjuvant. Three wk later they were bled and anti-OVA IgG was measured by ELISA (7). CMI was measured by eliciting a DTH reaction in the left hind footpad after intradermal injection of 100 μg OVA in saline (7).

Serum transfer procedure. Donor mice were fed by intragastric intubation with either 25 mg OVA dissolved in 0.2 ml saline or saline only. One h after feeding, the mice were bled out from the axillary vein and artery, serum pooled according to experimental groups and 0.8 ml injected i.p. into each recipient. Seven days later recipients were immunized with OVA and assessed for systemic immunity as described above.

Detection of OVA in mouse serum. An ELISA technique was used to detect immunoreactive OVA. Acrylic microtiter plates were coated with IgG anti-OVA. Standard and test samples were added and OVA was detected with alkaline phosphatase-conjugated rabbit IgG anti-OVA as previously described (8).

Absorption of serum with Sepharose-linked antibody. Rabbit anti-OVA was coupled to Sepharose 4B. The antigen binding capacity of the immunoadsorbent gel was 2.5 mg OVA per 100 μl of gel. Serum obtained from saline or OVA fed donor mice was incubated with S4B anti-OVA, twice, for 16 hours at room temperature, using fresh S4B-anti-OVA for the second incubation (8).

Serum fractionation. Serum proteins were fractionated by gel filtration through a column of Sephacryl S200 superfine (Pharmacia) in 0.25 M NaCl. Three pooled fractions of serum were selected; FI which contained all proteins with M.W. greater than 100,000 D; FII, which contained proteins within the approximate M.W. range of native OVA (43,500 D); and FIII which contained all proteins with lower M.Ws. Fractions were dialyzed and concentrated as described elsewhere (8).

Table 1. Systemic DTH and antibody responses of serum recipients three weeks after OVA/CFA immunization

Donor treatment	24 hr footpad increment (mm) (mean $\pm$ SE)	P	OD_{405} nm (mean $\pm$ SE)	P
Experiment 1[a]				
0.2 ml saline i.p.	0.12 $\pm$ 0.03	-	1.255 $\pm$ 0.06	-
10 μg OVA i.p.	0.22 $\pm$ 0.09	NS	1.31 $\pm$ 0.08	NS
Experiment 2[b]				
0.2 ml saline i.g.	0.12 $\pm$ 0.02	-	1.22 $\pm$ 0.31	-
25 mg OVA i.g.	0.02 $\pm$ 0.05	<0.005	1.27 $\pm$ 0.24	NS

[a]Experiment 1: Serum donors injected i.p. with OVA or saline.
[b]Experiment 2: Serum donors fed OVA or saline.
NS = not significantly different.

EXPERIMENTS AND RESULTS

Comparison of gut and systemic antigen processing

10 μg OVA dissolved in 0.2 ml saline was injected i.p. into mice. Control mice received saline only. One hour later the animals were bled out and their sera, containing systemically "filtered" OVA, pooled and transferred i.p. into recipient mice. The presence or absence of tolerance in recipients of this serum was established and results are shown in Table 1. It is clear that systemic processing of 10 μg native OVA for 1 h did not produce a serum tolerogen.

Properties of chemically altered OVA

Mice were injected i.p. with 0.1 μg, 1 μg or 10 μg of either native, denatured or deaggregated OVA. Seven days later all animals were immunized and the presence or absence of tolerance established. Results are summarized in Table 2. Mice injected i.p. with native or denatured OVA had identical antibody responses to mice injected with saline before systemic immunization. Deaggregated OVA suppressed the anti-OVA response over the entire test range of antigen doses. DTH responses of mice injected with saline, native OVA or denatured OVA were not suppressed, whereas there was suppression of DTH in mice which had received deaggregated OVA.

Antigenicity of circulating gut-processed OVA

Immunoreactive OVA was detected in the serum of OVA fed mice, and was not detected in the serum of saline fed mice. The effects of absorbing serum from OVA fed donor mice with immunoadsorbent IgG anti-OVA are shown in Table 3. Serum from OVA fed mice suppressed DTH responses of recipients. Following absorption with S4B-anti-OVA, immunoreactive OVA was no longer detected in the serum and this absorbed serum did not suppress DTH to OVA in recipients.

Molecular size of circulating gut-processed OVA

The presence of intact antibody binding sites on gut-processed OVA is not necessarily indicative of an intact molecule and the three fractions of the serum which had contained gut-processed OVA, were assayed for total protein content (Lowry), immunoreactive OVA (ELISA) and *in vivo* effect

Table 2. Systemic DTH and antibody responses of BDF_1 mice at three weeks after OVA/CFA immunization

Injected i.p.	24 hr footpad increment (mm) (mean ± SE)	P	OD_{405} nm (mean ± Se)	P
0.1 ml saline	0.15 ± 0.07	-	1.22 ± 0.1	-
0.1 μg OVA	0.16 ± 0.04	NS	1.23 ± 0.1	NS
1 μg OVA	0.07 ± 0.02	NS	1.19 ± 0.12	NS
10 μg OVa	0.09 ± 0.04	NS	1.02 ± 0.2	NS
0.1 μg den[a] OVA	0.08 ± 0.03	NS	1.25 ± 0.06	NS
1 μg den OVA	0.12 ± 0.05	NS	1.12 ± 0.32	NS
10 μg den OVA	0.11 ± 0.03	NS	1.2 + 0.1	NS
0.1 μg deag[b] OVa	-0.01 ± 0.03	<0.005	0.16 ± 0.08	<0.01
1 μg deag OVA	-0.01 ± 0.02	<0.001	0.22 ± 0.07	<0.01
10 μg deag OVa	-0.01 ± 0.03	<0.01	0.23 ± 0.08	<0.01

[a]den OVA = denatured OVA.

[b]deag OVA = deaggregated OVA.

Table 3. Immunoreactive OVA measured in pooled serum of saline or OVA fed donors before and after absorption with Sepharose-linked anti-OVA IgG and systemic DTH in serum recipients at three weeks after OVA/CFA immunization[a]

Donor feed (i.g.)	Serum OVA (ng/ml)	S4B-anti-OVA absorption	Subsequent serum OVA (ng/ml)	24 hr footpad increment (mean $\pm$ SE)	P
saline	neg[b]	-	-	0.13 ± 0.04	NS
saline	neg	x2	neg	0.08 ± 0.03	-
OVA	38	-	-	0.03 ± 0.03	<0.05
OVA	38	x1	neg	0.11 ± 0.03	NS
OVA	38	x2	neg	0.11 ± 0.02	NS

[a]Results were compared to recipients of twice-absorbed serum from saline fed mice.
[b]neg = negligible, below detectable levels.

Table 4. Total protein and immunoreactive OVA in serum and serum fractions of saline or OVA fed donors and systemic DTH response in recipients of serum fractions at three weeks after OVA/CFA immunization

Donor fed (i.g.)	Serum fraction	Serum protein (mg/ml)	Serum OVA (ng/ml)	24 hr footpad increment (mm), (mean ± SE)	P
-	-	32	neg	ND	-
OVA	-	52.6	38	ND	-
saline	I	6.4	ND[a]	0.08 ± 0.06	-
OVA	I	7.7	neg	0.03 ± 0.05	NS
saline	II	25	neg	0.1 ± 0.04	-
OVA	II	26.3	35	0.02 ± 0.05	<0.01
saline	III	neg	neg	0.14 ± 0.15	-
OVA	III	neg	neg	0.05 ± 0.05	NS
none[b]	-	-	-	0.07 ± 0.03	-

[a]ND = not done.

[b]None = a control group of mice which were untreated other than being immunized with OVA/CFA. Responses were compared between relevant serum fraction recipients.

on CMI (Table 4). All detectable protein was located in fractions I and II. Immunoreactive OVA was detected only in whole serum from OVA fed mice and in fraction II of this serum. Transfer of fraction II suppressed DTH responses in recipients and there was no statistically significant suppression of DTH in animals which received serum fractions I and III.

DISCUSSION

After absorption from the gut into the serum of mice, the immunological properties of OVA are altered. The experiments described above have shown that this is not merely the result of systemic processing of antigen after its absorption into the circulation from the gut. Alteration of OVA into tolerogenic form is different from the well established changes in immunogenicity and tolerogenicity that can be produced by physicochemical modification of the protein. High doses of urea-denatured OVA induced suppression of systemic antibody responses (9). However, at the low doses used in our experiments there was no suppression of systemic antibody or CMI. Denaturation with urea does not, therefore, expose pertinent tolerogenic portions of OVA. Monomeric forms of proteins are well known tolerogens (4,5,10) and the presence of native OVA in mouse serum following OVA feeding has been reported (11). Deaggregation suppresses both humoral and cell mediated limbs of the response to native OVA and this is not entirely similar to the action of gut-processed OVA which suppressed only CMI to native OVA.

One hour after an OVA feed, the serum of mice contained immunoreactive OVA. Absorption of tolerogenic serum with Sepharose-linked anti-OVA antibodies removed immunoreactive OVA and also removed the tolerogenicity associated with the serum. Thus tolerogenic OVA in serum possesses B cell recognition structures. These 3-dimensional structures may be important for the recognition of gut-processed OVA by suppressor T cells which share the same recognition repertoire as B cells (12).

Following fractionation of tolerogenic serum by gel filtration, tolerogenic immunoreactive OVA was found only in serum fraction II which contained proteins in a M.W. range including that of native OVA. Unfortunately the precise M.W. of the tolerogen could not be determined by our method and we have not eliminated the possibility that, in fraction II, immunoreactive OVA is present as a fragment in association with another molecule such as Ia antigen. Binding of antigen to intestinal Ia has been recently proposed as a mechanism of intestinal antigen processing (13). In addition, we have not ruled out the possibility that the small decrease in DTH (not statistically significant), produced by serum fraction I, is due to the presence of non-immunoreactive fragments of OVA either aggregated together or associated with mouse serum proteins.

We suggest that intestinal processing of OVA takes the form of a subtle alteration to the native protein with exposure of suppressor determinants on the molecule, such as those described for other antigens (14), and/or loss of immunodominant epitopes (15,16). This will profoundly alter the pattern of immune responses induced by the protein *in vivo*, and illustrates the relevance of digestive processes, and of the absorptive epithelium, in the precise regulation of immunity to fed antigen.

CONCLUSIONS

1. Gut processing of OVA is distinct from systemic antigen processing, and generates circulating tolerogenic OVA.

2. Gut processed OVA in serum is not tolerogenic by virtue of being denatured nor is its tolerogenicity a feature of the systemically available antigen dose. Protein deaggregation is probably not the reason for the phenomena associated with gut processing.

3. Suppression of systemic CMI by serum obtained one hour after feeding OVA is associated with the presence of immunoreactive gut processed OVA in the serum, recognized by rabbit IgG anti-OVA.

4. Tolerogenic gut processed OVA is located predominantly in the fraction of serum which contains proteins in a M.W. range including native OVA. We have not ruled out the possibility that antigen is present in the form of fragments of OVA lacking antibody epitopes and either aggregated together or associated with mouse serum protein.

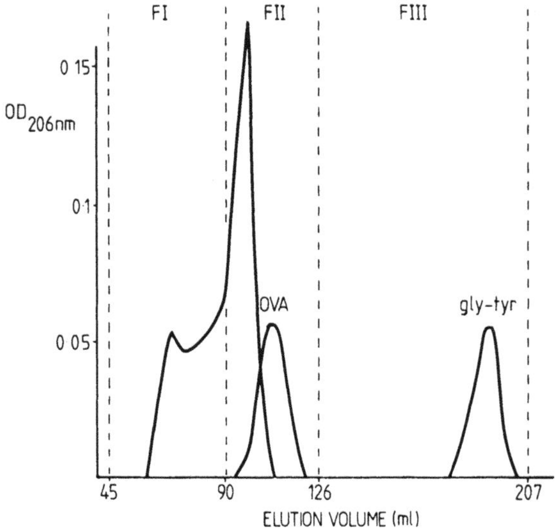

Figure 1. Elution profiles of normal mouse serum, OVA and glycyl tyrosine after gel filtration with Sephacryl S200. Fraction boundaries are indicated by broken lines.

ACKNOWLEDGEMENTS

This work has been supported by grants from the Medical Research Council and the National Fund for Research into Crippling Diseases. We thank Margaret Gordon, Hazel Drummond and staff of the Animal Unit, Western General Hospital, for their assistance. We also thank Dr. Donald G. Hanson and Dr. Allan McI. Mowat for gifts of antisera.

REFERENCES

1. Mowat, A.McI., Strobel, S., Drummond, H.E. and Ferguson, A., Immunology 45, 105, 1982.
2. Strobel, S., Mowat, A.McI., Pickering, M.G., Drummond, H.E. and Ferguson, A., Immunology 49, 451, 1983.
3. Frei, P.C., Benacerraf, B. and Thorbecke, G.J., Proc. Natl. Acad. Sci. 53, 20, 1969.
4. Lukic, M.L., Cowing, C. and Leskowitz, S., J. Immunol. 114, 503, 1975.
5. Colby, W.D. and Strejan, G.H., Eur. J. Immunol. 10, 602, 1980.
6. Chesnut, R.W., Endres, R.O. and Grey, H.M., Clin. Immunol. Immunopathol. 15, 397, 1980.

7. Bruce, M.G. and Ferguson, A., Immunology 57, 627, 1986.

8. Bruce, M.G. and Ferguson, A., Immunology 59, 295, 1986.

9. Takatsu, K. and Ishizaka K., Cell. Immunol. 20, 276, 1975.

10. Golub, E.S. and Weigle, W.O., J. Immunol. 102, 389, 1969.

11. Swarbrick, E.T., Antigen Handling by the Gut, MD Thesis. University of London, 1979.

12. Endres, R.O. and Grey, H.M., J. Immunol. 125, 1515, 1980.

13. Bland, P.W., in Topics in Gastroenterology, (Edited by Jewell, D.P. and Gibson, P.R.), 12, 225, 1985.

14. Sercarz, E.E., Yowell, R.L., Turkin, D., Miller, A., Araneo, B.A. and Adorini L., Immunol. Rev. 39, 108, 1978.

15. Berkower I., Matis, L.A., Buckenmeyer, G.K., Gurd, F.R.N., Longo, D.L. and Berzofsky, J.A., J. Immunol. 132, 1870, 1984.

16. Shimonkevitz, R., Colon, S., Kappler, J.W., Marrack, P. and Grey, H.M., J. Immunol. 133, 2067, 1984.

DELAYED RECOVERY OF ORALLY INDUCED TOLERANCE TO PROTEINS IN IRRADIATED AND SPLEEN-CELL RECONSTITUTED MICE

D.G. Hanson and T. Morimoto

Department of Pediatrics, Harvard Medical School and Combined Program in Pediatric Gastroenterology and Nutrition, Massachusetts General Hospital, Boston, MA USA; and Department of Medicine, Toneyama National Hospital, Osaka, Japan

INTRODUCTION

A single intragastric (i.g.) feeding of 20 mg of ovalbumin (OVA) or human gammaglobulin (HGG) to normal adult BDF1 mice produces specific tolerance to later parenteral immunization with the antigen. Previous work showed that the tolerance induced by feeding could subsequently be abolished by lethal whole-body irradiation. OVA-specific antibody responses were indistinguishable in normal and orally-tolerized mice that were irradiated and then injected with normal spleen cells immediately prior to immunization (1). In the present study, we examined the effects of irradiation and "reconstitution" with normal spleen cells on the induction of tolerance by OVA and HGG feeding.

MATERIALS AND METHODS

Normal adult female BDF1/J mice were irradiated from a ^{60}Co source (1000 R), reconstituted by i.v. injection of 20 million normal spleen cells between 3 h and 4 d later, and then fed saline or 20 mg of OVA in saline i.g at varied intervals thereafter. Other identically prepared mice were injected i.p. with deaggregated HGG (dHGG) (2) or fed HGG in saline. Tolerance was assessed by measurement of serum-antibody titers by Farr assays following i.p. immunization with OVA or DNP_4OVA in $Al(OH)_3$ adjuvant (1,3) or with aggregated HGG (aHGG) (2).

RESULTS

Mice that were fed OVA 1 or 2 days after irradiation and reconstitution did not develop tolerance (Fig. 1). However, OVA feeding after 3 days resulted in partial tolerance induction, and mice fed OVA after 7 days showed tolerance comparable in magnitude to that in OVA-fed normal animals. Capacity for effective tolerance induction by feeding, therefore, recovered over a period of days following irradiation and reconstitution.

We inquired whether the temporary failure of tolerance induction also applied to a parenterally injected tolerogen. Normal (non-irradiated) mice injected i.p. with 2.5 mg dHGG or fed 20 mg HGG developed similar degrees of tolerance (Fig. 2A). Mice injected with dHGG 1 day after irradiation + reconstitution developed tolerance (Fig. 2B), indicating that the reconstituting spleen cells were capable of supporting systemic tolerance within 1 day after transfer. However, irradiated + reconstituted mice did not develop tolerance after HGG feeding. The deficit in tolerance induction was, therefore, associted with exposure to antigen by the gastrointestinal route.

To determine whether recovery of tolerance was linked with reversible changes that occur in gastrointestinal mucosa after irradiation (4), the temporal relationships among irradiation, reconstitution and feeding were dissociated. Mice were reconstituted either 3 h or 4 d after irradiation, and then fed saline or OVA either 1 or 5 d after the cell transfers (Fig. 3). The results showed that recovery of tolerance was dependent upon a

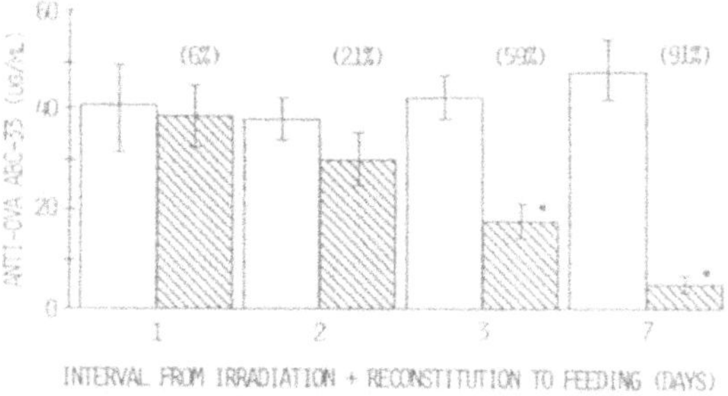

Figure 1. Recovery of orally induced tolerance following irradiation and reconstitution in BDF1 mice. Normal mice were irradiated, reconstituted within 3 h with normal spleen cells and fed saline (□) or 20 mg OVA (▨) i.g. 1, 2, 3 or 7 days later, as shown. All mice (n = 4-5/group) were immunized i.p. with 1 μg OVA + 1 mg $Al(OH)_3$ 9 and 37 days after feeding, and anti-OVA antibody titers were measured by Farr assay 2 wk after the secondary immunization. Numbers in parentheses indicate mean % suppression in OVA-fed mice. *$p < 0.01$ by planned orthogonal contrast analyses.

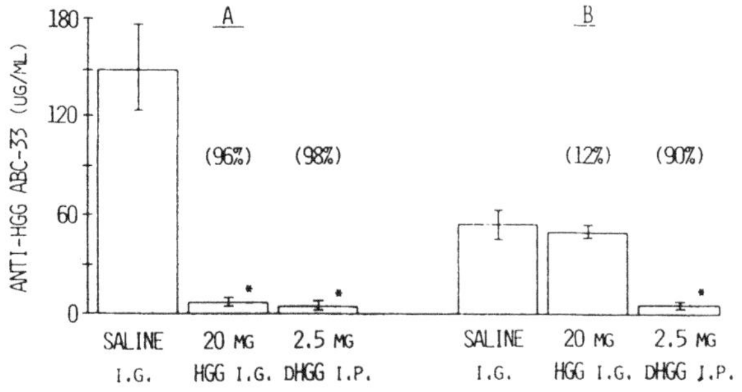

Figure 2. Comparison of orally and parenterally induced tolerance in normal mice (A) and in mice that were irradiated and reconstituted 1 day before antigen exposure (B). Mice were fed saline or 20 mg of HGG, or injected i.p. with 2.5 mg of dHGG (n = 5/group), immunized 9 and 37 days later with 400 μg aHGG, and bled for serum antibody titration after 2 wk. *$p < 0.01$, Student's _t_ test.

sufficient interval (> 1 day) between reconstitution and feeding. Allowing regeneration to proceed for 4 days in the absence of reconstitution did not reduce the additional requirement of 1 or more days for the appearance of orally induced tolerance after reconstitution. The additional time (4 days vs. 3 h) between irradiation and reconstitution did not affect the pattern of data, and accounted for less than 1% of the total variance in the experiment.

DISCUSSION

The induction of tolerance by feeding lethally irradiated mice, in addition to the need for functional lymphoid and accessory cells found in normal spleen, has critical prerequisite(s) that are not met within 48 h after those cells are supplied. Following that period the capacity for orally induced tolerance recovers gradually within approximately 5 d, and shows characteristics of the tolerance described in normal mice (5), including antigen specificity (data not shown), and depressed antibody responses to both the fed protein and an associated hapten (Fig. 3). Increasing the number of transferred spleen cells from 20 to 30 million did not improve tolerance induction by OVA feeding 2 days after irradiation + reconstitution (data not shown), indicating that the deficit was not simply due to insufficient numbers of reconstituting cells.

Whole-body irradiation produces acute degenerative changes in the intestinal mucosa as well as in other organ systems. Within 5 days following doses of irradiation comparable to that in the present study, the mucosa begins to regenerate in the absence of reconstitution with lymphoid cells (4). To determine whether a need for partial regeneration was responsible for the delay in reestablishment of orally induced tolerance (Fig. 1), we allowed 4 days for recovery after irradiation, and then tested by feeding either 1 or 5 days after reconstitution. We found that more than 1 day was required after reconstitution for induction of tolerance by feeding, irrespective of the interval between irradiation and reconstitution (Fig. 3). This observation does not rule out a role of gastrointestinal recovery in the reappearance of orally induced tolerance; however, if regeneration of the gastrointestinal or other systems is involved, then critical feature(s) of that process are dependent upon functional lymphoid cells.

Because tolerance was inducible by parenteral injection but not by feeding 1 day after reconstitution (Fig. 2), the deficiency in these animals is associated with gastrointestinal processing of antigen, and is not overcome until functional lymphoid cells are present for at least 2 days. The recovery of orally induced tolerance is, therefore, likely to be the result

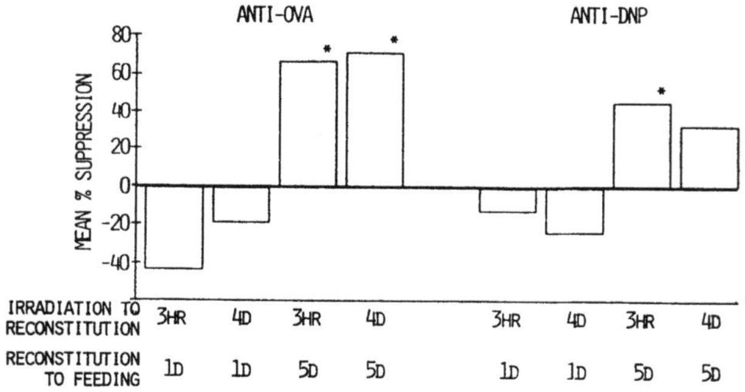

Figure 3. Effects of varying the intervals between irradiation and reconstitution, and between reconstitution and feeding, upon induction of tolerance by i.g. OVA. All mice were immunized with 1 μg DNP_4OVA in 1 mg $Al(OH)_3$ i.p. 1 wk after the feedings. Results were expressed as mean percent suppression in OVA-fed mice (n = 7/group) relative to saline-fed mice (control = 0% suppression in each test condition, n = 7/group), based on anti-OVA and anti-DNP serum antibody titers 4 wk after immunization. Separate three-way analyses of variance for anti-OVA and anti-DNP antibody responses showed no significant main effects or interactions involving the irradiation-reconstitution interval (p values > 0.18), indicating that this interval had little influence on the pattern of results. However, for both anti-OVA and anti-DNP responses there was a highly significant interaction between reconstitution-feeding interval and antigen feeding ($p < 0.01$), confirming that the effect of OVA vs saline feeding differed in mice reconstituted 5 days vs 1 day beforehand. *$p < 0.05$ by planned orthogonal contrast analyses comparing OVA-fed vs saline-fed mice.

of an interaction between irradiation-damaged gut and the reconstituting cells. The conditions that are necessary for this recovery may be related to (i) distribution of the injected cells, such as in repopulation of gut-associated lymphoid tissues (GALT), (ii) participation of (or acceleration by) spleen-derived cells in the recovery of gastrointestinal antigen-processing capabilities, and/or (iii) a direct contribution of lymphoid or reticuloendothelial cells to the processing of antigen encountered via the gut. Evidence in support of hypothesis (i) has been obtained in subsequent work showing that numbers of intraepithelial lymphocytes decreased progressively following irradiation, but remained stable in reconstituted animals. In addition, irradiation produced crypt and villous hypoplasia in the jejunum, followed by crypt hyperplasia and return to normal villous height in non-reconstituted mice. One hour after OVA feeding, the serum of irradiated + reconstituted mice contained an effective "tolerogen" capable of suppressing specific cell-mediated immune responses in normal recipients, whereas the serum of irradiated animals did not (6). These observations support the concept that "processing" of ingested OVA is an important step in the induction of tolerance by oral route, and demonstrate that spontaneous recovery of the intestinal mucosa alone is inadequate to support such processing in the absence of lymphoid cells.

CONCLUSIONS

1. Reconstitution with normal spleen cells is sufficient to restore the capacity for orally induced tolerance to proteins in lethally irradiated mice, but the restoration is not immediate: at least 3 days are required for partial recovery.

2. Spleen cells restore the expression of parenterally induced tolerance within 1 day under parallel conditions.

3. The time course of recovery of orally induced tolerance was associated with the interval between reconstitution and feeding rather than with the interval between irradiation and reconstitution.

4. Orally induced tolerance, therefore, depends upon direct or indirect contribution(s) by lymphoid/accessory cells to the processing or uptake of antigen encountered by the oral route.

ACKNOWLEDGEMENTS

This investigation was supported by U.S.P.H.S. research grants AI 13474 and AM 33506.

REFERENCES

1. Hanson, D.G., Vaz, N.M., Maia, L.C.S. and Lynch, J.M., J. Immunol. 123, 2337, 1979.
2. Chiller, J.M. and Weigle, W.O., J. Immunol. 106, 1647, 1971.
3. Hanson, D.G., J. Immunol. 127, 1518, 1981.
4. Quastler, H. and Hampton, J.C., Radiat. Res. 17, 914, 1962.
5. Hanson, D.G., Vaz, N.M., Maia, L.C.S., Hornbrook, M.M., Lynch, J.M. and Roy, C.A., Int. Arch. Allergy Appl. Immunol. 55, 526, 1977.
6. Bruce, M.G., Strobel, S., Hanson, D.G. and Ferguson, A., Intestinal antigen processing is eliminated following irradiation and is restored by normal spleen cells. (In preparation for publication)

MUCOSAL IMMUNITY AND TOLERANCE IN NEONATAL RABBITS

B.A. Peri and R.M. Rothberg

Pritzker School of Medicine
The University of Chicago
Chicago, Illinois USA

INTRODUCTION

It has been known for many years that neonatal rabbits are made tolerant by the feeding or injection of bovine serum albumin (BSA) (1-3). On the other hand, older (20+ days) orally immunized rabbit kits respond with anti-BSA production (4), primarily of the IgG subclass (5). Under some conditions, 20 d old kits from orally immunized dams are suppressed in their immune responses to either orally or parenterally administered BSA (4). A study of possible factors in milk that affect the responsiveness of neonates shows that anti-BSA of the IgG isotype is readily transferred into milk by the dam and subsequently is absorbed through the gut into the circulation of nursing kits (6). We now present further studies on the maternal regulation of the immune responses of rabbit kits to BSA and the factors involved.

MATERIALS AND METHODS

Rabbits

Cross-bred New Zealand White/Flemish rabbits from the University of Illinois "E" strain were maintained as a breeding colony in standard animal quarters and fed performance-blend Purina rabbit chow, free of bovine products. Litter size was reduced to 6-7 animals, kits began to consume food and water by 20 d of age and were weaned at 5 wk.

Antigens

Bovine serum fraction V (Sigma Chemical Corp., St. Louis, MO) was dissolved in tap water for feeding. Crystalline BSA (Reheis Chemical Co., Chicago, IL) was used for injection and was trace-labeled with ^{125}I by a modified chloramine T method for radioimmunoassay.

Immunization

Rabbits were given BSA solutions of various concentrations and at different times, as noted. Starting at 5 d of age, kits were fed BSA once daily by inducing suckling on a tubing-tipped syringe. Injection and blood sampling of 5 d old kits were performed via the intra-cardiac route. Older kits were bled from marginal ear veins. Kits were challenged 28 d after the first feeding with 5 mg BSA in incomplete Freund's adjuvant (IFA) injected intramuscularly.

Serologic determinations

Antibody was measured by precipitation with saturated ammonium sulfate and expressed as antigen binding capacity (ABC-33)/ml of serum using an ^{125}I-BSA concentration of 40 ng N/ml. The amount of BSA in samples was measured against a standard curve of the inhibition by BSA of the reaction of an anti-BSA serum and ^{125}I-BSA at 4 ng N/ml.

Statistics

All antibody determinations were done in replicate on individual samples and the mean $\pm$ SEM calculated for each group. The significance of differences between groups was determined by the Student's *t* test.

RESULTS

Effect of milk factors on immune responses on the kits

Dams were immunized by feeding 0.1% BSA for 10 days or more at various times before or during pregnancy and lactation. Kits were transferred immediately after birth between normal and immunized dams. At 20 d of age, 0.1% BSA was supplied ad libitum to both kits and dams, and kits were challenged with parenteral BSA at 48 d of age. Responses to oral BSA were variable within groups and were not significantly different when normal kits were compared with immunized kits suckled by their own dams (Fig. 1, A vs. B), in contrast to the suppression previously found in kits from orally immunized dams (4). Immunized kits suckled by normal dams (Fig. 1D) showed

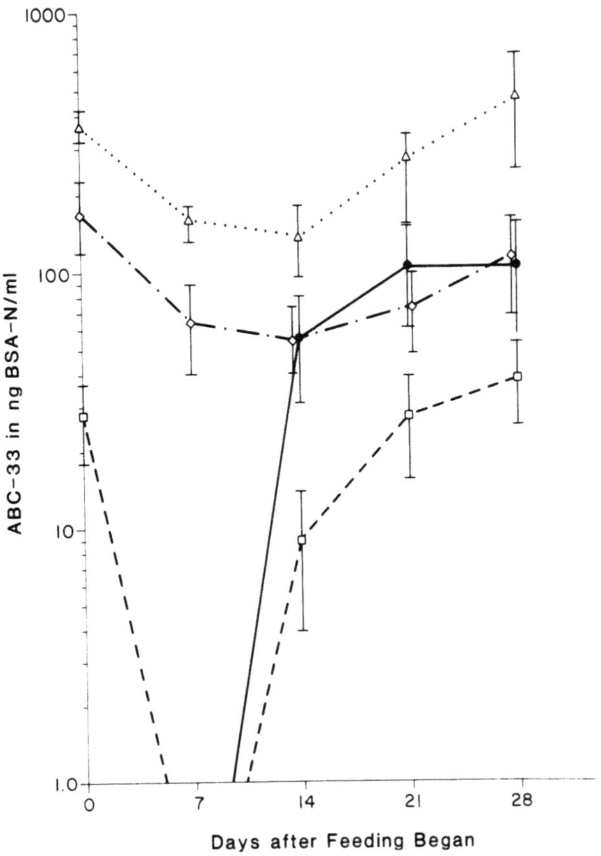

Figure 1. Anti-BSA in serum of kits fed 0.1% BSA from age 20-30 d. (A) (—•—•—) kits suckled by their own unimmunized dam (N=20); (B) (◇-•-◇) kits suckled by their own immunized dam; (C) (□---□) kits from unimmunized dams suckled by immunized dams (N=13); (D) (△....△) kits from immunized dams suckled by unimmunized dams (N=16).

significantly more antibody while the responses of normal kits were suppressed by suckling on immunized dams (Fig. 1C). Figure 2 shows responses after challenge of groups of 17-21 rabbits suckled either by their own dam or a foster dam. Significant suppression ($p < 0.05$) of the responses of the kits occurred only in the normal kits suckled by immunized dams (group B) on d 7 and 14 after challenge.

Antigen transfer into milk

Rabbit dams were fed 0.1% BSA ad libitum beginning either 3 days prepartum or 2 days postpartum. Normal adult rabbits are known to absorb a minimal amount of BSA (< 0.005 - 0.05 μg/ml of serum) (7) when similarly fed and most animals develop detectable circulating anti-BSA after 10 days.

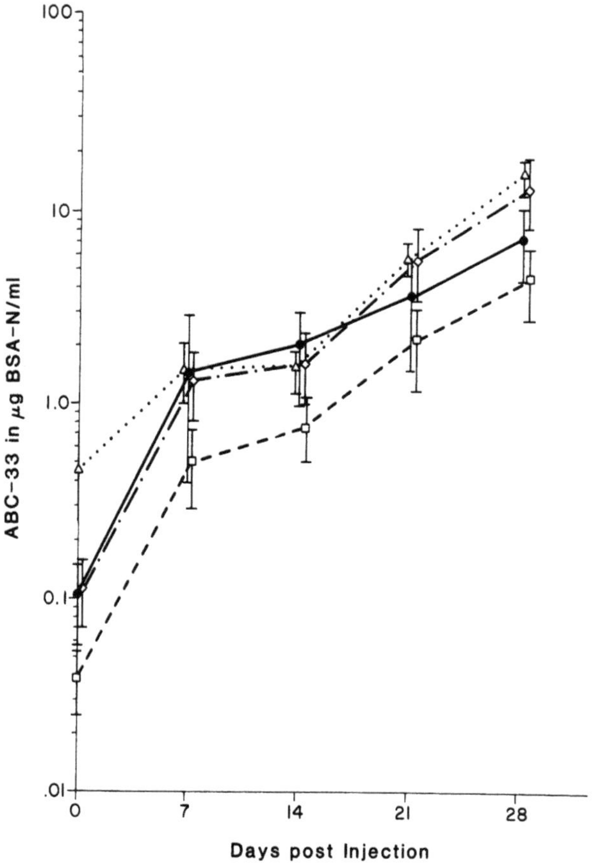

Figure 2. Anti-BSA in serum of kits fed and challenged with BSA. (A) (—•—•—) kits suckled by their own unimmunized dam (N=20); (B) (◇-·-◇) kits suckled by their own immunized dams (N=21); (C) (□---□) kits from unimmunized dams suckled by immunized dams (N=13); (D) (△....△) kits from immunized dams suckled by unimmunized dams (N=16). All kits fed 0.1% BSA from age 20-30 days, injected i.m. with 5 mg BSA in IFA at 48 days of age.

The present dams showed a similar response (Table 1) with the exception of one animal with higher BSA levels.

BSA was more concentrated in the milk than in the serum in all 5 rabbits. Since higher concentrations of BSA were desired in the milk to enable detection of small amounts of uptake by the kits, another series of dams were injected i.v. with BSA at various times postpartum. In this group (Table 2), serum BSA levels were consistently higher than those detected in milk.

<u>Antigen uptake by kits</u>

When kits were fed 0.1% BSA ad libitum between 20 and 30 d of age, BSA

Table 1. Transmission of ingested BSA into serum and milk

Dam	Day feeding began[a]	Day from delivery -2	0	2	4	6	8
592	+2		0/0[b]	0/0.3	0/0.3	0/3.0	0.01/1.0
585	+2		0/0	0/0	0/0	0/0	0.3/6.0
567	-3	0	0/0	0.01/0.2	0.08/0	0.04/0.01	0/0.01
573	-3	0.02	0/0.2	0.01/0.2	0.01/0.05	0/0	0/0
588	-3	0	0/0	0.02/0.8	0/0	0/0	0/0

[a]Dams were fed 0.1% BSA ad libitum continuously.

[b]BSA expressed as μg/ml of serum/milk; 0 = less than 0.01 μg/ml.

Table 2. Transmission of injected BSA from serum to milk

Dam[a]	1	2	3	4	5	6	8	9
589		250/53[b]			700/40	330/101		Ab/15
546		144/18		150/14			12/11	
547	240/34		170/17		110/11			22/3
549		26/5		Ab/Ab[c]				

[a]Dam 589 injected with 100 mg BSA i.v. on d 2 and 4 postpartum; Dam 546, 547, 100 mg BSA i.v. in d 6; Dam 549, 100 mg BSA i.v. on day -60 and 10 mg BSA i.v. on d 0.

[b]BSA expressed as μg/ml of serum/milk.

[c]Ab = anti-BSA detected.

concentration in the serum ranged from < 0.01 to 0.3 μg/ml, with a mean of 0.12 μg/ml, a level somewhat higher than that of the adults. To test the effect of an increased concentration of per-oral antigen on BSA uptake, kits were fed 2% BSA once daily for 10 days in an amount calculated to approximate the BSA intake of similar kits drinking 0.1% BSA ad libitum. With the 20-fold increase in concentration, 20 d old kits reached a serum level of BSA about 3-4 times that of kits fed 0.1% BSA (Table 3).

Table 3. Effect of age and peroral antigen concentration on BSA absorption

BSA fed	Age (days)	Days after feeding began			
		1	4	7	14
2%[a] daily	5-15		6.3 ± 0.75[b]	6.4 ± 0.92	2.6 ± 0.87
	20-30		0.41 ± 0.04	0.23 ± 0.11	0
single dose of 10% at 1 mg/gram body weight	5	7.8 ± 1.5			0.39 ± 0.16
	20	1.7 ± 0.6	0.27 ± 0.21	0	0

[a]5 d old kits were fed 0.5 ml, increasing gradually to 1.0 ml at 14 d; 20 d old kits were similarly fed 1.0-1.5 ml of the antigen solution.

[b]BSA expressed as μg/ml of serum: mean $\pm$ SEM of 5-8 kits, 0 = < 0.01.

However, when kits were fed the same 2% BSA at 5 d of age, the serum concentration of BSA increased greatly over that observed in the 20 d old kits. To enable comparison with similar studies in mice, another group of kits was given a single dose of BSA at either 5 or 20 d of age. Again (Table 3), the BSA absorption in 5 d old kits was much greater than in the 20 d old littermates.

Effect of age at BSA ingestion upon immune responses

Kits from the above group fed 2% BSA were challenged 28 days after BSA ingestion, starting with 5 mg BSA in IFA, injected i.m. When compared to kits given only the parenteral antigen challenge at the same age (Fig. 3A), kits fed at 20 days (Fig. 3B) responded as well, or slightly better. The anti-BSA responses of kits ingesting BSA at 5 d of age (Fig. 3D) were very significantly suppressed over those of control kits (Fig. 3C).

Effect of timing of i.v. immunization of the dam

Kits were fed 0.1% BSA from 20-30 d of age and parenterally challenged 28 days later. Anti-BSA responses following the injection were slightly increased when kits were fed before the challenge (Fig. 4, B vs. A). When the dam was given 100 mg BSA i.v. immediately postpartum, the kits were exposed to BSA in the milk for the first 10 days (Table 2). Anti-BSA was detected in milk after the period of known maximum antibody absorption by

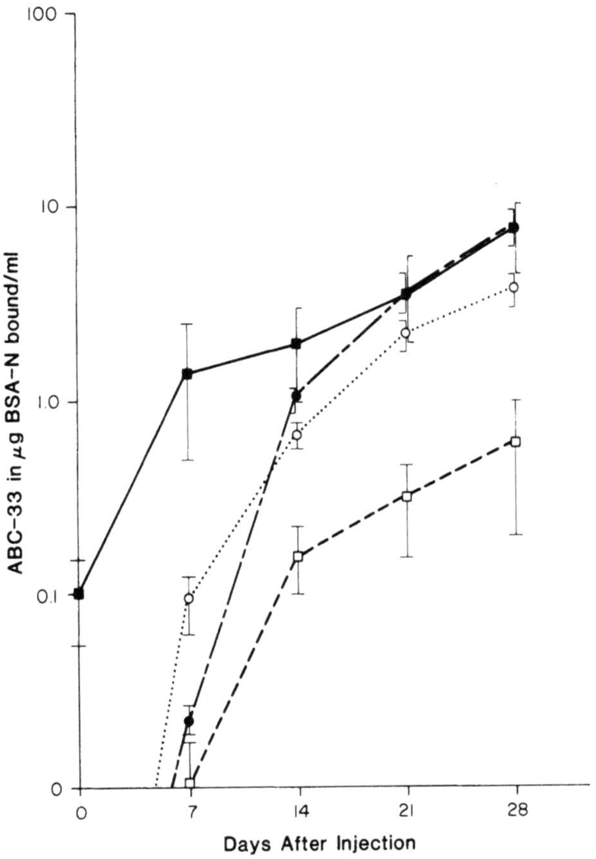

Figure 3. Effect of age at antigen ingestion. (A) (O....O) kits injected only at 48 d; (B) (■——■) kits fed age 20-30 d, injected age 48 d; (C) (●— - —●) kits injected only at 33 d; (D) (□---□) kits fed age 5-15 d, injected at 33 d. Kits 5 d old were fed 2% BSA once daily 10-20 mg/day, injected with 4 mg BSA: 20 d old kits were fed 2% BSA daily at 20-30 mg/day, injected with 5 mg BSA.

kits (6) and the responses of the kits were suppressed (Fig. 4C). A dam immunized i.v. with 100 mg BSA 2 months previously, followed by 10 mg i.v. at the time of delivery (Table 2, Dam #549) had very small amounts of BSA in milk for 4 days, followed by high levels of anti-BSA in the milk during the next 8 days, when kits could readily absorb antibody. These kits (Fig. 4D) responded significantly better than did the control animals (4B).

Effect of dam's immunization schedule on responses of the kits

In Figure 5, the relationship between the antibody concentrations of the dams and the responses of cross-suckled, unimmunized kits is examined (Experiment 1). The kits of group B absorbed little, if any, anti-BSA

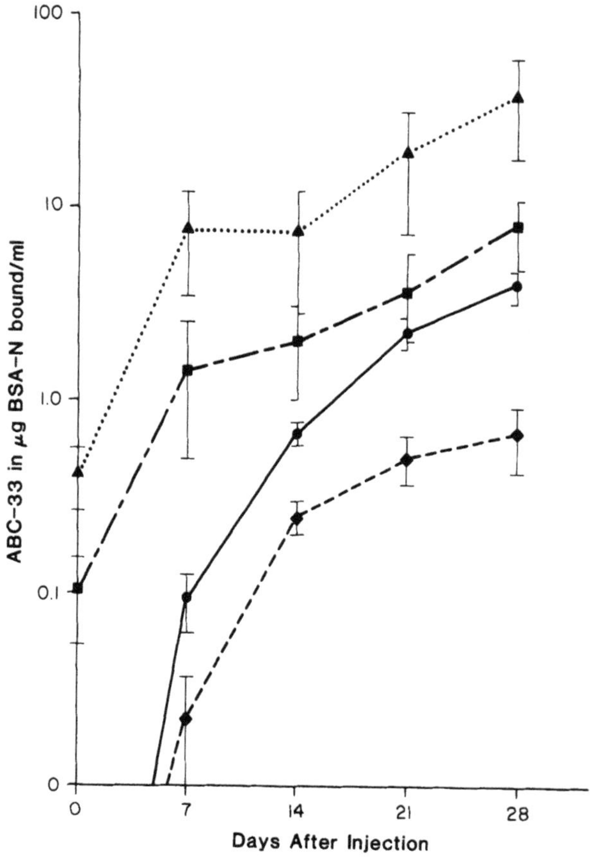

Figure 4. Immune responses of kits ingesting BSA transferred from their dam in milk. (A) (●——●) kits injected only (N=8); (B) (■— — —■) kits on normal dam (N=20); (C) (◆---◆) dam i.v. immunized at delivery (N=11); (D) (▲....▲) dam i.v. immunized before and at delivery (4). Kits B-D were fed 0.1% BSA from 20-30 d of age and injected i.m. with 5 mg BSA d 48.

from the foster dam's milk, only 2 of 7 kits made detectable anti-BSA after BSA ingestion and their responses to parenteral challenge were suppressed. The kits of group C had ingested more anti-BSA in the milk, still had detectable antibody when feeding began, and all kits showed increased anti-BSA levels after feeding. Their responses to the antigenic challenge were equal to those of control animals (A vs. C). Kits born to and suckled by their own highly immunized dam (Fig. 6B) had higher levels of anti-BSA derived both pre- and post-natally, and responded to feeding and challenge as well as control kits (Fig. 6A and Fig. 5C). However, kits from dams immunized orally during pregnancy, with lower antibody in milk (6C), showed the suppression previously observed with immunized dams (4).

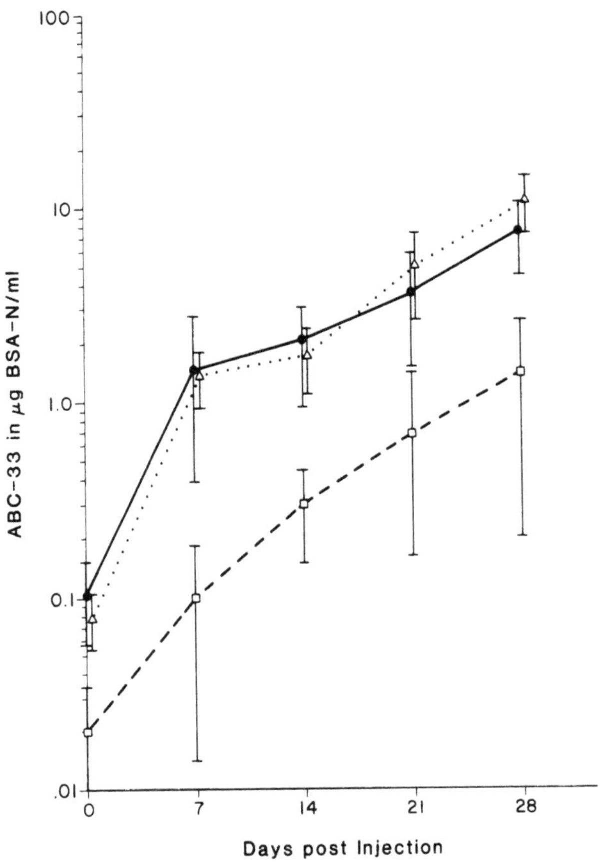

Figure 5. Immune responses of kits from unimmunized dams suckled by immunized dams. (A) (●——●) kits suckled by own unimmunized dam (N=20); (B) (□- -□) kits suckled by dams with low anti-BSA (N=7); (C) (Δ....Δ) kits suckled by a dam with high anti-BSA (N=5). All kits were fed 0.1% BSA at age 20-30 d, injected i.m. with 5 mg BSA in IFA at age 48 d.

DISCUSSION

The initial cross-suckling experients produced much less maternal regulation (Figs. 1A and 2A) than previously observed (4). Variable factors that might explain this discrepancy include antibody transfer, shown previously (6), and different degrees of antigen absorption by kits. Dams absorbing small quantities of BSA after ingesting 0.1% BSA concentrated the antigen from serum into milk, while animals given high serum BSA levels by injection had lower serum/milk ratios. This suggests an active transport mechanism which can be overloaded. Antigen uptake by kits from milk into serum was also affected by the concentration ingested, although not

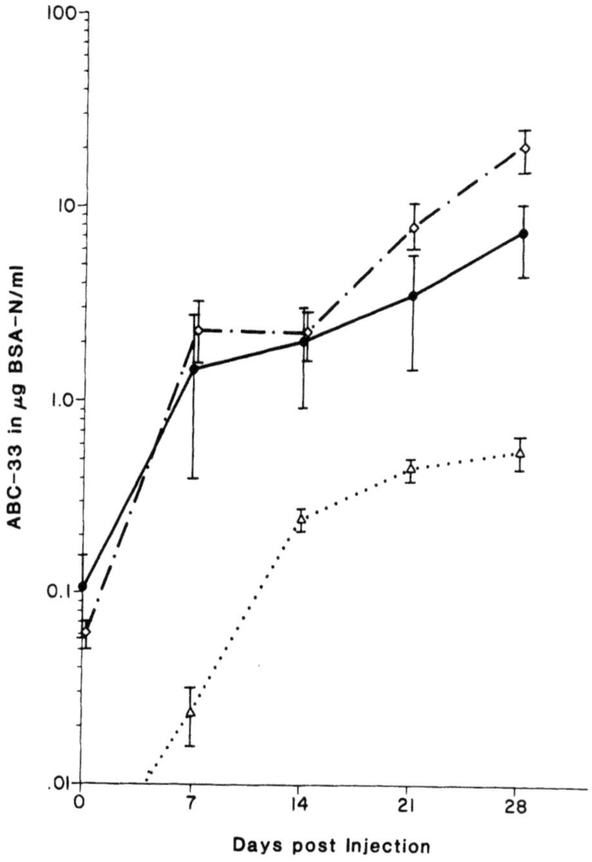

Figure 6. Immune responses of kits suckled by their own immunized dams. (A) (●——●) kits suckled on their own unimmunized dam (N=20); (B) (◇-·-◇) kits suckled by their own dam immunized orally 3 months previously and during pregnancy (N=5); (c) (△....△) kits suckled by their own dams immunized orally during pregnancy (N=10). All kits were fed 0.1% BSA at age 20-30 d and injected i.m. with 5 mg BSA in IFA at age 48 d.

proportionately. The age of the kit being fed had a major effect on the amount of antigenically active BSA absorbed through the gut. Five d old kits absorbed much more antigen than 20 d old animals, as had been the case with anti-BSA absorption (6). However, at given concentrations, much more antibody than antigen was absorbed (6), although the IgG molecule is larger, suggesting the possibility that different mechanisms of transport are involved.

When other factors were similar, the immune responses of kits ingesting BSA at 5 d of age were suppressed, as often reported by others (1-3).

This might be explained as a simple "high-dose tolerance," since more antigen is absorbed. When the effects of the presence of antibody in the milk are compared, this suppression appears to be overcome or prevented (Fig. 4D), depending on when antibody appears in the milk. Passive anti-BSA seems to have no effect on immune response in adult rabbits (8) or human infants (9). When kits from cross-suckling experiments were divided according to the amounts of anti-BSA ingested, dams with low antibody content in the milk suppressed their kits while milk with high titers appeared to enhance the immune responses (Figs. 5 and 6). Possible factors involved include the effect of antigen-antibody complexes, interference by antibody with antigen absorption (10), or unknown factors produced by dams during primary responses.

Immune responses to oral protein in mice appear to be rather different from those in rabbits (11) and man (12,13). Mice fed ovalbumin (OVA) during the first week after birth are primed, yet tolerance is produced by the same protocol at 3 or more weeks of age (14,15). Priming or tolerance in neonates is induced by varying dosage of human gammaglobulin (HGG) (14). Neonatal rabbits absorb less protein through the gut than do mice, and absorption of BSA or OVA in mice differs (16). Thus, it appears that generalizations from mouse models using different proteins are unwise and further concomitant study of the mouse and rabbit seem important.

CONCLUSIONS

Rabbit dams fed BSA absorb and transfer BSA into the milk, and rabbit kits absorb small amounts of ingested BSA during the first week after birth. Absorption is greatly decreased by 20 d of age. The immune responses of kits to feeding or parenteral challenge may be suppressed if antigen is ingested at 5 d; however, enhancement results if antibody is present in the milk at high levels. Maternal regulation of the responses of the kits appears to correlate with the anti-BSA concentration in the milk or other still unidentified factors involved in the immune responses of the dam.

REFERENCES

1. Filipp, G. and Boros, R., J. Allergy, 39, 167, 1967.

2. Pinckard, R.M., Halonen, M. and Meng, A., J. Allergy Clin. Immunol. 49, 301, 1972.
3. Rieger, C.H.L., Gulden, P. and Byrd, D.J., Immunobiology 160, 330, 1981.
4. Peri, B.A. and Rothberg, R.M., J. Immunol. 127, 2520, 1981.
5. Peri, B.A., Theodore, C.M., Losonsky, G.A., Fishaut, J.M., Rothberg, R.M. and Ogra, P.L., Clin. Exp. Immunol. 48, 91, 1982.
6. Peri, B.A. and Rothberg, R.M., Immunology 57, 49, 1986.
7. Rothberg, R.M., Kraft, S.C. and Farr, R.S., J. Immunol. 98, 386, 1967.
8. Rieger, C.H.L., Kraft, S.C. and Rothberg, R.M., J. Immunol. 124, 1789, 1980.
9. Muller, W., Lippmann, A. and Rieger, C.H.L., Pediatr. Res. 17, 724, 1983.
10. Harmatz, P.R., Bloch, K.J., Kleinman, R.F., Walsh, M.K. and Walker, W.A., Immunology 57, 43, 1986.
11. Silverman, G.A., Peri, B.A. and Rothberg, R.M., Develop. Comp. Immunol. 6, 737, 1982.
12. Rothberg, R.M. and Farr, R.S., Pediatrics 35, 571, 1965.
13. Rothberg, R.M., J. Pediatr. 75, 391, 1969.
14. Hanson, D.G., J. Immunol. 127, 1518, 1981.
15. Strobel, S. and Ferguson, A., Pediatr. Res. 18, 588, 1984.
16. Harmatz, P.R., Hanson, D.G., Walsh, M.K., Kleinman, R.E., Bloch, K.J. and Walker, W.A., Am. J. Physiol. E, 227-233, 1986.

ABNORMALITIES OF ORAL TOLERANCE IN NZB/W FEMALE MICE: RELATIONSHIP OF ANTIBODIES TO DIETARY ANTIGENS IN HUMAN SYSTEMIC LUPUS ERYTHEMATOSUS

R.I. Carr, D. Tilley, S. Forsyth and D. Sadi

Division of Rheumatology, Department of Medicine
Dalhousie University, Halifax, Nova Scotia
Canada B3H 2Y9

INTRODUCTION

We have found a significant increase in antibodies to bovine gamma globulin (BGG) in patients with systemic lupus erythematosus (SLE) (1). Conversely, their levels of antibodies to ovalbumin (OVA) are within the normal range (Table 1). Since both BGG and OVA are commonly ingested antigens, it was of interest to assess the levels of antibodies to bovine casein, an antigen which is the predominant protein of milk, and therefore is also a commonly ingested antigen. We discovered that SLE patients have a significant increase in anti-casein antibodies (Table 1). Thus, although they have normal levels of antibody to one dietary antigen they have high levels to two others. In view of the phenomenon of oral tolerance (reviewed in 2), which presumably would suppress the development of excess circulating antibodies directed against dietary antigens, these findings raised the possibility that an antigen specific failure of oral tolerance might occur in SLE. We decided to begin our assessment of the likelihood of defective oral tolerance in SLE by studying the responses of NZB/W mice, one of several murine models of SLE (3).

MATERIALS AND METHODS

Antigen

Bovine gamma globulin was purchased from Miles (Kankakee, IL) (Fraction II) and further purified by DEAE chromatography. ^{125}I-BGG was prepared

Table 1. Antibodies to OVA and casein in normal human controls and in patients with Systemic Lupus Erythematosus (SLE)

Ova Binding			
	Normal Sera	32.7 ± 21.8^a	
	SLE Sera	21.8 ± 17.3	$p > 0.05$
Casein Binding			
	Normal Sera	20.5 ± 9.2	
	SLE Sera	42.5 ± 15.5	$p < 0.05$

[a]Mean percentage binding of 25 ng ^{125}I-OVA or ^{125}I-Casein by 100 µl of a 1:10 dilution of 25 normal sera and 47 SLE sera.

using a standard chloramine-T labeling protocol. OVA (Sigma Chemical Co., St. Louis, MO) was labeled as described by Ishizaka and Okudaira (4). Cow's milk casein was purchased from Calbiochem-Behring (San Diego, CA) and used without further purification. The casein was labeled with ^{125}I using chloramine T.

Mice

BDF_1 (DBA/2 x C57BL/6) and NZB/W (NZB x NZW) females were bred in our animal care facilities using breeders purchased from Jackson Laboratories (Bar Harbor, ME). Age and sex matched females were used in all the studies reported.

Normal diet mice

Except for the casein free mice (see below), the mice used in these studies were bred and maintained on Rodent Laboratory Chow 5001 (Ralston Purina, Richmond, IN).

Casein free mice

Because most normal mouse chows contain casein, which interfered with experimental study of oral tolerance induction by casein (4), in these experiments, beginning one month prior to mating, parental mice were put on a chow free of bovine casein (Diet #TD 83109, Teklad, Madison, WI). During gestation, nursing, and throughout the experiment, the progeny were maintained on the same casein free diet. These mice were thus never exposed to bovine casein and will be referred to as casein-free mice.

Experimental induction of tolerance

Groups of 5-6 mice were given the proteins by gastric intubation. One month old mice were given 5 mg BGG or casein, or 10 mg OVA; 4 month old mice were given 10 mg BGG or casein, or 20 mg OVA. Some groups of mice, used as feeding controls, received saline alone. BDF_1 mice were used as a normal strain control. The tube feeding was performed once (OVA) or once daily for 3 days (BGG) or 4 days (casein).

Assessment of oral tolerance development

Seven days after the commencement of feeding, the mice were immunized with the appropriate antigen in Complete Freund's Adjuvant. Fourteen days later, they were bled and boosted and after another seven days the mice were exsanguinated.

Detection of circulating antibodies

Antibodies were detected with a standard radioimmunoassay (5) using ammonium sulphate as the precipitating agent for the anti-OVA assays, and PEG 6000 (Baker Chemical Co.) for the anti-casein and anti-BGG assays. Results were calculated as described by Minden and Farr (5).

Tests of significance

The Mann-Whitney non-parametric "U" test was used (6).

RESULTS

Attempts to induce oral tolerance in NZB/W females with BGG or OVA

As shown in Table 2, although 1 month old NZB/W females tolerized normally to BGG, 4 month old mice did not, and, in fact, were significantly primed by their oral exposure, since they had a 7 fold higher response to parenteral immunization than the saline fed controls. Conversely, with OVA as the test antigen, the NZB/W females tolerized normally at both 1 (data not shown) and 4 months of age.

Studies of casein

The study of oral tolerance with casein requires the mice to be on a special casein free diet, since normal mouse chow contains immunologically significant amounts of casein (7). The first question we asked was, will NZB/W mice, raised on the usual diet, be normally tolerized to casein? Indeed, both 1 month and 4 month old NZB/W female mice raised on the casein

Table 2. Antibodies to BGG or OVA in 1 and 4 month old NZB/W and BDF_1 mice after feeding followed by 2 i.p. immunizations

	Saline Fed Controls	Fed BGG
1 month old mice:		
BDF_1	43.6 ± 12.6[a]	8.3 ± 3.6
NZB/W	5.4 ± 2.8	1.1 ± 0.5

$p < .05$ for both strains and in the same direction (i.e. oral tolerance was induced in both).

	Saline Fed Controls	Fed BGG
4 month old mice:		
BDF_1	35.5 ± 16.4	3.9 ± 1.4
NZB/W	43.4 ± 14.1	204.8 ± 150

$p < .05$ for both strains but in opposite directions (i.e. oral tolerance was induced in the BDF_1's but the NZB/W's were primed).

	Saline Fed Controls	Fed OVA
4 month old mice:		
$C57Bl_6$	157 ± 50	58.2 ± 21.3
NZB/W	552 ± 254	88.7 ± 43.1

$p < .01$ for both strains and in the same direction (i.e. oral tolerance was induced in both).

[a]Results are expressed as μg antigen bound per ml of undiluted serum (ABC_{33}).

free diet showed a significantly higher response to parenteral immunization with casein, than those raised on the normal diet. As can be seen in Table 3, at both ages studied NZB/W females had been tolerized by the casein contained in the normal mouse chow. The second question assessed was, will casein-free NZB/W's orally tolerize using a protocol which tolerizes normal mice. As shown in Table 4, the results indicate that both at 1 and 4 months of age, casein-free NZB/W mice diet do not tolerize normally when fed casein experimentally. This could be due to a dose effect or to the fact that the normal diet mice are exposed to casein prior to one month of age. Preliminary studies suggest that it is the age of first exposure which is critical (data not shown) but further studies are required to verify this.

Table 3. Antibodies to casein after i.p. immunization in mice raised on normal mouse chow compared to those raised on casein-free chow

	Normal Diet	Casein free Diet
1 Month Old Mice		
BDF_1	2.8 ± 1.1[a]	11.0 ± 1.8[b]
NZB/W	1.8 ± 1.3	20.0 ± 13.9[b]
4 Month Old Mice		
BDF_1	1.8 ± 0.9	9.5 ± 2.4[c]
NZB/W	1.6 ± 1.2	13.3 ± 8.0[b]

[a]Results expressed as ABC_{33}.

[b]$P < 0.01$.

[c]$P < 0.05$.

Both BDF_1 and NZB/W females appear tolerized by the dietary content of casein when exposed to it prior to 1 month of age.

DISCUSSION

Abnormal levels of antibodies to dietary antigens are associated with a number of diseases. We have found that SLE patients have elevated antibodies to BGG and Casein, but normal levels of antibodies to OVA. We wondered whether this represented an antigen specific failure or oral tolerance in these patients. Directly studying oral tolerance to common dietary antigens in humans would not be readily possible because of prior dietary exposure and the undesirability of immunizing such individuals to assess orally induced suppression to common dietary substances. Therefore, we examined the development of oral tolerance in female NZB/W mice, which at about 4 months of age, uniformly develop a murine analog of human SLE. Indeed, we found that there is an antigen specific failure of oral tolerance in these mice, which is related to the age of first exposure, and which appears to parallel the abnormalities of anti-dietary antibodies we have found in the patients. Of considerable interest, while these studies were underway, Miller and colleagues reported antigen specific defective oral tolerance in NZB, BXSB and MRL/lpr/lpr mice, which are also considered to be models of human SLE. They did not study casein, but found abnormalities of oral tolerance to BGG and/or OVA depending on the mouse strain (8).

Table 4. Antibodies to casein after experimental feeding of casein to 1 and 4 month old casein-free mice, followed by i.p. immunization

	Saline Fed	Casein Fed
1 Month Old Mice		
BDF_1	11.5 ± 3.6^a	1.9 ± 0.9^b
NZB/W	20.0 ± 13.9	38.4 ± 10.2^c
4 Month Old Mice		
BDF_1	12.5 ± 2.2	2.3 ± 1.2^b
NZB/W	13.3 ± 8.0	21.5 ± 14.2

[a]Results expressed as ABC_{33}.

[b]$P < 0.01$.

[c]$P < 0.05$.

Although casein free BDF_1 mice are tolerized by the experimental feeding protocol, NZB/W females are primed at 1 month of age and, although the increase is not statistically significant when prefed at 4 months of age, they clearly do not orally tolerize at this time with casein.

CONCLUSIONS

Normally, there is an active mechanism to suppress systemic immune responses to ingested antigens, the phenomenon of oral tolerance. The results presented above are compatible with the possibility that there is an antigen specific failure of oral tolerance in human SLE. Further studies to understand the nature of the defect(s) in these mice might lead to a greater understanding of the abnormalities in SLE, and perhaps in other illnesses in which increased antibodies to dietary antigens have been detected. In addition, considering the fact that the gut is the body's major site of exposure to foreign antigens (many of which cross-react with an animal's self-antigens), a full examination of any defects in immune responses to ingested antigens may significantly contribute to our understanding of a number of auto-immune diseases.

ACKNOWLEDGEMENTS

This work was supported by grants from the Arthritis Society (Canada) and the Long Island, Louisiana, Michigan and New York City (SLE Foundation Inc.) chapters of The Lupus Foundation of America, Inc.

REFERENCES

1. Carr, R.I., Wold, R.T. and Farr, R.S., J. Allergy Clin. Immunol. 50, 18, 1974.
2. Stokes, C.R., in Local Immune Responses of the Gut (Edited by T.J. Newby and C.R. Stokes), p 97, CRC Press, Inc., Boca Raton, 1984.
3. Theofilopoulos, A. and Dixon, F.J., Adv. Immunol. 37, 269, 1985.
4. Ishizaka, K. and Okudaira, H., J. Immunol. 110, 1067, 1973.
5. Minden, P. and Farr, R.S., in Handbook of Experimental Immunology, Vol. I. Immunochemistry, (Edited by D.M. Weir), 3rd Edition, p 13.1, Blackwell Scientific Publications, London, 1978.
6. Siegel, S., Nonparametric Statistics for the Behavioral Sciences, McGraw-Hill, New York, 1956.
7. Carr, R.I., Hardtke, M.A., Katilus, J. and Sadi, D., Clin. Immun. Immunopath., 40, 497, 1986.
8. Miller, M.L., Cowdery, J.S., Laskin, C.A., Curtin, M.F. and Steinberg, A.D., Clin. Immunol. Immunopath. 31, 231, 1984.

EFFECT OF SUBSTANCE P ON HUMAN LYMPHOCYTE PROLIFERATION *IN VITRO*: A COMPARISON BETWEEN NORMAL AND BIRCH POLLEN ALLERGIC INDIVIDUALS

G. Nilsson, S. Rak and S. Ahlstedt

Department of Immunology, Pharmacia Diagnostics AB, Uppsala, Lung Clinic, Central Hospital, Västerås, and Department of Clinical Immunology, University of Gothenburg, Gothenburg, Sweden

INTRODUCTION

The hyperreactivity in allergic patients has been proposed to be a consequence of a wide range of effector mechanisms, including both the autonomous and the immune systems. In 1968, Szentivanyi proposed in his beta-adrenergic blockade theory that bronchial hyperreactivity and related atopic abnormalities might be caused by a decreased beta-adrenergic responsiveness (1). Such abnormality has also been found in the lymphocyte populations, which exhibit different reactivity to beta-adrenergic compounds compared with that of the cells of normal individuals (2). Lymphocytes from atopic patients also seem to have altered reactivity to mediators from inflammatory cells (3).

Besides the cholinergic and the adrenergic innervation of the airways there is a non-cholinergic, non-adrenergic, peptidergic system (4). Peptidergic innervation of the lower respiratory tract has been shown in a number of mammals including man (5). The peptidergic system can induce bronchoconstriction, bronchial mucosal oedema and mucus hypersecretion. The family of tachykinins, including Substance P and Substance K, has attracted interest as being possible transmittors of this system.

Substance P (SP) is present in the terminals of primary sensory neurones. These are distributed in the mucus membrane, adjacent to the mediator-releasing cells involved in allergy and immunity, including mast cells and lymphocytes. SP binds to both lymphocytes (6) and macrophages (7). The effect of binding to lymphocytes has been reported by some investigators to stimulate proliferation of human peripheral blood T cells (8) and mouse lymphoid cells (9). However, all investigators have not been able to confirm this effect (10). SP also binds to mast cells (11) and possesses a secretagogue effect. However, differences exist between mucosal mast cells and peritoneal mast cells in their responsiveness to the peptide (12). Thus, a firm link has been proposed between the sensory nerves in the mucosa and the immune system in evoking allergic inflammatory disorders.

This presentation deals with the effect of SP on the proliferation of peripheral blood lymphocytes from normal individuals and from patients suffering from atopic disease and hyperreactivity to birch pollen. The allergic patients were studied both before and during season.

MATERIALS AND METHODS

Peripheral blood lymphocytes (PBL) were prepared from venous blood from 15 normal individuals and 16 atopic individuals. The allergic patients with birch pollen induced rhinitis were documented with a skin prick test and a nasal provocation test. Blood was separated on Ficoll-Paque (Pharmacia AB) gradients. Lymphocytes were resuspended in RPMI 1640 (Dutch mod.) supplemented with 10% FCS, 2 mM Glutamine, 5×10^{-5} M 2-Mercaptoethanol and 100 µg/ml Garamycin (Flow). Cell cultures were established in flat-bottomed microtiter plates (Costar), 2×10^{5} cells in 200 µl per well, and stimulated with 3 µg/ml Con A (Pharmacia AB) and various concentrations, 10^{-9} - 10^{-6} M, of Substance P (Sigma). PBL were cultivated for 72 hours. Six hours prior to terminating the culture, 1 µCi/well of ^{3}H-Thymidine (New England Nuclear) was added and the incorporation of ^{3}H-Thymidine into cellular DNA was determined. The proliferative response of cells incubated with SP was expressed as a percent change of those incubated without SP. Statistical significance was assessed using the Chi-square test.

RESULTS

The median proliferation of PBL from normal individuals, simultaneously stimulated with Con A 3 µg/ml and SP 10^{-9} - 10^{-6} M, was close to +/- 10% of control. However, the response of the cells from 6 out of 15 individuals

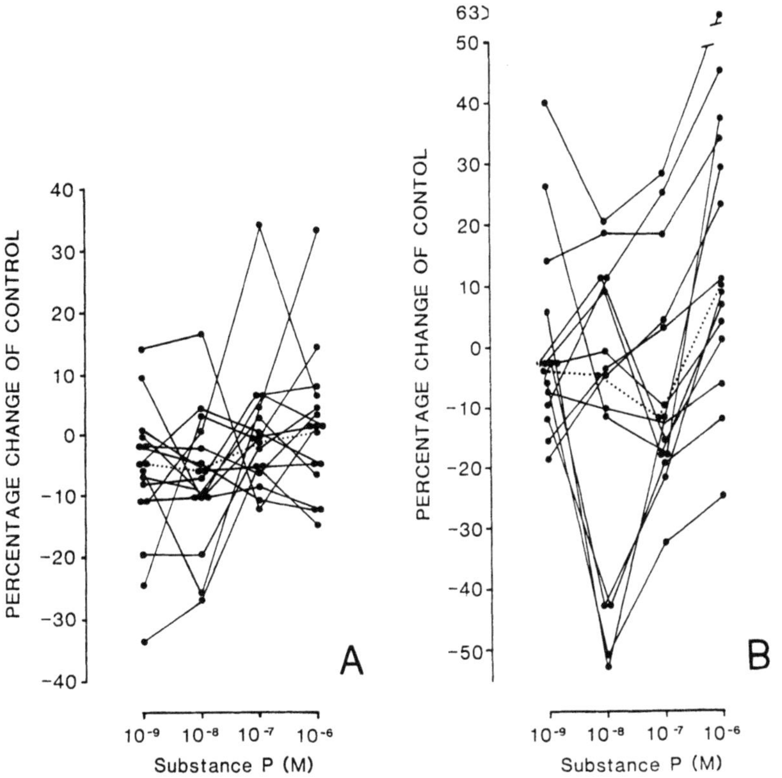

Figure 1. Proliferation of PBLs from normal individuals (a) and birch pollen allergic patients sampled during season (b), after stimulation with Con A 3 µg/ml and SP 10^{-9} - 10^{-6} M. The results are expressed as a percentage change of cells unexposed to SP. The dotted line represents the median value.

was more affected, either enhanced or depressed (Fig. 1A). The response of cells from atopics, sampled during birch pollen season, was even more affected than those of cells sampled before season and those cells from normal individuals (Fig. 1B). During birch pollen season the responses of the PBL from 4 out of 14 of the patients were profoundly depressed by SP at a concentration of 10^{-8} M and 6 out of 14 were substantially enhanced at a concentration of 10^{-6} M. Such alterations were never seen with cells from normal individuals.

When the concentration of SP was increased from 10^{-7} M to 10^{-6} M, the response of PBL from 8 out of 15 normal individuals showed an increased proliferation. In the other 7 cases there were decreased responses, giving an unchanged mean value, the mean ± SD being 2% ± 14 of the response without the addition of SP (Fig. 2A). The response of PBL from allergic patients showed a more enhanced proliferation rate when increasing the SP concentra-

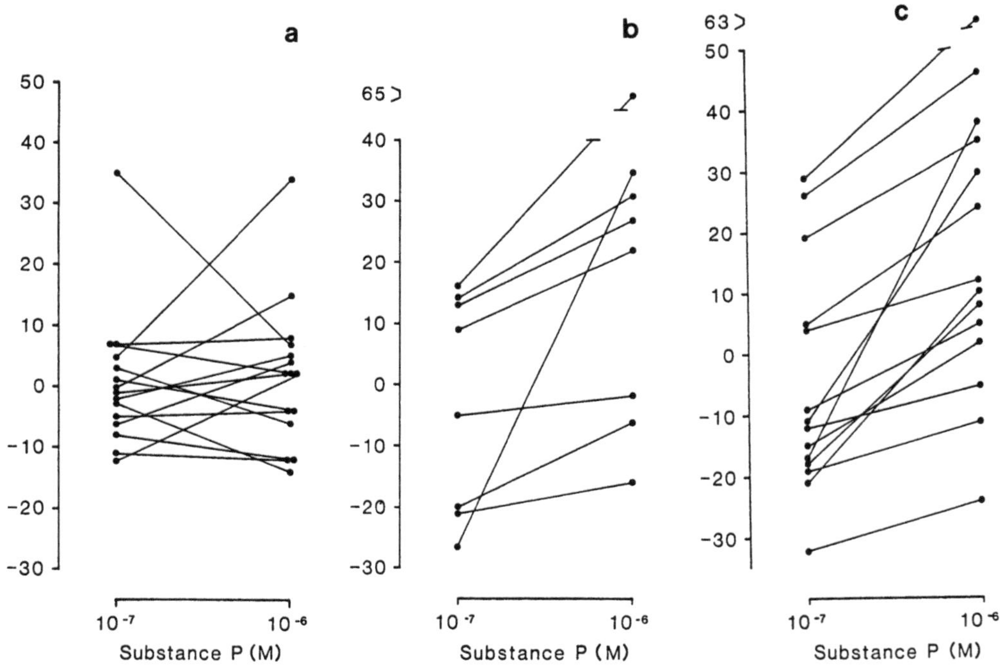

Figure 2. Proliferation rate to Con A 3 µg/ml and SP 10^{-7} or 10^{-6} M of PBLs from normal individuals (a), allergic patients sampled before season (b) and allergic patients sampled during season (c). The results are expressed as a percentage change of cells unexposed to SP. The difference between normal individuals and allergic patients, before and during season, in their responses to SP was statistically significant ($p < 0.05$, respectively $p < 0.01$).

tion. All 8 birch pollen allergics, sampled before season, had an increased proliferation response, the mean ± SD being 22% ± 21% (Fig. 2B). During season the same pattern was seen with all 14 patients that were investigated. The cells from them showed increasing proliferative response, the mean ± SD being 22% ± 14 (Fig. 2C). This alteration by SP on the response of PBL from allergic patients, before and during season, was significantly stronger than the effect of SP on the response of PBL from normal individuals ($p < 0.05$, respectively, $p < 0.01$).

DISCUSSION

Lymphocytes from allergic patients have been shown to respond to mediators involved in the allergic reaction. Thus, a change in the number of beta-adrenergic receptors has been demonstrated on lymphocytes from atopic subjects (2), and hence a change in their ability to respond to transmittors from the adrenergic system.

In this study, we found an increased sensitivity to Substance P of lymphocytes from allergic patients compared with normal individuals. Even though there was a great heterogeneity between the individuals in their proliferation response to SP, all of the allergic patients increased their proliferative rate when the SP concentration was increased from 10^{-7} - 10^{-6}M. The mean proliferation rate of lymphocytes from allergic patients sampled before and during season, respectively, differed little. Cells from four patients sampled during season, however, showed at a SP concentration of 10^{-8} M a suppression of their proliferation rate to about 50%. The results of SP effects on lymphocytes from normal individuals showed much weaker, and above all, more heterogeneous effects than reported by Payan et al. (8). The reason for this is not obvious, although influences of culture conditions and selection of patients cannot be excluded.

Release of SP from afferent neurones, innervating the mucosal membranes, results in a modulation of the immunity and hypersensitivity (13). Hence, when mucosal membranes are exposed to allergen, the neurones will be stimulated and SP released. Cells in the environment, e.g., lymphocytes and mast cells, will be affected by the peptide. This may be one mechanism which in concert with others may create the clinical symptomology seen in allergic patients suffering from hyperreactivity to birch pollen.

The firm link between such interplay between tachykinins and lymphocytes was not demonstrated in this study however. Thus, we could not demonstrate any relationship between the degree of the effect of SP on the lymphocyte proliferation and clinical symptoms of the individual patients. Nevertheless, the difference between allergic and non-allergic subjects, in their lymphocyte sensitivity to SP, may reflect that SP is involved in the mechanism of hyperreactivity in allergic patients, not only as a bronchoconstrictory agent but also as an immunologically active mediator.

REFERENCES

1. Szentivanyi, A., J. Allergy 42, 203, 1968.
2. Meurs, H., Koëter, G.H., de Vries, K. and Kauffman, H.F., J. Allergy Clin. Immunol. 70, 272, 1982.
3. Beer, D.J., Osband, M.E., McCaffrey, R.P., Soter, N.A. and Rocklin, R.E., N. Engl. J. Med. 306, 454, 1982.

4. Barnes, P.J., Thorax 39, 561, 1984.

5. Lundberg, J.M., Hökfeldt, T., Martling, C.-R., Saria, A. and Cuello, C., Cell Tissue Res. 235, 251, 1984.

6. Payan, D.G., Brewster, D.R., Missirian-Bastian, A. and Goetzl, E.J., J. Clin. Invest. 74, 1532, 1984.

7. Hartung, H.P., Wolters, K., Stoll, G. and Toyka, K.V., in Substance P: Metabolism and Biological Actions, (Edited by Jordan, C.C. and Oehme, P.) p. 237, Taylor and Francis, London and Philadelphia, 1985.

8. Payan, D.G., Brewster, D.R. and Goetzl, E.J., J. Immunol. 131, 1613, 1983.

9. Stanisz, A.M., Befus, D. and Bienenstock, J., J. Immunol. 136, 152, 1986.

10. Liping, Z., Dan, C., Shuzhen, Z. and Shilian, L., Immunol. Commun. 13, 457, 1984.

11. Piotrowski, W., Devoy, M.A.B., Jordan, C.C. and Foreman, J.C., Agents and Actions 14, 420, 1984.

12. Shanahan, F., Denburg, J.A., Fox, J., Bienenstock, J. and Befus, J., J. Immunol. 135, 131, 1985.

13. Payan, D.G., Levine, J.D. and Goetzl, E.J., J. Immunol. 132, 1601, 1984.

ENDOCRINE REGULATION OF THE OCULAR SECRETORY IMMUNE SYSTEM

D.A. Sullivan and L.E. Hann

Department of Ophthalmology, Harvard Medical School
and the Immunology Unit, Eye Research Institute
20 Staniford Street, Boston, MA USA

INTRODUCTION

Past research has demonstrated that androgens stimulate the accumulation of both IgA and secretory component (SC) in tears of rats (1,2). This hormone action appears to be due to an enhancement of the synthesis and/or secretion of IgA and SC by the lacrimal gland (2,3) and seems to underly the sexual dimorphism known to exist in the ocular secretory immune system (1-4). However, whether this hormonal effect is unique to the eye or is shared by other mucosal sites has not been determined.

More recently, it has been shown that absence of the pituitary gland completely inhibits the effect of androgens on mucosal immunity in the eye (5). This finding indicates that an intact hypothalamic-pituitary axis may either support, or mediate, the androgen regulation of the ocular secretory immune system.

The purpose of the present investigation was two-fold: (a) to assess whether androgen action on secretory immunity is unique to the eye or shared by other mucosal sites; and (b) to evaluate whether an intact hypothalamic-pituitary axis is in fact required for androgen control of the ocular secretory immune system.

MATERIALS AND METHODS

Animals and surgical procedures

Adult male Sprague-Dawley rats were obtained from Zivic-Miller Laboratories. Animals were housed in constant temperature rooms with light/dark intervals of 12 h duration. Surgical procuedures, including orchiectomy, hypophysectomy, anterior or posterior pituitary gland removal, pituitary transplant to under the kidney capsule, and appropriate sham-surgeries were all performed by Zivic-Miller Laboratories on 6 wk old rats. Depending upon the study, age-matched animals were allowed to recover for 12 to 14 days before experimental use. To compensate for pituitary gland ablation or transfer, hypophysectomized rats were given an electrolye solution containing sodium chloride (2.03 g/L), potassium chloride (0.083 g/L), magnesium chloride (0.017 g/L) and calcium chloride (0.035 g/L), as recommended by the surgical supervisor at Zivic-Miller Laboratories (6). To verify absence of the pituitary gland, serum from hypophysectomized animals, as well as their sham-operated controls, was tested for thyroxine content, according to reported techniques (6). Within the range of the radioimmunoassay (1 to 25 μg thyroxine/dL), no thyroxine could be detected in sera from hypophysectomized rats or animals without an anterior pituitary gland; serum thyroxine concentration were within normal limits in sham-operated controls and rats without a posterior pituitary gland.

General procedures

Tears were collected from the eyes of etherized rats as previously described (1,6). Saliva was obtained from pilocarpine-treated (1 mg/100 g BW, sc) rats under ether anesthesia. Secretions from the small intestine and lung were collected according to published procedures (7). Briefly, small intestinal secretions were obtained after rat sacrifice by clamping, removing and then flushing the first 10 inches of duodenum with 3 mls of 0.9% saline. Saline was introduced at the gastric end and gently massaged through the gut lumen into a collecting tube. Respiratory fluids were collected following excision of the lung/trachea complex, cannulation of the trachea with polyethylene tubing and suspension of the lung in a saline bath to permit equal lobular expansion. A syringe containing 10 mls of saline was attached to the tracheal tubing and lungs were lavaged five times with 5 ml saline under fairly constant pressure. Urine was withdrawn directly from the bladder lumen by puncture of the bladder wall with a 25 gauge needle and application of negative pressure through an attached syringe. Blood was obtained from the tail and allowed to clot at room temperature. All mucosal secretions and blood samples were centrifuged at 10,000 x g for 4 min and supernatants and sera were stored at -20°C until assay.

Protein levels in experimental samples were measured by the Hartree (8) method utilizing bovine serum albumin as the standard. Statistics were performed by using the Student's t test.

Immunological procedures

Levels of SC and/or IgA in mucosal secretions and sera were measured by specific radioimmunoassays, as previously described (7,9). The assay for SC detected primarily free SC (7). Radiolabeled antigens in these assays were affinity-purified rat IgA and rat SC (gifts from Dr. J.P. Vaerman, Brussels, Belgium) and unlabeled standards were a rat reference serum (Miles Laboratories), containing known amounts of IgA, and rat SC. Antisera included goat anti-rat IgA (Miles Laboratories) and rabbit anti-rat SC (a gift from Dr. C. Wira, Hanover, NH and prepared by Dr. B. Underdown, Tornoto, Canada) as first antibodies and rabbit anti-goat IgG (Miles Laboratories) and goat anti-rabbit IgG (Miles Laboratories) as second antibodies.

Steroid hormone preparations

Testosterone was purchased from Calbiochem-Behring and suspended in saline by glass-glass homogenization. Injections (200 μl volume) of testosterone or saline (controls) were administered subcutaneously and dosages and treatment schedules are described in the Results section.

RESULTS

Is androgen control of the ocular secretory immune system unique to the eye?

To determine whether androgen action on the ocular secretory immune system is unique to the eye or shared by other mucosal sites, we evaluated the effect of testosterone exposure on IgA and SC levels in various external secretions. Orchiectomized rats (n=5-8/group) were treated with saline or testosterone (2 mg/day) for 4 days and 24 h later, tears, saliva, respiratory and intestinal secretions, urine and serum were collected.

As shown in Table 1, testosterone administration significantly ($p < 0.001$) increased the level of IgA in tears of orchiectomized rats. This effect was found irrespective of whether IgA content was expressed in terms of concentration or as a percentage of total protein. Thus, tear IgA concentrations equalled 214 ± 21 and 839 ± 106 µg/ml in saline- (n=7) and hormone- (n=8) injected rats, respectively. In contrast, androgen treatment had no influence on the level of IgA in saliva, respiratory secretions, intestinal secretions, urine or serum.

Analysis of free SC content in these various mucosal secretions (10) demonstrated that tear SC levels, when expressed as a percentage of total protein, rose significantly ($p < 0.001$) following testosterone treatment. This increase was equivalent to a 3-fold elevation in tear SC concentration, compared to that of control animals. Secretory component levels in saliva and respiratory and intestinal secretions, however, were not significantly influenced by androgen exposure. We were unable to determine whether hormone treatment affected urinary free SC levels, because this protein could not be detected in the urine samples (sensitivity of the SC RIA = 0.44 ng). Of interest in the present studies was the finding that free SC content, when standardized to protein, was the highest in respiratory secretions of testosterone-injected rats. These free SC/protein percentages were

Table 1. Effect of testosterone exposure on IgA levels in mucosal secretions and serum

Sample	[IgA (µg)/Protein (µg)] - %	
	Saline	Testosterone
Tears	0.64 ± 0.11	1.82 ± 0.19*
Saliva	0.68 ± 0.05	0.81 ± 0.06
Respiratory secretions	11.7 ± 1.0	11.3 ± 1.4
Intestinal secretions	7.1 ± 0.6	6.7 ± 0.9
Urine	0.10 ± 0.01	0.09 ± 0.02
Serum	0.18 ± 0.01	0.20 ± 0.02

Mucosal secretions and serum were collected from age-matched and orchiectomized rats following 4 daily injections of saline or testosterone (2 mg/day). Numbers represent the mean ± SE of 5-8 determinations. *Significantly ($p < 0.001$) greater than saline-tested control. Data from (10).

as follows: respiratory secretions = 0.72 ± 0.12%; intestinal secretons = 0.18 ± 0.01%; tears = 0.101 ± 0.010%; and saliva = 0.033 ± 0.004%.

In the above study, no effect of androgen administration was found on the protein levels in mucosal secretions.

Does androgen regulation of the ocular secretory immune system require an intact hypothalamic-pituitary axis?

Recent research from our laboratory has shown that the androgen-induced accumulation of IgA and SC in tears is completely inhibited if rats are hypophysectomized (5). This finding suggest that an intact hypothalamic-pituitary axis may be required for the androgen regulation of the ocular secretory immune system. To evaluate this possibility, the following two studies were conducted.

In the first experiment, the effect of testosterone on tear IgA levels was determined in orchiectomized and hypophysectomized rats, which had undergone pituitary transplants to under the kidney capsule. Control animals in this study included those with orchiectomies, hypophysectomies and sham transplant surgery, as well as rats with orchiectomies, sham hypophysectomies and sham transplants. As shown in Table 2, testosterone exposure (2 mg/day for 4 days) significantly ($p < 0.001$) increased the tear content of IgA in animals with sham-hypophysectomies and sham-transplants, as compared to that of saline-injected controls. The tear IgA

Table 2. Influence of testosterone or tear IgA levels in hypophysectomized rats with pituitary transplants under the kidney capsule

Surgery		Tear IgA (ng)	
Hypophysectomy	Transplant	Saline	Testosterone
Yes	Yes	941 ± 308	555 ± 113
Yes	Sham	593 ± 82	409 ± 92
Sham	Sham	651 ± 194	2814 ± 327*

Age-matched rats underwent orchiectomies and hypophysectomies or sham-hypophysectomies and pituitary transplants to under the kidney capsule or sham-transplant surgery. Animals were then injected with either testosterone (2 mg/day; n = 6-8/group) or saline (n = 4-7/group) for 4 days and tears were collected 24 hours after the last injection. Numbers equal the mean ± SE. *Significantly greater ($p < 0.001$) greater than value of saline-treated controls. Data from (11).

Table 3. Effect of testosterone on tear IgA levels in orchiectomized rats with either anterior or posterior pituitary gland ablation

Surgical Group	(IgA/Protein) D 4 / (IgA/Protein) D 0	
	Saline	Testosterone
Anterior pituitary removal	1.07 ± 0.15	1.77 ± 0.30
Posterior pituitary removal	1.47 ± 0.52	1.25 ± 0.34
Sham pituitary surgery	1.22 ± 0.14	4.21 ± 0.71*

Aged-matched rats were orchiectomized and then underwent ablation of the anterior pituitary gland, the posterior pituitary gland or sham-pituitary surgery. Animals were administered 4 daily injections of either saline (n=6-7/group) or testosterone (2 mg/day; n=6-8/group) and tears were collected 24 h after the last treatment. Tear IgA data was standardized to total tear protein and expressed as a ratio of post-treatment (D 4) to pre-treatment (D 0) levels. Results cannot be accounted for by variations in total tear protein during the course of the experiment. Numbers represent the mean ± SE. *Significantly higher ($p < 0.01$) than value of saline treated controls. Data from (11).

concentrations in these animals equalled 176 ± 43 and 709 ± 71 µg/ml in saline- and androgen-treated controls, respectively. In contrast, testosterone administration had no effect on tear IgA levels in hypophysectomized rats, irregardless of whether they had received pituitary transplants or sham-transplant surgery.

In the second study, we examined whether the androgen modulation of tear IgA levels might be influenced by the selective removal of either the anterior or the posterior pituitary gland in orchiectomized rats. As demonstrated in Table 3, testosterone treatment (2 mg/day for 4 days) of orchiectomized rats (n = 7) with sham-pituitary surgery resulted in a significant ($p < 0.01$) elevation in tear IgA content, compared to that in saline-administered controls (n=6). The concentrations of tear IgA in these latter groups were 244 ± 30 (saline) and 871 ± 202 µg/ml (androgen). Removal of the anterior or posterior pituitary, however, blocked the effect of testosterone on tear IgA content. This absence of hormone action was evident irrespective of whether IgA data was expressed as a percentage of total tear protein or as concentration.

DISCUSSION

Hormones are known to stimulate or antagonize mucosal immunity in a variety of different sites, including lacrimal, salivary, mammary, respiratory, intestinal, hepatic, uterine, cervical and vaginal tissues (1-3,5, 10-30). However, these endocrine effects tend not to be generalized; rather, specific hormones (e.g. glucocorticoids, estrogens, progestins) appear to enhance or suppress only certain secretory immune systems (2,31). Thus, as shown in the present study, testosterone treatment of orchiectomized rats induced a marked elevation in the SC and IgA levels of tears, but had no effect on these parameters in saliva, respiratory and intestinal secretions, urine and serum. These findings were of interest, because androgens do have a significant impact on the morphology and/or function of salivary (32,33), intestinal (34,35) and respiratory (19) tissues. Yet, given the preceeding findings, it would appear that endocrine action on glandular development does not necessarily result in parallel immunologic effects.

With regard to the ocular secretory immune system, the regulatory influence of testosterone was most likely mediated through the lacrimal gland (2,3), which is the source of tear SC (3,36,37) and IgA (9,37-39) and a known target organ for androgens (40-44). In fact, androgens modulate both the structure and function of lacrimal tissue, including its morphology, biochemistry, histochemistry and genetic apparatus (40-44). One mechanism of hormone action of the lacrimal gland may involve binding to specific steroid receptors (45). However, our results with hypophysectomized rats raise the possibility that an intact hypothalamic-pituitary axis either supports, or mediates, androgen-induced changes in ocular immunity. Ablation of the pituitary gland, transfer of this tissue to the kidney capsule or selective removal of the anterior or posterior pituitary completely curtailed the effect of testosterone on tear SC (5) and/or IgA. These findings suggest that prolactin, a potent regulator of systemic immunity (46), is not involved in androgen action, because pituitary transplant to the kidney causes hyperprolactinemia (47). Further, given our findings with selective anterior/posterior pituitary ablation, it may be that multiple hormones from the pituitary, or specific components from the pars intermedia (e.g. alpha-melanocyte stimulating hormone) might be cooperating in androgen-associated immune effects in the eye. Of interest, certain androgen actions on peripheral tissues have been shown to be mediated through the pituitary (48), and hypophyseal hormones are known to influence both the immune system (13,27,46,47,49,50) and the lacrimal gland (51-53). Clearly, additional research is required to elucidate the mechanism of endocrine control of the ocular secretory immune system.

CONCLUSIONS

1. Androgen regulation of the ocular secretory immune system is unique to the eye and not shared by other mucosal sites.

2. Androgen control of the secretory immune system requires the presence of an intact hypothalamic-pituitary axis.

ACKOWLEDGEMENTS

We wish to thank Dr. J.-P. Vaerman (Brussels, Belgium) for his gift of purified polymeric IgA and secretory component, Dr. C.R. Wira (Hanover, NH) for supplying us with rabbit anti-rat SC and Dr. B. Underdown (Toronto, Canada) for preparing this antiserum. This research was supported by NIH grant EY 05612.

REFERENCES

1. Sullivan, D.A., Bloch, K.J. and Allansmith, M.R., J. Immunol. 132, 1130, 1984.
2. Sullivan, D.A. and Allansmith, M.R., J. Immunol. 134, 2978, 1985.
3. Sullivan, D.A., Bloch, K.J. and Allansmith, M.R., Immunology 52, 234, 1984.
4. Sullivan, D.A., Hann, L.E. and Allansmith, M.R., 1986 (This volume).
5. Sullivan, D.A. and Allansmith, M.R., Immunology, 1987 (in press).
6. Sullivan, D.A. and Allansmith, M.R., Exp. Eye Res. 42, 131, 1986.
7. Sullivan, D.A. and Wira, C.R., J. Immunol. 130, 1330, 1983.
8. Hartree, E.F., Anal. Biochem. 48, 422, 1972.
9. Sullivan, D.A. and Allansmith, M.R., Immunology 53, 791, 1984.
10. Sullivan, D.A. and Hann, L.E., 1987 (submitted).

11. Sullivan, D.A., 1987 (submitted).
12. Wira, C.R. and Sandoe, C.P., Nature 268, 534, 1977.
13. Weisz-Carrington, P., Roux, M.E., McWilliams, M., Phillips-Quagliata, J.M. and Lamm, M.E., Proc. Natl. Acad. Sci. USA 75, 2928, 1978.
14. Wira, C.R. and Sandoe, C.P., Endocrinology 106, 1020, 1980.
15. Wira, C.R., Hyde, E., Sandoe, C.P., Sullivan, D. and Spencer, S., J. Steroid Biochem. 12, 451, 1980.
16. McDermott, M.R., Clark, D.A. and Bienenstock, J., J. Immunol 124, 2536, 1980.
17. Schumacher, G.F.B., in Immunological Aspects of Infertility and Fertility Regulation, (Edited by Schumacher, G.F.B. and Dhinsa, D.S.), Elsevier/North Holland, New York, 1980.
18. Sullivan, D.A. and Wira, C.R., J. Steroid Biochem. 15, 439, 1981.
19. Manning, L.S. and Parmely, M.J., Int. Conf. Reprod. Immunol., Banff, Canada, 1981.
20. Murdock, A.J.M., Buckley, C.H. and Fox, H., J. Reprod. Immunol. 4, 23, 1982.
21. Canning, M.B. and Billington, W.D., J. Endocr. 97, 419, 1983.
22. Rachman, F., Casimiri, V., Psychoyos, A. and Bernard, O., J. Reprod. Fertil. 69, 17, 1983.
23. Sullivan, D.A. and Wira, C.R., Endocrinology 112, 260, 1983.
24. Wira, C.R., Sullivan, D.A. and Sandoe, C.P.,J. Steroid Biochem. 19, 469, 1983.
25. Wira, C.R., Sullivan, D.A. and Sandoe, C.P., Ann. N.Y. Acad. Sci. 409, 534, 1983.
26. Sullivan, D.A., Underdown, B.J. and Wira, C.R., Immunology 49, 379, 1983.
27. Weisz-Carrington, P., Emancipator, S. and Lamm, M.E., J. Reprod. Immunol. 6, 63, 1984.
28. Wira, C.R. and Colby, E.M., J. Immunol. 134, 1744, 1985.
29. Wira, C.R. and Sullivan, D.A., Biol. Reprod. 32, 90, 1985.
30. Halzonetis, T.D., Taubman, M.A., Mandel, I.D., Sullivan, D.A., Ebersole, J.L. and Smith, D.J., unpublished data.
31. Sullivan, D.A., in Hormones and Immunity, p. 54, MTP Press, Ltd., Lancaster, 1987.
32. Aloe, L. and Levi-Montalcini, R., Exp. Cell Res. 125, 15, 1980.
33. Chao, J. and Margolis, H., Endocrinology 113, 2221, 1983.
34. Carriere, R.M., Anat. Rec. 156, 423, 1966.
35. Carriere, R.M. and Buschke, M., Anat. Rec. 192, 407, 1978.
36. Allansmith, M.R. and Gillette, T.E., Am. J. Ophthalmol. 89, 353, 1980.

37. Gudmundsson, O.G., Sullivan, D.A., Bloch, K.J. and Allansmith, M.R., Exp. Eye Res. 40, 231, 1985.

38. Allansmith, M.R., Kajiyama, G., Abelson, M.B. and Simon, M.A., Am. J. Ophthalmol. 82, 819, 1976.

39. Brandtzaeg, P., Scand. J. Immunol. 22, 111, 1985.

40. Cavallero, C., Acta. Endocrinol. (Copenhagen) 55, 119, 1967.

41. Hahn, J.D., J. Endocr. 45, 421, 1969.

42. Paulini, K., Beneke, G. and Kulka, R., Gerontologia 18, 131, 1972.

43. Lauria, A. and Porcelli, F., Basic Appl. Histochem. 23, 171, 1979.

44. Shaw, P.H., Held, W.A. and Hastie, N.D., Cell 32, 755, 1983.

45. Ota, M., Kyakumoto, S. and Nemoto, T., Biochem. Intl. 10, 129, 1985.

46. Nagy, E., Berczi, I. and Freisen, H.G., Acta. Endocrinol. 102, 351, 1983.

47. Lotz, W. and Krause, R., J. Reprod. Fertil. 47, 385, 1976.

48. Norstedt, G. and Mode, A., Endocrinology 111, 645, 1982.

49. Besedovsky, H.O., Del Rey, A.E. and Sorkin, E., J. Immunol. 135, 750s, 1985.

50. Blalock, J.E., Harbour-McMenamin, D. and Smith, E.M., J. Immunol. 135, 858s, 1985.

51. Martinazzi, M. and Baroni, C., Folia. Endocrinol. 16, 123, 1963.

52. Ebling, F.J., Ebling, E., Randall, V. and Skinner, J., J. Endocr. 66, 407, 1975.

53. Jahn, R., Padel, U., Porsch, P.H. and Soling, H.D., Eur. J. Biochem. 126, 623, 1982.

THE EFFECTS OF MODERATE PROTEIN DEFICIENCY OR HIGH VITAMIN E ON INTESTINAL SECRETORY AND SERUM IgA LEVELS IN MICE

R.R. Watson and N. Messiha*

Department of Family and Community Medicine, University of Arizona, Tucson, AZ USA; and *Department of Food and Nutrition, Purdue University, West Lafayette, IN USA

INTRODUCTION

Vitamin E, which is a powerful antioxidant, also has a marked effect on resistance to bacterial infection through enhancing the humoral immune response to antigenic stimulation (1). Tanaka et al. (2), studied the effect of vitamin E on the humoral immune response by testing its influence on antibody production in mice using a hapten-carrier conjugate as an antigen. They found that although vitamin E supplementation does not augment either initial IgM or late IgG responses, it seems to facilitate the shift of antibody production from IgM to IgG. They suggested that vitamin E stimulates the helper activity of T lymphocytes. Tengerdy et al. (3) reported that the humoral immune response of mice against sheep red blood cells or tetanus toxoid antigens was increased by 30-40% when the food was supplemented by vitamin E (60-180 mg/kg). Similar results were reported by Nockels (4). Campbell et al. (5), demonstrated that the addition of vitamin E to the medium can stimulate the response of non-adherent spleen cells to sheep red blood cells in the relative absence of adherent cells. They also showed that vitamin E enhances *in vitro* immune responses by populations of spleen cells containing both adherent and nonadherent cells.

MATERIALS AND METHODS

Watson et al. (6) found that IgA in intestinal secretions was significantly lower and increased through the duration of their study, more slowly in malnourished mice than in the controls. They also observed that serum IgA levels were higher in malnourished mice and dropped significantly after week 24 approaching the lower control values. However, much less is known about the effects of high dietary protein on IgA levels (6). Therefore, the effects of high dietary protein or vitamin E were measured in young, growing mice.

Animals

Male inbred BALB/c mice were obtained from the Jackson Laboratories, Bar Harbor, ME. They were bred in the animal facilities in the Foods and Nutrition Department of Purdue University. Mice aged 3 weeks old are used in the study.

Experimental design

After weaning, 3 week old mice were fed either isocaloric control diet, or experimental diet containing 20 times control level of vitamin E, and water ad libitum. Mice were sacrificed by exsanguination at 3 weeks of age, and at various time periods after commencing their respective diets. Sera and intestinal washes are collected and then stored at -70°C until needed. After weaning, 3 week old mice were fed isocaloric diets of 20% protein (control), 50% protein (high protein), or 4% protein (low protein), or the high vitamin E supplemental diet (20 fold increase) and water ad libitum. The AIN synthetic diet has been described previously (7). Mice were sacrificed by exsanguination at 3 weeks of age and at various time periods after commencing their respective diets. Sera and intestinal washes were collected and then stored at -70°C until needed. Results for each point of time represent data obtained from 5-15 mice from each diet group that were randomly picked for the assay.

Collection samples

Serum. Whole blood was collected from decapitated mice, kept on ice for 1 h to be clotted, and then centrifuged at 800 x g for 10 min at 4°C. The serum was then aspirated into a small labeled vial and frozen at -70°C until tested for any of the parameters.

Intestinal wash. As soon as the animals were killed they were kept on ice for 5 min. Then the small intestines were gently separated both at the gastroduodenal and at the illeocoecal junctions. After separation each intestine was individually washed with 1.0 ml sterile (sodium azide) phosphate buffered saline (PBS) (pH 7.0-7.2) (4°C). The solution was then gently manipulated to wash the intestine out. These washes were then centrifuged at 800 x g for 10 min at 4°C. Supernatants were gently aspirated of debris with a pasteur pipette into a small vial, and frozen at -70°C until used for any of the assays.

Assay for IgA. Immunodiffusion plates were prepared with 3% nobel agar 1:10 dilution of goat anti-mouse IgA (alpha chain specific) (Cappel Laboratories, Cochranville, PA). Undiluted serum and supernatants of the intestinal washes were used for measurement of IgA concentrations (3.0 L for each well). Duplicate wells were set up for each sample. Plates were inverted and incubated for 48 h at 37°C in humid atmosphere. The precipitation ring diameters were measured to the nearest 0.1 mm using a Hyland precision viewer. Purified mouse myeloma obtained from Litton Bionetic Laboratories was used to develop the standard curve on which IgA levels were measured.

Statistical analysis. Statistical analysis of the results for animals at the same age and on different diets was done using the Student's *t* test for two groups with unequal numbers. The calculated *t* values were compared with the tabulated *t* values at probabilities of 95% and 99% and degrees of freedom (d.f.) equal to (n_1+n_2-2) where n_1 and n_2 represent the sample sizes.

RESULTS

Serum IgA concentrations. Our results indicated that the serum IgA levels measured as mg/ml of mouse serum were higher in animals fed the high vitamin E diet than in animals fed the control diet. Highly significant increase ($p < 0.01$) was found in serum IgA levels at the ages of 9.5 and 17 weeks. Also, a significant difference ($p < 0.05$) was detected in animals at the age of 12 weeks. By the 22nd week no significant difference was noticed (Fig. 1).

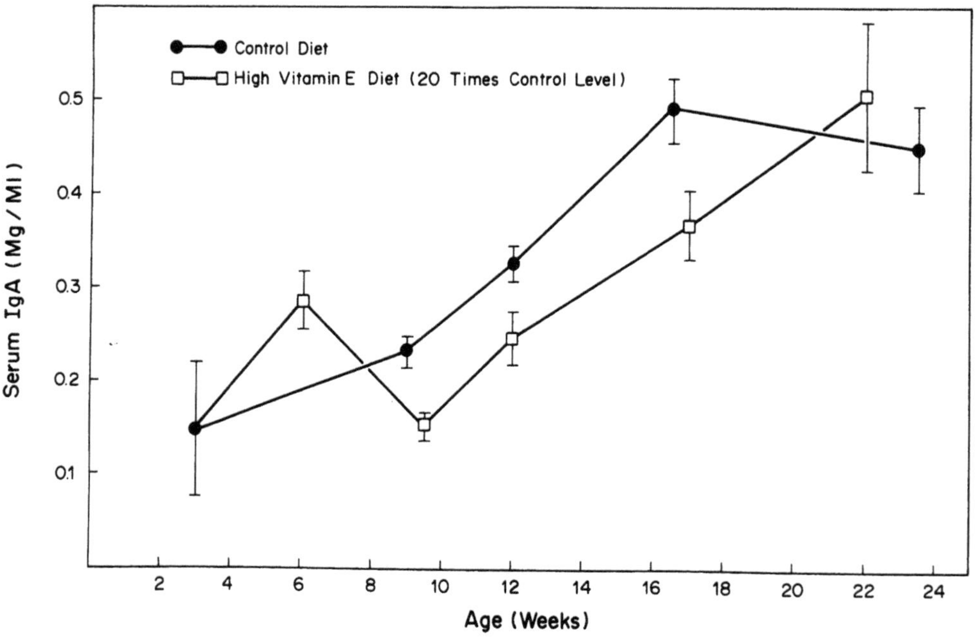

Figure 1. The effect of high vitamin E diet on the IgA concentrations in sera of growing BALB/c mice, measured as mg/ml.

In the animals fed the 50% protein diet, serum IgA concentration increased from 0.147 mg/ml in the third week of life up to 0.364 mg/ml in the ninth week. This is a highly significant difference from the control values ($p < 0.01$) (Fig. 2). The increase in IgA concentration continued up to 0.437 mg/ml in the 14th week, followed by a drastic drop to 0.241 mg/ml in the 17th week. This is a slightly significant difference from the control values (0.579 mg/ml). Then the IgA concentration in sera of animals fed 50% protein diet increased slightly up to 0.307 mg/ml in the 20th week. On the other hand, the 4% protein diet showed a very high increase in serum IgA concentration up to 2.38 fold from the control levels after 12 weeks (Fig. 2). Highly significant differences ($p < 0.01$) were found in serum IgA concentrations of animals fed 4% protein diet versus control animals.

Secretory IgA concentrations. The high vitamin E diet increased the concentration of IgA measured as mg recovered/small intestine in the intestinal secretions of mice throughout the course of the experiment (Fig 3). Statistical analysis of the results indicated that highly significant increase ($p < 0.01$) in the IgA concentration was reached at the 12th week.

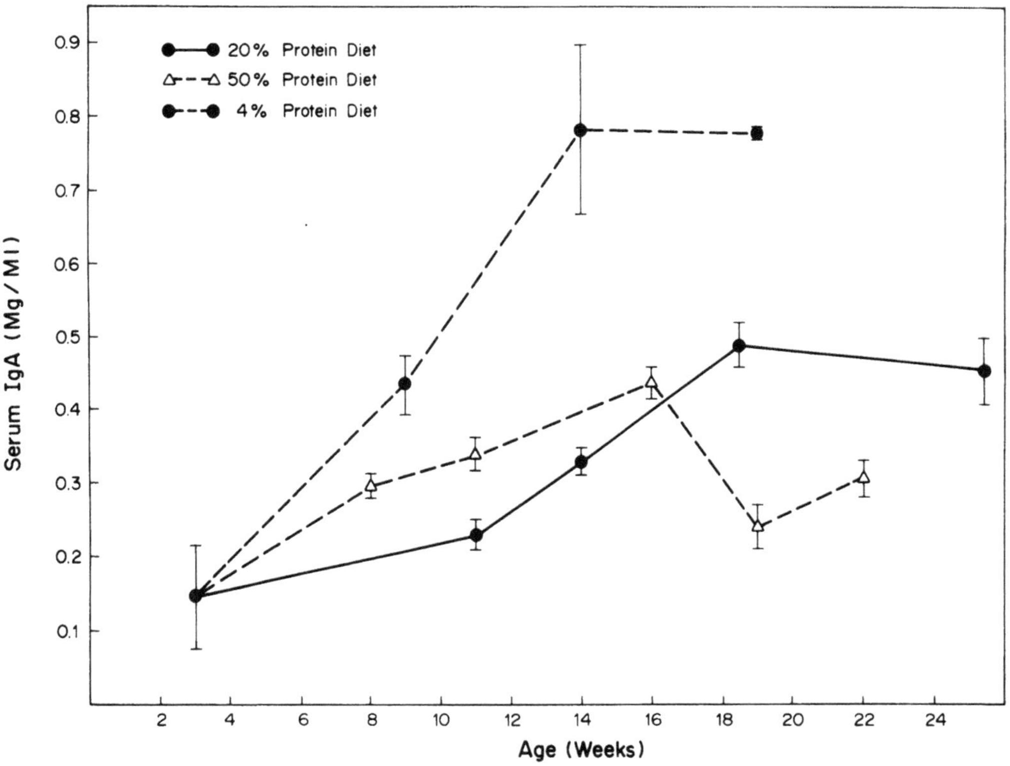

Figure 2. The effect of different protein diets on the IgA concentrations in sera of growing BALB/c mice, measured as mg/ml.

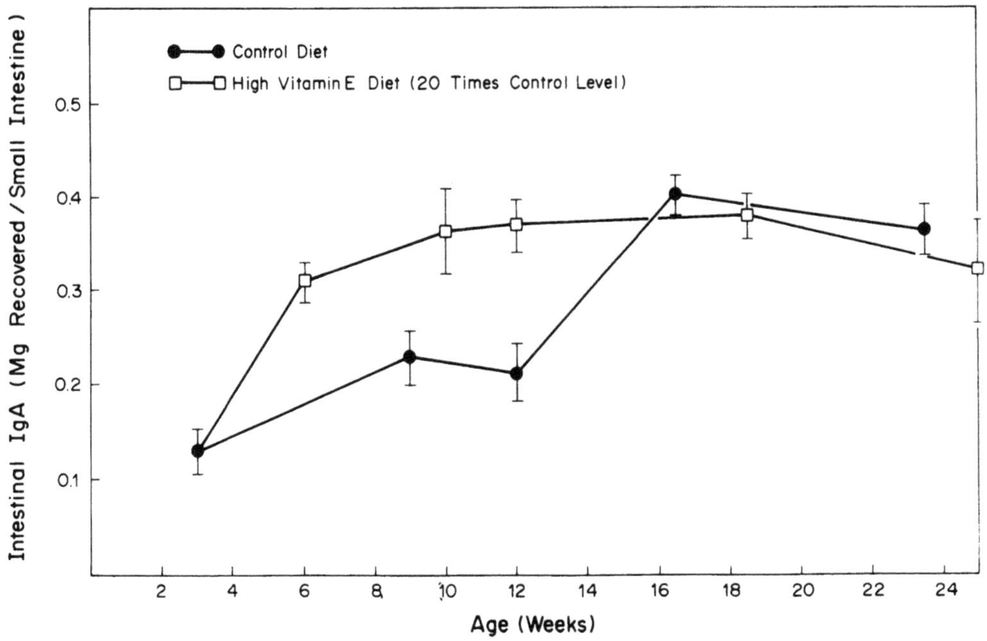

Figure 3. The effect of high vitamin E diet on the IgA concentrations in the intestinal secretions of growing BALB/c mice, measured as mg recovered/small intestine.

In Figure 4, the 50% protein diet exerted the following changes on the concentrations of IgA in the intestinal washes. The trend obtained with this diet was like the control with slightly higher levels in the beginning. A nearly constant level was obtained from the 9th to the 20th week, with a very slight rise in the 20th week. No marked drop was observed at the 17th week, compared to the drop in serum IgA level at the same age in the control group. Figure 4 also shows that the secretory IgA in the intestinal secretions of mice fed 4% protein diet was markedly lower than the control levels at all ages, conversely to the very high levels obtained in the serum of the same animals (Fig. 2).

CONCLUSIONS

Our results indicate that feeding mice on a high volume vitamin E diet (20 times the control level) increased the levels of IgA in the intestinal secretions over the control animals. The high levels of IgA in the intestinal secretions in animals fed on high vitamin E diet was accompanied by lower serum IgA levels. This indicates that vitamin E stimulates the selective transport of IgA across the intestines. The effect of high vitamin E in the diet on IgA levels seems to be specific for the secretory immune competence since we could not find similar effects of high vitamin E on

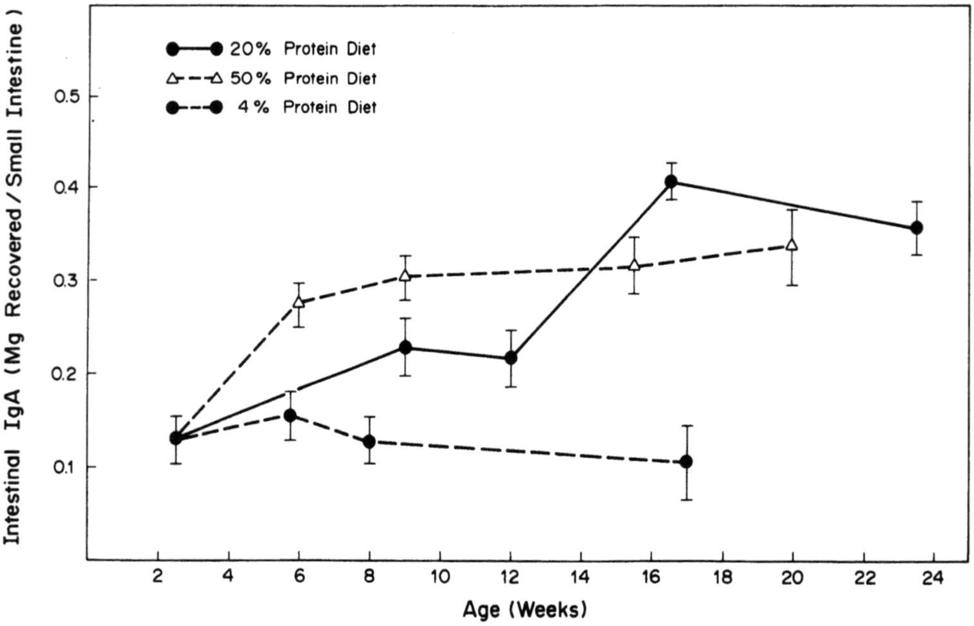

Figure 4. The effect of different protein diets on the IgA concentration in the intestinal secretions of growing BALB/c mice measured as mg recovered/ small intestine.

amylase activity which represents another secretory protein in the same animals (unpublished results). In general, the high vitamin E diet did not increase the total levels of IgA (serum and intestinal). These results agree with previous work reported by Tanaka et al. (2), who found that high vitamin E did not augment either the initial IgM or the late IgG responses.

Protein deficiency or hypoalbuminemia may occur primarily due to deficient protein intake or secondary to any disorder interfering with protein absorption. However produced, protein deficiency has a great influence on the function of the immune system. In our experiment we studied the effect of pure, primary protein deficiency on the immunocompetence of growing BALB/c mice. Our results showed that the secretory IgA (sIgA) in the intestinal at all ages after weaning (Figs. 2 and 4). These results agree with results from other studies in humans and guinea pigs. Conversely the serum IgA levels obtained from the same animals were markedly high. This would agree with previous work in humans and guinea pigs (8), where it was postulated that low protein diets cause suppression of IgA transport from tissues into secretions, leading to serum IgA in very high levels. On the other hand, the 50% protein diet slightly increased the IgA concentrations both in serum and in intestinal secretion. This slight increase represents the effect of high protein diet on the resting IgA levels, since the animals were not challenged with an antigen.

McMurray et al. (8) indicated that within 4-5 weeks of the application of high protein diet to malnourished Colombian children there was marked increases in the levels of serum IgA and Complement C_3. One year after discharge from the hospital, serum IgA levels declined especially with Kwashiorkor. Indicators of humoral and secretory immunity were within normal ranges. However, cell mediated immunity both in vitro and in vivo had begun to wane. In protein energy malnourished rats IgA levels and the ratio of IgA to IgG were decreased, and the decrease was related to the degree of malnourishment (3). They also reported that secretory IgA levels were decreased. However, IgA levels in bile were much higher than IgG levels.

Carlomagno et al. (9) reported that protein starvation in rats influenced the production of antibodies more than it did the number of antibody forming cells. They also stated that the nutritional impairment of immunoglobulin synthesis is reversible.

A significant reduction in the levels of IgA and complement C_4 was found in the colostrum of malnourished Colombian lactating mothers. The difference disappeared in mature milk due to improvement of the nutritional status.

Clearly, dietary materials including deficiency of protein and high vitamin E altered the levels of IgA in intestinal fluids and serum.

ACKNOWLEDGEMENTS

This work was supported by Wallace Genetics, Inc. and the National Livestock and Meat Board.

REFERENCES

1. Tengerdy, R.P., Heinzerling, R.H. and Nockels, C.F., Infect. Immun. 5, 987, 1972.
2. Tanaka, J., Fjuiwara, H. and Torisu, M., Immunology 38, 727, 1979.
3. Tengerdy, R.P., Heinzerling, R.H., Brown, G.L. and Mathias, M.M., Int. Arch. Allergy 44, 221, 1973.
4. Nockels, C.F., Fed. Proc. 38, 2134, 1979.
5. Campbell, P.A., Cooper, H.R., Heinzerling, R.H. and Tengerdy, R.P., Proc. Soc. Exp. Biol. Med. 146, 465, 1974.
6. Watson, R.R. and Safranski, D., CRC-Handbook Immunol. Aging. pp. 125-139, 1981.
7. Moriguchi, S., Werner, L. and Watson, R.R., Immunology 56, 169, 1985.
8. Watson, R.R., McMurray, D.N., Martin, P. and Reyes, M.A., Am. J. Clin. Nutr. 42, 281, 1985.
9. Carlomagno, M.A., Alito, A.E., Almiron, D.I. and Gemino, A., Infect. Immun. 38, 195, 1982.
10. Miranda, R., Saravia, N.G., Ackerman, R., Murphy, N., Berman, S. and McMurray, D.N., Am. J. Clin. Nutr. 37, 632, 1983.

IMMUNOLOGICAL AND IMMUNOPATHOLOGICAL CHARACTERIZATION OF A MUCOSAL ANTIGEN FROM GUINEA PIG SMALL INTESTINE

M.S. Nemirovsky and N. Desprès

Départment d'anatomie et de biologie cellulaire
Faculté de Médecine,
Université de Sherbrooke,
Sherbrooke, Québec, Canada J1H 5N4

INTRODUCTION

Ulcerative Colitis and Crohn's disease are non-specific inflammatory bowel diseases (IBD) with a worldwide geographic distribution. Epidemiological studies appears to indicate an increasing incidence of IBD in the industrialized world during the last decades (1).

The immunological status of patients with IBD has been extensively studied. Humoral immunity, including anti-colon antibodies (2) and those cross-reacting with a bacterial polysacchride (3) have been well characterized. The presence and the pathological implications of circulating antigen-antibody complexes in IBD patients are not yet resolved (4,5). Although the *in vivo* cell mediated hypersensitivity to bacterial and fungal antigens appears to be generally normal, as well as the response of circulating lymphocytes to mitogens, some degree of decrease can be observed (6). A specific cytotoxic reaction of circulating lymphocytes against colonic epithelial cells can be detected in patients with IBD. This cytotoxicity is complement independent and appears to be mediated by killer cells (7). Their implication in the pathogenesis of the disease is not clear, since no correlation can be established between their degree and the extension of the disease (8). The possibility of an immunoregulatory defect in these patients has been raised (9), although their conclusions has been contradicted by others (10).

The lack of a well characterized model of IBD in laboratory animals has impeded efforts to put together in a comprehensive way all the immunological implications of those unmistakable autoimmune features present in IBD patients. We have recently described (11) the immunopathology of guinea pig autoimmune enterocolitis induced by alloimmunization with a mucosal antigen extracted from small intestine that can become a useful model for the study of IBD.

The experiments presentedhere has been designed in order to further characterize the antigen implicated in autoimmune enterocolitis.

MATERIALS AND METHODS

The postmicrosomal supernatant of small intestine mucosal scrapings of outbred adult guines pigs was used for the preparation of the mucosal antigen (MA). After chromatography on Sephacryl S-200 Superfine (Pharmacia, Sweden) the major peak eluting immediately after the void volume was used as immunogen.

Adult male Hartley guinea pigs (300-350 g) received one or two doses of 5 mg N of MA emulsified in Complete Freund's Adjuvant (CFA) and were sacrificed at d 30 (single dose) or 60 (two doses). At that time, sera, spleen and lymph nodes were collected. The in vitro lymphocyte transformation test was used as a correlate of cell mediated immunity and the results expressed as Stimulatory Index (S.I.) in presence or in absence of MA in the cultures.

Heterologous rabbit anti-MA antisera was obtained by immunization with 5 doses of 6 mg N of the immunogen emulsified in CFA at 15 or 30 d intervals. The sera was collected at d 105. The globulin fraction was obtained by salt fractionation. The allo and heteroantisera were analyzed on immunodiffusion plates before and after absorption with saline extracts of normal liver, kidney and testis guinea pig as well as MA.

Representative pieces of the whole intestine as well as different organs of all alloimmunized and control animals were processes for histopathologic analysis. Guinea pigs non-immunized or injected with CFA were utilized as controls. The mucosal immunogen was analyzed by SDS-electrophoresis (12).

RESULTS

Only guinea pigs receiving two doses of MA develop precipitating antibodies (9/10). Some of the multiple precipitation bands gave identity reactions with those of heterologous anti-MA globulins. Rabbit anti-MA antibodies cross-react with saline extracts of liver and testis (Fig. 1). Absorption of the antisera with those saline extracts eliminate all cross-reactivity, leaving a few precipitation lines reacting only with MA (Fig. 1). Absorption with MA eliminate all reactivity.

When lymphocytes of spleen and lymph nodes were incubated for 72 h together with different concentrations of MA, a blastogenic response was found, as evaluated by ^{3}H-TdR incorporation (S.I. $\geq$ 3.0), in 9 out of 10 animals receiving a single dose of MA, whereas a reduced number of guinea pigs (6/10) gave a comparable response. However, lymphocytes of 2 out of 5 guinea pigs receiving a single dose of CFA alone, gave a slight increase in thymidine incorporation when cultured following the above mentioned conditions (S.I. = 1.5). No significant increase of the S.I. was recorded with cultures of non-immunized controls (0/5).

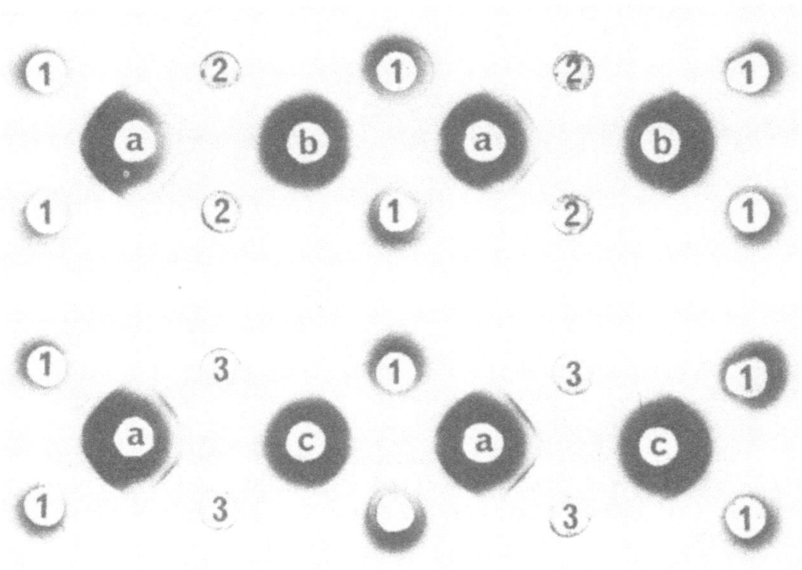

Figure 1. Immunodiffusion analysis of heterologous anti-MA antibodies. 1 = MA, 5 mg N/ml. 2 = Saline extract of guinea pig liver, 10 mg N/ml. 3 = Saline extract of guinea pig testis, 10 mg N/ ml. a = Rabbit anti-MA antibody, globulin fraction. b = Rabbit anti-MA antibody, globulin fraction absorbed with a lyophilized saline extract of guinea pig liver. c = Rabbit anti-MA antibody, globulin fraction absorbed with a lyophilized saline extract of guinea pig testis.

Histopathological alterations in alloimmunized guinea pigs were limited to the intestine. Thirty days after a single dose of MA, 7 out of 10 animals developed lesions, preferentially, but not exclusively, localized in the ileum and descending colon. They were characterized as showing vascular congestion of the lamina propria, superficial ulceration and microscopic hemorrhage. In some cases, there was an extensive loss of epithelium and lamina propria, including Lieberkhün glands. However, no evidence of blood loss was observed.

In animals receiving two doses of MA and sacrificed at d 60, similar lesions could be observed (8/10). However, some degree of mononuclear cell infiltration and destruction of the villous architecture were noted together with the above mentioned alterations, especially on the terminal ileum. Caecal lesions were more frequent than in single dose immunized animals.

Protein screening of MA by SDS-electrophoresis revealed three main bands present only in MA solutions (arrows, Fig. 2) and conspicuously absent in saline extracts of guinea pig liver, kidney and testis.

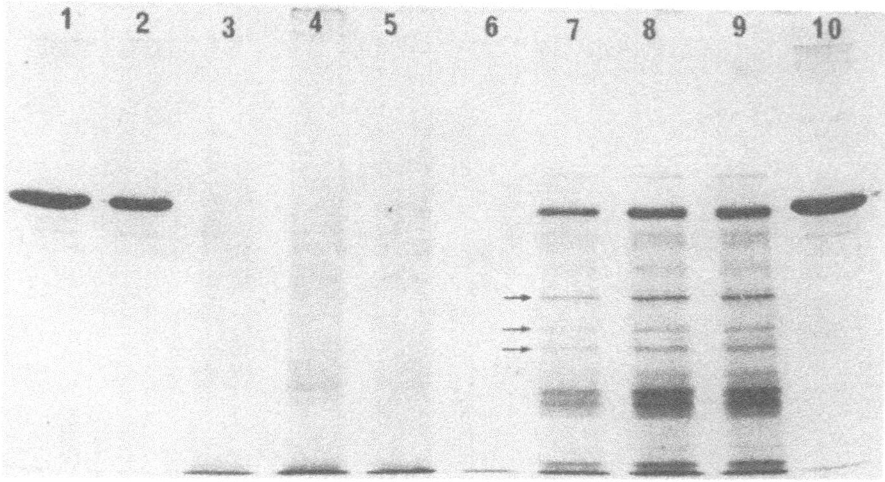

Figure 2. SDS-electrophoresis of mucosal antigen (MA). 1 = SAB 200 μg N. 2 = SAB 125 μg N. 3 = Saline extract of guinea pig testis, 200 μg N. 4 = Saline extract of guinea pig liver, 200 μg N. 5 = Saline extract of guinea pig kidney, 200 μg N. 6 = PBS. 7 = Pool 3, MA 100 μg N. 8 = Pool 3, MA 200 μg N.

DISCUSSION

The observations reported here are consistent with our previous study (11) as far as the immunological response and intestinal histopathology of MA alloimmunized animals were concerned.

The immunodiffusion analysis of allo and heteroanti-MA antisera with and without absorption with unrelated guinea pig organs extracts allowed us to demonstrate that, within the limits of this technique, some of the precipitating antibodies are organ-specific (i.e., to small intestine mucosa). Further analysis by SDS-electrophoresis of the mucosal antigen tentatively linked those organ-specific epitopes to three main bands of m.w. $<$ 60 Kd (m.w. probe:BSA).

Experimental autoimmune diseases can be elicitated mainly by immunization with myelin basic protein (13), thyroglobulin (14), spermatozoa (15), and uveal proteins (16). Those are characterized by array of humoral and cell-mediated autoimmune responses as well as lesions at the target organs. The latter are mainly the organs where the autoantigens can be obtained. This organ-specificity is characteristic of the experimental autoimmune models, whereas in some spontaneous models of autoimmune disease such as the spontaneously diabetic biobreeding Worcester rats (BBW rats), more than one organ can express histopathological alterations (17). It is of great interest to stress that when immunological manipulation is provoked, such as neonatal thymectomy in mice, multiple organs can become the target of autoimmune pathology (18).

The enterocolitis elicitated by alloimmunization with MA possess some of the basic requisites to be considered as an experimental autoimmune disease. Many of the models of IBD are obtained by ingestion of carragenen (19) or by irritation with diluted acid (20). As far as immunological methods of provoking intestinal lesions, cross-reacting bacterial antigens (21) and DNCB (22) has been more extensively used.

Our model of autoimmune enterocolitis possess some of the immunopathological features of IBD. Further studies will be useful in order to gain insight into the pathogenesis and eventually to immunological manipulations in ulcerative colitis and Crohn's disease.

CONCLUSIONS

1. Alloimmunization with a mucosal antigen (MA) provoke a humoral and cell-mediated autoimmune reaction together with lesions in the target organ (small and large intestine) of guinea pigs.

2. Some of the epitopes of MA are common to other guinea pig organs, but extensive absorptions allowed the identification of "true" mucosal epitopes.

3. Those mucosal epitopes can be tentatively linked to 3 main protein bands of m.w. of less than 60 Kd, as assessed by SDS-electrophoresis.

ACKNOWLEDGEMENT

This investigation has been supported by an MRC of Canada grant MA-9352. We are thankful to F. Navratil and R. Dumont for their skillful technical assistance.

REFERENCES

1. Kirsner, J.B. and Shorter, R.G., New England J. Med 306, 837, 1982.
2. Broberger, O. and Perlmann, P., J. Exp. Med. 117, 705, 1963.
3. Mattsby-Baltzer, I., Fasth, A. et al, Scand. J. Gastroenterol. 18, 305, 1983.
4. Hodgson, H.J.F., Potter, B.J., Jewell, D.P., Clin. Exp. Immunol. 29, 187, 1977.
5. Soltis, R.D., Hasz, D., et al., Gastroenterology 76, 1380, 1979.
6. Surrenti, C., Ramarli, D., et al., Hepato-gastroneterol. 28, 157, 1981.
7. Roche, J.K., Fiocchi, C. and Youngman, K., J. Clin. Invest. 75, 522, 1985.
8. Kemler, B.J. and Alpert, E., Gut 21, 353, 1980.
9. Ginsburg, C.H. and Falchuk, Z.M., Gastroenterology 83, 1, 1982.
10. MacDermott, R.P., Bradgon, M.J., et al, Gastroenterology 86, 476, 1984.
11. Nemirovsky, M.S. and Hugon, J.S., Gut, 27, 1434, 1986.
12. Takacs, B., in Immunological Methods, (Edited by Lefkovitz, I. and Pernis, B.), p. 81, Academic Press, 1979.
13. Rauch, H.C. and Roboz Einstein, E., Rev. Neurosci. 1, 283, 1974.
14. Rose, N.R. and Witebsky, E., J. Immunol. 76, 417, 1956.
15. Nemirovsky, M.S., Am. J. Reprod. Immunol. 2, 79, 1982.
16. Nussenblatt, R.B., Palestine, A.G. and Chan, C.C., Int. Ophthalmol. Clin. 25, 81, 1985.
17. Like, A.A. and Rossini, A.A., Surv. Synth. Pathol. Res. 3, 131, 1984.

18. Sakaguchi, S., Fukuma, K., Kuribayashi, K. and Masuda, T., J. Exp. Med. 161, 72, 1985.

19. Watt, J. and Marcus, R., Gut 12, 164, 1971.

20. Sharon, P. and Stenson, N., Gastroenterology 88, 55, 1985.

21. Mee, A.S., McLaughlin, J., et al Gut 20, 1, 1979.

22. Rabin, B.S. and Rogers, S.J., Gastroenterology 75, 29, 1978.

TRANSIENT DIETARY HYPERSENSITIVITY IN MICE AND PIGS

C.R. Stokes, T.J. Newby, B.G. Miller and F.J. Bourne

Department of Veterinary Medicine
University of Bristol, School of Veterinary Medicine
Langford House, Langford
Bristol BS18 7DU
ENGLAND

INTRODUCTION

In recent years, attention has focused upon the development of immune exclusion and oral tolerance as mechanisms that regulate and prevent damaging hypersensitivity reactions to dietary antigens. The significance of failure to develop these processes have similarly been investigated, it having been establshed that in the "mature response" to dietary antigens, local mucosal humoral immunity may co-exist with systemic tolerance, while both compartments of the cell mediated response are suppressed (1). It has long been known that following the introduction of a new dietary antigen, a transient serum response (2) may be induced; it is perhaps surprising, therefore, that the immunopathological significance of this early response to fed antigens has received little attention. Cell mediated responses may also be generated following feeding a wide range of antigens, including sheep red blood cells (SRBC) (3), ovalbumin (4) and contact sensitizing agents (5), as well as a wide range of infectious agents (6). In this study, we have induced transient cell mediated immune responses following feeding dietary antigens and determined the influence of "adjuvants" upon tolerance induction. The immunopathological consequence of this allergic response has been investigated in both mice and pigs.

MATERIALS AND METHODS

Animals

Groups of eight CBA male mice SPF grade 4 were used when aged between

2 and 3 months. Pigs, pregnant gilts, were obtained from a PHCA herd (Brockton Court, Shifnall, Shropshire). In all cases, except where indicated, piglets were weaned abruptly at 3 wk of age.

Diets

Mice were fed ad lib on Labsure diets throughout. The piglets were weaned onto a 22% protein diet which contained a heat-treated full fat soya (Trusoy; British Soya products) as the sole protein source. In one experiment, soya was replaced by either casein or hydrolysed casein.

Induction and elicitation of delayed hypersensitivity (DTH) to SRBC

Mice were given an intravenous (i.v.) injection of 1×10^5 SRBC. Five days later they were given a subcutaneous (s.c.) injection of 2×10^8 SRBC into the left hind footpad and either the increase in thickness of the footpad was measured after 24 h or the difference in weight between right and left feet measured (7).

Oral immunization

Mice were fed daily by gastric intubation with 2×10^9 SRBC in 0.2 ml.

Adjuvants

Dextran sulphate (m.w. 500,000) was added to the drinking water at a concentration of 0.1 mg ml^{-1}. Incomplete Freund's adjuvant was given as a single intraperitoneal injection of 0.1 ml of an oil and water emulsion.

Adoptive transfer

Suspensions of lymphocytes were prepared from donor spleens and mesenteric lymph nodes. Following washing in tissue culture medium, 5×10^7 lymphocytes were injected i.v. into each recipient which had (where indicated) been previously irradiated with 250 rads.

Xylose assays

Mice were fed a single feed of 10 mg xylose (0.2 ml) and were bled from the retro-orbital plexus 30 min later. Piglets were dosed with a 10% xylose solution (1 mg kg^{-1}) and bled 1 h later. Xylose concentration in serum was mesured by standard methods (8).

EXPERIMENTS AND RESULTS

Oral immunization of mice with SRBC

Mice were fed SRBC for 0, 5 or 14 days prior to footpad challenge 7 days later. Both the groups fed SRBC showed significantly greater increases in foot weight over the next 24 h (Table 1). In a further experiment, mice were similarly fed with SRBC and their immune responsiveness was then investigated by sensitizing them by i.v. injection 7 d later followed by footpad challenge after a further 5 days. The results indicate (Table 1) that while feeding for 5 days had no significant effect upon the ability to sensitize, feeding for 14 days reduced the response.

The effect of adjuvants upon oral tolerance induction. Mice were fed SRBC for 5 days. One group was also fed dextran sulphate during the oral immunization period, while another group received incomplete Freund's adjuvant one day before the start of oral immunization. The three groups were then sensitized by i.v. injection challenged into the footpad, and the 24 h increase in foot weights compared with a non-fed group. The results (Table 2) indicate that both dextran sulphate and incomplete Freund's adjuvant reduced the response (enhanced the development of tolerance).

TABLE 1. The effect of feeding SRBC on the induction of delayed type hypersensitivity and tolerance

Group	Days fed SRBC	i.v. SRBC	Footpad weight (mg)
1	0	-	1.9 ± 8
2	5	-	56 ± 26[a]
3	14	-	49 ± 2[b]
4	0	+	63 ± 22
5	5	+	65 ± 19[c]
6	14	+	31 ± 12[d]

[a] $t = 4.80$ $p < 0.001$ compared with group 1.

[b] $t = 5.02$ $p < 0.001$ compared with group 1.

[c] $t = 0.19$ $p > 0.1$ compared with group 4.

[d] $t = 3.61$ $p < 0.01$ compared with group 4.

Table 2. The effect of adjuvants on immune responsiveness to SRBC following oral immunization

Group	Adjuvant Dextran Sulphate	FIA	SRBC	Footpad weight
1	-	-	- i.v. + s.c.	75 ± 14
2	-	-	Fed.i.v. + s.c.	85 ± 16[a]
3	+	-	Fed.i.v. + s.c.	66 ± 11[b]
4	-	+	Fed.i.v. + s.c.	31 ± 13[c]

[a] $t = 1.3$ $p > 0.1$ compared with group 1.

[b] $t = 2.8$ $p < 0.02$ compared with group 2.

[c] $t = 7.4$ $p < 0.001$ compared with group 2.

The adoptive transfer of tolerance by spleen cells. Cell suspensions were prepared from the spleens of two groups of mice orally immunized with SRBC, one group of which was also injected with incomplete Freund's adjuvant as in the previous experiment. They were injected i.v. into irradiated (250 rads) recipients, which were then sensitized by i.v. injection of SRBC, challenged into the left hind pad and the 24 h increase in footpad thickness compared with the recipients of normal spleen cells. The recipients of lymphocytes from Freund's adjuvant treated mice had reduced responses (Table 3) compared with recipients of control lymphocytes, suggesting that these recipients received suppressor cells from the donors. In contrast, the recipients of lymphocytes from donors orally immunized without adjuvant showed an enhanced response.

Gastrointestinal effects. Groups of eight CBA male mice were sensitized by feeding 3×10^9 SRBC daily for two days. They were then challenged 10 days later on two consecutive days and their ability to absorb xylose measured one day later and compared with unsensitized mice, tolerized mice (i.e. previously fed SRBC for 14 days) and those sensitized with the non-cross-reacting antigen horse red blood cells (HRBC). The percentage reduction in xylose absorption, compared with non-sensitized/non-challenged mice, is shown in Table 4. Mice sensitized and challenged with SRBC absorbed significantly less xylose than non-sensitized mice, tolerized mice or those sensitized with HRBC. The xylose malabsorption was associated

Table 3. The effect of adjuvant upon adoptive transfer of oral tolerance to SRBC

Group	Treatment of Donors FIA	Treatment of Donors SRBC	Treatment of Recipients SRBC	Footpad Thickness
1	-	-	i.v. + s.c.	7.9 ± 1.5
2	-	Fed	i.v. + s.c.	10.4 ± 1.2
3	+	Fed	i.v. + s.c.	5.5 ± 1.4

with an increase in the rate of division of crypt cells (CCPR. h^{-1}) and number of intraepithelial lymphocytes (Table 4).

In subsequent experiments, we investigated the ability of spleen cells and mesenteric lymph node (MLN) cells from orally immunized mice at adoptive transfer (Table 5). Non-irradiated recipients of primed MLN cells and spleen cells both showed a reduced ability to absorb xylose by comparison with those mice receiving control cells.

Gastrointestinal changes in post-weaned pigs. Piglets from at least four litters were weaned abruptly at three weeks of age onto a diet in which the sole protein source was soya flour. Their ability to absorb xylose was measured at the time of weaning and 5 days post weaning and compared with a similar group of piglets which had eaten a large amount (greater than 750 g) of the post-weaning diet during the 7 days before weaning (tolerized). At weaning, there was no difference between the groups (1 and 2; Table 6) in their ability to absorb xylose. However, by five days post weaning, while those that had been toleized to soya still had a similar ability to absorb xylose, those that had not met the antigen before showed a marked reduction in their ability to absorb.

In a further series of experiments, piglets were weaned abruptly onto either casein or hydrolyxed casein based diets (groups 3 and 4, Table 6). By 5 days post weaning, while those pigs weaned onto the casein diet showed a markedly reduced ability to absorb xylose, those weaned onto the "antigen free" diet were not affected. Together, these studies indicate that antigenicity and previous exposure (tolerance) may influence the post weaning malabsorption.

Table 4. The effect of oral immunization with SRBC upon xylose absorption, crypt cell production rate (CCPR) and intraepithelial cell numbers (IELs)

Group	Days fed SRBC		% Reduction Xylose Absorption	CCPR (h^{-1})	IELs (per 100 epithelial cells)
	To Prime	Challenge			
1	0	0	0 ± 7	4.2	15.7 ± 3.1
2	0	2	9 ± 3	ND	ND
3	2	0	8 ± 5	ND	ND
4	(HRBC x 2)	2	4 ± 6	ND	ND
5	2	2	18 ± 4	11.7	23.4 ± 5.2
6	14	2	4 ± 5	4.3	ND

Table 5. The effect of adoptive transfer of spleen and mesenteric lymph node cells from orally immunized mice upon xylose absorption. All recipients were challenged with SRBC.

Group	Treatment of Recipients	% Reduction Xylose Absorption
1	control spleen cells	0
2	primed MLN cells	31 ± 10
3	primed spleen cells	42 ± 7

Table 6. The effect of weaning on the ability of piglets to absorb xylose

Group	Treatment		Xylose absorption	
	Pre-weaning	Post-weaning	At weaning	% Reduction (5d)
1	-	soya	1.14 ± 0.32	80.4 ± 10.6
2	soya(tolerized)	soya	1.23 ± 0.39[a]	8.6 ± 44.4[c]
3	-	casein	1.25 ± 0.20	57.8 ± 7.0
4	-	hydrolyzed casein	1.24 ± 0.18[b]	+1.2 ± 21.1[d]

[a] $t = 0.50$ $p > 0.1$ compared with group 1.
[b] $t = 0.10$ $p > 0.1$ compared with group 3.
[c] $t = 4.15$ $p < 0.001$ compared with group 1.
[d] $t = 7.49$ $p < 0.001$ compared with group 3.

DISCUSSION

We have shown that following the introduction of SRBC into the diet of mice, they pass through a brief phase of sensitivity, as indicated by their ability to mount DTH skin tests, prior to the development of tolerance. This pattern of hypersensitivity (cellular and/or humoral), before the development of tolerance is in agreement with the observations following feeding SRBC (3), contact sensitizing agents (5), ovalbumin (4) and microbial antigens (6). Further feeding of SRBC during this sensitive phase resulted in increases in the rate of division of crypt cells and in the number of IELs. These changes, together with a villus atrophy (data not shown), are identical to those changes reported during rejection of small intestinal allografts (9) and graft-versus-host reactions (10); such changes being shown to be compatible with a mucosal DTH reaction (see 11). In our studies, local sensitivity as indicated by a decreased ability to absorb xylose could be adoptively transferred by spleen cells and MLN cells from SRBC fed animals. These observations, together with the concurrent positive skin tests, would indicate that the gut changes observed following feeding erythrocytes may also be cell mediated.

Gut changes compatible with a DTH reaction to food antigens have also been reported in mice fed ovalbumin, but only those treated with cyclophosphamide (12), which apparently prevented the induction of oral tolerance.

In other studies of mice fed ovalbumin, strain differences have been observed in the expression of transient cell mediated sensitivity (13). Thus, the changes we describe here are likely to be of immunopathological significance beyond SRBC feeding. The experiments described here in the post-weaned pig would support this view. Further, in this species, we have shown that by dietary manipulation so as to induce tolerance or priming, damage may be prevented or promoted and these changes may influence the proliferation of enteropathogenic _E. coli_ (14,15).

Transient specific delayed hypersensitivity has been reported in CBA mice fed 25 mg ovalbumin for 2-4 days, prior to the development of tolerance (4). In addition to the local antigen specific effects of oral immunization reported here, we have earlier shown that during this period of sensitivity the response to non-related antigens is altered. These effects include the prevention of oral tolerance induction to a second antigen (HSA) introduced to the diet two days after the start of oral immunization with ovalbumin (4). The abrogation of tolerance induction has also been reported during graft-versus-host reactions and an enhanced presentation of antigen during this period implicated (16). Since we have shown that following a dietary change the rate of PVP clearance is enhanced (17), it is possible that a similar mechanism may be operating during oral immunization, possibly as a consequence of the DTH reaction.

It is established that following the start of oral immunization, a transient cell mediated immune response is generated and that this may be of immunopathological significance. In this context, it may therefore be important to enhance the development of tolerance and the observation of the effects of adjuvants in SRBC fed mice may, therefore, be of benefit in preventing these potentially damaging transient allergic responses.

CONCLUSIONS

1. Oral immunization with SRBC stimulates a transient DTH response that may be responsible for an altered gut morphology and a decreased ability to absorb xylose.

2. Adjuvants (dextran sulphate, incomplete Freund's adjuvant) may enhance the development of tolerance.

3. Similar changes occur in the gut of the post-weaned pig and may lead to the altered handling of microbial and non-microbial antigens.

ACKNOWLEDGEMENTS

This investigation was supported by the Agriculture and Food Research Council of the U.K.

REFERENCES

1. Newby, T.J. and Stokes, C.R., CRC Press, Boca Raton, U.S.A., 1984.
2. Lippard, V.M., Schloss, O.M. and Johnson, P.A., Am. J. Dis. Child. 5, 562, 1936.
3. Kagnoff, M.E., J. Immunol. 120, 1509, 1978.
4. Stokes, C.R., Newby, T.J. and Bourne, F.J., Clin. Exp. Immunol. 52, 309, 1983.
5. Asherson, G.L., Zembala, M., Perera, M.A.C.C., Mayhew, B. and Thomas, W.R., Cell. Immunol. 33, 145, 1977.
6. Newby, T.J., in Local Immune Responses of the Gut, (Edited by Newby, T.J. and Stokes, C.R.), p. 143, CRC Press, Inc., Boca Raton, USA, 1984.
7. Kitamura, K., J. Immunol. Meth. 39, 277, 1980.
8. Trinder, P., Analyst 100, 12, 1975.
9. MacDonald, T.T. and Ferguson, A., Gut 17, 81, 1976.
10. MacDonald, T.T. and Ferguson, A., Cell Tissue Kinet 10, 301, 1977.
11. Mowat, A.McI., in Local Immune Responses of the Gut, (Edited by Newby, T.J. and Stokes, C.R.), p. 199, CRC Press, Inc., Boca Raton, USA, 1984.
12. Mowat, A.McI. and Ferguson, A., Clin. Exp. Immunol. 43, 574, 1981.
13. Stokes, C.R., Newby, T.J., Miller, B. and Bourne, F.J., in Cell Mediated Immunity, (Edited by Quinn, P.J.), p. 249, CEC, Luxembourg.
14. Mille, B.G., Newby, T.J., Stokes, C.R. and Bourne, F.J., Res. Vet. Sci. 36, 187, 1984.
15. Miller, B.G., Newby, T.J., Stokes, C.R., Hampson, D.J., Brown, P.J. and Bourne, F.J., Am. J. Vet. Res. 45, 1730, 1984.
16. Strobel, S., Mowat, A.McI. and Ferguson, A., Immunology 56, 57, 1985.
17. Newby, T.J., Stokes, C.R. and Bourne, F.J., Clin. Exp. Immunol. 39, 349, 1980.

PASSAGE OF DIETARY ANTIGENS IN MAN: KINETICS OF APPEARANCE IN SERUM AND CHARACTERIZATION OF FREE AND ANTIBODY-BOUND ANTIGEN

S. Husby, S.-E., Svehag and J.C. Jensenius

Institute of Medical Microbiology
Odense University
DK-5000 Odense C, Denmark

INTRODUCTION

The passage of dietary antigens from the human gastrointestinal tract to the blood was indicated already in the 1920's, by experiments with passive cutaneous anaphylaxis (1). Quantitation of absorbed dietary antigens in healthy adults was later accomplished by the use of radioimmunological techniques (2). Further, dietary antigens have been reported in circulating immune complexes in atopic patients and in normals (3,4) and in patients with IgA-deficiency (5).

In order to elucidate the kinetics of appearance of dietary antigen in the blood, and the relation of antigen uptake to antibody levels, we have developed ELISA techniques for the quantitation of two dietary antigens, ovalbumin (OA) and beta-lactoglobulin (BLG). To ascertain the molecular form of absorbed antigen we have further combined these ELISA techniques with high performance gel permeation chromatography (HPLC) for the fractionation of serum samples. The present report summarizes these studies of antigen passage in healthy adults (6,7).

MATERIALS AND METHODS

ELISA for antigen determinations

Microplates were coated with affinity-purified rabbit $F(ab')_2$ anti-OA or $F(ab')_2$ anti-BLG antibody, with normal rabbit $F(ab')_2$ as control. Serum samples and standards (0.04-30 ng OA or BLG per ml of serum devoid of antibody), diluted 1:10, were incubated overnight in dupli- or triplicates. After washings, the wells were developed with biotin-labeled anti-OA or anti-BLG antibody, followed by avidin-β-galactosidase and substrate, with intermediate washings. The lower detection limit was about 0.3 ng/ml serum for both assays. The variability of the assays was evaluated with separate control samples at 1 ng/ml and at 10 ng/ml. The within-assay coefficient of variation (CV) ranged 0.10-0.16 for the OA-assay, and 0.02-0.12 for the BLG-assay, and the between-assay CV ranged 0.04-0.37 for the OA-assay and 0.10-0.29 for the BLG assay.

High performance gel permeation chromatography (HPLC) in combination with ELISA for the determination of OA

HPLC was carried out as described previously (6,8). Serum samples were centrifuged and pumped through a precolumn and a size separation column, either TSK G-3000 SW or TSK G-6000 PW. The separation characteristics were determined by the elution volumes (V_e) or purified protein markers: keyhole limpet hemocyanin (KLH), thyroglobulin (Tg), IgG, OA, BLG and myoglobin (Mg).

Microplate wells were coated with $F(ab')_2$ anti-OA antibody and fractions from the HPLC column were collected into the microplate wells. A standard curve was included in each plate, which was processed as described for the ELISA for OA.

HPLC in combination with ELISA for characterization of OA-containing immune aggregates

HPLC fractionation was performed into $F(ab')_2$ anti-OA coated wells as described above. After washings, the wells were incubated with biotin-labeled affinity-purified anti-IgG, IgA or IgM followed by development as described above. The lower detection limit of the assays was uniformly about 2 ng immunoglobulin per ml, as determined from a standard curve with purified IgG, IgA or IgM.

Antibody determinations

OA-binding capacity (titer at 10% binding) in serum was determined by a modified Farr assay (9). Serum IgG and IgA antibodies were quantitated by biotin-avidin amplified ELISA (10). The IgG antibody levels were related to a human serum with high antibody titers and expressed as mU/ml. IgA antibody titers were expressed as the highest dilution giving a signal above the background.

RESULTS

Eight healthy adults (age 22-38 years, 4 men and 4 women) with a range of serum antibody levels to OA and BLG abstained from food for 16 h before eating a mixture of 500 ml pasteurized buttermilk and 60 ml raw egg, with sugar added as flavor. Serial blood samples were taken from an indwelling cannula for 7 h after the meal, serum prepared and stored at -70°C. The test meal was repeated one year later with a 48 h egg-free diet before and after the test meal, in three individuals.

Antigen in serum after the test meal

No BLG was detected in any of the serum samples obtained after the test meal. OA as determined by ELISA was present in detectable amounts in 7/8 individuals (Fig. 1). The levels peaked at 1.7-10.5 ng OA/ml serum, in a monophasic pattern 120-300 min after the test meal. However, in two individuals no obvious peak was observed during the sampling period. Low levels of OA was observed in three sera, obtained before the meal (t_o).

The experiment was repeated one year later, for those three individuals who previously were found to have demonstrated OA levels at t_o (Fig. 2). In one case, a peak OA value was observed 24 h after the meal, and OA was

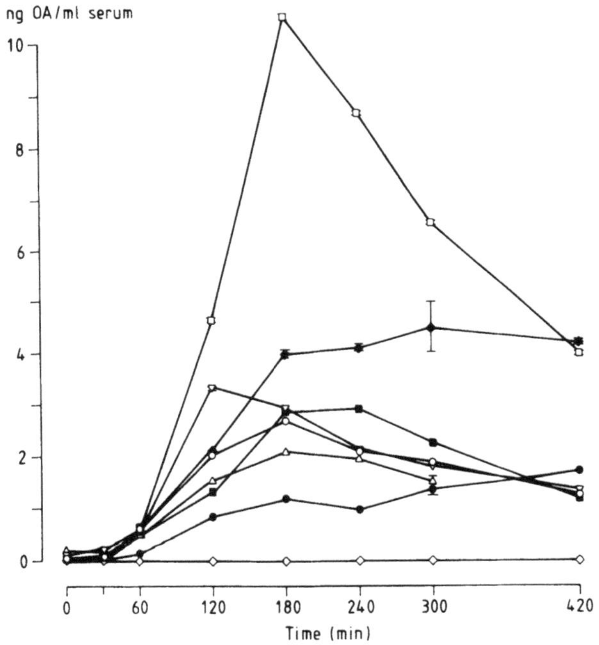

Figure 1. OA in the sera of eight healthy adults after a test meal. The test persons are denoted by: No. 1 (●), No. 2 (△), No. 3 (◇), No. 4 (○), No. 5 (▽), No. 6 (□), No. 7 (■) and No. 8 (◆). Bars denote range of triplicate determinations, when not indicated the ranges within the symbol. From Scand. J. Immunol. 22, 83, 1985, with permission.

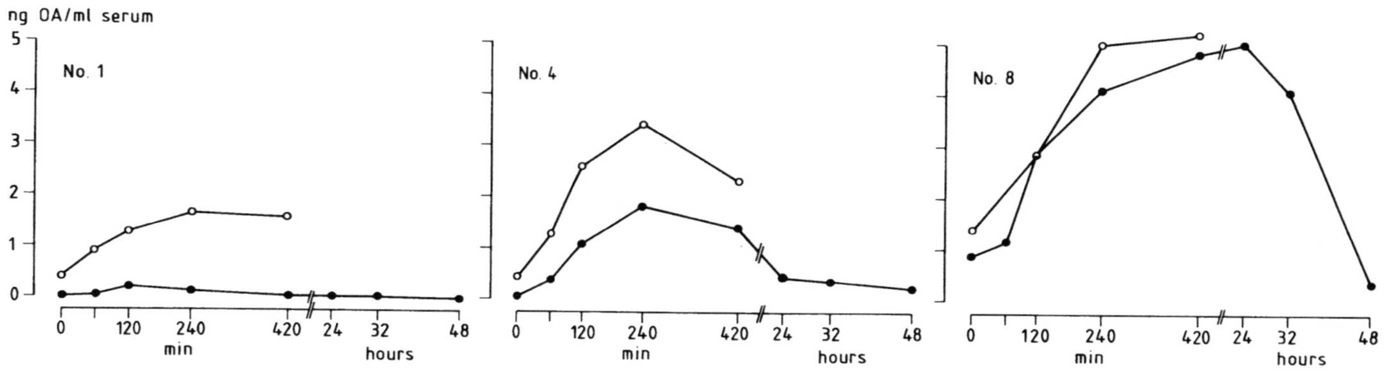

Figure 2. OA in the sera of three healthy adults after a test meal, after 16 h fast (○) or after 48 h of egg-free diet (●). Number of test subject is indicated in the figure. From Scand. J. Immunol., 24, 447, 1986.

detectable even in the 48 h sample. A clear repetition of the kinetics of OA appearance was present in two out of the three individuals.

Relation between OA and anti-OA antibody levels

Maximal OA levels, and antibody levels in serum and saliva are depicted in Table 1. The individual (No. 3) with no detectable OA had the highest serum IgG anti-OA antibody level (550 mU/ml), no serum IgA antibody, and intermediate anti-OA antibody in saliva. Conversely, the person (No. 6) with the highest OA level (10.5 ng/ml) had low IgG antibody in serum (4 mU/ml), no IgA antibody and no detectable antibody in saliva. Between these two extremes no obvious correlations between levels of antigen and antibody were noted.

Size distribution of OA in serum

Anti-OA antibody reactive material was detected by the combination of ELISA for OA and HPLC fractionation (TSK G-3000 SW) in all 8 individuals (Figs. 3-5). The antigen was found either at the V_e of native OA or in high MW fractions, mostly between V_e of IgG and V_o, which includes thyroglobulin at 660 kD. Three individuals with high IgG antibody levels had only high MW OA (Fig. 3). One of these test persons (No. 8) had a very slow metabolism of OA (Fig. 2).

Three individuals had comparable levels of native and high-MW OA, assuming full antigen-reactivity of OA-aggregates (Fig. 4). Two of these (No. 2 and No. 4) had intermediate serum IgG antibody levels, the third had a low IgG antibody level, but also low amounts of OA in the blood. The remaining two test persons had predominantly OA at the V_e of native OA (Fig. 5), and they had low IgG antibody levels in serum. No clear relation was noted between the molecular form of OA and IgM or IgA antibody levels in serum or saliva.

Isotype distribution of OA-immunoglobulin aggregates

Immune complexes between OA and antibody were determined with a combination of HPLC (TSK G-6000 PW) and ELISA, in the t_0 sera and the sera obtained 180 min after the meal. A significant difference between pre- and post-meal serum was observed in the IgG OA-aggregates in three individuals (Fig. 6). These sera contained high or medium IgG antibody levels. One of the persons with almost no high-MW OA was included as a negative control. No IgA or IgM containing OA aggregates were found.

Table 1. Maximal OA concentrations in serum and anti-OA antibody levels in serum and saliva of eight healthy subjects. From Scand. J. Immunol. 22, 83, 1985 (with permission)

Subject No.	Max. serum OA (ng/ml)	Serum anti-OA (% binding)[a]	Serum anti-OA IgG (mU/ml)[b]	Serum anti-OA IgA (titre)[c]	Saliva anti-OA (titre)[4]
1	1.7	100	336	310	8.2
2	2.2	<10	26	560	5.6
3	0	97	550	0	8.4
4	2.7	<10	24	90	12.0
5	3.3	<10	1	80	4.6
6	10.5	11	4	0	0
7	2.9	<10	4	250	9.2
8	4.5	87	160	190	3.2

[a]Measured by a modified Farr assay and expressed as percentage binding at a serum dilution of 1:2.

[b]Measured by ELISA and related to a high-titred human serum (100 mU/ml).

[c]Measured by ELISA: titre determined as the highest dilution giving a signal above background.

[d]Measured by a modified Farr assay, expressed as titre.

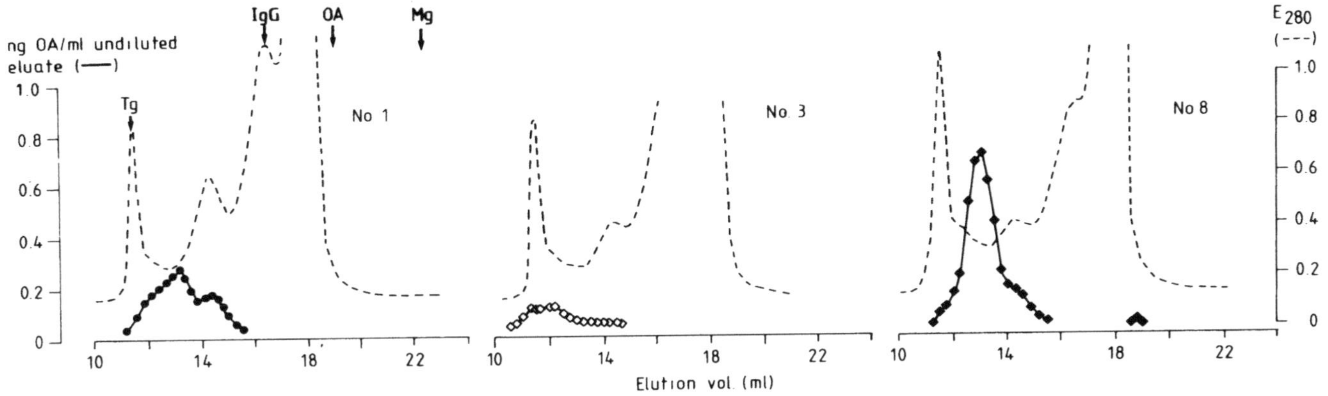

Figure 3. HPLC-fractionation (TSK G-3000 SW) followed by ELISA for determination of OA, in serum taken 180 min after the test meal, in three subjects with high MW anti-OA antibody reacting material only. Number of individual is indicated in the figure. Broken line denotes fractionation pattern of the sera (E_{280}) and full drawn line indicates OA detection. From Scand. J. Immunl 22, 83, 1985, with permission.

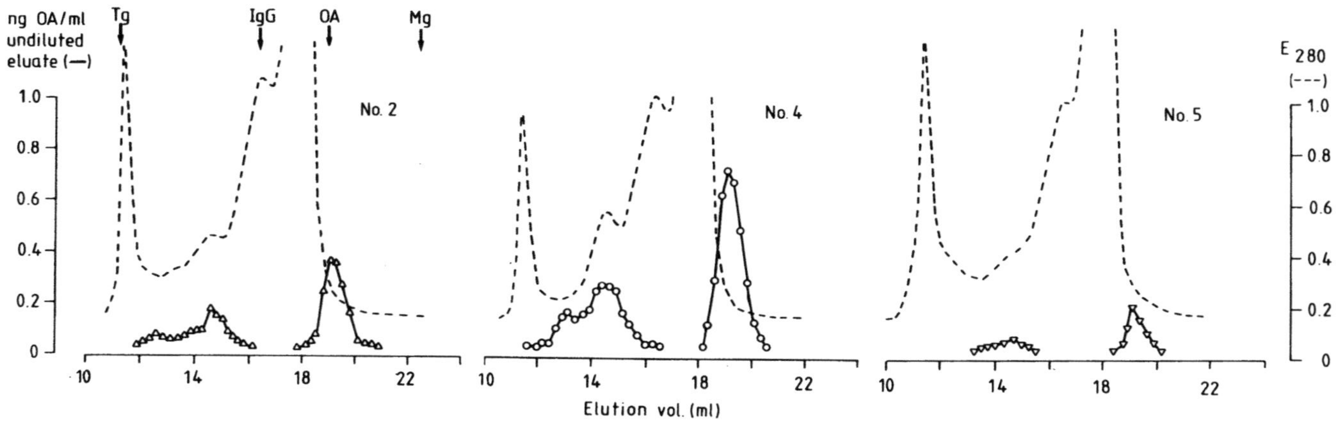

Figure 4. HPLC-fractionation followed by ELISA for OA, in 180 min-sera from three subjects with comparable amounts of high-MW OA and OA eluting as the native antigen. Number of the individual is indicated in the figure. From Scand. J. Immunol. 22, 83, 1985, with permission.

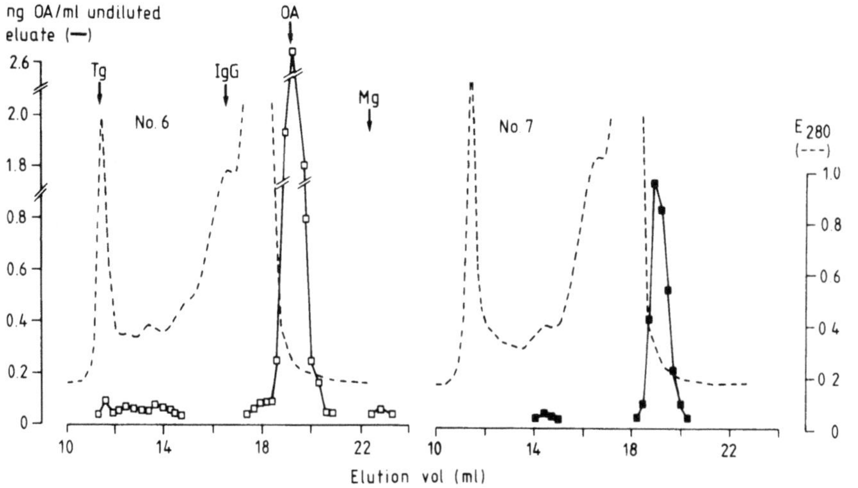

Figure 5. HPLC-fractionation followed by ELISA for OA, in 180 min-sera from two individuals with OA predominantly eluting at the M_r of native OA. Symbols as indicated in previous figures. From Scand. J. Immunol. 22, 83, 1985, with permission.

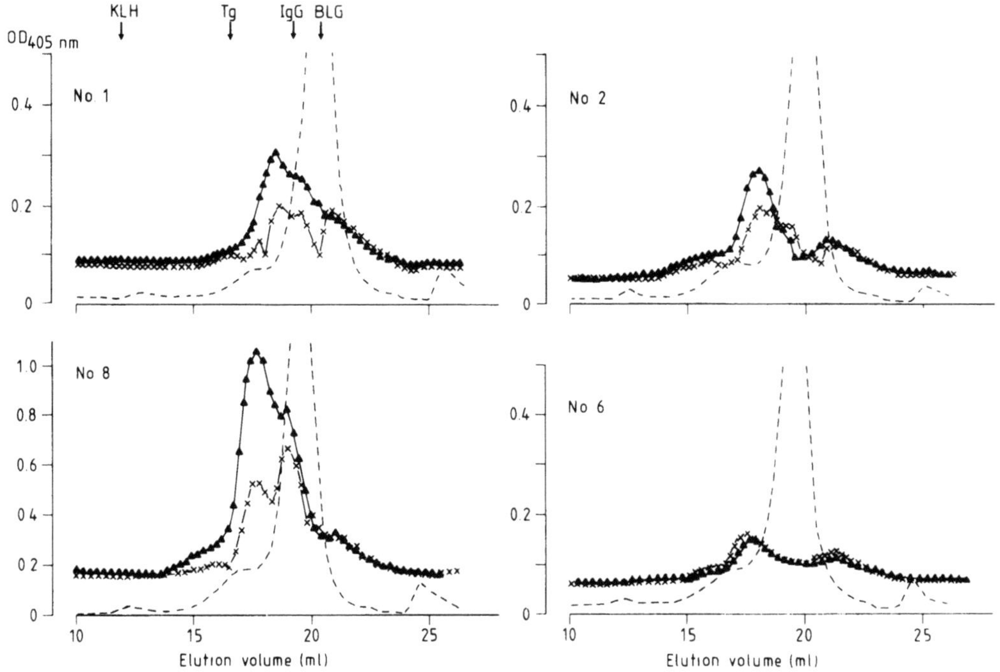

Figure 6. HPLC-fractionation (TSK G-6000 PW) followed by ELISA for IgG-containing OA aggregates, in the T_o (x) and the 180 min sera (▲) of three individuals. Number of test subject is shown in the figure. From Scand. J. Immunol. 24, 447, 1986 with permission.

DISCUSSION

The present results confirm data indicating that dietary antigens may pass the mucosal barrier of the gastrointestinal tract and appear in the circulation of healthy adults. We could only detect OA in serum after a test meal, but not BLG, in contrast to the results of Paganelli and Levinsky (2), possibly due to lack of antibody recognition of BLG-fragments in the present studies, in combination with more efficient enzymatic breakdown of BLG than of OA (6).

OA was demonstrated in serum already 30 min after the meal, indicating passage rather early in the gastrointestinal tract. The antigen was detectable in up to two days in one individual, suggesting a variable, but slow clearance of OA, seemingly without any deleterious effects in the individual. Little is otherwise known about the metabolism of soluble antigens in man, whereas the clearance ($T_{1/2}$) of heat-damaged or antibody-coated red blood cells occurs within one hour in normals, to some extent depending on the experimental conditions (11).

The size distribution of the absorbed OA was dominated by antigencally intact OA in the V_e of the native protein, and of high-MW anti-OA reacting material, which was shown to be antigen-antibody aggregates. No fragments of OA were observed, possibly because of lack of recognition by the antibodies raised against intact OA.

The OA aggregates mainly eluted within the fractionation range of the column (V_o includes Tg at 660 kD), and thus, were of a limited composition: Ag_4Ab_2, Ag_3Ab_3 or below. Such discrete complexes are probably not or weakly complement-fixing, and this may explain the sustained presence of OA in complexed form in some individuals. The complexes tended to become more heterogeneous in size after a few hours (7).

The OA aggregates in serum contained IgG in three subjects, and the presence of high-MW OA related to IgG antibody levels only, whereas no IgA or IgM was detected in the aggregates. IgA is generally regarded as the major non-phlogistic immunoglobulin isotype. Whether the SC-mediated transport of IgA-antigen complexes from blood to bile in rodents (12) is of significance in man seems at present unclear (13). The human IgG subclasses have variable complement fixing and cell activating properties (14,15). Thus, IgG antibodies, both in the lamina propria of the gut and in the circulation, may participate in the physiological disposal of harmless antigens, without any tissue damage. To this end, we have demonstrated a preponderance of the non-complement fixing IgG4 antibodies to dietary antigens in normal human sera (16).

Orally induced immunological tolerance (17), that is, the induction of secretory immunity concomitant with systemic tolerance, has in experimental animals been indicated to prevent the absorption of soluble antigen from the gut (18,19). When present, serum-derived antibody may retard antigen penetration and/or enhance the absorption of unrelated by-stander antigen (20). Orally induced tolerance is currently believed to be the physiological reaction of the immune system to antigens presenting at the mucous membranes, thus avoiding a systemic hypersensitivity. The present studies indicate that immunization (subject Nos. 2,4,5 and 7) and possibly anergy (subject No. 6) may occur in healthy humans without any deleterious effects. Thus, the physiological reactions of the human immune system to dietary antigens seems regulated in a more complex way, probably involving cellular as well as antibody-isotype specific immune responses.

CONCLUSIONS

1. Dietary antigens such as OA may, in minute amounts (ng/ml serum) pass into the human circulation of healthy adults. The clearance rates vary from hours to days.

2. OA was observed in serum either of a MW size corresponding to the native protein, or as high MW anti-OA reacting material, containing small sized (< 660 kD) immune complexes.

3. The presence of OA immune aggregates was related to the levels of IgG antibodies in serum. IgG, but not IgA or IgM was detected in the OA aggregates.

REFERENCES

1. Walzer, M., J. Immunol. 11, 249, 1926.
2. Paganelli, R. and Levinsky, R.J., J. Immunol. Meth. 37, 333, 1980.

3. Paganelli, R., Levinsky, R.J., Brostoff, I. and Wraith, D.G., Lancet 1, 1270, 1979.
4. Paganelli, R., Levinsky, R.J. and Atherton, D.J., Clin. Exp. Immunol. 46, 44, 1981.
5. Cunningham-Rundles, C., Eur. J. Immunol. 11, 504, 1981.
6. Husby, S., Jensenius, J.C. and Svehag, S-E., Scand. J. Immunol. 22, 83, 1985.
7. Husby, S., Jensenius, J.C. and Svehag, S-E., Scand. J. Immunol. 24, 447, 1986.
8. Holmskov-Nielsen, U., Erb, K. and Jensenius, J.C., J. Chromat. 297, 225, 1984.
9. Husby, S., Oxelius, V-A., Teisner, B., Jensenius, J.C. and Svehag, S-E., Int. Archs. Allergy Appl. Immunol. 77, 416, 1985.
10. Husby, S., Schultz Larsen, F., Hyltoft Peterson, P. and Svehag, S-E., Allergy, 41, 379, 1986.
11. Frank, M.M., Lawley, T.J., Hamburger, M.J. and Brown, E.J., Annals Int. Med. 98, 206, 1983.
12. Socken, D.J., Simms, E.S., Nagy, B.R., Fischer, M.R. and Underdown, B.J., J. Immunol. 127, 316, 1981.
13. Brandtzaeg, P., Scand. J. Immunol. 22, 111, 1985.
14. Spiegelberg, H.L., Adv. Immunol. 19, 259, 1974.
15. Unkeless, J.C., Fleit, H. and Mellman, J.S., Adv. Immunol. 31, 247, 1981.
16. Husby, S., Jensenius, J.C. and Svehag, S-E., J. Immunol. Meth. 82, 321, 1985.
17. Chase, M.S., Proc. Soc. Exp. Biol. Med. 61, 257, 1946.
18. Swarbrick, E.T., Stokes, C.R. and Soothill, J.F., Gut 20, 121, 1979.
19. Lim, P.L. and Rowley, D., Int. Archs. Allergy Appl. Immunol. 68, 41, 1982.
20. Tolo, K., Brandtzaeg, P. and Jonsen, J., Immunology 33, 733, 1977.

DETECTION OF FOOD ANTIGEN-SPECIFIC IgA IMMUNE COMPLEXES IN HUMAN SERA

M.W. Russell, M.F. Spotswood, B.A. Julian, J.H. Galla and J. Mestecky

Departments of Microbiology and Medicine, The University of Alabama at Birmingham, Birmingham, Alabama USA

INTRODUCTION

The functions of immunoglobulins in disposal of antigens and immune complexes (IC) depends critically upon the isotype of Ig involved. In particular, the fate of IC containing IgA differs from that of IC containing IgG or IgM, because in contrast to the latter two, IgA does not readily activate complement or promote phagocytosis (1). Deposits of IgA, thought to represent IgA-IC, occur in skin or kidneys in certain disease states such as dermatitis herpetiformis, and IgA nephropathy (2). IgA antibodies are induced by gut antigens including food materials, and may be involved in limiting both the absorption of enteric macromolecules and the immune response to them (3). Investigation of these possibilities in human subjects necessitates a means of detecting IgA-IC containing specific antigens. We have developed a method of detecting IgA-IC containing bovine milk proteins, and have used it to detect such IC in sera of normal subjects as well as patients with IgA nephropathy.

METHODS

A pool of rabbit antisera having high levels of precipitating antibodies to bovine milk proteins, including bovine γ-globulin (BGG), casein and other whey proteins, was used to prepare the reagent. The IgG fraction of this serum, prepared by DEAE-cellulose chromatography, was cleaved with pepsin at pH 4.0 and chromatographed on Ultrogel AcA 34 to yield $F(ab')_2$ fragments. These were then passed sequentially over columns of CNBr-activated Sepharose conjugated with human serum protein, staphylococcal protein A, BGG, casein, and whey protein (prepared from milk by precipitation of casein with acetic acid). The latter three columns were eluted separately with 0.5 M acetic acid/0.15 M NaCl to obtain affinity-purified $F(ab')_2$ antibody fragments, which were neutralized and dialyzed against borate-buffered saline. For control purposes, $F(ab')_2$ of normal rabbit IgG was also prepared.

An enzyme-linked immunosorbent assay (ELISA) was developed to detect IC containing both a specific antigen, which would bind to $F(ab')_2$ antibody-coated plates, and IgA, which would be detected by an anti-IgA reagent. Plastic microtiter plates were coated with 1 μg/ml of $F(ab')_2$ anti-BGG, anti-casein, anti-whey protein, or normal rabbit $F(ab')_2$ and blocked with 5% horse serum. Human serum samples, or polyethylene glycol (PEG) precipitates, were diluted 1:10 in 5% horse serum and incubated for 6 h on the coated plates in quadruplicate. Bound IgA-IC were detected by means of biotin-conjugated $F(ab')_2$ affinity-purified goat anti-human IgA (Tago, Inc., Burlingame, CA) diluted 1:1000, followed by avidin-peroxidase (Sigma) (1 μg/ml). The color developed with 2,2'-azinobis-(3-ethylbenzthiazoline sulfonic acid) plus H_2O_2 was measured after 0.5 h.

Immune complexes were precipitated from human sera by means of PEG 8,000 (3.5% w/v), washed and redissolved to 10 times the original volume in 0.075 M tris.HCl pH 7.4, 0.01 M ethylenediamine tetracetic acid, and 1% bovine serum albumin.

Ultracentrifugation was performed in linear 10-50% (w/w) sucrose gradients (5 ml) spun at 30,000 rpm for 16 h in a Beckman SW 50.1 rotor. Fractions of 0.5 ml were assayed for IgA-IC by the ELISA described above.

RESULTS

Specific antigen-containing IgA-IC were putatively detected significant ly above the values obtained on the control plate, coated with normal rabbi $F(ab')_2$, in 7 of 8 normal human sera tested (Table 1). IC were most often detected, and at higher levels, on plates coated with $F(ab')_2$ anti-BGG.

Table 1. Milk protein-specific IgA-IC in 8 normal sera and PEG precipitates

Sample		Level of IgA-IC detected[a] on plates coated with:		
		anti-whey	anti-BGG	anti-casein
1.	Serum	0	0.275[b] ± 0.020	0
	PEG	0	0.200[b] ± 0.014	0
2.	Serum	0.001 ± 0.007	0.048[b] ± 0.005	nd[c]
	PEG	0	0.061[b] ± 0.008	nd
3.	Serum	0.040 ± 0.033	0.853[b] ± 0.045	nd
	PEG	0	0.109[b] ± 0.012	nd
4.	Serum	0.011 ± 0.042	0	nd
	PEG	0	0	nd
5.	Serum	0	0.069[b] ± 0.009	0.051[b] ± 0.010
	PEG	0	0.030[b] ± 0.012	0.031 ± 0.012
6.	Serum	0.112[b] ± 0.022	0.405[b] ± 0.010	0.275[b] ± 0.015
	PEG	0.035[b] ± 0.010	0	0
7.	Serum	0	0	0
	PEG	0	0	0
8.	Serum	nd	0.221[b] ± 0.017	nd
	PEG	nd	0.018[b] ± 0.005	nd

[a]Mean difference (absorbance at 414 nm) above controls [normal rabbit $F(ab')_2$] ± SED, quadruplicate determinations.
[b]Significant at $p < 0.05$ (Student's *t* test).
[c]nd, Not determined.

In most instances, when a significant value was recorded for serum, a corresponding value was obtained with the PEG precipitate from the same serum.

To simulate the possible effect of antigen absorption from the gut on IC formation, bovine skim milk was added to these sera (5 µl/ml), and the ELISA test repeated on serum and PEG precipitates (Table 2). In most

Table 2. Formation of milk protein-specific IgA-IC by addition of milk (5 µl/ml) to normal sera

Sample		Level of IgA-IC detected[a] on plates coated with:		
		anti-whey	anti-BGG	anti-casein
1.	Serum	0.031[b] ± 0.015	0.312[b] ± 0.014	0
	PEG	0	0.321[b] ± 0.012	0.004 ± 0.011
2.	Serum	0.008 ± 0.008	0.073[b] ± 0.008	nd[c]
	PEG	0	0.050[b] ± 0.007	nd
3.	Serum	0.025 ± 0.034	0.435[b] ± 0.030	nd
	PEG	0.029 ± 0.020	0.586[b] ± 0.016	nd
4.	Serum	0.068[b] ± 0.014	0.041 ± 0.044	nd
	PEG	0.051[b] ± 0.024	0.180[b] ± 0.024	nd
5.	Serum	0	0.050[b] ± 0.010	0.039[b] ± 0.010
	PEG	0.003 ± 0.025	0.043[b] ± 0.014	0.059[b] ± 0.023
6.	Serum	0.044[b] ± 0.016	0.283[b] ± 0.016	0.147[b] ± 0.016
	PEG	0.047[b] ± 0.011	0.075[b] ± 0.017	0
7.	Serum	0	0	0
	PEG	0	0	0
8.	Serum	nd	0.441[b] ± 0.007	nd
	PEG	nd	0.627[b] ± 0.014	nd

[a]Mean difference (absorbance at 414 nm) above controls [normal rabbit $F(ab')_2$] ± SED, quadruplicate determinations.
[b]Significant at $p < 0.05$ (Student's *t* test).
[c]nd, Not determined.

cases, there was an increase in the values obtained for putative BGG-containing IgA-IC, and two additional subjects (#1 and #4) appeared to display IgA-IC containing whey protein. The individual (#7) whose serum did not reveal IgA-IC either before or after the addition of milk had previously been found to have undetectable levels of IgA antibodies to milk proteins.

To examine the molecular behavior of the putative IgA-IC, the serum and PEG precipitates from one subject (#3), who was known to have high levels of serum IgA antibodies to BGG and casein, were subjected to ultracentrifugal analyses (Fig. 1). The serum alone (panel A) revealed a peak of ELISA-positive material at approximately 7S, but there was no corresponding peak in the PEG precipitate. After addition of milk, the serum and PEG precipitate revealed peaks of IgA-IC heavier than 19S (panel B). These IC were eliminated by treatment of the serum and PEG precipitates at pH 3.0, and running on gradients at pH 4.0 (panel C).

Sera of 12 normal subjects and 27 patients with IgA nephropathy were screened for the presence of milk protein-specific IgA-IC (Table 3). No significant difference was found between the two groups.

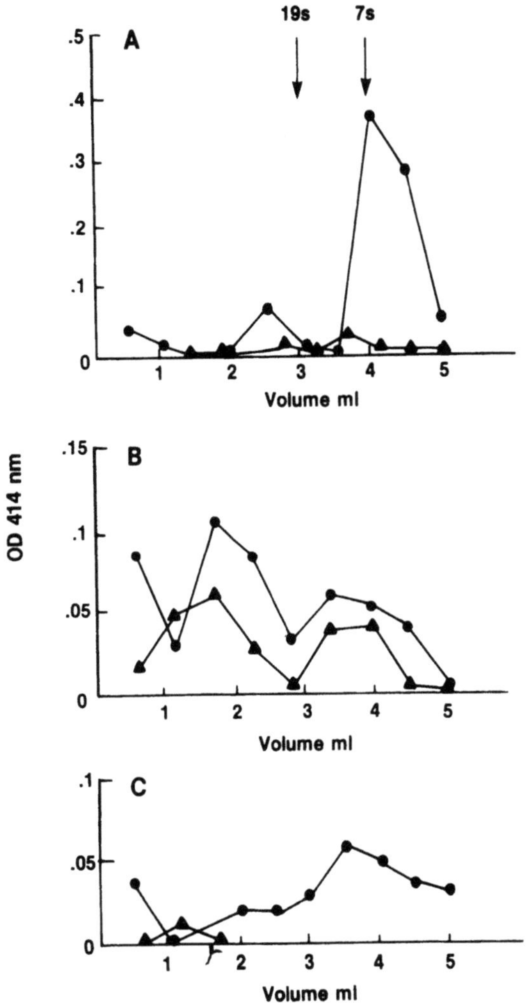

Figure 1. Ultracentrifugal analysis of BGG-containing IgA-IC in serum (●) and PEG precipitates (▲). (A), Serum and PEG precipitate; (B), Serum and PEG precipitate after the addition of milk (5 μl/ml); and (C), Serum and PEG precipitate after the addition of milk (5 μl/ml), samples dissociated in 0.5 M acetate pH 3 and run on gradients at pH 4.

Table 3. Milk protein-specific IgA immune complexes in sera of patients with IgA nephropathy

Group	Level of IgA-IC detected[a] on plates coated with: anti-whey	anti-BGG	anti-casein
IgA-nephropathy (N = 27)	0.229 ± 0.277	0.094 ± 0.123	0.085 ± 0.101
Normal subjects (N = 12)	0.203 ± 0.211	0.179 ± 0.234	0.077 ± 0.114
p (Student's *t*)	0.69	0.14	0.68

[a]Mean ± SD absorbance at 414 nm.

DISCUSSION

A large number of tests have been devised for the measurement of IC in human sera (4). Frequently, these depend on the ability of complexed Igs to fix complement, a property that is not well developed in IgA (1). While IgA may be detected in, for example, IC bound to anti-C3 or Raji cells (5,6), it is likely that these IC are mixed Ig isotype, since these assays detect IC by virtue of bound C3b. Even detection of IC-aggregated IgA is complicated because of the occurrence of polymeric forms of IgA, which may be present in serum at up to about 10% of total IgA.

The ELISA described here was designed to detect IgA bound to specific antigens. $F(ab')_2$ reagents were used in order to obviate interference by IgA rheumatoid factors, which have been found in the sera of rheumatoid arthritis and IgA nephropathy patients (5). Nevertheless, sera revealed a variable ability to bind to normal rabbit $F(ab')_2$ used to coat control plates, and therefore, values so obtained were subtracted from those given by $F(ab')_2$ antibody-coated plates. Several normal sera then revealed putative IgA-IC, especially on plates coated with anti-BGG. In most, though not all cases, PEG precipitates which would be expected to contain complexed or aggregated Igs, including IgA (7), showed parallel ELISA values. However, the sera were obtained without regard to food ingestion, and it was known from previous studies that some of the subjects had high levels of serum IgA antibodies to milk proteins. After addition of small amounts of milk to the sera, several then revealed increased ELISA values, especially in PEG precipitates.

Ultracentrifugal analysis of one serum known to have high levels of IgA antibodies to milk proteins, however, showed a substantial peak of ELISA-reactivity at about 7S that was not present in the PEG precipitate. Although addition of milk antigen appeared to generate heavier IgA-IC that were susceptible to acid dissociation, this 7S peak does not agree with normal concepts of IC material. One possibility is that it represents anti-idiotypic antibody against the rabbit $F(ab')_2$ anti-BGG. Anti-idiotypic antibodies against milk-specific antibodies have been reported in human sera (8), though not of the IgA isotype. The possibility that the rabbit $F(ab')_2$ anti-BGG also binds human Ig is unlikely, because the reagent was absorbed on a column of human serum protein, and not all sera gave positive results on this coating. Alternatively, IC could be formed in situ in the assay, from dissociated BGG and IgA anti-BGG, which would co-sediment at 7S.

In conclusion, the ELISA for milk antigen-containing IgA-IC appears capable of detecting such IC in human sera. However, interference from other unknown factors remains to be eliminated.

ACKNOWLEDGEMENTS

This investigation was supported by U.S.P.H.S. grants AI 18745 and AM 28537.

REFERENCES

1. Heremans, J.F., in The Antigens, (Edited by Sela, M.), p. 395, Academic Press, New York, 1974.
2. Russell, M.W., Mestecky, J., Julian, B.A. and Galla, J.H., J. Clin. Immunol. 6, 74, 1986.

3. Mestecky, J., Russell, M.W., Jackson, S. and Brown, T.A., Clin. Immunol. Immunopathol. 40, 105, 1986.
4. Lambert, P.H., Dixon, F.J., Zubler, R.H., Agnello, V., Cambiaso, C., Casali, P., Clarke, J., Cowdery, J.S., McDuffie, F.C., Hay, F.C., Maclennan, I.C.M., Masson, P., Müller-Eberhard, H.J., Penetinen, K., Smith, M., Tappeiner, G., Theofilopoulos, A.N. and Verroust, P., J. Lab. Clin. Immunol. 1, 1, 1978.
5. Czerkinsky, C., Koopman, W.J., Jackson, S., Collins, J.E., Crago, S.S., Schrohenloher, R.E., Julian, B.A., Galla, J.H. and Mestecky, J., J. Clin. Invest. 77, 1931, 1986.
6. Hall, R.P., Lawley, T.J., Heck, J.A. and Katz, S.I., Clin. Exp. Immunol. 40, 431, 1980.
7. Jensenius, J.C., Siersted, H.C. and Johnstone, A.P., J. Immunol. Meth. 56, 19, 1983.
8. Cunningham-Rundles, C., J. Exp. Med. 155, 711, 1982.

FLOW CYTOMETRY: A NEW APPROACH TO THE ISOLATION AND CHARACTERIZATION OF KUPFFER CELLS

J.N. Udall, R.A. Moscicki, F.I. Preffer, P.D. Ariniello,
E.A. Carter, A.K. Bhan and K.J. Bloch

Departments of Pediatrics, Pathology and Medicine, Harvard Medical School; Combined Pediatric Gastroenterology and Nutrition Units of Massachusetts General Hospital and Children's Hospital; Immunopathology and Clinical Immunology and Allergy Units of Massachusetts General Hospital, Boston, MA USA

INTRODUCTION

Kupffer cells clear portal blood of absorbed proteases, endotoxins and other noxious substances. These cells are well positioned to do so, they reside in the sinusoids of the liver and lie on the luminal side of the sinusoidal endothelium with cytoplasmic processes which insert focally between endothelial cells. Numerically, Kupffer cells comprise approximately 10% of all liver cells (1). Despite their relative abundance, it has been difficult to obtain pure suspensions of Kupffer cells. Cell suspensions containing 40-85% Kupffer cells have been obtained by treating the rat liver in situ with collagenase and subjecting the resulting cell suspension to centrifugal elutriation.

In this report we describe the application of flow cytometry to the further purification of Kupffer cell suspensions. This application depends upon the distinctive light scattering properties of Kupffer cells. Flow cytometry permitted us to obtain cell suspensions containing approximately 98% Kupffer cells.

MATERIALS AND METHODS

Collagenase perfusion technique

The abdomen and chest of anesthetized rats were opened and the portal vein was cannulated (2). The inferior vena cava was cut to allow free efflux of perfusate from the liver. The liver was perfused (17 ml/min/100 gm body weight), via the portal vein, initially with a calcium-free Krebs-Ringer bicarbonate (KRB) modified buffer (pH 7.6; 37°C) for ten minutes. Oxygenation of the perfusate with 95% O_2/5% CO_2 was accomplished with a simple oxygenator. After ten minutes, the perfusate was changed to a KRB (pH 7.6; 37°C) buffer containing 5 mM calcium chloride, 0.001% DNAse (Sigma Chemical Co., St. Louis, MO), soybean trypsin inhibitor (Sigma) and 0.5 mg collagenase/ml (Cooper Biomedical Inc., Malvern, PA). Perfusion was continued for an additional 10 min. Thereafter, the liver was removed and teased apart. The resulting cell suspension was centrifuged to remove the majority of hepatocytes and clumps of cells. The supernatant consisted of small hepatocytes, sinusoidal cells (endothelial cells, Kupffer cells) and erythrocytes. The erythrocytes were lysed using ammonium chloride. After washing, the cell suspension was adjusted to 40.0 ml and infused into a centrifugal elutriator.

Centrifugal elutriation

A Beckman J2-21 centrifuge, JE-6B elutriator rotor and a standard elutriator system was used to enrich the liver cell suspension for Kupffer cells (3). The system was first equilibrated with elutriation buffer (calcium- and magnesium-free Hanks' solution, Gibco Laboratories, Grand Island, NY) containing 0.75% BSA (Sigma) and 0.002% DNAse (pH 7.4); the temperature of the buffer was maintained at 20°C. The Beckman JE-6B elutriator rotor was set precisely at 2000 RPM, and the circulation pump (Masterflex model 900-197, Barnant Co., Barrington, IL) was set at a flow rate of 9.0 ml/min. The 40 ml cell suspension was infused into the sample mixing chamber.

After infusing the cells into the sample mixing chamber of the rotor, 200 ml of elutriation buffer was collected and discarded. The flow rate was then increased to 18 ml/min and 150 ml of the eluent collected. This fraction contained most of the endothelial cells. The flow rate was then increased to 28 ml/min and a second fraction of 150 ml of eluent containing mostly Kupffer cells, was collected. The cells in this fraction were concentrated by centrifugation at 500 x g for 7 min. The cell pellets were pooled and resuspended in 1-2 ml of elutriation buffer and used for flow cytometric analysis and further purification.

Flow cytometry

Flow cytometric analysis was performed using a 440 Fluorescence Activated Cell Sorter (Becton-Dickinson Immunocytometry Systems, Mt. View, CA) equipped with an argon laser (Spectra-Physics, Mt. View, CA) tuned to emit a 488 nm beam (4). The instrument was calibrated and aligned with stable fluorescent polystyrene beads (Polysciences, Inc., Warrington, PA). Reproducible scatter calibration was obtained by having these beads fall in the same peak scatter channel after optimal laser peaking and mechanical alignment of the optical bench at fixed amplification and photomultiplier voltages.

Cell preparations were examined by simultaneous measurement of two linear parameters, foward angle and 90 degree side angle scatter. For two parameter analysis, data from 4,000 cells per test were collected and stored in list-mode with a Consort 30 Hewlett-Packard computer system (Becton-Dickinson Immunocytometry Systems). The sorting of hepatic sinusoidal cell subpopulations was performed from a 50 μm diameter stream at a frequency of 39 $\pm$ 1 KHz and an amplitude of 5 volts. Coincidence circuitry was employed to abort any deflections containing unwanted cell combinations. Both analysis and sorting were done at relatively low flow rates (1-2000 cells/sec), which reduces the chance of two cells entering the same micro-droplet. After an initial sorting, purified populations of cells were immediately analyzed to ascertain their purity.

Peroxidase staining

Peroxidase staining was performed on samples of cells obtained at various steps throughout the isolation procedure. This staining was employed to differentiate Kupffer cells from endothelial cells by light microscopy. Kupffer cells stain for endogenous peroxidase activity, whereas endothelial cells do not. Two staining techniques were used (5). Air-dried cells adhered to glass slides were immersed in a buffered diaminobenzidine (DAB)-hydrogen peroxide solution (pH 7.6) for 30 min. Staining was followed by a 3 min wash in 0.01 M phosphate buffered saline (PBS; pH 7.1). The cells were counterstained with 2% methyl green for 3 min, for better visualization, and rinsed 2 times with tap water and examined for peroxidase staining with a light microscope. Cells to be stained in suspension were first centrifuged at 500 x g for 7 min. The pellet was resuspended in buffered DAB solution (pH 7.6) for 25 min, and the suspension was centrifuged at 500 x g for 7 min and the pellet resuspended in PBS (pH 7.1) After another centrifugation step at 500 x g for 7 min, cells were resuspended in elutriation buffer. The cells were then placed in a hemocytometer chamber and examined using a light microscope or analyzed using flow cytometry.

RESULTS

Centrifugal elutriation

We used centrifugal elutriation to obtain enriched populations of Kupffer cells (3). A cell suspension obtained following collagenase perfusion, initial centrifugation and lysis of erythrocytes consisted mainly of endothelial cells, Kupffer cells and small hepatocytes. This suspension was loaded into the sample mixing chamber of the elutriator system and infused at a low flow rate (9 ml/min) into the cell separation chamber of the centrifugal elutriator rotor. As the flow rate was increased, cells were eluted according to their size and specific gravity. Smaller cells (endothelial cells) were eluted at lower flow rates and larger, more dense cells (Kupffer cells, small hepatocytes) were eluted at higher flow rates. Maximal enrichment for Kupffer cells was obtained at a flow rate of 28 ml/min. In this fraction, 40-85% of the cells stained for endogenous peroxidase, a marker for Kupffer cells.

Flow cytometry

The 28 ml/min centrifugal elutriation fraction was examined using flow cytometry. Based on the unique light scattering properties of Kupffer cells, it was possible to distinguish them from other cells, i.e., endothelial cells, present in this fraction. As illustrated in Figure 1, two distinct cell populations are seen in a graphic representation of forward angle and 90 degree side angle light scatter. These populations fall separately into areas defined by region 1 and region 2. Approximately 42% of the cells analyzed fell within region 1 and 43% in region 2. Fifteen percent of the cells fell outside regions 1 and 2.

In a second approach to cell separation by means of the FACS, mixed hepatic sinusoidal cells obtain by elutriation (flow rate fraction 28 ml/min) were stained for the presence of peroxidase activity. The stained cell suspension was examined by flow cytometry. Uptake of stain induced

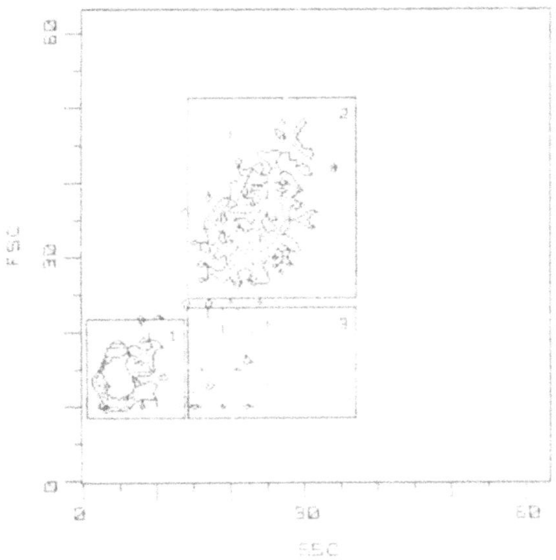

Figure 1. Graphic representation of forward angle (FSC) versus 90 degree side angle (SSC) light scatter of hepatic sinusoidal cells obtained after elutriation. Region 1 contained endothelial cells. Region 2 contained primarily Kupffer cells.

a change in light absorption of cells as manifested by a shift of the light scatter of all cells formerly in region 2. These cells were now found in region 3. No change in light absorption or scatter was shown by cells in region 1. Following analysis, another sample of the stained, mixed hepatic sinusoidal cells (flow rate fraction 28 ml/min) were sorted utilizing flow cytometry. In the sorting mode, the FACS was used to collect, separately, region 1 cells and region 3 cells. Microscopic analysis of the sorted cells of region 3 revealed that more than 98% were positive for endogenous peroxidase. Only 1-2% of the cells in region 1 were positive for peroxidase activity.

DISCUSSION

In this study, we report that Kupffer cells have light scattering properties different from those of endothelial cells. On the basis of these properties, Kupffer cells can be examined and isolated as a highly purified population.

The light scattering properties of individual cells are determined in part by their size, plasma membranes, cytoplasm, mitochondria, pinocytotic vesicles and lysosomes (4,6). It is of interest that cell organelles are quantitatively different in Kupffer and endothelial cells. Kupffer cells have less plasma membrane, pinocytotic vesicles and total cell cytoplasm compared to endothelial cells, whereas the lysosome content of Kupffer cells is greater than that of other sinusoidal cells (7).

Kupffer cells are macrophages adapted to the hepatic environment. There is precedence for studying macrophages using flow cytometry. Haskill and Becker used flow cytometric analysis to evaluate cell volume, phagocytic activity and enzyme markers in cultured macrophages and monocytes (8). Furthermore, Zahlten et al. (9) suggested that flow cytometry would be useful in the isolation and study of liver cell populations (9).

In our study of Kupffer cells, the cell population of region 2, but not region 1, dramatically changed its forward angle light scatter after staining for peroxidase activity. Presumably, staining altered the light absorption and changed the light scattering properties of these cells. Alternatively, staining of cells for peroxidase activity resulted in cell death or alteration of the plasma membranes resulting in a change in light scattering properties. In either case, our findings suggest that the cells of region 2, but not region 1, uniformly stain for peroxidase activity and, hence, are Kupffer cells. Examination of region 2 cells by light microscopy confirmed the uniform staining of this cell population.

CONCLUSIONS

It is evident from these preliminary studies that flow cytometry permits the isolation of Kupffer cells from mixed hepatic sinusoidal cell suspensions on the basis of the light scattering properties of the Kupffer cell. Highly purified Kupffer cell suspensions can be achieved by this method.

ACKNOWLEDGEMENTS

This research was supported in part by grants HD 12437 and AM 33506 from the National Institutes of Health.

REFERENCES

1. Jones, E.A. and Summerfield, J.A., in The Liver: Biology and Pathobiology, (Edited by Anias, I., Popper, H., Schacter, D. and Shafritz, D.A.), p. 507, Raven Press, NY, 1982.
2. McGowan, J.A. and Bucher, N.L.R., J. Tissue Culture Meth. 9(2), 49, 1985.
3. Zahlten, R.N., Hagler, H.K., Nejter, M.E. and Day, C.J., Gastroenterology 75, 80, 1978.
4. Saltzman, G.G., Mullaney, P.F. and Price, B.J., in Flow Cytometry and Sorting, (Edited by Melamed, H.R., Mullaney, P.F. and Mendelsohn, M.L.), p. 105, John Wiley, NY, 1979.
5. Wisse, E., J. Ultrastruct. Res. 46, 393, 1974.
6. Herzenberg, L.A. and Herzenberg, L.A., in Handbook of Experimental Immunology, (Edited by Weir, D.M.), p. 22.1, Blackwell Scientific Publications, London, 1978.
7. Blouin, A., Bolender, R.P. and Weibel, E.R., J. Cell. Biol. 72, 441, 1977.
8. Haskill, S. and Becker, S., RES: J. Reticuloendothelial Soc. 32, 273, 1982.
9. Zahlten, R.N., Rogoff, T.M. and Steer, C.J., Fed. Proc. 40, 2460, 1981.

BARRIER DEFENSE FUNCTION OF THE SMALL INTESTINE: EFFECT OF ETHANOL AND ACUTE BURN TRAUMA

E.A. Carter, P.R. Harmatz, J.N. Udall and W.A. Walker

Combined Gastroenterology and Nutrition Unit, Massachusetts General Hospital, Children's Hospital, Shriner Burns Hospital and Harvard Medical School, Boston, MA USA

INTRODUCTION

Nonspecific barriers to the passage of infectious and/or potentially toxic macromolecules exist in the small intestine. They include the "unstirred water layer," a zone of retarded diffusion which would slow the movement of macromolecules toward the mucosal epithelium; a layer of intestinal mucus which would interfere with macromolecule penetration; and finally, the glycocalyx, anchored in the plasmalemma of the epithelial cell (1).

We have become increasingly interested in the effect of various materials in the diet as well as the effect of stress on small intestinal gut sac nutrient absorption (2-4). For this reason, we undertook an examination of gut permeability changes under these conditions. The present report details our initial observations.

METHODS

Female rats (150-200 grams, Charles River Breeding Labs, Wilmington, MA) were used throughout these studies. Rats were sacrificed by cervical dislocation without previous anesthesia.

Gut sacs were prepared as described previously (5). Briefly, eight cm sections of the small intestine were removed, rinsed with 20 ml of ice cold saline, everted and the ends tied to form closed sacs. Gut sacs were filled with 1 ml of buffer which contained 125 mM sodium choloride, 10 mM fructose and 30 mM Tris buffer, pH 7.5. The filled gut sacs were placed in 10 ml of the same buffer as that inside the sac except that the outer buffer contained 10 mM polyethylene glycol 4000 (PEG 4000) containing 10,000 DPM per ml of 14C-PEG 4000 or 10 micromolar horse radish peroxidase (type VI, 300 units per mg solid, Sigma Chemical Co., St. Louis, MO).

Assessment of gut sac permeability was achieved by incubating the gut sacs prepared as described above under 100% oxygen atmosphere using a Dubnoff metabolic shaking incubator for varying periods of time, removing the sacs from the buffer, blotting them lightly and then extracting the contents by means of a 1 cc tuberculin syringe equipped with a 27 gauge needle. The contents from the 14C-PEG experients were added to 10 ml of Aquasol 2, and the radioactivity measured by liquid scintillation spectrometry using a Searle Trianylser (Searle, Chicago, IL). The contents from the horse radish peroxidase (HRP) experiments were analyzed for HRP activity spectrophotometrically as described previously (6).

Rats were subjected to cutaneous thermal injury by the method of Walker and Mason (7) as modified here at the SBI (4).

RESULTS

As can be seen in Table 1, there was a steady increase in the radioactivity or HRP found inside the gut sac as the length of the incubation at 37°C continued. Constantly more radioactivity or HRP was detected in the middle segment of the rat small intestine (defined by taking the entire small intestine, folding it in half and then taking 4 cm on either side of the bend).

The addition of ethanol to a final concentration of 2% significantly increased ($p < 0.01$) the radioactivity or HRP inside the upper, middle or lower gut sacs (Table 2).

Application of acute burn trauma to rats 6 h prior to experimentation, significantly increased ($p < 0.01$) the radioactivity or HRP inside the upper small intestinal gut sacs, and especially the middle and lower sacs (Table 3).

Table 1. Time course for the gut sac permeability assay using ^{14}C-PEG HRP

Time of incubation	PEG -4000[a]			HRP[b]		
	Upper	Middle	Lower	Upper	Middle	Lower
15 minutes	8	11	11	3	7	4
30 minutes	13	21	20	6	13	5
45 minutes	19	32	19	11	26	21
60 minutes	18	61	26	18	52	26

[a]DPM/100 microliters of serosal fluid corrected for background.

[b]Nanomoles of HRP per liter found in the serosal fluid.

DISCUSSION

A major function of the small intestine is to act as a defense barrier to the penetration of macromolecules which may have toxic and/or immunological consequences. Thus, the small intestinal luminal surface contains various components which serve to prevent the penetration of macromolecules (1). However, dietary and/or stress related alterations of this barrier could result in the enhanced uptake of macromolecules. In the present communication, we have examined the use of the gut sac model to study small intestinal barrier function, in particular, macromolecule permeability.

The gut sac model allows the direct addition of substances to the system in the absence of in vivo factors such as gastric empyting, motility, etc. Thus, we were able to demonstrate that ethanol, at concentrations found in the lumen of humans ingesting moderate amounts of alcohol, could definitely increase the permeability of PEG-4000 or HRP, whose molecular weight is 40,000. It is interesting to note that the ethanol effects the permeability of all three segments of the small intestine, even though the middle small intestine in the normal rat appeared to be more permeable than the upper or lower intestine. Previous work has demonstrated that 2% ethanol addition inhibits the transport of nutrients by small intestinal gut sacs (EAC, unpublished data). It has also been observed that the different segments of the small intestine transport nutrients differently in the rat, with gut sacs from the upper small intestine transporting calcium,

Table 2. Effect of ethanol addition on small intestinal permeability to ^{14}C-PEG or HRP

Segment	PEG-4000[a]			HRP[b]		
	Control	2% Ethanol	P	Control	2% Ethanol	P
Upper	15	30	0.05	11	26	0.01
Middle	30	65	0.01	27	74	0.001
Lower	17	31	0.01	20	54	0.01

[a]Gut sacs from normal rats were used for determining permeability to PEG-4000 or HRP as described in Methods using a 45 min incubation period. There were four rats in each group. Activity in the PEG groups was expressed as DPM/100 microliters of serosal fluid (corrected for background).

[b]Activity in the HRP groups was expressed nanomoles of HRP per liter found in the serosal fluid after the 45 min incubation.

the middle small intestine transporting glucose and the lower small intestine transporting amino acids (3).

It is also interesting to note that acute burn trauma effected gut sac permeability but more in the middle and lower small intestine. Rhodes and Karnovsky (8) demonstrated previously that there was a loss of macromolecular barrier function associated with surgical trauma to the guinea pig small intestine. The mechanism(s) for the alteration produced by the acute burn trauma are not clear, but previous work has demonstrated that altered small intestinal nutrient transport, small intestinal DNA synthesis, and reduced small intestinal mucosal mass occur at this same time point (3). In data not shown, we have observed that the increased permeability is still present 18 hr after burn trauma, but not detectable 72 hr later.

In conclusion, we have explored the use of the evert gut sac technique to study alterations in small intestinal barrier function. Our data suggests that the addition of ethanol (2%) or the application of acute burn trauma to rats 6 hr prior to sacrifice, significantly alters the uptake of ^{14}C-PEG 4000 and HRP. It may be possible to elucidate the mechanism(s) whereby these manipulations produce these alterations, and in so doing, better understand the workings of the small intestinal barrier function.

Table 3. Effect of acute burn trauma on small intestinal permeability to PEG-4000 or Horse Radish Peroxidase (HRP)[a]

Segment	PEG-4000			HRP		
	Control	Burn	P	Control	Burn	P
Upper	16	26	0.05	11	52	0.01
Middle	30	44	0.05	26	94	0.01
Lower	18	59	0.01	21	152	0.01

[a]Rats were subjected to acute burn trauma as described in Methods and sacrificed 6 h later. Permeability to PEG-4000 or HRP was determined using everted gut sacs and a 45 min incubation period. There were three rats in each group. The bathing media (mucosal side) contained the ^{14}C-PEG or HRP while the media inside (serosal side) the everted gut sac did not. Activity of the PEG-4000 groups expressed as DPM/100 microliters of serosal fluid (corrected for background) while activity in the HRP groups expressed as nanomoles of HRP per liter found in the serosal fluid after 45 min incubation.

REFERENCES

1. Cantey, J.R., Am. J. Med. 78(6B), 65, 1985.
2. Stern, M., Carter, E.A. and Walker, W.A., Digest. Dis. 31, 1242, 1986.
3. Carter, E.A., Udall, J.N., Kirkham, S.E. and Walker, W.A., J. Burn Care and Rehab. 7, 469, 1986.
4. Carter, E.A., Kirkham, S.E., Udall, J.N., Jung, W., and Walker, W.A., J. Burn Care and Rehab. 7, 475, 1986.
5. Carter, E.A., Bloch, K.J., Cohen, S., Isselbacher, K.J. and Walker, W.A., Gastroenterology 81, 1091, 1981.
6. Walker, W.A., Cornell, R., Davenport, L.M. and Isselbacher, K.J., J. Cell. Biol. 54, 195, 1972.
7. Walker, H.L. and Mason, A.D., J. Trauma 8, 1049, 1968.
8. Rhodes, R.S. and Karnovsky, M.J., Lab. Invest. 25, 220, 1971.

INTESTINAL ABSORPTION OF BACTERIAL CELL WALL POLYMERS IN RATS

R.B. Sartor, T.M. Bond, K.Y. Compton and D.R. Cleland

Department of Medicine and Core Center for Diarrheal Diseases, University of North Carolina School of Medicine
Chapel Hill, North Carolina USA

INTRODUCTION

Bacterial cell wall polymers initiate and sustain chronic granulomatous inflammation and characteristic immunological changes in animal models after local and systemic injection (1,2). The component of the cell wall responsible for the inflammation and immunodulation is the covalently bound peptidoglycan-polysaccharide (PG-PS) complex, which is found in nearly all bacterial species, including the normal enteric flora. Purified aqueous suspensions of PG-PS can induce granulomatous enterocolitis that persists for 6 months in rats after intramural injection and chronic relapsing synovitis, uveitis, vasculitis with skin lesions, hepatic granulomas, carditis and anemia after systemic injection (3). PG-PS activates macrophages and the alternate complement pathway and has mitogenic, adjuvant and immunogenic properties for B cells (4). Because the histologic appearance, immunologic response and location of systemic inflammation of PG-PS-induced inflammation resembles that seen in Crohn's disease and because high concentrations of bacteria are found in the distal intestine, we postulate that PG-PS from intestinal bacteria may be important in the pathogenesis of Crohn's disease However, to be etiologically significant, PG-PS must cross the intestinal epithelium. The purpose of these experiments is to investigate absorption of gavage-fed PG-PS by measuring systemic uptake and serum antibody response in rats.

METHODS

Purified PG-PS was prepared from group A, type 3, strain D-58 streptococci (5). Cells were mechanically disrupted, treated with sodium dodecyl sulfate, suspended in phosphate buffered saline (PBS), sonicated and centrifuged at 1000 x g for 30 min to yield PG-PS polymers ranging from 5×10^6 to 5×10^8 molecular weight (6). Covalently radiolabeled PG-PS was created by mixing benzimidate-substituted PG-PS and $Na^{125}I$ with lactoperoxidase, then dialyzing for 72 h to remove unbound ^{125}I (5).

To measure systemic absorption, 10 Sprague-Dawley female rats, mean weight 250 gms, were gavage-fed 1.5 ml radiolabeled PG-PS (1.28×10^7 cpm, 18.8 mg), the 5 rats were killed after 4 h and 5 rats killed after 24 h. Four control rats fed $Na^{125}I$ (1.28×10^7 cpm) were sacrificed 4, 24, 48 and 72 h after feeding. Radioactivity was measured in the livers, spleens, mesenteric lymph nodes, ankle joints, cardiac blood and cecal contents. Selected organs were homogenized, sonicated, then their supernatants were assayed for PG-PS by micro ELISA technique using affinity purified antibody to either group A streptococcal PG or the terminal D-alanyl-D-alanine $(D\text{-}ala)_2$ of the PG pentapeptide.

To measure the serum antibody response to PG-PS, 10 Sprague-Dawley rats were fed 1 ml (13.2 mg) PG-PS by gastric intubation and 10 rats were fed 1 ml PBS, then the rats were fed 0.5 ml PG-PS or PBS twice weekly for 3 weeks. Serum was collected before feeding and at weekly intervals for 3 weeks. Antibody to PG-PS was measured by micro-ELISA technique using either purified PG, PG-PS or $(D\text{-}ala)_2$ and affinity-purified goat anti-rat IgM or IgG antibody.

RESULTS

Higher amounts of radioactivity were present in the livers, spleens, mesenteric lymph nodes, cardiac blood and joints of rats fed radiolabeled PG-PS than in control rats fed $Na^{125}I$ (Table 1).

To demonstrate whether the organs contained ^{125}I-PG-PS or simply free ^{125}I, PG-PS immunoreactivity was measured in selected homogenated tissues. Tissue PG-PS concentrations were consistently higher in the PG-PS fed rats (Table 2).

Table 1. Radioactivity of organs in rats fed PG-PS or ^{125}I

	mean CPM/gram + SEM			
	4 h PG-PS	4 h ^{125}I	24 h PG-PS	24 h ^{125}I
liver	16,297 ± 2,086	9,749	14,186 ± 1,505	2,891
spleen	10,991 ± 8,657	8,657	6,829 ± 638	1,042
mesenteric LN	10,055 ± 4,121	4,121	5,640 ± 738	743
blood (cpm/ml)	31,376 ± 21,321	21,321	17,702 ± 1,496	2,643
ankle joint	15,175 ± 2,174	8,741	8,390 ± 704	897
cecal contents	206,833 ± 97,779	5,343	151,813 ± 31,615	2,663

Table 2. Immunoreactive PG-PS within tissue homogenates (ng/ml, mean ± SEM)

	Group A PS		$(D\text{-}ala)_2$	
	PG-PS fed	Controls	PG-PS fed	Controls
liver	272 ± 10	[a]60.5 ± 6.5	3180 ± 170	[a]1090 ± 150
mesenteric LN	222 ± 105	46.7 ± 7.8	1570 ± 560	[b]113 ± 69

[a]$P < 0.01$ PG-PS fed compared with controls.

[b]$P < 0.03$ PG-PS fed compared with controls.

Table 3. Serum IgM antibody to PG and $(D\text{-}ala)_2$, μg/ml (Mean ± SEM)

Material	Anti-PG		Anti-$(D\text{-}ala)_2$	
fed	0 day	21 days	0 day	21 days
PG-PS	5.48 ± 0.26	6.93 ± 0.48[a]	5.34 ± 0.25	6.43 ± 0.21[a]
PBS	6.03 ± 0.24	4.40 ± 0.23	5.69 ± 0.18	4.62 ± 0.33

[a]$P < 0.01$ vs. 0 day. $P < 0.001$ vs. PBS-fed.

Serum IgM antibody to PG and $(D\text{-ala})_2$ were significantly elevated by 3 weeks after beginning PG-PS feedings compared with initial and control values (Table 3). Anti-PG-PS IgM levels of PG-PS-fed rats were higher than baseline and control values, but were not statistically significant ($P = 0.06$). IgG antibody to cell wall epitopes were not reproducibly different between the groups.

DISCUSSION

These results suggest that small, but immunologically significant amounts of bacterial cell wall are absorbed from the normal rat intestine. While much of the radioactivity within the liver, spleen, mesenteric lymph nodes, blood and joints of rats fed ^{125}I-labeled PG-PS is free ^{125}I absorbed from the intestines after intraluminal cleavage of the ^{125}I-PG-PS bond, the presence of immunoreactive cell wall within tissue indicates systemic absorption of PG-PS polymers. The concentrations of $(D\text{-ala})_2$ are higher than PS because the $(D\text{-ala})_2$ immunoassay measured PG from all bacterial species while the PS assay measured only group A streptococcal carbohydrate antigen. The induction of a serum antibody response confirms absorption of antigenically intact PG. The observations that all rats had detectable anti-PG serum antibodies prior to gavage feeding of PG-PS and that control rats have PG within tissues suggest uptake of naturally occurring PG, possibly absorbed from their intestines. We have previously demonstrated increased levels of serum anti-PG IgA in Crohn's disease patients compared with normals and other patients with diarrhea (7). Collectively, these studies support the concept that enteric bacterial PG-PS crosses the intestinal epithelia in an immunologically active form. We speculate that PG-PS derived from the enteric bacterial flora is important in regulation of the normal mucosal immune response and can initiate and/or perpetuate intestinal and systemic inflammation in susceptible hosts.

ACKNOWLEDGEMENTS

This investigation was supported by grants AM 01112 and AM 25733 from the National Institute of Arthritis, Diabetes and Digestive and Kidney Diseases. We thank Shirley Willard for secretarial assistance.

REFERENCES

1. Sartor, R.B., Cromartie, W.J., Powell, D.W. and Schwab, J.H., Gastroenterology 89, 587, 1985.
2. Cromartie, W.J., Craddock, J.G., Schwab, J.H., Anderle, S.K. and Yang, C., J. Exp. Med. 146, 1585, 1977.
3. Stimpson, S.A., Schwab, J.H., Janusz, M.J., Anderle, S.K., Brown, R.R. and Cromartie, W.J., in Biological Properties of Peptidoglycan, (Edited by Seidl, H.P. and Schleifer, K.H.), p. 273, Walter de Gruyter, Berlin, 1986.
4. Chetty, C. and Schwab, J.H., in Handbook of Endotoxin Vol. 1: Chemistry of Endotoxin, (Edited by Reitschel, E.T.), p. 376, Elsevier Science Publishers, 1984.
5. Esser, R.E., Stimpson, S.A., Cromartie, W.J. and Schwab, J.H., Arthritis and Rheumatism 28, 1402, 1985.
6. Fox, A., Brown, R.R., Anderle, S.K., Chetty, C., Cromartie, W.J., Gooder, H. and Schwab, J.H., Infect. Immun. 35, 1003, 1982.
7. Sartor, R.B., Cleland, D.R., Catalano, C.J. and Schwab, J.H., Gastroenterology 88, 1571, 1985.

SIZE DISTRIBUTION OF SERUM IgA ANTIBODIES TO FOOD PROTEINS: BOVINE BETA-LACTOGLOBULIN (BLG), BOVINE SERUM ALBUMIN (BSA) AND GLIADIN (GL)

F. Mascart-Lemone, D.L. Delacroix*, S. Cadranel**, J.P. Vaerman* and J. Duchateau

Departments of Immunology and **Pediatric Gastroenterology, St. Pierre University Hospital, U.L.B.; and *International Institute of Cellular and Molecular Pathology, U.C.L., Brussels, Belgium

INTRODUCTION

As IgA is the main immunoglobulin of mucosal surfaces, IgA antibodies are formed in response to antigens encountered in the gastrointestinal tract, such as food substances. Previous studies have shown that the sera of normal individuals often contain antibodies of IgA, as well as IgG and IgM isotypes, against a variety of dietary substances (1,2). Such antibodies (particularly antibodies to gluten), are also often detected in sera of patients with coeliac disease (3).

In the present study, we have analyzed the incidence and the levels of serum IgA antibodies to 3 food proteins in children presenting a gastrointestinal pathology and compared their results to those obtained in controls with a healthy intestinal barrier and in children allergic to cow's milk. Serum IgA antibodies were assayed against bovine beta-lactoglobulin (BLG), bovine serum albumin (BSA) and gliadin (GL). As IgA occurs in two molecular forms, monomeric for $\pm$ 90% of serum IgA and polymeric for $\pm$ 90% of secretory IgA, the size distribution of the serum IgA antibodies was further determined in the different groups.

PATIENTS AND METHODS

The control population included 40 adult clinically healthy blood donors evenly distributed between 20 and 60 years, and 47 pediatric controls, between 0 and 19 years, hospitalized for various reasons other than allergy, gastrointestinal pathology or an auto-immune disorder. Patients consisted of 17 children allergic to cow's milk (positive RAST) (0 to 2 years), 5 suspected coeliac children (12 to 18 months) and 59 with severe acute gastroenteritis (0 to 2 years). Campylobacter jejuni, Salmonella, Shigella or rotavirus were isolated from the stools, and blood samples were taken during the first week of symptoms.

Serum titers of IgA antibodies were measured by solid phase radioimmunoassay. BLG (Koch-Light) was dissolved at 25 μg/ml in carbonate-buffered saline, pH 9.6. BSA (Sigma) and crude wheat GL (Sigma) were dissolved in phosphate-buffered saline, pH 7.2 (PBS), respectively at 5 and 25 μg/ml; GL was prediluted in 70% ethanol. Polystyrene cups were coated with the antigens overnight at room temperature. After blocking cups with 10% horse serum in PBS and washing with PBS, serum samples, diluted 1/50 in PBS supplemented with 10% horse serum, were incubated overnight at room temperature. After further washing, cups were filled with ^{125}I-labeled mouse monoclonal IgG1 anti-human alpha chain for 16 h, and bound radioactivity was then counted after a last washing. All samples were tested simultaneously on wells without antigen and these non-specific counts were subtracted from counts bound to antigen-coated wells. Antibody titers were expressed in arbitrary units (arb. u.) by reference to standard curves established by serial dilutions of reference sera. Specificity was assessed by absorption of positive sera on BLG-, BSA- and GL-sepharose. The antibody titer dropped significantly only after absorption with the corresponding antigen. Sensitivities were 7, 5 and 4 arb. u., respectively, for BLG, BSA and GL, as defined by the mean + 3 SD of results obtained for 15 positive sera after specific absorption. Monomeric (m-) and polymeric (p-) IgA distribution in sera was determined by density gradient ultracentrifugation (sucrose 5%-21%) measuring both total and specific IgA on each fraction. Anti-gliadin IgG was measured similarly, using ^{125}I-labeled, affinity purified goat IgG anti-human gamma chain antibodies.

RESULTS

IgA antibodies to food proteins were common in serum of controls (Fig. 1), especially in young children (BLG) and in adults between 40 and 60 years (GL). Titers were always low (BLG < 25, BSA < 17, GL < 27 arb. u.).

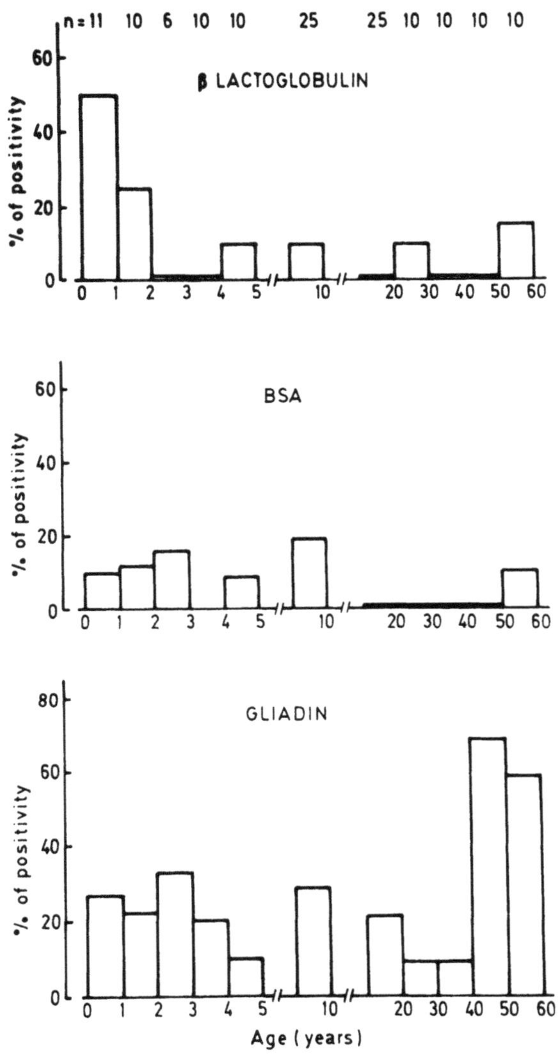

Figure 1. Incidence of serum IgA antibodies to food antigens in a control population (n = number of controls tested).

Positive sera most often contained IgA antibodies to only one antigen. Both the prevalence and titers of IgA to BLG and BSA were higher in cases of alterations of the intestinal mucosa such as acute gastroenteritis (GE) and coeliac disease (CD) (Fig. 2, Table 1). The IgA response to GL was, however, higher in CD than in GE, whereas the IgA responses to BLG and BSA were similar in both conditions. The incidence of serum anti-BLG IgA was also elevated in children allergic to cow's milk, but titers were not different from those of controls. However, patients (allergic - GE - CD) often had antibodies to several antigens, which was not obvious in the control group.

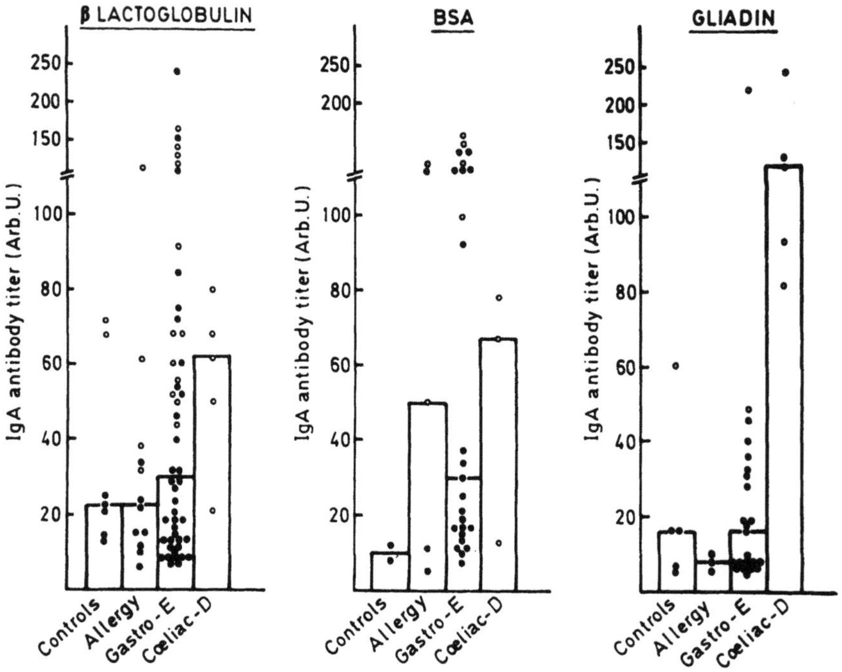

Figure 2. Serum IgA antibody titers to food antigens in young children (0 - 2 years). Columns represent medians of the results; (o) are the sera which were further centrifuged on sucrose gradients.

The size distribution of serum anti-BLG and anti-BSA was also not discriminant between controls and allergic children, and/or acute GE and/or CD (Fig. 3). Whatever the group, there was roughly equal representation of p- and m-IgA antibodies. For GL, however, results suggested that serum anti-GL IgA was mainly p-IgA in CD, whereas it was mainly m-IgA in the only positive control and the positive acute GE. The same results were obtained when samples were run at acid pH indicating that anti-GL p-IgA were not IgA immune complexes in untreated CD.

Finally, kinetics of titer decrease were followed in CD patients at the start of the gluten-free diet. Anti-GL IgA titers quickly dropped to zero after 3 to 5 months, whereas IgG titers decreased more slowly, reaching undetectable levels only after about 12 months.

DISCUSSION

Our incidence of serum IgA antibodies to food proteins in healthy individuals confirms previous reports (1,2) but interestingly, analyzing the

Table 1. Incidence of serum IgA antibodies to food antigens in young children (0 - 2 years)

	Bovine beta-lactoglobulin				Bovine serum albumin				Gliadin			
	C	A	GE	CD	C	A	GE	CD	C	A	GE	CD
Nr of sera tested	19	17	59	5	19	17	59	5	21	14	51	5
Nr of positive sera	7	12	46	5	2	5	25	3	5	3	23	5
Positivity	37%	71%	78%	100%	10%	29%	42%	60%	24%	21%	45%	100%

C = controls; A = allergy; GE = gastroenteritis; CD = Coeliac disease.

results in function of the age, we noted two peaks of high prevalence of these antibodies: one for BLG in children between 0 and 2 years, and the other for GL in adults between 40 and 60 years. The presence of serum antibodies to food antigens in sera of young children is generally interpreted as reflecting an increased food antigen absorption from the gastrointestinal tract (4). The higher prevalence of serum IgA anti-GL antibodies in adults between 40 and 60 years was not correlated to the increase of total IgA with age. It might be related to modifications of the immune functions with age (1,5) or to increased incidence of absorptive disorders such as subclinical local inflammation of the intestinal mucosa.

The incidence and the titers of IgA antibodies to food antigen were higher in cases of important alterations of the intestinal mucosa. Local inflammation during infection or untreated CD could increased the absorption of low molecular weight allergen through the mucosa, allowing an immune response to develop (6). The higher incidence of antibodies to BLG compared to BSA and GL might be due to differences in molecular weights and epitope densities between the antigens (7). These results suggest that the presence of serum IgA antibodies to food antigen in CD probably reflects an increased intestinal permeability secondary to mucosal damage. The IgA response to GL is, however, quantitatively (high titers) and perhaps qualitatively (mainly p-IgA) different between patients with CD and others with gastrointestinal mucosa disease. Therefore, determination of serum IgA anti-GL titers appears to have a diagnostic value for CD, whereas IgA anti-BLG and anti-BSA responses remain less discriminant.

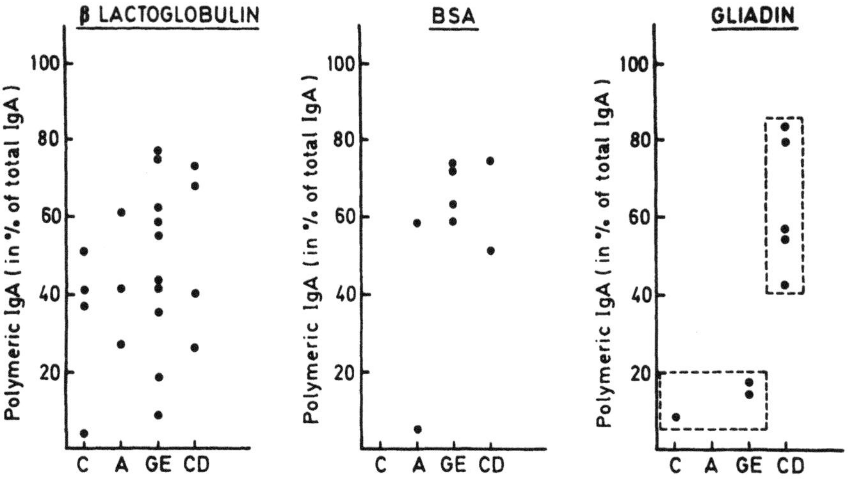

Figure 3. Polymeric IgA in percentage of total IgA antibodies to food antigens.

ACKNOWLEDGEMENTS

This work was supported by grant 1.5.235.87F of the Fonds Nationeal de la Recherche Scientifique, Brussels, Belgium.

REFERENCES

1. Russell, M.W., Hammond, D., Radl, J., Haaijman, J.J. and Mestecky, J., Prot. Biol. Fluids 32, 77, 1985.
2. Russell, M.W., Mestecky, J., Julian, B.A. and Galla, J.H., J. Clin. Immunol. 6, 74, 1986.
3. Scott, H., Ek, J. and Brandtzaeg, P., Int. Archs. Allergy Appl. Immun. 76, 138, 1985.
4. Kleinman, R.E., Harmatz, P.R. and Walker, W.A., in Gastrointestinal Immunity for the Clinician, (Edited by Shorter and Kirsner), p. 23, 1985.
5. Holt, P.R., in Nutritional Approaches to Aging Research, (Edited by Shorter and Kirsner), p. 157, 1982.
6. Gruskay, F.L. and Cooke, R.E., Pediatrics 16, 763, 1955.
7. Mayrhofer, G., Local Immune Response of the Gut, (Edited by Neuby, T.J. and Stokes, C.R.), p. 11, 1984.

IMPAIRMENT OF IgA EXPRESSION AND CELL MEDIATED IMMUNITY OBSERVED ON PEYER'S PATCHES OF PROTEIN-DEPLETED RATS AT WEANING AND THEN FED ON 20% CASEIN

M.E. Roux and M. del Carmen Lopez

Experimental Nutrition and Food Science Department
Cellular Immunology Division, Faculty of Pharmacy and
Biochemistry, University of Buenos Aires
Buenos Aires, Argentina

INTRODUCTION

The gastrointestinal immune system has many unique structural and functional features, that include the Peyer's patch and the secretory IgA system (1). Precursors of the IgA plasma cells are first recognizable as bone marrow-derived B cells in the Peyer's patches (1-3). IgA committed Peyer's patch cells, that bear surface IgA, leave Peyer's patches to mesenteric lymph nodes, where they further maturate and acquire the capacity to seed the intestinal lamina propria as IgA plasma cells (2,4).

The progeny that express IgA is selected through successive C_H rearrangements and DNA deletions involved in the switch of surface immunoglobulins (3). Its clonal expansion in Peyer's patches, apparently occurs by environmental antigens entering from the gut by way of specialized epithelium (4-9). Further, Peyer's patches contain IgA class-specific T cells (switch T cells) that preferentially induce IgA B cell development or T cells which preferentially support IgA responses (10-13).

It is known that secretory immunity is induced, in part, by sensitized cells from gut associated lymphoid tissues that migrate to secretory sites; and, that nutritional stresses such as protein deprivation alter mucosal surfaces and cell mediated immunity (1,2,6,9,14-18).

Therefore, Peyer's patches damaged by protein depletion at weaning should present a breakdown in B cell differentiation. Is it possible to revert this impairment by refeeding? In this report we are going to define, at the Peyer's patch level, the impairment of IgA expression caused by severe protein deficiency and we are going to present results which suggest the possibility that the precursor B cell population left in Peyer's patches could be recruitable for IgA synthesis after protein-refeeding.

MATERIALS AND METHODS

Weaning rats (21-23 d of age) of the Wistar strain (closed colony from the breeding unit kept at the Department of Experimental Nutrition and Food Science) were depleted by being fed a protein-free diet. Animals that lost about 25% of the initial weight were killed, or housed individually receiving a 20% casein diet (19).

Peyer's patches were removed, placed in RPMI 1640 medium plus 10% fetal calf serum (RPMI 1640/FCS). Organ weight was determined. Peyer's patches were minced with scissors before pressing through a nylon sieve in the above medium. All cell suspensions were filtered through nylon wool before use. Cell recovery and viability was determined by trypan blue exclusion (0.05% saline) using a haemocytometer counting chamber (20).

Surface antigenic determinants were characterized in a suspension of living cells by immunofluorescence staining, as previously described (21).

Cells bearing T cell markers were labeled in a indirect assay using the mouse monoclonal antibodies: W3/13, W3/25 and MRC OX8 (Seralab Ltd., Crawly Down Sussex). Cells binding these antibodies were subsequently labeled with fluorescein-conjugated anti-mouse IgG.

B cells with surface immunoglobulins were labeled in an indirect assay using the following affinity purified antibodies (1) goat anti-rat IgM (μ chain specific) and the fluorescein conjugated IgG fraction of rabbit anti-goat IgG (Cappel Lab) or (2) sheep anti-rat IgA (α chain specific) and the fluorescein conjugated IgG fraction of rabbit antisheep IgG (Cappel Lab).

Delayed type hypersensitivity (DTH) to diet antigens (dextrin and casein) and sheep red blood cells (SRBC) was assessed by the degree of footpad swelling elicited by challenge with the specific antigen (22-25).

RESULTS

Peyer's patch weights and numbers of cells are markedly affected by severe protein deficiency at weaning (32.0 vs. 134.4; 1.3×10^6 vs. 2.9×10^6; $P < 0.001$). When rats were fed n a 20% casein diet during 9 and 21 days, neither Peyer's patch weight nor Peyer's patch numbers of cells reached age-matched control values even though normal development of Peyer's patches tends to be restored (Table 1).

The protein-free group was divided into two groups according to the different percentage of membrane Ig-bearing cells (IgM or IgA bearing cells) (Table 2). The absolute number of membrane Ig bearing lymphocytes were calculated from an estimate of the total number of Peyer's patch cells per rat and the percentage of these which were positively stained for surface IgM or surface IgA. The degree of decrease of the B cell population in the protein-free group was four- to seven-fold smaller than that of

Table 1. Weights and numbers of cells in the Peyer's patches

Control and experimental groups	n[a]	Mean weight ± SE (mg)	No. of cells ± SE x 10^{-6}/ml
control 39 days	5	140.7 ± 11.5	1.3 ± 0.2
	5	134.4 ± 18.4	2.9 ± 0.4
control 45 days	8	107.6 ± 19.7	2.3 ± 0.4
	8	141.6 ± 20.2	2.6 ± 0.6
control 60 days	8	214.0 ± 17.9	6.2 ± 1.2
PFG[b]	14	32.0 ± 7.1[e]	1.3 ± 0.2[e]
(34-38 days)	15	37.5 ± 3.5[e]	1.3 ± 0.2[e]
PFG + 9 d 20% Cas.	9	107.2 ± 5.4	1.8 ± 0.2
(43-47 days)	7	88.8 ± 3.8[c]	1.6 ± 0.1
PFG + 21 d 20% Cas.	10	140.9 ± 13.9[c]	2.5 ± 0.4[c]
(55-60 days)	11	131.5 ± 9.3[d]	1.3 ± 0.2[e]

[a] n=number of observations.

[b] PFG: protein-free group.

[c] Significantly different from age-matched controls $P < 0.05$.

[d] Significantly different from age-matched controls $P < 0.01$.

[e] Significantly different from age-matched controls $P < 0.001$.

the age-matched control population (4.2×10^5 and 0.3×10^5 vs. 9.4×10^5 and 1.8×10^5 vs. 4.9×10^5; $P < 0.001$). When rats were fed on a 20% casein diet by the oral route the proportion and the absolute number of membrane Ig bearing cells were partially restored (Table 2). Normal values for absolute numbers of membrane IgA bearing cells could not be reached even after rats were fed on 20% casein for 21 days (5.0×10^5 vs. 15.4×10^5; $P < 0.001$).

There was a decrease in the percentge and the absolute number of $W3/13^+$ T lymphocytes (Table 3). Also, there was a decrease in the absolute number of $W3/25^+$ T lymphocytes (2.6×10^5 vs. 5.3×10^5; $P < 0.01$). When rats were fed on a 20% casein diet by the oral route the absolute number of $W3/13^+$ and $W3/25^+$ T lymphocytes, were partially restored. But normal values could not be reached (5.0×10^5 vs. 17.2×10^5 and 4.2×10^5 vs. 12.5×10^5; $P < 0.05$) (Table 3).

A diminished DTH reaction to dextrin and SRBC was observed in the protein depleted rats and in the refed animals (Table 4). The experimental groups mentioned above presented a DTH reaction to casein similar to that of the control group.

Table 2. The proportion and absolute numbers of IgM containing lymphocytes and of IgM and IgA bearing lymphocytes in the Peyer's patches

	Mean % stained cells ± SE			No. lymphocytes ± SE $\times 10^{-5}$		
control and experimental grp.	$\mu+$ cit	$\mu+$ s	$\alpha+$ s	$\mu+$ cit	$\mu+$ s	$\alpha+$ s
control 39 days	N.D.	44.9±1.9	23.7±4.4	N.D.	9.4±0.9	4.9±0.9
control 60 days	29.4±5.0	15.3±4.0	47.6±2.4	5.6±1.5	5.4±2.0	15.4±1.9
PFG[a]	35.0±4.0	36.6±5.0	14.8±1.4	3.8±0.6	4.2±0.6[c]	1.8±0.1[b]
		4.5±1.4[c]	5.8±1.2[c]		0.3±0.1[c]	0.7±0.1[c]
PFG+21d 20%Cas.	41.4±11.2	44.9±5.1[b]	27.9±2.4[c]	14.2±4.6	7.9±1.5	5.0±0.7[c]

[a]See abbreviations in Table 1.

[b]Significantly different from age-matched controls $P < 0.01$.

[c]Significantly different from age-matched controls $P < 0.001$.

Table 3. The proportion and absolute numbers of T lymphocytes labeled by the monoclonal antibodies: W3/13, W3/25 and MRC OX8 in the Peyer's patches

Control and Experimental groups	Mean % stained cells ± SE			No. of lymphocytes ± SE x10^{-5}		
	W3/13+	W3/25+	MRC OX8+	W3/13+	W3/25+	MRC OX8+
control 45 d	28.0±4.7	20.4±4.5	13.4±1.3	7.3±1.2	5.3±1.2	3.5±0.3
control 60 d	28.0±4.7	20.4±4.5	13.4±1.3	17.2±2.9	12.5±2.8	8.2±0.8
PFG[a]	11.4±1.7[c]	19.8±2.7	16.7±2.4	1.5±0.2[d]	2.6±0.4[c]	2.2±0.3[b]
PFG+21d 20%Cas.	38.0±7.2	31.7±7.4	38.6±8.1[c]	5.0±1.0[b]	4.2±1.0[b]	5.1±1.1

[a]See abbreviations in Table 1.

[b]Significantly different from age-matched controls P ≤ 0.05.

[c]Significantly different from age-matched controls P ≤ 0.01.

[d]Significantly different from age-matched controls P ≤ 0.001.

Table 4. DTH to diet antigens (dextrin, casein) and to SRBC

Control and Experimental groups	Delayed-type hypersensitivity to		
	Dextrin[c]	Casein[c]	SRBC[c]
control[b]	0.42 ± 0.07 (11)	0.41 ± 0.05 (10)	0.39 ± 0.05 (8)
PFG[a]	0.12 ± 0.03 (20)[d]	0.36 ± 0.07 (13)	0.06 ± 0.02 (13)[d]
PFG+21d 20%Cas.	0.15 ± 0.03 (18)[d]	0.41 ± 0.09 (18)	0.06 ± 0.02 (10)[d]

[a]See abbreviations in Table 1.

[b]Control rats were sensitized: (1) to dextrin by injecting 10 μg dextrin i.p.; (2) to SRBC by injecting 0.5 ml from 0.5% suspension i.p.; (3) to casein by injecting 50 μg casein in CFA subcutaneously. 5 days following sensitization (dextrin or SRBC) and 7 days following sensitization (casein) rats were footpad challenged with the specific antigen (dextrin: 7.5 μg; SRBC: 0.05 ml from 0.001% SRBC suspension; casein: 600 μg).

[c]The increase in thickness of the antigen-challenged footpad was determined, X ± SE (n) represents the mean value between footpad thickness before and 24 h after the antigen challenge.

[d]Significantly different from control, P ≤ 0.001.

DISCUSSION

Evidence from several laboratories indicates that the differentiation pathway of IgA plasma cell precursors starts in Peyer's patches (1-4). The effect of severe protein deficiency on IgA B cell differentiation at the Peyer's patches level is presented in this paper by means of an experimental model. Previous reports have shown that Wistar rats fed on a protein-fed diet at weaning presented an impairment of IgA plasma cell precursors (19,21). Now, we demonstrate in the Peyer's patches that B lymphocytes of the IgA isotype are not found, whereas IgM containing cells together with cells bearing little or no surface IgM predominated (Table 2). It thus appears that most Peyer's patch B cells display an immature phenotype that suggests the presence of a pre-B cell population.

Is it possible to restore the immunocompetence of the secretory immune system? Some reports present data indicating that the impairment of the mucosal immune system is reversed by refeeding (26,27). In this report, we deal with the possibility that the precursor B cell population present in protein-depleted Peyer's patches could be recruitable for IgA synthesis after the oral administration of a 20% casein diet. Our results indicate a low percentage and absolute numbers of cells bearing surface IgA in Peyer's patches (Table 2).

Moreover, there was a three-fold decrease in the absolute numbers of the W3/13$^+$ lymphocytes of these rats when compared to age-matched controls (Table 3). This population may comprise regulatory T cells that in rats can be labeled by the monoclonal antibodies W3/25 and MRC OX8. Our data indicates that the decrease observed in the W3/13$^+$ cell population could be ascribed to cells expressing the W3/25 phenotype.

It has been pointed out that germinal centers begin to appear in Peyer's patches by days 14 to 28, which is paralleled by the population of the interfollicular areas with recirculating T cells (28). Therefore, it could be assumed that there exists partial histological damage, which is irreversible, and accounts for the low number of W3/13$^+$ cells. Besides, it is thought that IgA class-specific regulatory T cells selectively expand B cell population (10-13).

Recent _in vitro_ studies carried on by the group of W. Strober provided evidence of the existence of an IgA class-specific "switch T cell" in Peyer's patches. This group of cells directs the early differentiation of B cells towards IgA B cell development (29). Our findings in vivo, of a low number of cells bearing surface IgA in association with a low number of W3/25^{+} cells seem to confirm what has been observed in vitro. It would be of great interest to ascertain if regulatory T cells, recognized by the monoclonal antibody W3/25, are IgA-specific switch T cells and/or IgA class-specific T helper cells.

An impairment of cell mediated immunity was observed but only to new antigens (dextrin and SRBC). Results obtained with casein in protein-depleted rats, indicate the existence of some memory T cells, due to the fact that the antigen has been presented via colostrum. This situation would inhibit the appearance of even partial tolerance when feeding the rats on a 20% casein diet for a long period of time.

Besides, the unresponsiveness to dextrin, even after feeding the rats on a 20% casein diet for a long period of time could be comparable with the unresponsiveness observed in antigen-pretreated nude mice (30).

The diminished number of T cells would account for the impairment in IgA B cell differentiation as confirmed by the observed low number of cells expressing IgA in refed animals; and also for the inability to mount a cell mediated immune response to new antigens.

CONCLUSIONS

1. Malnutrition provokes a breakdown in B cell differentiation which is recognizable at the level of Peyer's patches. B lymphocytes of the IgA isotype were not found. Only IgM containing cells together with cells bearing little or no surface IgM predominated, suggesting the presence of a pre-B cell population.

2. Casein feeding to rats protein-depleted at weaning indicates that the precursor B cell population that exists in their Peyer's patches is recruitable for IgA synthesis. The findings in vivo of a low number of cells bearing surface IgA in association with a low number of W3/25^{+} cells seems to confirm the necessity of IgA class-specific "switch T cells" in Peyer's patches in order to obtain good IgA B cell development.

3. An impairment of cell-mediated immunity was observed only to new antigens.

ACKNOWLEDGEMENTS

This investigation was supported by CONICET grant PID 0212.

REFERENCES

1. Bienenstock, J., Befus, A.D. and McDermott, M., Monog. Allergy 16, 1, 1980.
2. Lamm, M.E., Adv. Immunol. 22, 223, 1976.
3. Cebra, J.J., Fuhrman, J.A., Gearhart, P.J., Hurwitz, J.L. and Shahin, R.D., in Recent Advances in Mucosal Immunity, (Edited by Strober, W., Hanson, L.A. and Sell, K.W.), p. 155, Raven Press, New York, 1982.
4. Roux, M.E., McWilliams, M., Phillips-Quagliata, J.M. and Lamm, M.E., Cell. Immunol. 61, 141, 1981.
5. Bockman, D.E. and Cooper, M.D., Amer. J. Anat. 136, 455, 1973.
6. Pierce, N.F. and Gowans, J.L., J. Exp. Med. 142, 1550, 1975.
7. Owen, R.L., Gastroenterology 72, 440, 1977.
8. Husband, A.J. and Gowans, J.L., J. Exp. Med. 148, 1146, 1978.
9. Andre, C., Andre, F., Druget, M. and Fargier, M.C., Adv. Exp. Med. Biol. 107, 583, 1978.
10. Kiyono, H., McGhee, J.R., Mosteller, L.M., Eldridge, J.H., Koopman, W.J., Kearney, J.F. and Michalek, S.M., J. Exp. Med. 156, 1115, 1982.
11. Kawanishi, H., Saltzman, L.E. and Strober, W., J. Exp. Med. 157, 433, 1983.
12. Kawanishi, H., Saltzman, L. and Strober, W., J. Exp. Med. 158, 649, 1983.
13. Kiyono, H., Cooper, M.D., Kearney, J.F., Mosteller, L.M., Michalek, S.M., Koopman, W.J. and McGhee, J.R., J. Exp. Med. 159, 798, 1984.
14. Roux, M.E., McWilliams, M., Phillips-Quagliata, J.M., Weisz-Carrington, P. and Lamm, M.E., J. Exp. Med. 146, 1311, 1977.
15. Weisz-Carrington, P., Roux, M.E., McWilliams, M., Phillips-Quagliata, J.M. and Lamm, M.E., J. Immunol. 123, 1705, 1979.

16. Beisel, W.R., in Nutrition, Disease Resistance and Immune Function, (Edited by Watson, R.R.), p. 3, Marcel Dekker Inc., New York, 1984.

17. Chandra, R.K., Br. Med. Bull. 37, 89, 1981.

18. Watson, R.R. and McMurray, D.N., CRC Crit. Rev. Food Nutr. 12, 113, 1979.

19. López, M.C., Roux M.E., Langini, S.H., Rio, M.E. and Sanahuja, J.C., Nutr. Rep. Int. 32, 667, 1985.

20. McWilliams, M., Lamm, M.E. and Phillips-Quagliata, J.M., J. Immunol. 113, 1326, 1974.

21. Roux, M.E., Rio, M.E., Slobodianik, N.H., Cosarinsky, R., Langini, S. and Sanahuja, J.C., Comunicaciones Biolögicas 2, 175, 1983.

22. Titus, R.G. and Chiller, J.M., J. Immunol. Methods 45, 65, 1981.

23. Mongini, P.K.A., Longo, D.L. and Paul, W.E., J. Immunol. 132, 1647, 1984.

24. Karch, H. and Nixdorff, K., J. Immunol. 131, 6, 1983.

25. Mattingly, J.A. and Waskman, B.H., J. Immunol. 121, 1878, 1978.

26. Barry, W.S. and Pierce, N.F., Nature 281, 64, 1979.

27. Chandra, R.K., Ann. N.Y. Acad. Sci. 409, 345, 1983.

28. Anderson, A.O., Anderson, N.D. and White, J.D., in Animals Models of Immunological Processes, (Edited by Hay, J.B.), p. 25, Academic Press, London, 1982.

29. Kawanishi, H., Ozato, K. and Strober, W., J. Immunol. 134, 3586, 1985.

30. Bösing-Schneider, R., Cell. Immunol. 61, 245, 1981.

ISOLATION AND ENUMERATION OF ISOTYPE SPECIFIC PLAQUE FORMING CELLS FROM THE MURINE INTESTINE TO STUDY THE DEVELOPMENT OF THE INTESTINAL B CELL BACKGROUND RESPONSE

A.T.J. Bianchi, Ph.J. van der Heijden, W. Stok, J.W. Scholten and B.A. Bokhout

Dept. of Immunology, Central Veterinary Institute
P.O. Box 65, 8200 AB Lelystad, The Netherlands

INTRODUCTION

Quantification of (specific) IgA in faeces using the ELISA technique (1,2) and localization of antibody containing cells (ACC) by immunohistology (3,4) are important methods to investigate the *in vivo* expression of the enteric humoral immune response. These methods have improved our knowledge of the expression of the mucosal immune system, but they have several restrictions. Immunohistological studies give a direct insight in the *in vivo* expression of the mucosal immune system itself, but quantitative data are very difficult to obtain and the number of ACC does not reflect the number of B cells secreting antibodies (5) contributing to the intestinal IgA response. Moreover, IgA measured in faeces is not merely a reflection of locally (intestinally) produced and secreted IgA, since systemically produced IgA can also contribute to the IgA levels in faeces (6). Knowledge about the quantitative expression of the enteric humoral immune response can be obtained by isolation of lymphocytes from the intestine which can be tested subsequently for their capacities to secrete (antigen-specific) IgA.

Isolation of lamina propria (LP) lymphocytes is relatively easy for large species (7-10). Since the mouse is the best documented model for immunological studies, the importance of an adequate isolation procedure of LP lymphocytes from the murine intestine that can be tested in functional assays is evident. Although isolation procedures of LP lymphocytes of rat (11) and mouse (12,13) have been described, most of these investigations deal with the characterization of the isolated LP lymphocytes (11-13) and do not study the functional activity of the LP B lymphocytes. In an earlier study (14) we described an isolation procedure of murine LP lymphocytes that enabled us to quantitate antigen- and isotype-specific antibody secreting B cells in the murine intestine. In this paper this isolation procedure has been used to study the age dependent development of the intestinal B cell background response. To enable comparison of our data with data from studies of the systemic background response (6), and to investigate the contribution of the intestinal mucosal immune system to the total B cell background response in the mouse, the B cell background response of several other lymphoid organs was quantitated as well.

MATERIALS AND METHODS

Mice. Female C3H/He mice were purchased from Harlan-Olac, Ltd., Bicester, United Kingdom and used at different ages.

The isotype specific protein A-plaque forming cell (PFC) assay has been described previously (15). Rabbit-anti-mouse-IgM, -IgG and -IgA were obtained commercially (Nordic, The Netherlands).

Isolation of intestinal antibody secreting cells (ASC). Mice were killed with carbon dioxide. Immediately thereafter, the intestine was isolated and thoroughly rinsed with physiological saline. All visible Peyer's patches (PP) were removed. Subsequently, the intestine was opened longitudinally and the resulting tissue strip was cut in 0.5-1 cm pieces per mouse. These tissue pieces were first incubated during 10 min in 25 ml of Ca- and Mg-free balanced salt solution supplemented with DTT (0.145 mg/ml) and EDTA (0.37 mg/ml). The supernatant containing primarily epithelial cells was discarded. The remaining debris was rinsed once with RPMI 1640 (containing 5% FCS and HEPES) and thereafter incubated during 75 min in 25 ml of RPMI 1640 containing 5% FCS, HEPES and collagenase (0.15 mg/ml, Serva). The supernatant of this incubation mixture was decanted and the cells washed once in RPMI 1640 [containing 5% FCS, HEPES and DNA-se (0.1 mg/ml, Sigma)] and squeezed through nylon gauze filters (100 mesh followed by 50 mesh) to obtain a single cell suspension (nr. 1). The pieces of intestine remaining after decantation were also squeezed through nylon gauze filters (200, 100 and 50 mesh) to produce a second single cell suspension (nr. 2). The cell suspensions number 1 and 2 were pooled, washed in RPMI 1640 (containing 5% FCS, HEPES and DNA-se), and counted in a haemocytometer. Viability of leukocytes was determined by nygrosine exclusion. To avoid bacterial growth, penicillin and streptomycin were added to all the RPMI 1640 solutions used during the isolation procedure and during culture of antibody secreting cells.

Preparation of cell suspensions of other organs. Cell suspensions from spleen, mesenteric lymph nodes (MLN) and PP were prepared in balanced salt solution as described before (15). Bone marrow (BM) was collected from femora.

RESULTS

The distribution of ASC along the murine intestine. From an earlier study (14) it appeared that more than 99% of ASC isolated from the intestine of adult mice secrete IgA. Therefore, in this study only the distribution of IgA secreting cells along the murine intestine was investigated. The intestine of adult mice was divided in five parts; duodenum, jejunum 1, jejunum 2, ileum, and colon with caecum. After isolation of LP lymphocytes from each part of the intestine, the number of IgA secreting cells was determined using a protein-A PFC assay. The relative distribution of IgA secreting cells along the intestine is shown in Fig. 1. The percentages shown in Fig. 1 represent the mean values calculated from 3 experiments. These results (Fig. 1) demonstrate that more than 95% of the IgA secreting cells of the gut are localized in the small intestine (SI). So, for studies of the expression of the intestinal IgA background response one can confine to study the SI. In the SI itself the number of IgA secreting cells declined from cranial to caudal. The average number of IgA secreting cells isolated per complete intestine was 6.8×10^6 on a total number of 1.5×10^8 isolated, living LP cells. Consequently, 4 percent of the LP cells in adult mice appeared to be IgA secreting B cells.

The isotype distribution of ASC over a number of organs including the SI of mice of different ages. The number of IgM, IgG and IgA secreting cells in spleen, MLN, PP and SI was determined in mice of 2.5, 4 and 20 weeks of age using the protein-A PFC assay. The relative distribution of IgM, IgG and IgA secreting cells at different age over a number of organs is presented in Fig. 2. The total number of ASC per mouse isolated from the various organs is shown in Table 1. From these results (Fig. 2 and Table 1) it appeared that in young mice at 2.5 wk of age, just before weaning at 3 wk of age, the ASC are mainly localized in the spleen, while

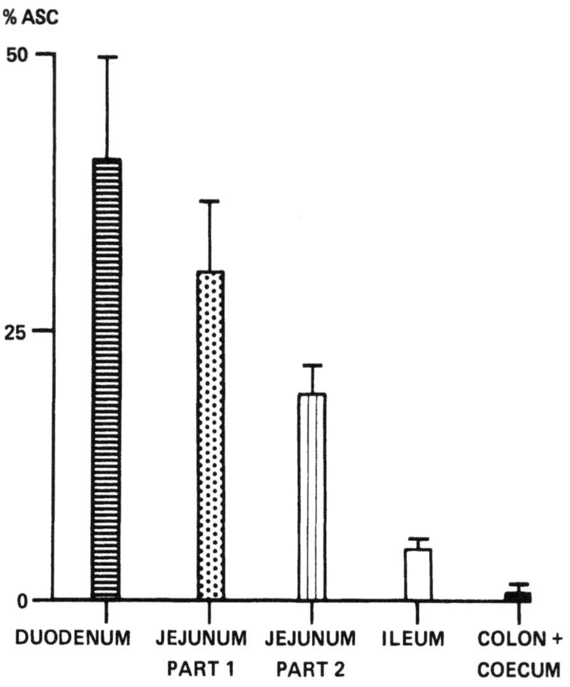

Figure 1. Relative distribution of IgA PFC along the murine intestine.

IgM at that age is the predominant isotype. After weaning, most IgA secreting cells are localized in the SI. In adult mice most of the IgG secreting cells are localized in the BM. At 20 wk of age, more than 80% of all ASC isolated from the principal (lymphoid) organs of mice are producing IgA.

DISCUSSION

Useful procedures for isolation of functional intestinal lymphocytes (IL) have been described for human IL (7,8) first. From these studies (7,8) it appeared that the isolation procedure which makes use of EDTA-collagenase treatment is superior over the mechanical isolation procedure (by cell-scraping) of IL. The only quantitative data of murine, intestinal, antigen specific ASC were obtained by André et al. (16) after mechanical isolation of IL. Unfortunately, these authors hardly described the isolation procedure, while from our experience and from that of other investigators (12,17) it appeared that appropriate single cell suspensions necessary for quantitative, functional studies can hardly be obtained using a mechanical isolation method. Cebra et al. (17) and Davies and Parrott (12) further demonstrated that, after some modifications the enzymetical

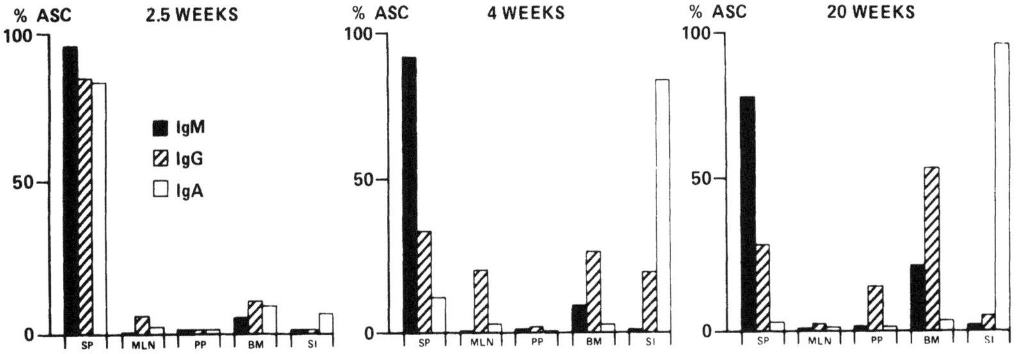

Figure 2. The relative isotype distribution of ASC over a number of (lymphoid) organs in mice of distinct age. SP-spleen, MLN-mesenteric lymph nodes, PP-Peyer's patches, BM-bone marrow, SI-small intestine.

EDTA-collagenase procedure is the method of choice to obtain viable, functionally active single cell suspensions from the murine intestine.

To be able to quantitate the murine intestine (background) ASC, we developed an isolation procedure, which is based on the EDTA-collagenase isolation method described by Davies and Parrott (12). The results presented in this paper show that ASC can be isolated from the murine intestine by this isolation procedure and subsequently quantitated using a protein-A PFC assay. The cell suspensions obtained with our isolation method contain 50-60% living cells. In our studies, the ASC were quantitated using a protein-A PFC assay directly after the EDTA-collagenase isolation procedure, while in most of the other studies (12,13,17,20) the LP cells were characterized after an extra gradient purification step. Therefore, direct comparison of our data with data obtained by other investigators of murine LP cells is not possible.

Cebra et al. (17) and Tseng (13) presented data which indicate that 10^7 cells/mouse, almost totally devoid of dead cells, could be obtained after gradient purification of LP cells isolated with the EDTA-collagenase procedure. Fluorescence studies (13) demonstrated that gradient purified suspensions of LP cells contained an average of 22% Ig containing cells and 18% B cells (13). Studies (6) comparing the number of ASC determined with either a protein-A PFC assay or with immunofluroescence in various lymphoid organs demonstrated that the protein-A PFC assay always gives a higher frequency of Ig-producing cells than does fluorescence. So, it can be expected that after gradient centrifugation at least 20% of the

Table 1. The total number ($\times 10^{-3}$) of ASC per mouse

Age	IgM	IgG	IgA
2.5 weeks	608	10	53
4 weeks	990	80	1,081
20 weeks	833	182	7,152

isolated LP cells will respond in the protein-A PFC assay. Preliminary data from gradient purification experiments (data not shown) done after our isolation procedure showed a 4-5 fold increase of the percentage of protein-A PFC in the obtained LP cell suspension. Twenty percent of the 10^7 gradient purified LP cells isolated per mouse appeared to be protein-A PFC. From these figures it can be calculated that more than half of the ASC (protein-A PFC) recovered after EDTA-collagenase isolation were lost during gradient purification. Therefore, it can be concluded that gradient purification is unnecessary for quantification of the ASC in the SI and should be omitted for a good quantification of all intestinal ASC.

Our study of the intestinal ASC was restricted to LP cells since the intestinal intra-epithelial cell population hardly contains any B cell (18-20) or ASC (14). Moreover, the results shown in Figure 1 demonstrated that more than 95% of the ASC are localized in the SI. Consequently, for studying murine intestinal ASC one can confine to study the LP cells isolated from the SI. The average number of living LP cells per adult C3H/He mouse was 1.5×10^8, while 4% of these cells appeared to be IgA secreting B cells.

The results concerning the distribution of ASC of different Ig classes in spleen, PP, MLN and BM at distinct ages (Fig. 2 and Table 1) in general confirm the results described in the studies of Benner et al. (6,21,22). Our results (Fig. 2 and Table 1) also demonstrate that the response of ASC in the murine spleen is almost at its normal level a few weeks after birth, while the ASC response in BM increases constantly at increasing age. This is the first time that quantitative data concerning the ASC in the SI are presented. These results (Fig. 2 and Table 1) demonstrate that just like in the BM the number of ASC in SI increases enormously at increasing age. Already at 4 wk after birth 50% of all ASC were localized in the SI. Moreover, the absolute and relative contribution of the intestinal ASC to the total pool of background ASC in mice increased at least up to 20 wk after birth. From these results, it can be concluded that especially the ASC response in the SI and probably in all mucosal tissues is exclusively dependent on exogenous antigenic stimulation. It is obvious that the importance of the mucosal immune system for the total background ASC response until now is always underestimated.

An interesting phenomenon is the 50 fold increase of the ASC response in the SI during 10 d between 2.5 and 4 wk after birth. This phenomenon, that may depend on the sudden variability of consumed food antigens or a sudden termination of the intake of maternal antibodies caused by weaning at 3 wk of age, will be one of the major subjects for further study.

CONCLUSIONS

1. Antibody secreting cells (ASC) can be isolated from the murine intestine using the EDTA-collagenase isolation procedure and subsequently quantitated with the isotype-specific protein-A PFC assay.

2. The number of ASC along the intestine of adult mice declines from cranial to caudal. More than 95% of the intestinal ASC (mostly IgA secreting cells) are localized in the small intestine.

3. In young mice (2.5 wk of age just before weaning) the ASC are mainly localized in the spleen, while in adult mice most IgA secreting cells are localized in the SI and most IgG secreting cells in the bone marrow.

4. In adult mice the majority of <u>all</u> ASC are localized in mucosal tissues.

REFERENCES

1. Elson, C.O., Ealding, W. and Lefkowitz, J.J., Immunol. Meth. 67, 101, 1984.
2. Zaane, van D. and IJzerman, J., Immunol. Meth. 72, 427, 1984.
3. Sminia, T., Delemarre, F. and Janse, E.M., Immunology 50, 53, 1983.
4. Pierce, N.F., Infect. Immun. 43, 341, 1984.
5. Benner, R., van Oudenaren, A., Björklund, M., Ivars, F. and Holmberg, D., Immunol. Today 3, 243, 1982.

6. Solari, R. and Kraehenbuhl, J.P., Immunol. Today 6, 17, 1985.
7. Bull, D.M. and Bookman, M.A., J. Clin. Invest. 59, 966, 1977.
8. Bartnik, W., Remine, S.G., Cluba, M., Thayer, W.R. and Shorter, R.G., Gastroenterology 76, 976, 1980.
9. Rudzik, O. and Bienenstock, J., Lab. Invest. 30, 260, 1974.
10. Watson, D.L., Bennell, M.A. and Chaniago, T.D., Am. J. Vet. Res. 40, 61, 1979.
11. Lyscom, N. and Brueton, M.J., Immunology 45, 775, 1982.
12. Davies, M.D.J. and Parrott, D.M.V., Gut 22, 481, 1981.
13. Tseng, J., Cell. Immunol. 73, 324, 1982.
14. van der Heijden, P.J., Bianchi, A.T.J., Oenema, R.G., Scholten, J.W., Stok, W. and Swart, R.J., Proc. 4th Int. Symp. Vet. Lab. Diagnosticans 745, 1986.
15. van der Heijden, P.J., Bokhout, B.A., Bianchi, A.T.J., Scholten, J.W. and Stok, W., Immunobiology 171, 143, 1986.
16. André, C., André, F., Druget, M. and Fargier, M.C., Adv. Exp. Med. Biol. 107, 583, 1978.
17. Cebra, J.J., Gearhart, P.J., Kamat, R., Robertson, S.M. and Tseng, J., Abstracts of Communications, BSI Meeting 5, 1565, 1977.
18. Ernst, P.B., Befus, A.B. and Bienenstock, J., Immunol. Today 6, 50, 1985.
19. Dillon, S.B. and Macdonald, T.T., Immunology 52, 501, 1984.
20. Tagliabue, A., Befus, A.D., Clark, D.A. and Bienenstock, J., J. Exp. Med. 155, 1785, 1982.
21. Benner, R., Rijnbeek, A.M., Bernabé, R.R., Matinez-Alonso, C. and Coutinho, A., Immunobiology 158, 225, 1981.
22. Benner, R., The Immune System, (Edited by Steinberg and Lefkovits), S. Karger, Basel, 1981.

SERUM IgG AND IgE ANTIBODY AGAINST AEROSOLISED ANTIGENS FROM *NEPHROPS NORVEGICUS* AMONG SEAFOOD PROCESS WORKERS

C. McSharry and P.C. Wilkinson

University Department of Bacteriology and Immunology
Western Infirmary, Glasgow G11 GNT, Scotland

INTRODUCTION

Occupation-related asthma and dermatitis among seafood process personnel in a local factory prompted a study of their immune response to antigens in the factory environment, especially those antigens aerosolized during the processing of prawns. A similar clinical syndrome has already been reported (1,2), but the present study examined the nature and extent of the antibody class response to definable inhaled antigens, and assessed the value of this serology as a clinical adjunct in the investigation of hypersensitivity. The effects of intrinsic parameters such as age, gender and atopy, as well as environmental factors such as the extent of antigen exposure and smoking history was also examined in relation to symptoms and the antibody response.

SUBJECTS AND METHODS

Twenty-six female process workers in a seafood factory of 400 employees approached the factory medical officer with complaints of various degrees of respiratory symptoms which they attributed to their working environment. Each was clinically examined, performed simple spirometry and donated a blood sample. A control groups of females individually matched for age and work history were contacted. They had no symptoms and agreed to donate a blood sample. Serum IgE and IgE antibody to house dust mite, grass pollen and prawn antigens were measured by PRIST and RAST (Pharmacia, Ltd.) according to the manufacturers instructions. IgG was measured by radial immunodiffusion, and IgG antibody to saline soluble prawn antigens by enzyme immunoassay, ELISA, on microtiter plates, using known positive and negative sera from a previous investigation (1). Significance testing was by Wilcoxon's Sum of Ranks analysis.

RESULTS

The symptomatic and control groups were individually matched for age and years of antigen exposure in the work place, but the incidence of atopy was higher in the symptomatic group, as was the total IgE and prawn antigen specific IgE antibody (p less than 0.04 and 0.002, respectively, Table 1). There was no significant difference between the two groups for either IgG or IgG antibody titers to prawn antigens. These serological parameters were compared between the current smokers and never-smokers irrespective of symptoms (Table 2). There was a significantly higher titer of IgE and IgE antibody in the smokers and a significantly higher titer of IgG and IgG antibody in the non-smokers.

Table 1. Comparison of age and antigen exposure (mean + S.D.), smoking and atopic history, and serology between symptomatic and asymptomatic workers

	Symptomatic	Asymptomatic
Number	26	26
Age (years)	33.7 (11.4)	32.7 (11.9)
Exposure (years)	6.5 (4.9)	6.7 (5.1)
Smokers (number)	14	14
Atopic (number)	9	3
IgE (i.u./mL)	180.5 (187)	88 (129)
IgG (mg/mL)	11.9 (2.9)	11.4 (3.1)
prawn RAST (units)	3.78	0.13
prawn ELISA (units)	472	452

IgE and IgG expressed in mean (+S.D.), RAST in RAST units and ELISA in optical density units.

Table 2. Comparison of serology between smoking and non-smoking process workers irrespective of symptoms

	Smokers	Non-Smokers	p
Number	28	20	
IgE	174.4	75.6	0.029
IgG	10.6	12.9	0.003
prawn RAST	2.8	0.3	0.012
prawn ELISA	291	673	0.001

DISCUSSION

The serological parameters of these seafood process workers at risk of hypersensitivity pneumonitis (extrinsic allergic alveolitis) and occupational asthma would suggest that an atopic predisposition is three fold more common in subjects who develop respiratory symptoms. In keeping with this, the subjects with serum IgE antibody to prawn antigens all had symptoms and this may be a useful clinical adjunct, perhaps by appropriate skin testing. The IgG antibody response was predominant among non-smokers but the IgE antibody response to the same antigens was predominant among smokers. This segregation of antibody class response to the same inhaled antigen according to smoking habit has not, to our knowledge, been reported previously. These observations suggest that smoking has a modulating influence on the antibody class response to inhaled antigens, the study of which may provide a useful probe into how the respiratory tract processes antigen.

SUMMARY

Employees in a seafood factory developed high titers of serum IgE and IgG antibody to antigens from prawn (N. norvegicus) which were aerosolized during processing. Significant serum IgE antibody titers occurred only among those subjects with occupation-related respiratory symptoms, and this serological parameter may be a useful clinical adjunct in the investigation of this disease. Serum IgG antibody was detected with equal frequency and titer in symptomatic and asymptomatic workers. There was no significant correlation between either antibody class response and the individual's age or years of work exposure. Cigarette smoking, however, was positively associated with the IgE antibody response, and negatively associated with the IgG antibody response to the same inhaled antigen. Investigating the effects of smoking at the mucosal level in the lung may provide insight into how the lung processes and responds to inhaled antigens.

REFERENCES

1. Gaddie, J., Legge, J.S., Friend, J.A.R., Reid, T.M.S., Lancet ii, 1350, 1980.
2. Cartier, A., Malo, J.-L., F., Lafrance, M., Pineau, L., St. Aubin, J.-J., Dubois, J.-Y., J. Allergy Clin. Immunol. 74, 261, 1984.

THE EFFECT OF EXERCISE ON SECRETORY AND NATURAL IMMUNITY

L.T. Mackinnon, T.W. Chick, A. van As and T.B. Tomasi

Department of Cell Biology, University of New Mexico
School of Medicine and Department of Medicine, VA Medical
Center, Albuquerque, NM USA

INTRODUCTION

The high frequency of recurrent respiratory infections following "over-training" in competitive athletes prompted this study to examine the effects of intense prolonged exercise on mucosal immunoglobulins (Ig). In a previous study from this laboratory, it was shown that in elite athletes (US National Nordic ski team) resting salivary IgA levels are lower than in age-matched control subjects, and that IgA levels decrease further after two to three hours of exhaustive exercise (1981 US National Nordic ski competition) (1). It was unclear whether the decreases in IgA were due to the effects of exercise, to the effects of cold (1°C), to the stress of competition, or to a combination of factors. To further elucidate the role of exercise, we studied competitive bicyclists in a controlled environment and noncompetitive laboratory setting. We followed secretory Ig levels for two days after exercise in order to study the time course of suppression and return to baseline levels following cessation of exercise. In addition, we measured NK cytotoxic activity before and after exercise in order to study whether severe exercise alters other immune parameters.

METHODS

Eight well-trained male competitive bicyclists, ages 20 to 31 were studied during the competitive season (August to September). Each subject exercised on a bicycle ergometer for two hours at 90% of his anaerobic threshold. This workload is an exhaustive exercise, corresponding to approximately 70 to 75% of each cyclist's maximum exercise capacity. Saliva, nasal washes, and venous blood were sampled at five time points: immediately before and after exercise, and one hour, 24 hours, and 48 hours after exercise. Parotid saliva was collected with a Curby cap placed over the duct of the parotid salivary gland and salivation was stimulated with a sour hard candy. For comparison, saliva samples were obtained from age-matched, untrained control subjects who did not exercise regularly. Nasal washes were obtained by rinsing the nostrils with sterile saline and collecting the effluent. Venous blood was obtained by venipuncture of the antecubital vein.

Serum and salivary Ig (IgA, IgM, IgG) levels were measured by direct competitive ELISA. Serum antibody titers to specific pathogens were measured by complement fixation for the following: adenovirus, influenza A and B, parainfluenza, cytomegalovirus, varicella-Zoster, herpes simplex, chlamydia, Mycoplasma pneumoniae, and rubeola. In order to study whether exercise influences the production and secretion of Ig by circulating lymphoid cells, PBL were obtained from blood drawn at the five time points, and were grown for seven days in the presence of 10 µl/ml PWM. Supernatant IgA and IgG levels were measured by ELISA. In order to study whether severe exercise alters other parameters of immunity, natural killer (NK) activity of PBL taken at the five time points was measured by a standard four hour ^{51}Cr release assay. PBL were stained with various commercially available cell markers to identify lymphocyte subpopulations by flow cytometry using a fluorescence-activated cell sorter (FACS).

RESULTS

In the athletes, salivary IgA, IgM and IgG levels were not different from corresponding levels in age-matched, untrained control subjects (Table 1). Immediately after the two hour exercise, both IgA and IgM concentrations decreased in all athletes (65% and 55% decreases, respectively; $p < .01$ for each Ig, t test for repeated measures). One hour after exercise, both IgA and IgM levels had begun to increase, but were still lower than at rest (53% and 37% lower, respectively; $p < .025$). IgA and IgM levels returned to pre-exercise values by 24 hours after exercise. Salivary IgG levels were unchanged after exercise.

Table 1. The effect of exercise on salivary Ig concentrations

Time	IgA	IgM	IgG
Controls	22.4 ± 8.4 (5)	2.0 ± 0.8 (5)	0.6 ± 0.2 (3)
Pre-exercise	27.5 ± 6.9 (6)	3.0 ± 0.6 (5)	0.8 ± 0.3 (3)
Post-exercise	9.5 ± 2.8[a] (6)	1.3 ± 0.3[a] (5)	0.6 ± 0.2 (3)
One h Post-	13.8 ± 3.7[b] (6)	1.8 ± 0.8[b] (5)	0.9 ± 0.4 (3)
24-48 h Post-	32.2 ± 11.2 (6)	3.3 ± 1.2 (5)	1.1 ± 0.5 (3)

Values are mean μg of Ig/mg protein ± SEM. No. subjects in parentheses.
[a]$p<.01$ vs. pre-exercise, *t* test for repeated measures;
[b]$p<.025$ vs. pre-exercise, *t* test for repeated measures, Bonferroni's method.

Salivary IgA levels decreased regardless of whether the data are expressed as μg of IgA per mg protein or μg of IgA per ml saliva. The concentration of IgA in nasal washes was unchanged by exercise. *In vitro* secretion of IgA and IgG by PWM-stimulated PBL also was not altered by exercise. Serum IgA, IgM and IgG levels, and serum antibody titers to specific antigens were unchanged after exercise.

Total NK lytic activity, as measured by ^{51}Cr release, was unchanged immediately after exercise, but decreased 35% one hour after exercise (Fig. 1). NK activity returned to pre-exercise levels by 24 hours after exercise. There were no differences between any of the slopes, but the intercept at one hour post-exercise was significantly lower than at the other time points ($p < .005$, analysis of covariance).

Flow cytometry showed that the percentage of PBL which were positive for the NK markers Leu-7 and Leu-11a decreased both immediately and one hour after exercise (Table 2). By one hour after exercise, when NK activity had decreased by 35%, the percentage of Leu-7 and Leu-11a positive cells had decreased 47% and 71%, respectively.

Since the percentage of PBL expressing the NK cell markers decreased after exercise, but the total number of PBL in each well of the ^{51}Cr release assay remained constant, the numbers of NK cells in each well also decreased. To adjust for different numbers of NK cells in the assay, cytotoxic activity per NK cell was calculated by dividing total lytic activity by NK cell

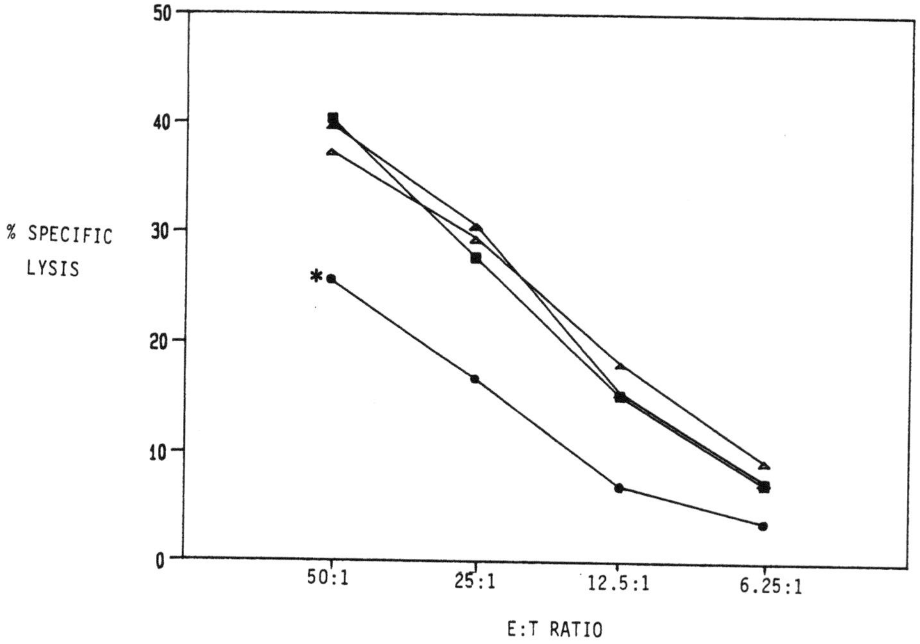

Figure 1. The effect of exercise on NK activity. N=4; * $p < .01$, analysis of covariance; pre-exercise ▲; post-exercise ■, one h post- ●, 24-48 h post- △.

number (Leu-11a$^+$) in each well (Table 3). When cytotoxic activity is expressed on a per cell basis, NK activity was higher both immediately and one hour after exercise, and returned to pre-exercise levels by 24 hours.

DISCUSSION

The results of the present study on bicyclists confirm previous data which show decreased salivary IgA levels after a cross country ski race (1), and extend these findings to include IgM levels as well. The bicycle ergometer test was an exercise of similar duration and intensity to the ski race, but held under controlled laboratory conditions. Thus, it appears that intense endurance exercise by itself suppresses salivary IgA and IgM levels. The exercise-induced suppression of secretory Ig was transitory, since IgA levels remained low for one hour and return to pre-exercise values by 24 hours after exercise. In other mucosal secretions (e.g., nasal fluids, lung washings), the levels of secretory antibodies of the IgA class are related to resistance to respiratory infection (2-6). The secretory IgA in saliva specifically inhibits attachment of several bacterial strains

Table 2. Flow cytometry with NK cell markers

Marker	Pre-exercise	Post-exercise	1 h Post-	24-48 h Post-
Leu-7	13.8 ± 2.0	9.3 ± 1.7	7.4 ± 1.2[a]	14.5 ± 2.6
Leu-11a	10.6 ± 2.0	5.8 ± 2.5	3.1 ± 1.6[a]	10.5 ± 3.1

Values are mean percentage of PBL positive for each marker ± SEM. N=4.
[a]$p < .025$ *t* test for repeated measures, Bonferroni's method.

Table 3. NK cytotoxic activity per NK cell

Total lytic activity, % specific lysis	39.7	40.2	25.6	37.4
% Leu 11a$^+$ cells	10.6	5.8	3.1	10.5
#Leu 11a$^+$ cells/well x 10^4	5.3	2.9	1.6	5.2
Activity per cell x 10^{-4}	7.5	13.9	16.0	7.2

Values are for an E:T ratio of 50:1, with 5 x 10^5 PBL per well.

to human buccal epithelial cells (7). Thus, if the level of IgA in saliva is also related to resistance to infection caused by microorganisms that colonize the oral mucosa, the data presented here suggest that an athlete may be susceptible to upper respiratory diseases for at least several hours after intense prolonged exercise.

It is unclear as to why salivary IgA levels decreased, while nasal wash IgA levels remained unchanged, after exercise. One possible explanation is that exercise influences IgA-secreting cells of the oral and nasal mucosae differently, perhaps involving local and/or circulating factors. Differences in the volumes of air flow through the two regions may also be involved. For example, ventilation increases dramatically during endurance exercise (up to 115 l/minute in these athletes). Epithelial transport of secretory Ig and/or the function of IgA-secreting cells residing beneath the oral mucosae may be altered by the large volumes of air moving rapidly over the mucosal surfaces. Alternatively, IgA-secreting cells of the nasal and oral mucosae may respond differently to circulating factors, such as stress hormones, which are released during exercise.

In our previous study (1), world class athletes had lower resting salivary IgA levels compared to age-matched, untrained control subjects, suggesting a possible chronic suppression of secretory Ig. However, in the present study, there were no differences between resting salivary Ig levels in athletes and age-matched control subjects These differences may be due to variations in season and/or location of the studies. The skiers study was done during the winter in New York, whereas the bicyclist study was performed in the summer in New Mexico.

The decreases in salivary IgA levels observed immediately after exercise were of similar magnitude regardless of whether the data are expressed as μg of IgA per mg protein or as μg of IgA per ml saliva (65% and 70% decreases, respectively). Protein concentration of saliva increased approximately 20% immediately after exercise, reflecting the slight dehydration often observed with exercise. However, this increase in protein concentration cannot account for the decreases in salivary IgA and IgM concentrations. Although the best way to express Ig secretion would be to measure the actual rate of secretion over time, collection of unstimulated saliva would have required 30 to 60 minutes. Since many of the exercise-induced changes in immune parameters are transitory, it was felt that any changes in secretory Ig occurring immediately after exercise would have been obscured by pooling saliva collected over one hour. Thus, salivation was stimulated and Ig concentration expressed per mg protein.

Only salivary IgA and IgM levels decreased after exercise. Salivary IgG, serum IgA, IgM and IgG and serum antibodies to specific antigens were not influenced by exercise. These data indicate that prolonged intense exercise has a specific effect on the secretory immunoglobulins, and suggest that the secretory process may be inhibited by severe exercise.

The mechanism(s) by which salivary Ig levels are depressed after exercise are unclear at present. Intense exercise may alter plasma cell secretion of secretory Ig or the secretory component-dependent transport of secretory Ig or both. Alternatively, plasma cell precursor migration to the oral mucosa may be altered by exercise. The observation that *in vitro* secretion of IgA and IgG by PWM-stimulated PBL was not influenced by exercise suggests that exercise does not alter the ability of circulating lymphocytes to synthesize and secrete Ig.

In order to study whether severe exercise alters other parameters of immune function we measured NK activity of PBL taken at the five time points.

We chose to study NK function because NK activity has been shown to be sensitive to the effects of stress and moderate exercise. Total NK activity was suppressed by 35% one hour after exercise. The decrease in activity was accompanied by decreases in the percentages of Leu-7 and Leu-11a positive cells. Since the percentge of NK cells was lower at both time points after exercise, lytic activity was adjusted arithmetically for the decrease in NK cell number in the assay system. When activity is expressed on a per cell basis, cytotoxic activity actually increased both immediately and one hour after exercise. These data suggest that NK activity is stimulated during and perhaps after intense endurance exercise, and are consistent with previous reports showing a stimulation of NK activity and an increase in the number of effector to target interactions following moderate and intense exercise of short duration (8,9). The mechanisms responsible for the exercise-induced stimulation of NK cells are unknown at present, but may involve one or more of the lymphokines or hormones known to modulate NK function, such as interferons, IL-1, IL-2, or the opioid peptides. Plasma levels of several of these molecules (e.g., IL-1, interferon-α, β-endorphin, and met-enkephalin) increase during exercise (10-14).

SUMMARY

Secretory immunity

1. Intense endurance exercise suppresses salivary immunoglobulins. The exercise-induced decrease is specific for the secretory antibodies IgA and IgM.

2. The suppression of secretory Ig is transitory, lasting at least one hour, and returning to pre-exercise levels by 24 hours after a single bout of severe exercise.

These results suggest that anecdotal statements by athletes and their coaches of an increased susceptibility to upper respiratory infection afte severe exercise could be related to changes in secretory immunity.

Natural immunity

1. Natural killer activity of PBL is suppressed one hour after intense endurance exercise. This effect is transitory, since activity returns to pre-exercise levels by 24 hours after a single bout of exercise.

2. The decrease in NK lytic activity is due to a decrease in the percentage of NK cells (Leu-11a$^+$ cells). When NK cell activity is expressed on a per cell basis, it appears that activity is enhanced after exercise.

CONCLUSIONS

These results indicate that prolonged intense exercise alters parameters of both mucosal and natural immunity, and suggest that severe exercise may be a form of stress associated with changes in immune reactivity.

REFERENCES

1. Tomasi, T.B., Trudeau, F.B., Czerwinski, D. and Erredge, S., J. Clin. Immunol. 2, 178, 1982.
2. Cate, T.R., Rossen, R.D., Douglas, R.G., Butler, W.T. and Couch, R.B., Am. J. Epidemiol. 84, 352, 1966.
3. Liew, F.Y., Russell, S.M., Appleyard, G., Brand, C.M. and Beale, J., Eur. J. Immunol. 14, 350, 1984.
4. Murphy, B.R., Nelson, D.L., Wright, P.F., Tierney, E.L., Phelan, M.A. and Chanock, R.M., Infect. Immun. 36, 1102, 1982.
5. Perkins, J.C., Tucker, D.N., Knopf, H.L.S., Wenzel, R.P., Kapikian, A.Z. and Chanock, R.M., Am. J. Epidemiol. 90, 519, 1969.
6. Smith, C.B., Purcell, R.H., Bellanti, J.A. and Chanock, R.M., New Engl. J. Med. 275, 1145, 1966.
7. Williams, R.C. and Gibbons, R.J., Science 177, 697, 1972.
8. Brahmi, Z., Thomas, J.E., Park, M. and Dowdeswell, I.R.G., J. Clin. Immunol. 5, 321, 1985.
9. Targan, S., Britvan, L. and Dorey, F., Clin. Exp. Immunol. 45, 352, 1981.
10. Cannon, J.G. and Kluger, M.J., Science 220, 617, 1983.
11. Cannon, J. and Dinarello, C., Fed. Proc. 43, 462, 1984.
12. Viti, A., Muscettola, M., Paulesu, L., Bocci, V. and Almi, A., J. Appl. Physiol. 59, 426, 1985.
13. Farrell, P.A., Gates, W.K., Maksud, M.G. and Morgan, W.P., J. Appl. Physiol. 52, 1245, 1982.
14. Howlett, T.A., Tomlin, S., Ngahfoong, L., Rees, L.H., Bullen, B.A., Skrinar, G.S. and McArthur, J.W., Br. Med. J. 288, 1950, 1984.

AUTHOR INDEX

SUBJECT INDEX

GPSR Compliance
The European Union's (EU) General Product Safety Regulation (GPSR) is a set of rules that requires consumer products to be safe and our obligations to ensure this.

If you have any concerns about our products, you can contact us on

ProductSafety@springernature.com

In case Publisher is established outside the EU, the EU authorized representative is:

Springer Nature Customer Service Center GmbH
Europaplatz 3
69115 Heidelberg, Germany

www.ingramcontent.com/pod-product-compliance
Ingram Content Group UK Ltd.
Pitfield, Milton Keynes, MK11 3LW, UK
UKHW050647051126
16351UKWH00012B/63
* 9 7 8 1 4 6 8 4 5 3 4 5 4 *